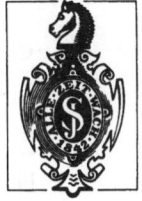

Alfred Breit (Editor-in-Chief)

Advanced Radiation Therapy

Tumor Response Monitoring and Treatment Planning

Andreas Heuck, Peter Lukas,
Peter Kneschaurek, Manfred Mayr (Co-Editors)

With 241 Figures and 71 Tables

Springer-Verlag
Berlin Heidelberg New York
London Paris Tokyo
Hong Kong Barcelona Budapest

Editor-in-Chief
Professor Dr. A. Breit
Institut und Poliklinik für Strahlentherapie,
Klinikum rechts der Isar, Ismaninger Straße 15,
8000 München 80, FRG

Co-Editors
Dr. med. A. Heuck
PD Dr. med. P. Lukas
PD Dr. med. P. Kneschaurek
Dr. med. M. Mayr
Institut für Strahlentherapie und Radiologische Onkologie,
Klinikum rechts der Isar, Ismaninger Straße 22,
8000 München 80, FRG

ISBN 978-3-540-54783-9   ISBN 978-3-642-48681-4 (eBook)
DOI 10.1007/978-3-642-48681-4

Library of Congress Cataloging-in-Publication Data
Tumor response monitoring and treatment planning: advanced radiation
therapy/Alfred Breit (editor-in-chief); Andreas Heuck [et al.]
(co-editors). p. cm. Includes index.
ISBN 978-3-540-54783-9
1. Cancer—Radiotherapy. 2. Cancer—Prognosis. 3. Cancer-
-Diagnosis. 4. Tumors—classification.   I. Breit, Alfred.
II. Heuck, Andreas. III. Title: Advanced radiation therapy.
[DNLM: 1. Monitoring, Physiologic—methods. 2. Neoplasms-
-radiotherapy. 3. Patient Care Planning.   QZ 629 T925]
RC271.R3T85 1992   616.99'40642—dc20   DNLM/DLC
for Library of Congress 92-2182 CIP

The use of general descriptive names, registered names, trademarks, etc. in this publication
does not imply, even in the absence of a specific statement, that such names are exempt from
the relevant protective laws and regulations and therefore free for general use.

Product liability: The publishers cannot guarantee the accuracy of any information about
dosage and application contained in this book. In every individual case the user must check
such information by consulting the relevant literature.

Typesetting; Macmillan India Ltd., Bangalore-25

25/3020–543210-Printed on acid-free paper

Preface

Medical imaging has progressed to a standard undreamt of not very many years ago. The advances are due to continuous development of radiological techniques and the introduction of magnetic resonance imaging. With the improved and new methods three-dimensional target volumes for radiation therapy can be defined with hitherto unknown precision. This leads to an improvement in irradiation techniques and, as a consequence, to a higher likelihood of tumor control and a lower risk of normal tissue complications.

Beside the improvement in irradiation techniques the new imaging methods may enable great strides in tumor response monitoring, not only in the detection of morphological alterations but also by showing physiological changes in the tumor during and after treatment by means of MRI and PET. This not only leads to better prognostic information but may also allow early evaluation of the response to treatment. It may then be possible to individualize not only the radiation dose but also the alternative treatment for nonresponders. This is certainly a future direction for radiation oncology.

The scientific value of the ART Symposium on Tumor Response Monitoring and Treatment Planning was further increased by the satellite EORTC high-LET particle group meeting. The new imaging modalities may have a particularly great influence on the application of these types of radiation.

We sincerely hope that the publication of this volume will throw light on interesting new aspects of radiation oncology and lead to improvement in the management of our patients.

Andreas Heuck, Peter Lukas,
Peter Kneschaurek, Manfred Mayr

Foreword

The International Symposium of the W. Vaillant Foundation on Tumor Response Monitoring and Treatment Planning took place in Munich in the spring of 1991 under the banner "Advanced Radiation Therapy ART 91". The aim of the conference was to provide a forum where scientists from all over the world could contribute their knowledge and experience to the improvement of radiation therapy treatment. Exact planning of radiation therapy, an essential prerequisite for optimized treatment results, demands cooperation between radiation therapists and diagnostic radiologists, physicists, engineers, and scientists from other related fields. The major new technologies for tumor imaging (e.g., computed tomography, magnetic resonance imaging, and positron emission tomography) and for image processing allow more precise definition of tumor volume and target volume and the selection of adequate portals to ensure optimal tumor control and protection of normal tissue. These imaging and processing technologies have also proved to be excellent tools for monitoring the tumor response to therapy during and after the treatment course and are able to provide early information about the effectiveness of treatment regimens.

The meeting of organizers and editors have attempted to integrate in this volume all the relevant new information on advanced treatment planning and tumor response monitoring. Renowned researchers from the fields of radiology, medical physics, and engineering have contributed numerous articles on both topics, resulting in a comprehensive survey of the latest developments and newest trends in radiation oncology. A satellite symposium of the EORTC Heavy Particle Therapy Group was part of the ART 91 meeting and this volume contains an appendix with contributions related to this type of therapy.

We hope we have succeeded in presenting a topical and comprehensive survey on advances in tumor response monitoring and treatment planning.

Munich, August 1992   Alfred Breit

Contents

Tumor Response Monitoring: Brain

Tumor Response Monitoring: Head and Neck

Tumor Response Monitoring: Thorax and Breast

Magnetic Resonance Relaxometry

Part 2

Treatment Planning

Introductory Contribution

Treatment Planning: New Tools

Treatment Planning: Biological Models

Treatment Planning: Mathematical Models

**Treatment Planning: Treatment Volume Definition
and Three-Dimensional Treatment Planning**

Part 3

Advances in Neutron Theory
(Contributions of the EORTC Heavy Particle Therapy Group)

Part 1

Tumor Response Monitoring

Introductory Contribution

Diagnostic Imaging in Oncology: Present and Future

A.R. Margulis

Oncologic imaging has undergone revolutionary changes during the 1980s; a number of cross-sectional techniques introduced in the 1970s and some adopted in the 1980s have matured, permitting diagnosis, staging, and follow-up of therapy for cancer. Digital gray scale ultrasound, computed tomography (CT) with contrast media enhancement, and magnetic resonance imaging (MRI) have become indispensable in clinical centers and have made diagnostic radiology one of the mainstays of oncologic medicine. Oncologic imaging also involves interventional radiology, which in the treatment of tumors may involve introduction of catheters into terminal arteries in order to permit tolerance of higher doses of chemotherapeutic agents with infusion pumps. Needle biopsies under imaging localization have practically eliminated exploratory laparotomies in the industrial world.

Conventional Radiology and Mammography: Advances in Imaging Modalities

Conventional radiography, except for portable radiography to follow post-operative patients and those in intensive care units, is being significantly impinged upon by ultrasound, CT, and even MRI. Another such technique is mammography, the use of which has increased significantly in the United States and western Europe. Small, nonpalpable lesions are being discovered by screening, and although still no reliable criteria exist to differentiate between highly invasive and noninvasive tumors by mammography alone, the discovery of these small, nonpalpable lesions has led to less disfiguring yet equally successful therapy [1–3].

Computed Tomography. Modern CT continues its dissemination in the United States, Japan, and western Europe. In oncology it is the indispensable modality for the examination of the lungs and upper abdomen. CT is also indispensable for the examination of kidney masses; it is excellent in the retroperitoneum, and

University of California, San Francisco, CA 94143-0292, USA

Advanced Radiation Therapy Tumor Response
Monitoring and Treatment Planning
Breit (Editor-in-Chief)
© Springer-Verlag, Berlin Heidelberg 1992

although it can depict large lymph nodes, it suffers from the same handicaps as MRI, as large nodes sometimes may be inflammatory, and nodes smaller than 1 cm can still harbor cancer. The new fast CT units permit rapid data acquisition without gaps, providing three-dimensional information, which permits display of images in any of the orthogonal or even curved oblique planes [4, 5].

Ultrasound. The basic screening procedure for the whole abdomen is ultrasound, and although its spatial resolution is continuously improving, it does have lower signal-to-noise ratios than either CT or MRI. As it requires greater operator skills, its performance and accuracy in diagnosis vary from satisfactory to outstanding. With the addition of color Doppler, ultrasound is capable of evaluating blood flow and is indispensable after surgery in the evaluation of patency of major vessels. It is readily available and relatively inexpensive and brings the physician into contact with the patient, thus permitting better targeting of the examination. Ultrasound is therefore widely embraced, not only by radiologists but also by other specialists. Its enthusiastic acceptance is reflected in the wide spectrum of sophistication in equipment, and this, again, is mirrored in a great variety of prices. Intracavitary transducers, such as transrectal, transvaginal, transesophageal, or intragastric ultrasound are continuously progressing and are being accepted as an excellent staging approach assessing invasion of the organ wall and immediate adjacent lymph nodes [6, 7].

Magnetic Resonance Imaging. With the introduction of gadolinium DTPA, MRI has increased its scope in oncology. It is the modality of choice for the diagnosis of brain, cord, and face tumors. It is outstanding for the detection and evaluation of tumors of the heart chambers, the mediastinum, and various studies show it to be a slight improvement over CT in the diagnosis of hepatic primary and metastatic tumors. With the introduction of new contrast media, such as manganese DPDP, it may vastly surpass the utility of CT. In the staging of pelvic tumors, both in men or in women, MRI is showing a definite superiority over other modalities. In tumors of the bladder, the endometrium, and ovaries, the use of gadolinium DTPA further improves the sensitivity, specificity and accuracy of the examination. In the musculoskeletal system, including the spine, MRI is supreme because of its significant soft tissue contrast resolution. Future advances in MRI will include the introduction of new contrast media targeted to receptors; these may be tumor specific and may enhance MR spectroscopy. Spectroscopic imaging (chemical shift imaging) with simultaneous recording of spectra of many voxels over the field of view and computer selection of peaks localized on a superimposed proton image, promises better tissue characterization of tumors, hopefully leading to improved selection and follow-up of treatment [8–16].

Imaging of Tumors of the Brain, Cervix, and Rectum

To illustrate the changes that have occurred with the new developments in imaging, it is helpful to show what has occurred in the diagnosis of tumors of the brain, rectum, and cervix.

Brain Tumors. Ventriculography, as a procedure to evaluate the effect of brain tumors on ventricles, has, along with pneumoencephalography, disappeared from practice with the advent of CT. Skull radiography plays no role anymore in the evaluation of patients suspect for central nervous system tumors. Angiography is rarely employed except in a few cases which demonstrate findings or are suggestive of vascular malformation on CT or MR. In these cases, angiography is used for preoperative embolization and for surgical planning. CT, which first came into clinical use in early 1974, had been the primary approach for screening patients suspect for brain tumors and for lesion characterization until the advent of MRI. In recent years, MRI has surpassed CT in sensitivity and specificity and is presently the least invasive technique for the detection and characterization of CNS neoplasms. Its use for this purpose is influenced only by the relatively limited access to this modality (more so in Europe than in the United States). The use of gadolinium DTPA has further refined the use of MRI in brain tumors and has been particularly valuable in the diagnosis and study of meningiomas. It is hoped that, in the future, MR spectroscopy will further contribute to the diagnosis, localization, characterization, and posttherapeutic follow-up of brain tumors [17–19].

Carcinoma of the Cervix. As the prognosis of cervical cancer is determined by the volume of the tumor and the stage of the disease at the time of diagnosis, imaging is of great importance in the handling of this neoplasm. Because the clinical FIGO staging is inaccurate, and because the stage of the disease alone is no longer the exclusive parameter used in selecting therapy, the role of imaging in the evaluation of carcinoma of the cervix is of paramount importance. MRI is, at the moment, the imaging approach of choice as it allows the precise delineation of tumor location, depth of cervical stromal invasion, and extension of tumor to the uterine cavity. The use of gadolinium DTPA, while not improving tumor depiction, is helpful in demonstrating and assessing invasion of the adjacent organs. The value of MRI rises in proportion to the volume and stage of the disease, as well as the presence of concomitant uterine or adnexal tumor masses [20–23].

Carcinoma of the Rectum. The superiority of MRI over CT or transrectal ultrasound in the evaluation of carcinoma of the rectum has not been established as yet. Continuous advances and increased experience suggest that transrectal ultrasound is an excellent modality for evaluation of the intramural extent of carcinoma of the rectum. As CT does not demonstrate the tissue layers of the rectum, transrectal ultrasound and transrectal MRI, performed with an endorectal coil, appear to be superior to CT. For extrarectal extent, MRI and CT appear to be equally accurate, with MRI having the advantages of multi-planar depiction. Multicoil surface techniques for the evaluation of the rectum show great promise and, because they are less invasive, would be more readily applied than the endorethal MRI approach. As carcinoma of the anal canal spreads to inguinal lymph nodes, both CT and MRI are of value in diagnosing their enlargement, but neither of them can provide specific tissue diagnosis. Carcinoma of the rectum frequently spreads to the liver. At present, MRI appears to be somewhat superior to CT in the detection of metastatic in-volvement of the liver. Neither is very efficient at present in the detection of lesions smaller than 1 cm. The introduction of contrast media will most likely improve the versatility of MRI in this field. MR spectroscopy of the liver also holds the promise of improved tissue specificity [24–30].

Summary

Oncologic imaging is indispensable for the diagnosis of the malignancy, its staging, and its posttherapy follow-up. Rapid advances in cross-sectional imag-ing, in the development of contrast media for MRI and further breakthroughs in MR spectroscopy promise a bright future for diagnostic imaging.

References

1. Sickles EA (1986) Mammographic features of 300 consecutive nonpalpable breast cancers. AJR 46: 661
2. Sickles EA (1989) Combining spot-compression and other special views to maximize mammo-graphic information. Radiology 173: 571
3. Mendelson EB, Harris KM, Doshi N, Tobon H (1989) Infiltrating lobular carcinoma: mammo-graphic patterns with pathologic correlation. AJR 153: 265
4. Lee JKT, Sagel SS, Stanley RJ (eds) (1989) Computed body tomography with MRI correlation, 2nd edn. Raven, New York
5. Boyd DP, Couch JL, Napel SA, Peschmann KR, Rand RE (1987) Ultrafast cine CT: where have we been? What lies ahead? Am J Cardiac Imaging 1: 175–185
6. Mendelson EB, Bohm-Velez M, Joseph N, Neiman HL (1988) Gynecologic imaging: com-parison of transabdominal and transvaginal sonography. Radiology 166: 321
7. Merritt CRB (1987) Doppler color flow imaging. J Clin Ultrasound 15: 591
8. Stark DD, Bradley WG Jr (eds) (1988) Magnetic resonance imaging. Mosby, St. Louis
9. Saini S, Stark DD, Rzedzian RR et al. (1989) Forty-millisecond MR imaging of the abdomen at 2.0 T. Radiology 173: 111–116
10. Henrich D, Hasse A, Mattael D (1990) 3-D snapshot flash NMR imaging of the human heart. Magn Res Imaging 8: 377
11. Stehling MK, Charnley RM, Blamire AM et al. (1990) Ultrafast magnetic resonance scanning of the liver with echo-planar imaging. Br J Radiol 63: 430

12. Maudsley AA, Twieg DB, Sappey Marinier D, Hubesch B et al. (1990) Spin echo P-31 spectroscopic imaging in the human brain. Magn Res Med 14: 415–422
13. Brasch RC (1983) Work in progress: methods of contrast enhancement for NMR imaging and potential applications. Radiology 147: 781
14. Runge VM, Clanton JA, Lukehart CM, Partain CL, James AE (1983) Paramagnetic agents for contrast enhanced NMR imaging: a review. AJR 141: 1209–1215
15. Englestad BL, Wolf GL (1988) Contrast agents. In: Stark DD, Bradley WG (eds) Magnetic resonance imaging. Mosby, St. Louis, pp 161–181
16. Vigneron DB, Nelson SJ, Murphy-Boesch J, Kelley DAC, Kessler HB, Brown TR, Taylor JS (1990) Chemical shift imaging of human brain; axial, sagittal and coronal P-31 metabolite images. Radiology 177: 643–649
17. Russell EJ, George AE, Kricheff II, Budzilovich G (1980) Atypical computed tomographic features of intracranial meningioma. Radiology 135: 673–682
18. Claussen C, Laniado M, Schorner W, Niendord HP, Weinmann JJ, Fiegler W, Felix R (1985) Gadolinium-DTPA in MR imaging of glioblastomas and intracranial metastases. AJNR 6: 669–674
19. Spagnoli MV, Goldberg HI, Grossman RI, Bilaniuk LT, Gomori JM, Hackney DB, Zimmerman RA (1986) Intracranial meningiomas: high-field MR imaging. Radiology 161: 369–375
20. Hricak H (1986) MR of the female pelvis: review. AJR 146: 1115–1122
21. Hricak H, Lacey CG, Sandles LG, Chang YCF, Winkler ML, Stern JL (1988) Invasive cervical carcinoma: comparison of MR imaging and surgical findings. Radiology 166: 623
22. Burghardt E, Hofmann HM, Ebner F, Haas J, Tamussino K, Justich E (1989) Magnetic resonance imaging in cervical cancer: a basis for objective classification. Gynecol Oncol 33: 61–67
23. Kim SH, Choi BI, Lee HP et al. (1990) Uterine cervical carcinoma: comparison of CT and MRI finds. Radiology 175: 45–51
24. Hricak H, Hamm B, Semelka R et al. The use of Gd-DTPA in gynecologic oncology. Radiology (in press)
25. Beynon J, Foy DM, Roe AM, Temple LN, Mortensen NJ (1986) Endoluminal ultrasound in the assessment of local invasion in rectal cancer. Br J Surg 73: 474–477
26. Beynon J, Mortensen NJ, Foy DM, Channer JL, Virjee J (1986) Preoperative assessment of local invasion in rectal cancer digital examination, endoluminal sonography or computer tomography? Br J Surg 73: 1015–1017
27. DeLange EE, Fechner RE, Wanebo HJ (1989) Suspected recurrent rectosigmoid carcinoma after abdominaoperineal resection: MR imaging and histopathologic findings. Radiology 170: 323–328
28. Stark DD, Wittenberg J, Butch RJ, Ferrucci JT (1987) Hepatic metastases: randomized, controlled comparison of detection with MR imaging and CT. Radiology 165: 399–406
29. Moss AA (1989) Imaging of colorectal carcinoma. Radiology 170: 308–310
30. Rifkin MD, Ehrlich SM, Marks G (1989) Staging of rectal carcinoma: prospective comparison of endorectal US and CT. Radiology 170: 319–322

New Tools in Tumor Response Monitoring

Magnetic Resonance Relaxometry and Tumors*

P.A. Rinck[1], R.N. Muller[2], and H. W. Fischer[2]

Introduction

Outstanding soft-tissue contrast is among the main characteristics of magnetic resonance imaging (MRI) which enabled the technique to be developed so rapidly. This contrast is basically the result of the relaxation phenomena T1 and T2. Following the impulse given by a radio frequency burst, the process of returning to a state of equilibrium from an excited state is called the longitudinal or spin-lattice relaxation process. This is characterized by the T1 relaxation time, which commonly lies in the range of several hundred milliseconds. The T2 relaxation time characterizes the dephasing of the spins; therefore, it is called the spin-spin or the transverse relaxation process. In fluids, T2 equals T1; in tissues, however, T2 times are shorter than T1 times. For example, at a magnetic field strength of 0.5 T, human kidney tissue has a T1 relaxation time of approximately 500 ms and a T2 of approximately 80 ms.

History

The use of relaxation times for medical applications was first proposed, attempted, and patented in 1974 by Damadian and collaborators [1, 2]. Originally, Damadian did not intend to use the relaxation times for imaging but for tissue characterization. The method was aimed at screening humans for cancer cells. This idea has since occupied the minds of many researchers, as the ultimate goal of diagnostic medicine is noninvasive tissue characterization and the external identification of malignant cells within the human body without touching the body. Damadian's claim that relaxation-time changes highlight cancer cells seemed to be the pivotal step in medical progress. Thus, it is

[1] University of Trondheim, Medical Faculty, MR Center, Medical Section, 7006 Trondheim, Norway
[2] Université de Mons-Hainaut, Faculté de Médecine, Laboratoire de RMN, 7000 Mons, Belgium
* The relaxometry research was supported by a Collaborative Research Program grant of the North Atlantic Treaty Organization, Scientific Affairs Division, Brussels, Belgium.

Advanced Radiation Therapy Tumor Response
Monitoring and Treatment Planning
Breit (Editor-in-Chief)
© Springer-Verlag, Berlin Heidelberg 1992

understandable that relaxation has been described as the Holy Grail of magnetic resonance. Damadian's assertion that nuclear magnetic resonance can detect cancer has proven partly true, but in a different way: MRI with images based on relaxation times has become one of the main medical technologies applied in cancer diagnosis and follow-up.

Problems

The original idea of replacing hospital pathology departments by MRI equipment did not materialize. In vivo relaxation-time measurements based on MRI have been tried over the years by a large number of researchers who have used relaxation-time values for tissue characterization in the brain, body, muscles, and bones. The task proved to be in vain because all efforts to characterize or even to type tissues largely failed. The reasons are manifold and include systematic measurement errors, inaccuracy of two-point plotting methods of relaxation curves, inherent variability of tissue composition, partial volume effects, and interobserver variability. Researchers realized that it is futile to measure a point or a region of interest within a tumor because too many different components, such as tumor and necrotic cells, small vessels, calcifications, and other structures, can be found within a volume of interest. In addition, T1 and T2 values overlap with those of other pathologies and sometimes of normal tissue, and T1 and T2 values of normal tissue change with age and hormonal cycles, breast tissue being a good example.

In 1985 we demonstrated that even carefully performed in vivo T2 measurements are nondiagnostic in cancer detection, characterization, or typing [3]. After absolute T1 or T2 values had been used unsuccessfully by researchers, combinations of T1 and T2, histogram techniques, and more sophisticated three-dimensional display techniques of factor representations were used [4]. However, the heterogeneity of normal tissues, as well as that of pathological benign and malignant tissues, did not allow the pathologist's view through the microscope to be replaced with MRI techniques. Thus, for tissue characterization new techniques have been proposed which are not based upon relaxation time measurements [5].

Damadian also claimed that T1 values of tumorous tissue are always higher than those of normal tissue. His dream of MRI becoming the perfect screening method for cancer tissue in the human body was finally shattered when this claim was refuted. T1 values depend on the magnetic field strength, i.e., they increase with the magnetic field. Some tumor values can be lower than the values of normal tissue at certain fields; some are even the same at certain fields so that they cannot be distinguished [6].

Applications

Every year, the literature announces new attempts to exploit relaxation time measurements in vivo. There are some positive reports about the successful use of relaxation-time measurements in vivo. These all concern follow-up of therapy with the patient being his own reference. Recent publications include, for instance, the report that relaxation times from leucemic bone marrow can be used for the differential diagnosis of this disease [7]. Similar results in high-grade gliomas were published by another research group [8]. Another quite interesting relaxation-time study is the measurement of "noninvolved" white brain matter in multiple sclerosis (MS) patients. Not only MS plaques but also the unconspicuous-looking white matter is also changed by the disease. Relaxation-time measurements revealed longer T2 values than in normal subjects. This is not enough to diagnose MS, but it may be of use in follow-up therapy or in helping in differential diagnosis [9].

Field-Cycling Relaxometry

An area of relaxometry which developed specific medical applications in the second half of the 1980s is field-cycling relaxometry. This technique requires a special NMR machine, the field-cycling relaxometer. With this machine, ex vivo or in vitro measurements of the relaxation behavior of tissue samples or contrast-enhancing compounds can be performed at any field strength. The advantages of this methods are obvious: (a) identical samples can be examined at identical conditions; (b) there is no interference by motion, diffusion, perfusion, flow, imaging artifacts, partial volume effects, or interindividual variations in region-of-interest/volume-of-interest delineation; (c) exact multiple-points fit are possible; (d) the entire field range used for MRI can be covered; and (e) the standard error is less than 3%. Field-cycling relaxometry showed that T1 increases nonuniformly with field, leading to specific finger-prints of T1 increase for different tissues. It also showed that T1 contrast for brain tissues is best at low/medium field [6, 10]. The pivotal benefit of such relaxation-time or relaxation-rate (1/T1 or 1/T2) measurements allows the prediction of image contrast and the development of more specific contrast agents [11]. A field-cycling data bank with more than 20 000 data points has been built up to facilitate this kind of research.

Conclusion

From a physician's point of view, in vivo relaxometry, at its present stage, is suited neither to characterize nor to type or grade diseases in the human body; it is possibly useful in the follow-up of therapy, but other methods seem more feasible in clinical surroundings. From a scientist's point of view, relaxometry is a challenging area of research, (a) in vivo, to try monitoring therapy; (b) ex vivo or in vitro, to try characterizing tissues and understanding contrast behavior. The optimum method for the latter is field-cycling relaxometry.

References

1. Damadian R (1971) Tumor detection by nuclear magnetic resonance. Science 171: 1151–1153
2. Damadian R, Zaner K, Hor D, Dimaio T (1973) Human Tumors by NMR. Physiol Chem Physics 5: 381–402
3. Rinck PA, Meindl S, Higer HP, Bieler EU, Pfannenstiel P (1985) MRI of brain tumors: discrimination and attempt of typing by CPMG sequences and in vivo T2-measurements. Radiology 157: 103–106
4. Skalej M, Higer HP, Meves M, Brückner A, Bielke G, Meindl S, Rinck P, Pfannenstiel P (1985) T2-Analyse normaler und pathologischer Strukturen des Kopfes. Digitale Bilddiagn 5: 112–119
5. Alaux A, Rinck PA (1990) Multispectral analysis of magnetic resonance images: a comparison between supervised and unsupervised classification techniques. In: Higer HP, Bielke G (eds) Tissue characterization in MRI imaging. Springer, Berlin Heidelberg New York, pp 165–169
6. Rinck PA, Fischer HW, Vander Elst L, Van Haverbeke Y, Muller RN (1988) Field-cycling relaxometry: medical applications. Radiology 168: 843–849
7. Jensen KE, Grundtvig Sørensen P, Thomsen C, Christoffersen P, Henriksen O, Karle H (1990) Magnetic resonance imaging of the bone marrow in patients with acute leukemia during and after chemotherapy. Changes in T1 relaxation. Acta Radiol 31: 445–448
8. Boesiger P, Greiner R, Schoepflin RE, Kann R, Kuenzi U (1990) Tissue characterization of brain tumors during and after pion radiation therapy. Magn Reson Imaging 8: 491–497
9. Rinck PA, Appel B, Moens E (1987) Relaxationszeitmessungen der weißen und grauen Substanz bei Patienten mit multipler Sklerose. Fortschr Rontgenstr 147: 661–663
10. Fischer HW, Rinck PA, Van Haverbeke Y, Muller RN (1990) Nuclear relaxation of human brain gray and white matter: analysis of field dependence and implications for MRI. Magn Reson Med 16: 317–334
11. Muller RN, Vander Elst L, Rinck PA, Vallet P, Maton F, Fischer HW, Roch A, Van Haverbeke Y (1988) The importance of nuclear magnetic relaxation dispersion (NMRD) profiles in MRI contrast media development. Invest Radiol 23: S229–231

Clinical ^{31}P Magnetic Resonance Spectroscopy of Cancers

D.J. Meyerhoff and M.W. Weiner

Phosphorus magnetic resonance spectroscopy (^{31}P MRS) is currently being evaluated as a clinical tool for improved diagnosis and treatment of human cancers. Its ability to obtain metabolic information from the malignancy in repeated examinations noninvasively and without known harm to the patient make it a potentially useful tool to monitor ^{31}P metabolites in cancers and their response to therapy. We discuss here the use of ^{31}P MRS first in studies of animal tumors and then in various types of human cancers.

Animal Studies

Early ^{31}P MRS studies on animal tumors demonstrated that the level of the high-energy phosphates adenosine triphosphate (ATP) and phosphocreatine (PCr; if the latter is detected at all in tumors) are lower in tumors than in normal tissue close to the tumor, and that inorganic phosphate (Pi) and phosphomonoesters (PME) are relatively high [1, 2]. ^{31}P MRS was also used to detect metabolic changes in animal tumors in response to radiation, chemotherapy, and hyperthermia (for a review see e.g., [3]). Experiments performed in this laboratory included injection of tumor necrosis factor (TNF) into tumor-bearing mice, which caused tumor ATP to diminish rapidly. Simultaneous histological evidence of focal thrombosis, hemorrhage, and early necrosis suggested that TNF produced tumor ischemia leading to tumor necrosis [4]. A significant fall in blood flow was measured with the D_2O "wash-in" method prior to decreased ATP. These results demonstrate that a major action of TNF is to produce tumor ischemia, resulting in death of cancer cells.

In maneuvers designed selectively to inhibit glycolysis and oxidative metabolism of experimental brain tumors, insulin-induced hypoglycemia produced a significant reduction in tumor ATP with no change in brain PCr or ATP [5]. Injection of 2-deoxyglucose had the same effect as insulin, suggesting that insulin inhibits tumor glycolysis by lowering blood glucose levels. Rhodamine

Magnetic Resonance Unit, DVA Medical Center, 4150 Clement St. 11M, San Franciso CA 94121, USA

Advanced Radiation Therapy Tumor Response Monitoring and Treatment Planning
Breit (Editor-in-Chief)
© Springer-Verlag, Berlin Heidelberg 1992

123, an inhibitor of oxidative phosphorylation also selectively reduced tumor ATP [5].

Brain Tumors

^{31}P MRS has recently been used to investigate human tumors and to monitor their response to therapy, and its potential in clinical applications has been reviewed [6]. With regard specifically to brain tumors, ^{31}P MR spectra appear generally to vary with type and grade. Highly malignant glioblastomas have low PME, whereas low-moderate grade astrocytomas have moderate PME levels, and meningiomas and pituitary adenomas have high amounts. Thus, PME levels alone do not simply correlate with rapid cellular growth or grade of malignancy; however, PME levels may be indicative for certain brain tumors. Upon successful tumor treatment, the ratio of PME to ATP (PME/ATP) often decreases. We performed quantitative ^{31}P ISIS spectroscopy on patients with astrocytomas and meningiomas [7], using a metabolite quantitation method developed in this laboratory [8]. All ^{31}P metabolite concentrations in these brain tumors were reduced by 20%–70%, with the exception of Pi, which was almost unchanged compared to normal brain. This overall reduction of metabolites is most likely due to decreased numbers of cells, necrosis, ischemia, and edema. The relative increase in Pi may be due to ischemia and necrosis of cancer regions. T_1 studies of two patients showed that T_1 values are increased by only about 50%, so that increased T_1 values are only partly responsible for the calculated low concentrations. Because MR signals were obtained from a relatively large volume, heterogeneity of different zones and subcellular heterogeneity were obscured. As is true for most brain tumors, intracellular pH in these tumors was significantly higher than in normal brain (7.12 versus 6.99) [7, 9, 10].

Recent studies [11] suggested that ^{1}H MRS which detects, for example, lactate, glutamate, gamma-aminobutyric acid, N-acetyl-aspartate, and other amino acids [12] may specifically characterize the type of brain tumor; in particular, glioblastomas had high levels of lactate in contrast to other brain tumors, while N-acetyl-aspartate was absent or diminished in many brain tumors [11].

Magnetic resonance spectroscopic imaging (MRSI) is conceptionally a combination of MRI and MRS, thus providing both biochemical and anatomical information [13, 14]. MRSI data can be reconstructed in a flexible manner *after* acquisition as spectra from any chosen volume within the brain and as low-resolution metabolite images from the head reflecting anatomy and metabolic heterogeneity. After initial results in animals [15, 16], preliminary ^{31}P and ^{1}H MRSI data have been obtained from human brain cancers [17, 18]. Metabolic images and spectra reflect metabolic variations across tumors, lactate in tumors, and increased PME in gliomas.

Superficial Tumors Outside CNS

Studies of human tumors outside of the brain have suggested that most of these cancers are characterized by large amounts of PME (primarily consisting of the phospholipid precursors phosphorylcholine and phosphorylethanolamine) and/or increased levels of phosphodiesters (PDE; composed predominantly of the phospholipid breakdown products glycero-phosphorylcholine and glycero-phosphorylethanolamine), and that PME/ATP decreases as these tumors respond to therapy.

Superficial squamous cell carcinomas and lymphomas, a Ewing's sarcoma, and an adenocarcinoma were studied in this laboratory using single-pulse experiments with surface coils placed directly over the tumor [19]. The average PME/ATP in four lymphomas (1.8 $\pm$ 0.5), which appear to have the highest level of PME of all examined tumors, was greater than that of seven other superficial tumors (1.0 $\pm$ 0.24) and much higher than that of the underlying skeletal muscle (PME/ATP = 0.2). Response of tumors to therapy correlated with a decrease in PME/ATP [19]. PME/ATP increased in two nonresponders (whose tumors increased in size) and decreased or remained constant in all responders (whose tumors decreased in size). These data suggest that changes in ^{31}P MR spectra correlate with tumor regression or progression. However, in one case the PME/ATP of one responder did not change, suggesting that these metabolic changes may not be highly specific indicators of response to therapy. Our results show that changes in MRS parameters during therapy did not reliably *precede* changes in tumor size.

Liver Tumors

Extensive studies of liver tumors have been hampered by the lack of suitable localization techniques for use with surface coils. A ^{31}P ISIS localization technique, modified for use with surface coils, has been used in this laboratory on patients with hepatic adenocarcinomas and metastases from colon cancer [20]. Serial ^{31}P MRS measurements were performed before and after a combined chemotherapy/embolization treatment of the cancerous liver (chemo-embolization) [20]. Again, it was the PME/ATP ratio that was significantly elevated in these cancers compared to healthy liver parenchyma in normal controls, and molar metabolite concentrations were significantly reduced. As an acute effect of chemoembolization, ATP, PME, and PDE levels decreased dramatically while Pi slightly increased consistent with necrosis and tissue ischemia due to embolization. In a clinically successful chemoembolization, ATP, PDE, and Pi levels recovered to at least prechemoembolization values (usually 60%–80% of normal), whereas PME decreased with time. These early results suggest that localized, serial ^{31}P MRS may provide direct evidence of the success of chemoembolization that cannot be obtained otherwise. For instance, serial computed tomography, ultrasound, and MRI did not show immediate changes in the appearance of tumors with therapy and were only in-direct measures of therapeutic outcome, as were serial alpha-fetoprotein measurements.

Prostate Tumors

There is no clinical technique that can detect prostatic cancer noninvasively and sensitively, and that can distinguish it from benign prostatic hypertrophy (BPH). Prostatic cancers and BPH have been studied in this laboratory with a ^{31}P transrectal surface coil [21]. Both diseases were associated with increased PME/ATP, whereas PCr/ATP was significantly decreased in prostatic cancer compared to normal controls and BPH.

Conclusion

To summarize, tumors have unique ^{31}P and ^{1}H MR spectra compared to normal tissue, and metabolic alterations of high-energy and amino acid meta-bolism during therapy can often be monitored *before* established imaging modalities such as computed tomography, ultrasound, and MRI detect any metabolic changes. To improve the role of MRS in the diagnosis and treatment of human cancers, large-scale clinical studies on homogeneous patient popula-tions are necessary. MRSI will be important in the study of heterogeneous disease such as cancer because it is or will become appealing to the clinician because it provides images of metabolite distribution in the tumor and from adjacent noncancerous tissue [17, 22]. Technically, increased spatial resolution and better molar quantitation techniques are required to make MRS a more useful clinical tool.

References

1. Evanochko WT, Ng TC, Glickson JD (1984) Application of in vivo NMR spectroscopy to cancer. Magn Reson Med 1: 508–534
2. Griffiths JR, Iles RA (1982) NMR studies of tumors. Biosci Rep 2: 719–725

3. Steen RG (1989) Response of solid tumors to chemotherapy monitored by in vivo ^{31}P nuclear magnetic resonance spectroscopy: a review. Cancer Res 49: 4075–4085
4. Shine N, Palladino MA, Patton JS et al. (1989) ^{31}P NMR defects early response to tumor necrosis factor in mouse sarcoma. Cancer Res 49: 2123–2127
5. Arbeit JA, Toy BJ, Karczmar GS, Hubesch A, Weiner MW (1988) Inhibition of tumor high-energy phosphate metabolism by insulin combined with Rhodamine 123. Surgery 104: 161–170
6. Daly PF, Cohen JS (1989) Magnetic resonance spectroscopy of tumors and potential in vivo clinical applications: a review. Cancer Res 49: 770–779
7. Hubesch B, Sappey-Marinier D, Roth K, Meyerhoff DJ, Matson GB, Weiner MW (1989) P-31 MR spectroscopy of normal human brain and brain tumors. Radiology 174: 401–409
8. Roth K, Hubesch B, Meyerhoff DJ et al. (1989) Non-invasive quantitation of phosphorus metabolites in human tissue by NMR spectroscopy. J Magn Reson 81: 299–311
9. Segebarth C, Balerieaux D, Arnold DL, Luyten PR, Den Hollander JA (1987) MR image-guided 31-P MR spectroscopy in the evaluation of brain tumor treatment. Radiology 165: 215–219
10. Arnold DL, Shoubridge EA, Feindel W, Villemure JG (1987) Metabolic changes in cerebral gliomas within hours of treatment with intra-arterial BCNU demonstrated by phosphorus magnetic resonance spectroscopy. Can J Neurol Sci 14: 570–575
11. Bruhn H, Frahm J, Gyngell ML et al. (1989) Noninvasive differentiation of tumors with use of localized H-1 MR spectroscopy in vivo: initial experience in patients with cerebral tumors. Radiology 172: 541–548
12. Weiner MW, Hetherington HP (1989) The power of the proton. Radiology 172: 318
13. Maudsley AA, Hilal SK, Perman W, Simon HE (1983) Spatially resolved high resolution spectroscopy by "four-dimensional" NMR. J Magn Reson 51: 147–152
14. Brown TR, Kincaid BM, Ugurbil K (1982) NMR chemical shift imaging in three dimensions. Proc Natl Acad Sci USA 79: 3523–3526
15. Maudsley AA, Hilal SK, Simon HE, Wittekoek S (1985) In vivo MR spectroscopic imaging with P-31. Radiology 153: 745–749
16. Haselgrove JC, Subramanian VH, Leigh JS, Gyulai J, Chance B (1983) In vivo one-dimensional imaging of phosphorus metabolites by phosphorus-31 nuclear magnetic resonance. Science 220: 1170–1173
17. Hugg JW, Matson GB, Twieg DB et al. (1992) ^{31}P spectroscopic imaging of normal and pathological human brain. Magnetic Resonance Imaging 10: 227–243
18. Luyten PR, Marien AJH, Heindel W et al. (1990) Metabolic imaging of patients with intracranial tumors: H-1 MR spectroscopic imaging and PET. Radiology 176: 791–799
19. Karczmar GS, Meyerhoff DJ, Boska MD et al. (1991) ^{31}P MRS study of response of superficial human tumors to therapy. Radiology 179: 149–155
20. Meyerhoff DJ, Karczmar GS, Venook AP et al. (1992) Hepatic cancers and their response to chemoembolization therapy: Quantitative image-guided ^{31}P Magnetic Resonance Spectroscopy. Investigative Radiology 27 (in press)
21. Kurhanewicz J, Thomas MA, Jajodia P et al. (1991) Spectroscopy of the human prostate gland in vivo using a transrectal probe. Magn Res Med 22: 404–413
22. Meyerhoff DJ, Maudsley AA, Schaefer S, Weiner MW (1992) Phosphorus-31 magnetic resonance metabolite imaging in the human body. Magnetic Resonance Imaging 10: 245–256

Monitoring of Tumor Response After Chemo- and Radiotherapy by In Vivo Magnetic Resonance Spectroscopy

W. Semmler, P. Bachert, and G. van Kaick

Introduction

At present, in vivo magnetic resonance spectroscopy (MRS) is the only method that allows the detection of metabolites in vivo, noninvasively, and at real time in the intact tissue. Further development of MRS may well increase the specificity of the method and lead to improved insight into the cell metabolism. Experimental studies — in vitro and in vivo — demonstrated that MRS is capable of detecting different stages of tumor growth, monitoring therapy response, and observing the tissue metabolism. Accordingly, extensive studies of muscle, liver, kidney, brain tissue and of tumors in human subjects were carried out (for a review, see [1]). Tumor characterization by means of in vivo MRS is controversial [2, 6]; however, it seems that ^{1}H and ^{31}P MRS are not able to differentiate between various tumor types. One feasible clinical application of MRS is tumor therapy control [4, 9, 11–14].

Materials and Methods

Good spectral resolution is mandatory; hence MRS requires a much higher magnetic field homogeneity than MRI. This should be in the order of about 0.1–0.3 ppm in a $5 \times 5 \times 5\,cm^3$ volume in the tissue. The minimum detectable volumes in humans are about $1\,cm^3$ for ^{1}H MRS and $30\,cm^3$ for ^{31}P MRS. In our clinical studies we used a 1.5-T whole-body MR system. Fast MR images for control of the position of the coil and the volume of interest were obtained using the spectroscopy coil. In the standard ^{1}H and ^{31}P MRS examinations, a total acquisition time of not more than 8 min for a single MR spectrum is used. The time needed for a MRS patient examination was generally less than 60 min; follow-up studies lasted up to 3 h. Long-term and short-term follow-up protocols were defined for tumor patients after chemo- and radiotherapy. In general, the long-term study lasted 2 weeks, including the acquisition of baseline

Institute of Radiology and Pathophysiology, German Cancer Research Center, Im Neuenheimer Feld 280, 6900 Heidelberg, FRG

Advanced Radiation Therapy Tumor Response
Monitoring and Treatment Planning
Breit (Editor-in-Chief)
© Springer-Verlag, Berlin Heidelberg 1992

spectra, examinations on the 1st, 2nd, and 3rd day after beginning of therapy and a control experiment after 2 weeks. In these types of studies, changes in different cell populations can be observed, for example, an increase in necrotic cell mass and a decrease in the number of cells with aerobic metabolism [12, 13]. During short-term follow-ups MR spectra are obtained before, during, and after administration of the chemotherapeutic drug. These examinations allow the monitoring of immediate metabolic and physiological changes upon chemotherapy.

Clinical Applications

In the past, most of the effort of in vivo MRS has been directed to biochemical studies, and especially spectroscopy of the muscle has been of major interest [8]. However, these studies are not clinical routine. In contrast to the sophisticated experimental arrangements and data evaluation used in biochemistry and in vivo animal experiments, the demand on MRS by the clinician is much simpler.

The monitoring of tumor response to therapy is a routine oncological procedure and is performed predominantly by imaging modalities. The tumor size is used as the main indicator of tumor response; however, most of its reduction is not observed before the 1st or 2nd week after onset of therapy. As a consequence, the success of therapy — that is, the differentiation of responders and nonresponders — can be assessed only very late with these methods. If MRS could detect therapy effects at an earlier stage, the resulting time advantage would provide a more effective therapy, and an optimization of tumor therapy could be possible.

Most clinical MRS investigations were performed using surface coils, because this is a simple technique and a high signal-to-noise ratio is achieved. In a recent study, Ross et al. [10] compared surface coil localization and chemical shift imaging (CSI) when monitoring a patient after chemotherapy. Although contamination from muscle signal was present in the spectra obtained with surface coils, the changes in phosphomonoester (PME) intensity were observed as in the CSI experiment.

Short-term follow-up examinations are performed within the first hours of therapy. In these studies no changes in tumor size or relaxation behaviour were observed. However, shortly after the start of infusion, a change in ^{31}P MRS spectral parameters was seen, but no change in pH. Whether these effects are due to an immediate therapeutic response or to physiological reactions is an open question.

Long-term studies have been performed by several groups [4, 9, 11–14, 17]. Ross et al. [10] monitored chemotherapy in a patient with osteosarcoma. In the course of the treatment they observed a decrease in phosphodiester (PDE) and adenosine triphosphate signal intensities. In patients with bone sarcomas our group found similar changes in spectral parameters [13]. These examinations demonstrate that changes in the tumor metabolism after administration of chemotherapeutic drugs can be detected and monitored by ^{31}P MRS. Similar observations were made by Ng et al. [5], who observed changes in the PDE/ATP ratio after radiation therapy in a patient with a lymphoma.

In patients with lymph node metastases, the ^{31}P MRS spectra show elevated PME and PDE resonances after chemotherapy. PDE and PME have a steep increase and drop later. Inorganic phosphate is increased immediately after chemotherapy. The pH value drops initially and rises later [3]. The tumor diameter measured in the MR images was usually constant the first 3–4 days after onset of therapy.

At present it is not yet clear whether ^{31}P MRS can differentiate responders from nonresponders, although Gademann et al. [3] and Sostman et al. [17] observed a high correlation between the pH value measured by ^{31}P MRS and the clinical response measured by the reduction in tumor size and the amount of necrosis, respectively. The first follow-ups after fractionated radiotherapy were performed using ^{1}H MRS. Significant increases in the signal intensities of phosphocreatine, inositole, and choline resonances were observed after the first fractions [15].

In contrast to positron emission tomography, MRS can measure labeled drugs and their metabolites separately. For example, using in vivo ^{19}F MRS, not only the chemotherapeutic drug 5-fluorouracil (5-FU), but also its catabolite α-fluoro-β-alanine (FBAL) and in one case the cytotoxic anabolites (5-FUranuc) were detected in tumor patients undergoing 5-FU therapy [7, 16, 18]. The observed time courses for 5-FU and FBAL intensities in the patients with liver metastases vary significantly. The correlation of these data with the clinical outcome cannot be established at present because of the small number of patients and different pretreatments.

Conclusion

The results discussed here can be summarized as follows:

- Immediate effects of chemotherapeutic drugs on the tumor metabolism can be observed.
- Metabolic changes caused by therapy can be observed earlier than with conventional methods.
- Discrimination of responders from nonresponders may be possible; however, the number of cases is too low, and the changes in the spectral parameter are only moderate, so this must be verified in a greater number of patients.
- ^{31}P MRS may be a suitable tool for monitoring of tumor therapy.
- ^{19}F MRS can be employed for therapy monitoring during 5-FU administration. The cytotoxic 5-FU nucleotides can be observed in patients.

References

1. Bottomley PA (1989) Human in vivo NMR spectroscopy in diagnostic medicine: clinical tool or research probe? Radiology 170: 1–15
2. Bruhn H, Frahm J, Gyngell M, Merbold KD, Hänicke W, Sauter R, Hamburger C (1989) Noninvasive differentiation of tumors using localized H-1 MR spectroscopy in vivo: initial experience in patients with cerebral tumors. Radiology 172: 541–548
3. Gademann G, Semmler W, Bachert-Baumann P, Gückel F, Zabel H-J, Lenarz T, van Kaick G (1988) ^{31}P MR spectroscopy and ^{1}H MR tomography of cervical lymh node metastases under chemotherapy in short term follow-up studes. Soc Magn Reson Med, San Francisco, p 715 (book of abstracts)
4. Karczmar GS, Meyerhoff DJ, Boska MD, Hubesch B, Matson GB (1989) Response of superficial human tumors to therapy studied by ^{31}P MRS. Soc Magn Reson Med, Amsterdam, p. 432 (book of abstracts)
5. Ng TC, Vijayakumar S, Majors AW, Thomas FJ, Meaney TF, Baldwin NJ (1987) Response of a non-Hodgkin lymphoma to ^{60}Co therapy monitored by ^{31}P MRS in situ. Int J Rad Oncol Biol Phys 13: 1545–1551
6. Ott D, Ernst T, Hennig J (1990) Clinical value of ^{1}H spectroscopy of brain tumors. Soc Magn Reson Med, New York, p. 105 (book of abstracts)
7. Presant CA, Wolf W, Albright MJ, Servis KL, Ring III R, Atkinson D, Ong RL, Wiseman C, King M, Blayney D, Kennedy P, El-Tahtawy A, Singh M, Shani J (1990) Human tumor fluorouracil trapping: clinical correlations of in vivo ^{19}F nuclear magnetic resonance spectroscopy pharmacokinetics. J Clin Onc 8: 1868–1873
8. Radda GK (1986) Control of bioenergetics: from cells to man by phosphorus nuclear-magnetic-resonance spectroscopy. Biochem Soc Trans 14: 517–525
9. Redmond O, Stack JP, Scully M, Dervan P, Carney D, Ennis JT (1988) Tissue characterisation and spectral analysis of malignant tumours following chemotherapy. Soc Magn Reson Med, San Francisco, p 432 (book of abstracts)
10. Ross B, Helsper JT, Cox IJ, Young IR, Kempf R, Makepeace A, Pennock J (1987) Osteosarcoma and other neoplasms of bone: magnetic resonance spectroscopy to monitor therapy. Arch Surg 122: 1464–1469
11. Semmler W (1988) Monitoring tumor response to chemotherapy in patients with ^{31}P MR spectroscopy. Tumor Diagn Ther 9: 167
12. Semmler W, Gademann G, Bachert-Baumann P, Bier V, Zabel H-J, Lorenz WJ, van Kaick G (1988) In vivo ^{31}Phosphor-Spektroskopie von Tumoren: prä-, intra- und posttherapeutisch. ForstchrGeb Rontgenstr 149: 369–377
13. Semmler W, Gademann G, Bachert-Baumann P, Zabel H-J, Lorenz WJ, van Kaick G (1988) Monitoring human tumor response to therapy by means of P-31 MR spectroscopy. Radiology 166: 533–539
14. Semmler W, Gademann G, Schlag P, Bachert-Baumann P, Zabel H-J, Lorenz WJ, van Kaick G (1988) Impact of hyperthermic regional perfusion therapy on cell metabolism of malignant melanoma monitored by ^{31}P MR spectroscopy. Magn Reson Imaging 6: 335–340
15. Semmler W, Bachert-Baumann P, Gademann G, Bellemann M, Gückel F, Lorenz WJ, van Kaick G (1990) In-vivo-Tumortherapieverlaufskontrolle mit Hilfe der ^{1}H-MR-Spektroskopie unter Teilhirnbestrahlung. Zentralb Radiol 141: 421
16. Semmler W, Bachert-Baumann P, Gückel F, Ermark F, Schlag P, Lorenz WJ, van Kaick G (1990) Realtime follow-up of 5-fluorouracil metabolism in the liver of tumor patients by means of F-19 spectroscopy. Radiology 174: 141–145
17. Sostman D, Dewhirst M, Charles C, Leopold K, Moore D, Burn R, Tucker A, Harrelson J, Oleson (1990) Prognostic evaluation and therapy monitoring in human soft tissue sarcomas with ^{31}P MRS. Soc Mag Reson Med, New York, p. 319 (book of abstracts)
18. Wolf W, Presant CA, Servis KL, El-Thataway A, Albright MJ, Barker PB, Ring III R, Atkinson D, Ong R, King M, Singh M, Ray M, Wiseman C, Blayney D, Shani J (1990) Tumor trapping of 5-fluorouracil: in vivo ^{19}F NMR spectroscopic pharmacokinetics in tumor-bearing humans and rabbits. Proc Natl Acad Sci USA 87: 492–496

Positron Emission Tomography for Therapy Management

L.G. Strauss

Tumor Perfusion and Metabolism

Colorectal Tumors. Positron emission tomography (PET) was used in the follow-up of patients with colorectal malignancies to differentiate recurrent colorectal tumor and scar. The tumor perfusion was evaluated with ^{15}O-labeled water while [^{18}F]fluorodeoxyglucose (FDG) was used for the assessment of tumor metabolism. FDG is transported like glucose, but it is trapped after phosphorylation. Therefore, FDG provides information about regional glucose metabolism. The tracer concentration was evaluated quantitatively by means of a region-of-interest (ROI) technique and standardized for both injected dose and body volume. Twenty-seven patients had a recurrent colorectal malignancy, and 13 had a nonmalignant mass. Quantitative evaluation of the data demonstrated rapid FDG uptake by the tumor followed by a slight decrease in uptake values for up to 40 min after FDG administration (Fig. 1). Of the 27 tumors, 25 were correctly identified using the standardized concentration values 1 h after FDG injection, while all 13 benign lesions were correctly classified. Perfusion imaging with ^{15}O-labeled water gave no additional information.

Lung Tumors. The metabolism of lung tumors was determined by PET using FDG. Furthermore, ^{15}O-labeled water and [^{13}N] glutamate were used in selected patients to evaluate tumor perfusion and metabolism. PET studies were performed prior to therapy ($n = 23$) and during chemotherapy ($n = 8$). The change in tumor volume was compared to the change in tumor metabolism during chemotherapy. All tumors showed a significant FDG uptake prior to therapy. Involved lymph nodes were correctly identified in three patients. We noted no correlation between FDG uptake in the tumor and histology of the lesions. The change in FDG uptake was a more sensitive parameter for therapy response than the change in tumor volume. The FDG uptake prior to therapy was correlated with survival.

Hypopharyngeal Tumors. PET studies were performed in patients with hypopharynx carcinoma to determine the metabolism of the tumor and the involved

German Cancer Research Center, Im Neuenheimer Feld 280, 6900 Heidelberg, FRG

Advanced Radiation Therapy Tumor Response
Monitoring and Treatment Planning
Breit (Editor-in-Chief)
© Springer-Verlag, Berlin Heidelberg 1992

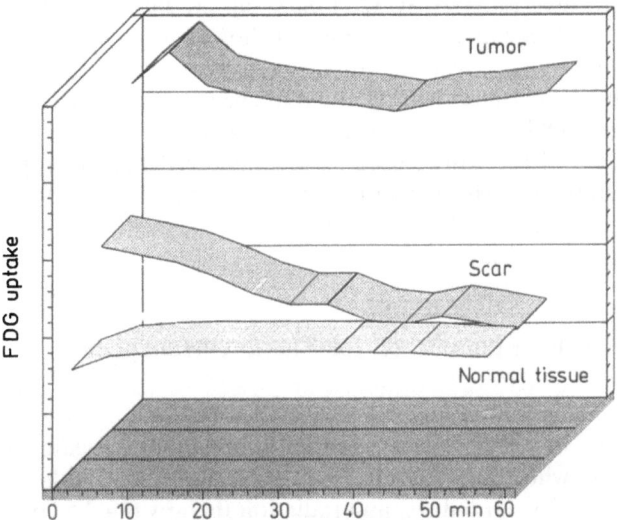

Fig. 1. FDG uptake (mean values) up to 60 min after radiotracer injection

lymph nodes prior to and after chemotherapy. Furthermore, computed tomography (CT) was used to measure the change in tumor volume during chemotherapy. Tumor proliferation was evaluated with biopsy and one-dimensional flow cytometry. All patients ($n = 6$) were directed to chemotherapy with cisplatin shortly after the first PET study. A second PET examination was performed after the first chemotherapeutic cycle. We noted a high tracer uptake in all malignancies, indicative of high tumor metabolism. Furthermore, a high FDG accumulation was found in involved lymph nodes and bone metastases. The FDG uptake in the lesions decreased in four patients and was constant in two. A correlation was found between the change in tumor volume as measured by CT and the change in FDG uptake. The proliferative index, as determined by one-dimensional flow cytometry, was correlated with the FDG uptake in the malignant lesions.

Malignant Melanoma. Different chemotherapeutic protocols are used for the treatment of patients with metastatic melanomas. We used PET in these patients to quantify the metabolic activity in metastases prior to and after therapy. The evaluation included ten PET studies in five patients. CT examinations preceded PET in each patient to determine the target area. PET studies were performed with intravenously injected FDG (370–444 MBq) followed by sequential imaging for 60 min. Standardized uptake values (SUV) were calculated from the iteratively reconstructed cross-sections using a ROI technique. The FDG uptake in lymph node metastases was 2.1–13.1 SUV prior to therapy. Lower values were observed in bone metastases (1.3 SUV) while FDG uptake was 2.5–3.0 SUV in metastases of the adrenal gland. Comparable results were obtained in liver metastases (2.5–3.4 SUV). Follow-up studies after chemo-therapy with fotemustine (200 mg, 30-min infusion) showed a 3% decrease in tumor metabolism 90 min after chemotherapy. The decrease in FDG uptake was 9% and 26% 1 and 2 days after therapy and remained constant for 1 week. The median decrease in FDG uptake following chemotherapy was 27.5%. Our results show that PET with FDG can be used to quantify early chemotherapeu-tic effects on tumor metabolism. The duration of the cytostatic effect can also be demonstrated by PET. Therefore, different chemotherapeutic protocols may be compared on the basis of PET studies.

Evaluation of Radiolabeled Fluorouracil for Therapy Management

Primary and Recurrent Colorectal Tumors. We examined eight patients with colorectal malignancies who were directed to intraarterial chemotherapy (Fluorouracil, FU, 750 mg/m^2 for 5 days) and radiation therapy (4 ∗ 2.5 Gy per cycle). A scanning device and/or two-ring PET was used to evaluate the distribution of intraarterially injected FU and [^{13}N] glutamate. Single-photon emission computed tomography (SPECT) with ^{99m}Tc-labeled microaggregated albumin (MAA) was performed to quantify tumor perfusion and shunting. The median shunting fraction of the tumor was 10.1% of the intraarterially injected activity and exceeded even the median perfusion value (7.5%). The FU accumu-lation increased with blood flow until optimal flow values were reached. Increasing the flow further resulted in decreased FU uptake. A linear correlation existed between glutamate uptake and FU accumulation.

Chemotherapy of Liver Metastases from Colorectal Tumors

Standard Intravenous FU Chemotherapy. [^{18}F] FU was used to obtain informa-tion about the time-dependent accumulation of the cytostatic agent; ^{15}O-labeled water was used to evaluate the perfusion pattern. Normalized tracer concentra-tions were determined for the metastases, liver parenchyma, and aorta. Data were evaluated from 52 metastases of 27 patients. Maximum liver activity was noted 28 min (median value) after FU infusion, and this was three times higher than after 2 h. The ^{18}F activity in the metastases 2 h after FU infusion was 33% of the liver activity. A low correlation was noted for the FU uptake and the perfusion of the lesions. Only 20% of the metastases showed a high tracer uptake. Furthermore, different metastases in the same patient sometimes showed different ^{18}F concentrations.

Intraarterial FU Chemotherapy. FU has found use in both intravenous and intraarterial chemotherapy. The evaluation comprised 26 double examinations (intravenous and intraarterial studies) in 13 patients with surgically implanted catheters in the gastroduodenal artery. The FU concentrations 2 h after tracer application were higher in 10 of 18 metastases using the intraarterial approach. We observed a higher systemic toxicity in 33% of patients. While the accumulation of the perfusion tracer ^{15}O-labeled water was up to ten times higher in the metastases after intraarterial injection, the FU uptake was not significantly increased by the regional application. Therefore, perfusion studies alone cannot be used to evaluate the chemotherapy outcome. The results of the ongoing study demonstrate that PET with $[^{18}F]$ FU should find preferential use in optimizing regional chemotherapy and in selecting those patients who do profit from the intraarterial approach.

FU Uptake and Tumor Growth. Tumor response to chemotherapy necessitates the accumulation and metabolism of the cytostatic agent in the target area. PET examinations were performed in 12 patients prior to chemotherapy, and the ^{18}F concentrations in the metastases ($n = 18$) were determined. Sequential CT scans were used to calculate the tumor growth rate during chemotherapy. The FU accumulation in the lesions prior to therapy was compared to the growth rate of the lesions. The correlation coefficient for the standardized FU concentration values and the growth rates exceeded 0.8. A decrease in tumor volume requires FU concentrations higher than 3.5. The polynomial regression function between FU concentration values and tumor growth rate can be used for therapy planning and optimization.

[157]Gd-Labeled Monoclonal Antibody: A Tumor-Specific Contrast Medium for Magnetic Resonance Imaging

S. Göhr-Rosenthal, H. Schmitt-Willich, W. Ebert, H. Gries, H. Vogler, and J. Conrad

The development of Gd-DTPA (Magnevist®) as a contrast-enhancing agent for magnetic resonance imaging (MRI) was a major breakthrough in contrast media research. Gd-DTPA, the first of a new generation of imaging agents was launched in 1988 in several countries, including the Federal Republic of Germany, the United States, and Japan as a contrast medium for the diagnosis of brain tumors. Contrast medium uptake by the tumor is attributed to disruption of the blood-brain barrier and is, in principle, nonspecific. In recent years several approaches for increasing the specificity of MRI contrast has been tried. One possibility for retaining a higher local concentration is the use of tissue-specific contrast agents such as Mn-DPDP, Gd-BOPTA, Gd-EOB-DTPA. Gd complexes with increased lipophilicity are eliminated not only by glomerular filtration but also by a hepatocellular transport mechanism which transfers them to the intracellular compartments of the hepatocytes, thus shortening their relaxation times. Such compounds become tissue specific as a result of this additional excretory mechanism. Implanted tumors or metastases do not show any uptake. They appear as low-signal structures and can be visualized better because of the increased contrast between the enhanced healthy liver parenchyma and the pathological area. Because of their protein-binding facility these compounds show much greater relaxivity in plasma than in water, a fact that increases the efficiency by a factor of 2. Another approach for increasing the specificity of MRI contrast is to couple Gd-DTPA to a monoclonal antibody (MAb) that is specific for a particular tumor line. We started this project despite the fact that the authors of several publications concluded that this approach would be less successful [1, 2].

The aim of our study was to link about 100 Gd atoms to one MAb molecule without significant loss of immunoreactivity. As it is not possible to retain the immunological activity of MAbs by attaching 100 Gd-DTPA molecules to the MAb, the immunoconjugates were formed by site-specific attachment of polymeric chelators to the carbohydrate moiety of the MAb far away from the antigen-binding region. This approach necessitated the development of new polymeric Gd complexes to enable us to reach measurable signal enhancement by MRI. A large number of polymeric Gd complexes were synthesized in our chemical laboratory. This study focuses on two types.

Institut für Diagnostikforschung, Freie Universität, Klinikum R. Virchow, Spandauer Damm 130, 1000 Berlin 19, FRG

Advanced Radiation Therapy Tumor Response Monitoring and Treatment Planning
Breit (Editor-in-Chief)
© Springer-Verlag, Berlin Heidelberg 1992

The first one is the so-called polychelon. This consists of a polyethylenimine backbone substituted with bromoacetic acid. Since there are no chelating subunits per se, the complex is formed by the addition of Gd. The second type consists of a polylysine backbone with DTPA molecules as chelating subunits. The preparation of conjugates was performed by periodate oxidation of the MAb followed by covalent coupling of the hydrazide derivative of the poly-chelates to the oxidized carbohydrate residue of the MAb [3]. MAb RA96 defines a mucinlike glycoprotein, extracted from a human pancreatic adeno-carcinoma [4]. The conjugate was separated from excess chelator by means of protein A or by ion-exchange chromatography. Finally, the conjugate was labeled with Gd. The Gd content was specified by atom emission spectroscopy. In the case of the polychelon type we were able to attach up to 130 Gd atoms per MAb, depending on the molecular size of the polychelate. The immunological activity was reduced to 50%. We used a cell enzyme linked immunosorbent assay (CELISA) with immobilized cells in microtiter plates to determine the immunological activity of the conjugate. The principle of this method was a competitive protein binding assay using MAb RA96 labeled with biotin as tracer.

For the second type of polymeric Gd complex, polylysine poly-DTPA, we concentrated our studies on a derivative that chelates about 50 Gd atoms per molecule. The in vitro studies showed that we could covalently attach one or two polylysine poly-DTPA molecules per MAb. These results were confirmed by atom emission spectroscopy (AES) studies which demonstrated that we labeled about 50–100 Gd atoms per MAb. The immunological activity was reduced to about 60%. Since this result was not an effect of the periodate oxidation, we see steric, and associated with this hydrophobic, interactions of the bound polychelate with the MAb as the possible reason for this reduced binding to the antigen.

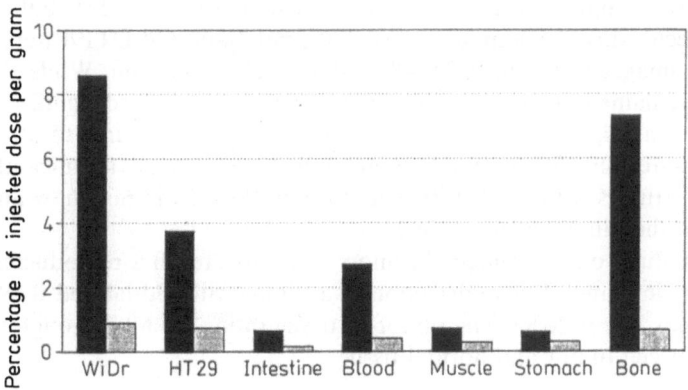

Fig. 1. In vivo distribution of RA96 polylysine ^{153}Gd-DTPA (*dark bars*) and polylysine ^{153}Gd-DTPA (*light bars*) 48 h after injection

Our relaxivity studies were performed with a 0.47-T Bruker spectrometer and demonstrated that the T_1 relaxivities of the Gd-labeled immunoconjugates were significantly higher than those of Gd-DTPA (3.84 ± 0.021 mmol^{-1} s^{-1}). This increases the efficiency of imaging in the case of Gd-polychelon by a factor of 8 and of polylysine Gd-DTPA$_{50}$ by a factor of 4.

The biodistribution studies were performed in nude mice with subcutaneously implanted colon carcinomas in the flanks. We used the WiDr cell line as specific tumor and the HT29 cell line as control tumor. We injected 222 kBq and 30 µg MAb 14–17 days after tumor implantation. The radiolabeled contrast agent was injected via the tail vein. The distribution of radioactivity was expressed as a percentage of the injected dose per gram. The animals were sacrificed 24 or 48 h after injection.

When we started these studies with the Gd-polychelon immunoconjugate, we recognized two major problems: (a) due to the poor stability of the complex we found high uptake into bone and bone marrow; (b) due to the large size (approximately 400 kDa) we did not find specific tumor uptake. Although we were able to attach up to 130 Gd atoms per MAb, we could not target the tumor with these Gd-polychelon immunoconjugates. The uptake of polylysine Gd-DTPA immunoconjugate into the specific WiDr tumor was nearly 9% of the administered dose per gram and twice as high as that into the control tumor, whereby 4% is not sufficient to constitute specific enhancement (Fig. 1). Control studies with the unbound Gd-polychelate and an unspecific immunoconjugate also showed no specific enhancement in the tumors. The WiDr tumor to tissue ratios of RA96 polylysine Gd-DTPA 48 h after injection were high enough to differentiate between tumor and normal tissue. Exceptions were liver, spleen, and kidneys.

The imaging studies were performed with two different MRI scanners (GE CSI, 1.95 T; Bruker, 2.35 T) but the technical parameters did not differ considerably. The T_1 weighted images were taken with a spin-echo sequence with a repetition time of $T_R = 400$ ms and an echo time of T_E 30 ms or 25 ms. The tumor-bearing animals were the same as those used for the biodistribution studies. The injected doses of nonradioactive RA96 polylysine Gd-DTPA were 2 and 3 mg. The images were taken 24, 48, and 72 h after injection. While the control tumor remained unaltered the specific WiDr-tumor showed significant signal enhancement 24, 48, and 72 h after injection (Fig. 2). Compared to other tissues the measurements for the WiDr tumor were nearly always significantly higher. Control studies with Gd-DTPA and Gd-polychelate did not show any enhancement in the tumors at these times.

The present study on experimental tumors demonstrates in a reproducible manner that the immunoselective detection of a tumor with Gd-labeled RA96 polychelate is possible in MRI. The tumor-to-tissue ratios are high enough to differentiate between tumor and normal tissue.

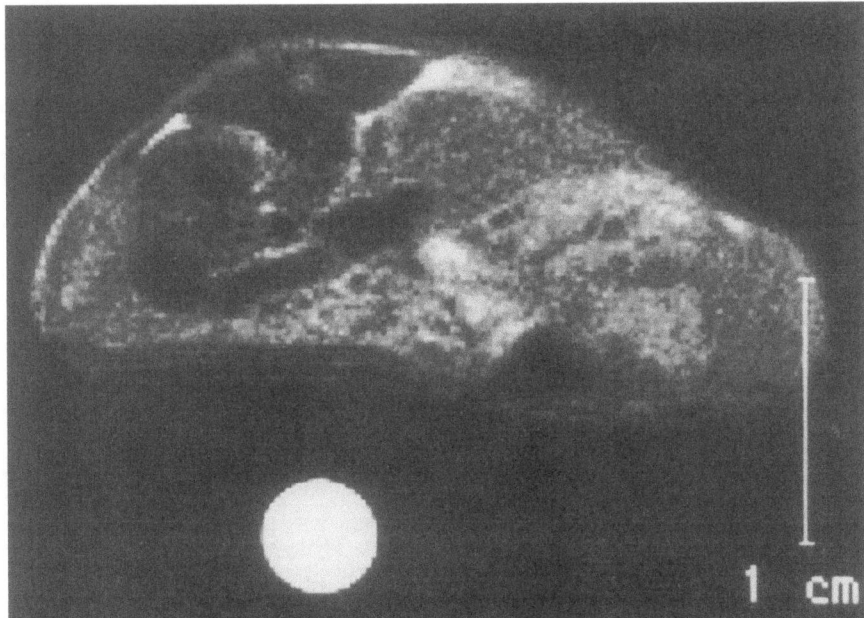

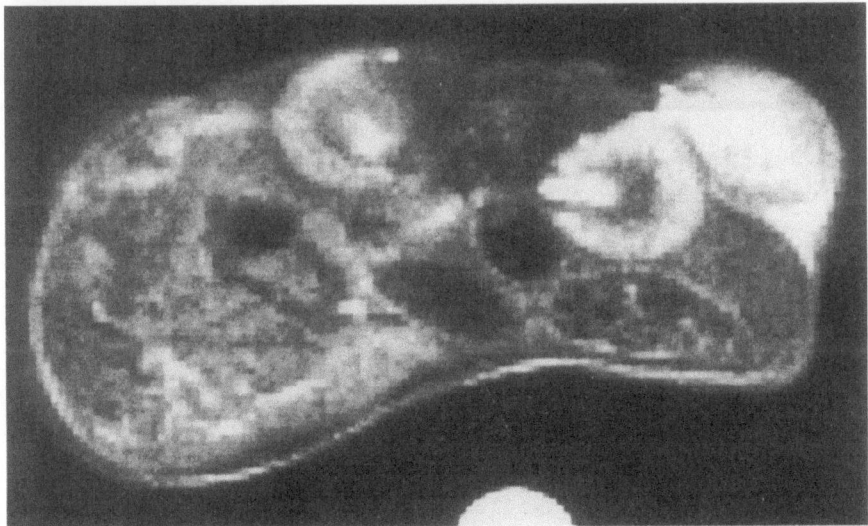

Fig. 2a, b. T1-weighted magnetic resonance images of a nude mouse. **a** Contrast enhancement of the implanted WiDr tumor (*right*) before injection of 3 mg RA96 polylysine Gd-DTPA. **b** Image 24 h after injection. The kidneys are also enhanced

References

1. Shreve P, Aisen AM (1986) Monoclonal antibodies labelled with polymeric paramagnetic ion chelates. Magn Reson Med 3: 336–340
2. Unger C, Totty WG, Neufeld DM, Otsuka FL, Murphy WA, Welch MJ, Connett JM, Philpott CW (1985) Magnetic resonance imaging using gadolinium labelled monoclonal antibody. Invest Radiol 20: 693–700
3. Shannessey DJ, Anarles RH (1985) Specific conjugation reactions of the oligosaccharide moieties of immunoglobulins. J Appl Biochem 7: 347–355
4. Kalthoff H, Holl K, Schmiegel W, Klöppel G, Arndt R, Matzku S (1987) A new mucine reacting monoclonal antibody for serum diagnosis and immunscintigraphy of pancreatic cancer. J Tumor Marker Oncol 2: 75

Present Status and Future Prospects in Application of Radiolabeled Monoclonal Antibodies in Diagnosis and Therapy

R. Senekowitsch

Tumor localization trials with radiolabeled polyclonal antibodies began 40 years ago based on the idea that antibodies against tumor-associated antigens could bring sufficient radioactivity to the tumor for efficient diagnosis and therapy of cancer [5, 11]. The development of the hybridoma technique by Köhler and Milstein for production of monoclonal antibodies (MAb) was an important contribution to further applications in the field of immunoscintigraphy and radioimmunotherapy [8]. Despite promising results concerning the accumulation of MAb to tumor-associated antigens in xenotransplanted human tumors in nude mice, with uptake values of 70% of injected dose per gram of tissue [18], the results in clinical application did not fulfill the expectations. In most clinical trials very tiny amounts of the injected dose, usually between 0.001% and 0.05%, were taken up per gram of tumor tissue, with the rest circulating in blood or localized in normal tissue such as liver and kidney [9]. Therefore tumor-to-background ratios of radioactivity, essential for scintigraphic imaging of the tumor and for radioimmunotherapy, remain too low.

A great number of factors have been demonstrated to affect the uptake of MAb by tumor and normal tissue, factors that are related to the characteristics of the tumor, the antibody itself, the tumor antigen expression, the availability of the antibody to the antigen, or the radiolabel of the MAb. Concerning these factors some major problems at present limit the application of MAb for routine clinical investigations. Essential limitations are presented by the physiological barriers to delivery of the MAb in the tumor. Three physiological barriers responsible for the poor localization of MAb in tumors have been identified; heterogeneous blood supply, elevated interstitial pressure, and long transport distances in the interstitium [7]. Radiolabeled MAb with a molecular weight of 150 kDa and even the F(ab')$_2$ fragments and Fab fragments with 100 and 50 kDa are large molecules compared to drugs and hormones. To bind specifically to a solid tumor antigen the molecule must pass out of the vascular compartment into the interstitial space. The vasculature of the tumor, though more permeable than that of normal organs, still represents a significant barrier for intact MAb and the fragments. The tumor interstitium is characterized by a large interstitial space, high collagen, low proteoglycan content, and the absence

Nuklearmedizinische Klinik und Poliklinik, Technische Universität München, Ismaninger Str. 22, 8000 Munich 80, FRG

Advanced Radiation Therapy Tumor Response
Monitoring and Treatment Planning
Breit (Editor-in-Chief)
© Springer-Verlag, Berlin Heidelberg 1992

of anatomically well-functioning lymphatic vessels [3]. These structural differences are responsible for the high interstitial pressure that influences the convection of the MAb. Increases in interstitial pressure lead to decreased extravasation of the MAb and reduce the rate of MAb movement in the interstitium. Because of the heterogeneous vasculature the antibody molecule may have to move a great distance. The vascular density has been shown to be high in the periphery of the tumor and markedly reduced in the tumor core. Therefore the MAb can hardly reach the central region of the tumor to bind to the antigen.

Another limitation stems from the fact that the current generation of MAb is largely of murine origin, and they are therefore immunogenic to the patient. The development of human anti-mouse antibody (HAMA) is a frequent problem in the repetitive administration of mouse antibodies to patients. Circulating HAMA can form high molecular weight complexes with the injected MAb, resulting in rapid blood clearance, high hepatic and/or splenic uptake, and reduced tumor targeting of the MAb. The rapid complex formation has been demonstrated in mice experiments and in vitro complex formation studies of MAb with sera of patients who had received the MAb earlier [13, 17]. The level of HAMA is correlated with the degree of complex formation. The larger molecular weight complexes have a more important role in altering the serum clearance of the radioactivity conjugated to the MAb.

The degree of immunoreactivity of MAb following radiolabeling is an important determinant of the success of binding to the antigen. MAb may be inactivated during the radiolabeling procedure due to the attachment of the label near the antigen binding site. This effect increases with increasing specific activity of the labeling and is more probable for the smaller antibody fragments. Depending on the method of labeling and the radionuclide used, there is a discrepancy between the radiolabel distribution and antibody distribution. Since the injection of MAb labeled with ^{131}I has resulted in dehalogenation or release of the radiolabel from the tumor, ^{111}In has gained more importance for MAb labeling. The radionuclide ^{99m}Tc is most suitable for labeling concerning energy and availability. The new labeling method — with the label attached directly to the protein via endogenous groups, and available as commercial kit — will be the method of the future [1, 16]. Radionuclides that can be used for immunoscintigraphy are listed in Table 1.

Table 1. Radionuclides for immunoscintigraphy

Nuclide	$t_{1/2}$	Radiation	E_γ (keV)
^{99}Tc	6.0 hours	IT	141
^{111}In	2.8 days	EC	171, 245
^{123}I	13.3 hours	EC	159
^{131}I	8.0 days	β	364
^{97}Ru	2.9 days	EC	216, 325
^{67}Ga	3.3 days	EC	93, 184

A number of metallic radionuclides are good candidates for labeling of MAb used for radioimmunotherapy, including ^{186}Re, ^{67}Cu, and ^{90}Y. The principal method of attaching these radionuclides to the MAb by chelation has suffered from the decrease in immunoreactivity and cleavage of the radionuclide from the MAb with accumulation in liver, bone, and kidney. ^{186}Re and ^{67}Cu provide good properties for radioimmunotherapy, but little experience in their use is currently available. The major problems are the chemistry of their conjugation to the MAb and their low specific activity. In radioimmunotherapy the heterogeneous binding pattern of MAb due to the heterogeneity of the antigen expression as well as the delivery of the MAb can be overcome with radionuclides of appropriate radiation properties. In solid tumors even cells which do not bind the MAb can be exposed to radiation that can kill cells several cell diameters away from the MAb bound to an antigen-positive cell. Table 2 lists the radionuclides already used for radioimmunotherapy with promising radiation properties, including α-emitters.

Many attempts have been made to improve the tumor-to-background ratio by increasing the accumulation of the MAb or the blood clearance. Increasing blood flow by external beam radiation, hyperthermia, and pharmacologic interventions with α-adrenergic stimulants failed to change tumor uptake significantly [14]. An alternative approach to the problem of low and heterogeneous antigen expression is to increase the number of antigenic sites available for binding of the radiolabeled MAb. It has been shown that recombinant α-interferon [15] and tumor-necrosis factor [12] can up-regulate the expression of tumor-associated antigens.

An important step toward the unfavorable whole-body radioactivity compared to the tumor is given by in vivo labeling of bifunctional antibodies, where one arm recognizes a tumor antigen and the other a radiolabeled chelate. The "cold" bispecific MAb is first targeted to the tumor antigen. After allowing a suitable period of time for the nonbound antibody to be cleared from the circulation, the radionuclide compound, which is recognized by the second free specificity of the MAb is injected, leading to a specific localization of the radiolabel on the tumor. Bispecific MAb can be produced from quadromas obtained after fusion of two hybridomas [2]. Another approach to in vivo labeling is the injection of a cold biotin- or streptavidin-conjugated MAb

Table 2. Radionuclides for radioimmunotherapy

Nuclide	$t_{1/2}$	Radiation	E_{av} (keV)
^{131}I	8.0 days	β	192
^{90}Y	2.7 days	β	1045
^{186}Re	3.8 days	β	386
^{67}Cu	2.6 days	β	152
^{153}Sm	2.0 days	β	230
^{212}Bi	1.1 hours	β, α	1032, 6009
^{211}At	7.2 hours	α	5900

[6, 10]. After waiting an appropriate time, the second injection of radiolabeled streptavidin or biotin leads to a rapid tumor localization of the radiolabel, taking advantage of the high affinity of streptavidin to biotin.

To overcome the problem of the patients' immune response to murine MAb several chimeric antibodies have been generated using the variable region of the murine MAb fused with a human constant region of an immunoglobulin. Recombinant/chimeric MAb use variable regions of the murine MAb with human constant-region sequences. Different recombinant human constant regions can be used for selection of optimal pharmacokinetics and effector cell interaction.

Recent advances in genetic engineering have lead to the development of recombinant single-chain antigen-binding proteins (SCA) consisting of the variable light-chain amino acid sequence of the immunoglobulin and the variable region sequence of the heavy chain [4]. The two sequences representing the antigen binding region of an antibody are connected by an amino acid linker, which can be designed especially for labeling of the molecule. The small size of the SCA, with a molecular weight of only 25 kDa, enables a more rapid diffusion across the capillary barriers and a better penetration through the tumor, therefore resulting in an improved contrast of tumor-to-normal tissue for imaging. The first experimental results indeed demonstrated a very rapid plasma clearance and an extremely rapid whole-body clearance. Despite its rapid clearance SCA showed a significant uptake in human tumor xenografts and the in vivo stability of the molecule. Since SCAs are synthesized from recombinant genes in bacterial cell systems, the potential contamination of the substance with mammalian oncogenes and viruses and also HAMA induction does not represent a further problem. If the rapid whole-body clearance and tumor targeting, as these experimental results show, is valid also for patients, it may be possible to label these molecules with positron-emitting radionuclides. The application of positron emission tomography allows the detection of smaller lesions because of its high resolution and also permits quantitative imaging.

An ideal MAb or parts of a MAb for immunoscintigraphy and radio-immunotherapy must show a high and rapid tumor accumulation and a fast excreation from nontumor tissue, providing high target-to-nontarget ratios. Successful in vitro or in vivo conjugation of radionuclides, even of α- and β-emitters with high specific activity to chimeric/recombinant or "humanized" antibodies as well as the application of recombinant antigen-binding proteins, may lead to a new generation of tailored molecules with more desirable characteristics. The possible innovations listed below demonstrate that there are different ways to modify the MAb for more efficient diagnosis and treatment of human cancer:

- Use of recombinant/chimeric or "humanized" MAb
- Use of recombinant small antigen-binding molecules that can penetrate into the tumor more efficiently
- Enhancement of antigen expression

- Use of appropriate radionuclide and new chemistry for conjugation to the MAb with high specific activity
- In vivo labeling of bispecific MAb
- Two- or multi-step labeling procedures, for example, by using the streptavidin-biotin system.

References

1. Baum R, Hertel A, Lorenz M, Schwarz A, Encke A, Hör G (1989) Tc99-m labelled anti CEA monoclonal antibody for tumour immunoscintigraphy. Nucl Med Commun 10: 348–354
2. Bosslet K, Steinsträsser A, Hermentin P, Kuhlmann L, Bruynck A, Magerstädt M, Seemann G, Schwarz A, Sedlacek HH (1991) Generation of bispecific monoclonal antibodies for two phase radioimmunotherapy. Br J Cancer 63: 681–686
3. Cobb LM (1989) Intratumor factors influencing the access of antibody to tumor cells. Cancer Immunol Immunother 28: 235–240
4. Colcher D, Bird R, Roselli M, Hardman KD, Johnson Syd, Pope S, Dodd SW, Pantoliano MW, Milenic DE, Schlom J (1990) In vivo tumor targeting of a recombinant single-chain antigen-binding protein. JNCI 82: 1191–1197
5. Goldenberg DM, De Land F, Kim E et al. (1978) Use of radiolabeled antibodies to carcino-embryonic antigen for the detection and localization of diverse cancers by external photo-scanning. N Engl J Med 298: 1384–1388
6. Hnatowich DJ (1990) Antibody radiolabeling, problems and promises. Nucl Med Biol 17: 49–55
7. Jain RK (1990) Physiological barriers to delivery of monoclonal antibodies and other macro-molecules in tumors. Cancer Res [suppl] 50: 814s–819s
8. Köhler G, Milstein C (1975) Continuous cultures of fused secreting antibody of predefined specificity. Nature 256: 495–497
9. Larson SM (1991) Radioimmunology. Cancer 67: 1253–1260
10. Oehr P, Westermann J, Germer U, Biersack HJ (1988) Scintigraphic imaging of tumors by in vivo application of biotin-conjugated antibodies and radiolabeled streptavidin. In: Höfer R, Bergmann H (eds) Radioactive isotopes in clinical medicine and research. Schattauer, Stuttgart, pp 38–43
11. Pressman D, Korngold L (1953) The in vivo localization of anti-Wagner-osteogenic-sacroma antibodies. Cancer 6: 619–623
12. Römer W, Senekowitsch R, Pabst HW (1991) Experimental studies on the use of anti-EGF-receptor MAb 425 for the tumor therapy. Eur J Nucl Med 15: 411
13. Sakahara H, Reynolds JC, Carrasquillo JA, Lora ME, Maloney PJ, Lotze MT, Larson SM, Neumann RD (1989) In vitro complex formation and biodistribution of mouse antitumor monoclonal antibody in cancer patients. J Nucl Med 30: 1311–1317
14. Sands H (1990) Experimental studies of radioimmunodetection of cancer: an overview. Cancer Res [suppl] 50: 809s–813s
15. Schlom J, Hand PH, Greiner JW, Colcher D, Shrivastav S, Carrasquillo JA, Reynold JCF, Larson SM, Raubitshek A (1990) Innovations that influence the pharmacology of monoclonal antibody guided tumor targeting. Cancer Res [suppl] 50: 820s–827s
16. Schwarz A, Steinsträsser A (1987) A novel approach to Tc-99m-labeled monoclonal antibodies. J Nucl Med 28: 221
17. Senekowitsch R, Bode W, Reidel G, Glässner H, Möllenstädt S, Kriegel H, Pabst HW (1987) Improved radioimmunoscintigraphy of human mammary carcinoma xenografts after injection of an anti-antibody. Nucl Med 26: 13
18. Senekowitsch R, Reidel G, Möllenstädt S, Kriegel H, Pabst HW (1989) Curative radio-immunotherapy of human mammary carcinoma xenografts with iodine-131-labeled mono-clonal antibodies. J Nucl Med 30: 531–537

Tumor Response Monitoring:
Brain

Nuclear Magnetic Resonance Spectroscopy of Low- and High-Grade Human Gliomas

S.R. Felber, G.J. Stockhammer, G.G. Birbamer, H. Kostron, and F.T. Aichner

Introduction

Magnetic resonance imaging (MRI) is most sensitive in detecting intracranial tumors but lacks specificity concerning histopathology and the malignant versus benign nature of the lesion. Since in vivo magnetic resonance spectroscopy (MRS) became available, several experimental and clinical investigations have suggested that MRS provides useful information for biochemical tumor characterization (Tanaka et al. 1986; Heindel et al. 1988; Bruhn et al. 1989; Gill et al. 1990). Monitoring of therapy effects (Naruse et al. 1986; Segebarth et al. 1987) may become an even more important application of MRS. The purpose of this study was to evaluate the clinical value of MRS for the diagnosis of low- and high-grade gliomas.

Patients and Methods

Combined MRI/MRS examinations were performed in 25 patients (12 women, 13 men), aged 7–68 years (mean, 47) with intracerebral gliomas of at least 3 cm diameter. Histology (WHO classification; Zülch 1980) was available in 15 patients with grade III or IV tumors and in 5 patients with grade II astrocytomas. Five patients were not operated on and were considered to be suffering from low-grade gliomas based on clinical follow-up (3–11 years) and neuroradiologic findings. Group 1 consisted of the nonoperated low-grade gliomas and grade II astrocytomas ($n = 10$); proton spectroscopy of the tumors was performed in all patients, and four underwent additional ^{31}P MRS. Group 2 consisted of the cases of high-grade glioma ($n = 15$); MRS was performed prior to surgery in 13 patients, and recurrent tumor was investigated on two occasions.

Sequential MRS studies (in two patients up to five times) were obtained in four patients of group 1 and two patients of group 2. Two patients with

Departments of Magnetic Resonance, Neurology, and Neurosurgery, University of Innsbruck, Anichstr. 35, Innsbruck, Austria

Advanced Radiation Therapy Tumor Response
Monitoring and Treatment Planning
Breit (Editor-in-Chief)
© Springer-Verlag, Berlin Heidelberg 1992

recurrent glioblastoma underwent MRS immediately before and after intravenous administration of ACNU 100 mg/m^2. All MR examinations were performed on a 1.5-T imaging/spectroscopy system (Siemens). The protocol consisted of T1- and T2-weighted spin-echo sequences in orthogonal orientations, followed by localized spectroscopy without repositioning of the patients. Additional T1-weighted images after administration of intravenous contrast agent (Gd-DTPA 0.1 mmol/kg BW) were acquired if necessary. For localized proton spectra a recently described stimulated echo sequence was used (Frahm et al. 1989). The volume of interest (16–27 ml) was targeted from routine T2-weighted images and positioned to fit as close to the tumor as possible. Sequence parameters were TR = 1500 ms, TE = 270 ms, and NEX = 256–512. Phosphorous spectra were obtained from 64- to 125-ml volumes of interest in four low-grade gliomas using ISIS with a TR of 4 s.

High-resolution localized spectra were obtained in all patients. The resonances of the phosphorous spectra were assigned to phosphomonoesters, inorganic phosphate, phosphodiesters, phosphocreatine, and adenosine

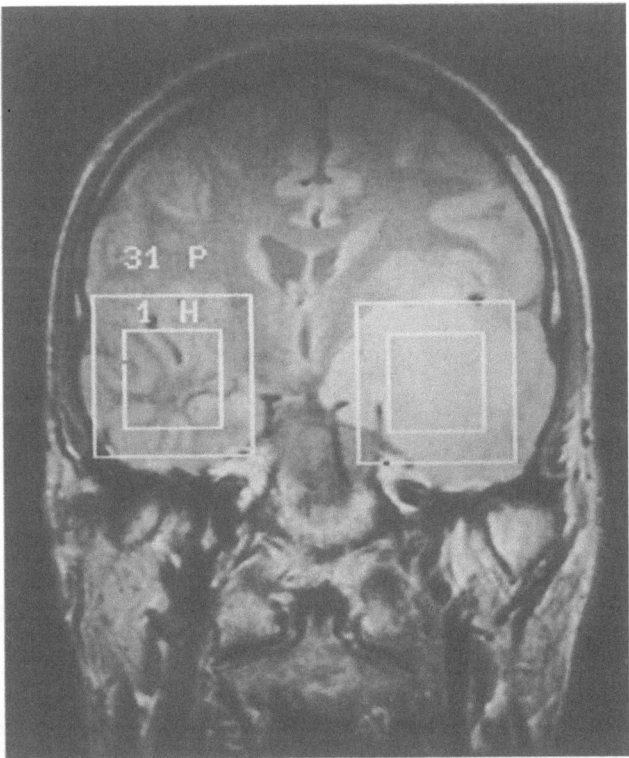

Fig. 1. Coronal long TR, short TE MR image of a 54-year-old patient with a huge left temporal low-grade glioma known since 1981. *Boxes*, Volumes of interest for ^{31}P MRS (125 ml) and water-suppressed ^{1}H MRS (27 ml)

triphosphate. In the water-suppressed proton spectra cholines, creatine/ phosphocreatine, N-acetyl-aspartate (NAA), and lactate were measured (Frahm et al. 1989).

Results

In group 1, phosphorous spectra of four low-grade gliomas (see Fig. 1) did not show significant differences to spectra of normal brain tissue (Fig. 2a); however, proton spectra always revealed significant changes in tumors (Fig. 2b). These changes consisted of increased choline relative to creatine/phosphocreatine and reduced NAA. In four patients there was also evidence of lactate at 1.3 ppm. Four patients had follow-up proton MRI/MRS at 6-month intervals. None had signs of tumor progression on MRI, and proton spectra showed constant changes over periods of 1–2.5 years.

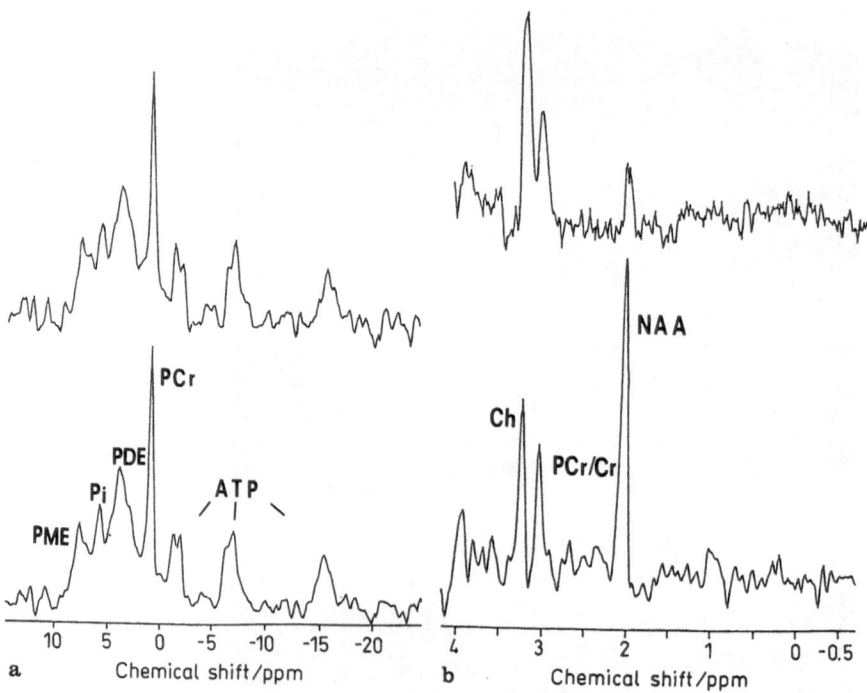

Fig. 2. a Localized phosphorous spectra of the tumor (*above*) showed no significant differences to the ³¹P spectrum of the contralateral hemisphere (*below*). **b** Proton spectra from the tumor (*above*) and the contralateral normal hemisphere (*below*). The tumor spectrum shows increase in choline compounds and marked decrease in NAA signal. *PME*, Phosphomonoesters; P_i, inorganic phosphate; *PDE*, phosphodiesters; *PCr*, phosphocreatine; *ATP*, adenosine triphosphate, *Ch*, cholines; *PCr/Cr*, phosphocreatine/creatine; *NAA*, N-acetyl-aspartate

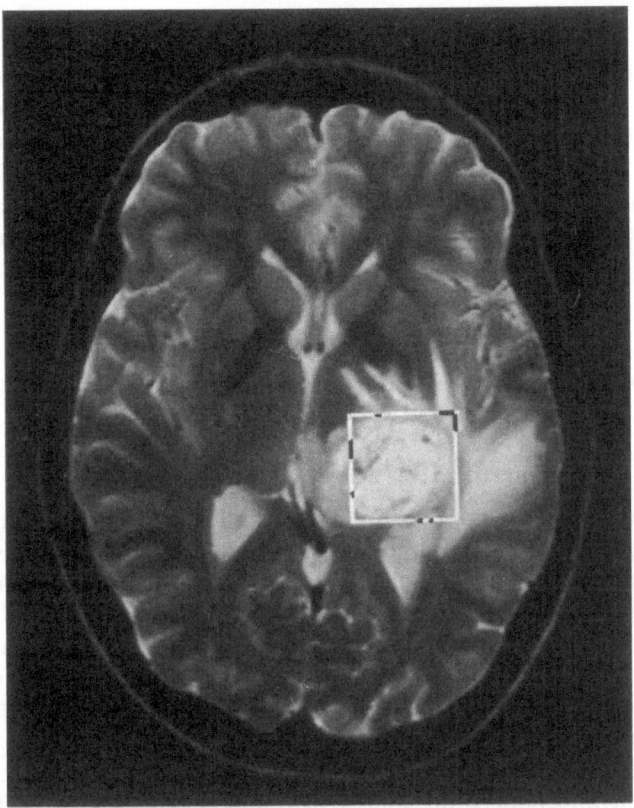

Fig. 3. Axial T2-weighted MR scan of a central glioblastoma located in the thalamus and surrounded by edema, extending along the white matter tracts. Contrast-enhanced scans (not shown) revealed ring enhancement, confirming that the volume of interest (*box*) contains central tumor necrosis

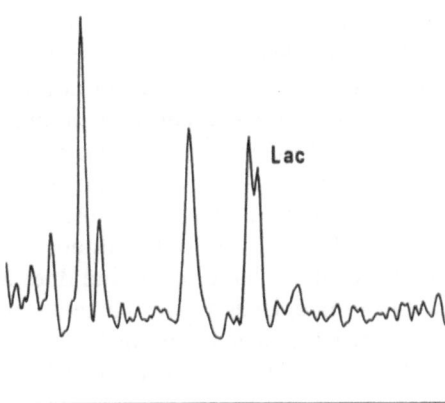

Fig. 4. The water-suppressed proton spectrum is characterized by increased cholines and reduced NAA together with a strong signal from lactate at 1.3 ppm. *Lac*, lactate

In group 2, proton spectra were obtained in 13 patients with high-grade gliomas (see Fig. 3) prior to surgery. All spectra were abnormal and revealed changes which were more pronounced than those seen in low-grade tumors. Lactate was present in all high-grade tumors and was higher than that observed in low-grade tumors (Fig. 4). Two patients with recurrent grade IV tumors were examined immediately before and after intravenous administration of 100 mg $ACNU/m^2$. On one occasion a slight increase in lactate after chemotherapy was noted.

Discussion

MRS was conducted in the routine imaging protocol of 25 patients suffering from intracerebral gliomas. In the group of low-grade gliomas proton MRS of the tumors was more sensitive than phosphorous MRS and revealed significant biochemical differences compared to normal brain tissue. This is partially explained by smaller volumes of interest and minimal partial volume averaging between tumor tissue and normal brain in proton MRS. The normal ^{31}P spectra may also reflect the fact that the metabolism of low-grade tumors closely resembles that of normal brain (Jeske et al. 1989).

The most apparent changes in proton MRS were increased choline signals and decreased creatine/phosphocreatine and NAA resonances. This agrees with previous in vivo studies (Bruhn et al. 1989; Demaerel et al. 1991) and is further supported by in vitro studies (Gill et al. 1990). Assuming that NAA is located predominantly in viable neurons (Koller et al. 1984), and that cholines originate from membrane structures, proton spectra reflected the infiltrating nature of gliomas.

These changes were more pronounced in high-grade tumors, as was expected from previous in vitro investigations (Gill et al. 1990). However, in our series spectral abnormalities overlapped between the two groups and did not allow accurate prediction of dignity in all cases. Lactate was a constant finding in grade III and IV tumors and was highest when MRI suggested tumor necrosis (Figs. 3 and 4). Lower levels of lactate were also seen in four homogeneous-appearing grade II astrocytomas. Presently, ^1H MRS cannot distinguish lactate accumulation in necrosis from anaerobic glycolysis in viable tumor cells. Furthermore, MRS at 1.5 T is restricted to relatively large voxels and does not provide access to the microheterogeneities of neoplastic tissue. Therefore it is not surprising that in vivo MRS did not provide definite specificity, but the trends observed here and by others (Bruhn et al. 1989; Demarel et al. 1990) will improve diagnosis of gliomas in future.

Follow-up spectroscopy in low-grade gliomas revealed constant changes correlating with stable clinical and MRI features. Sequential proton MRS was also performed in two patients before and after chemotherapy. In one patient with recurrent glioblastoma (confirmed at autopsy) a rise in lactate immediately after chemotherapy was observed. This preliminary observation cannot be explained by the pharmacological effects of ACNU and needs further substantiation.

In conclusion, we have shown that MRS can be integrated into a routine MR examination protocol of patients with brain tumors. Proton spectroscopy was more sensitive than phosphorous spectroscopy using ISIS in detection of tumor-associated biochemical alterations. Differences between tumor tissue and normal brain in proton MRS tended to be more pronounced in high-grade tumors, but the findings overlapped with those in low-grade tumors. In future it will be necessary to confirm further the role of proton MRS in therapy monitoring, but initial results are promising.

References

Bruhn H, Frahm J, Gyngell ML et al. (1989) Noninvasive differentiation of tumors with use of localized H-1 MR spectroscopy in vivo: initial experiences in patients with cerebral tumors. Radiology 172: 541–548

Demaerel P, Johannik K, van Hecke P et al. (1991) Localized 1H NMR spectroscopy in fifty cases of newly diagnosed intracranial tumors. J Comput Assist Tomogr 15/1: 67–76

Frahm J, Bruhn H, Gyngell ML et al. (1989) Localized high resolution H-1-NMR spectroscopy using stimulated echoes: initial applications to human brain in vivo. Magn Reson Med 9: 79–93

Gill SS, Thomas DGT, Van Bruggen N et al. (1990) Proton MR-spectroscopy of intracranial tumors: in vivo and in vitro studies. J Comput Assist Tomogr 14/4: 497–504

Heindel, W, Bunke J, Glathe S et al. (1988) Combined 1H-MR imaging and localized 31-P spectroscopy of intracranial tumors in 43 patients. J Comput Assist Tomogr 12/6: 907–916

Jeske J, Herholz K, Heinckl W et al (1989) Stoffwechseluntersuchungen an Gliomen mit der Positronen-Emissiiounstomographie und der Phosphor 31-MR Spektroskopie in Diagnostik und Therapieplanung. Onkologie 12: 42–45

Koller KJ, Zaczek R, Coyle JT (1984) N-Acetyl-aspartate-glutamate: regional levels in rat brain and the effects of brain lesions as determined by a new HPLC method. J Neurochem 43: 1136–1142

Naruse S, Horikawa Y, Tanaka C (1986) Evaluation of the effects of photoradiation therapy on brain tumors with in vivo P-31 MR spectrscopy. Radiology 160: 827–830

Segebarth C, Baleriaux D, Arnold D (1987) MR-image-guided P31 MR spectroscopy in the evaluation of brain tumor treatment. Radiology 165: 215–219

Tanaka C, Naruse S, Horikawa Y et al. (1986) Proton nuclear magnetic resonance spectra of brain tumors. Magn Reson Imaging 4: 503–508

Zülch KJ (1980) Principles of the new World Health Organization (WHO) classification of brain tumors. Neuroradiology 19: 59–66

^{31}P Magnetic Resonance in the Follow-Up of Astrocytomas

T.E. Southon, U. Sonnewald, I.S. Gribbestad, G. Nilsen, G. Unsgård, and P.A. Rinck

Introduction

The feasibility of using ^{31}P nuclear magnetic resonance spectroscopy (MRS) on living brain was demonstrated by Chance et al. (1978), and a considerable amount of data has since been published (for references see Glickson 1989). Particular effort has been directed at the diagnosis of brain tumor (Arnold et al. 1990). Metabolic studies of brain tumors have revealed that the pH of the tumor is either the same as that of the surrounding tissue or is slightly more alkaline, the phosphocreatine/nucleoside triphosphate (PCr/NTP) ratio is usually decreased, and the phosphomonoester/NTP (PME/NTP) ratio is increased relative to normal brain (Glickson 1989). Statistical analysis by Segebarth et al. (1989) has revealed that significant differences in ^{31}P MR spectra only exist between populations of normal brains and intracranial tumors. Interindividual differences are too large to unambiguously identify a particular spectrum as coming from normal or diseased brain. However, monitoring human tumor response to therapy by means of ^{31}P MRS is showing some promise. Response to chemotherapy and radiation treatment has been demonstrated in five and three patients, respectively (Semmler et al. 1988; Segebarth et al. 1987). Quantification of these changes has proven difficult, and the general applicability is questionable.

We present here the results on seven tumor patients monitoring the effect of radiation treatment and correlate the MRS data to the tumor response. Summing the signal intensities of the tumor volume and comparing this to the total intensities after treatment make it possible to distinguish between responders and nonresponders.

Materials and Methods

The examinations were performed on a Philips Gyroscan S15 at 1.5 T. The ^{1}H head coil was used to produce the images, and a ^{31}P earphone coil for the spectroscopy. The experimental procedure was image-guided volume selective

MR Center and Department of Neurosurgery, University of Trondheim, 7006 Trondheim, Norway

Advanced Radiation Therapy Tumor Response
Monitoring and Treatment Planning
Breit (Editor-in-Chief)
© Springer-Verlag, Berlin Heidelberg 1992

spectroscopy. A sagittal scout view was followed by 16 T_2-weighted transverse slices (TE = 30/90, TR = 2100). These images were used to select a volume of interest for spectroscopy, which closely matched the volume of the tumor. A second volume of interest of the same size was also selected in the noninfiltrated hemisphere. Shimming was performed on a single large volume which encompassed the two volumes of interest. The ^{31}P pulse length was measured and the acquisition performed using 90° adiabatic excitation pulses. Volume selection was by the ISIS method. Normally 512 scans were performed with a 3-s TR. The time-sharing version of ISIS used on this equipment means that effectively 364 scans were obtained for each volume. The FIDs were filtered with a convolution difference procedure and an exponential function of 15 Hz prior to Fourier transformation. Peak frequencies, line widths, and areas were determined by fitting the spectra to a series of Lorentzian peaks using the Gyroscan computer. In calculating the total phosphorus signal the intensities of PME, PDE, PCr, and ATP are included; inorganic phosphate is omitted because of difficulties in quantification. All intensities are set to 100% for the first examination, and subsequent intensities are calculated as a percentage of this value. This allows division of the patients into responders and nonresponders.

Patients were selected on the basis of previous computed tomography and MR imaging studies. The histological diagnosis was made on biopsy samples obtained either by resection in the course of surgical treatment or by stereotactic biopsy.

For in vitro studies the resected tissue was frozen within 30 s of removal. The frozen tissue was weighed and then pulverized with mortar and pestle under liquid nitrogen. Perchloric acid (PCA) 7% in D_2O was added to the tissue powder (3 ml PCA/g tissue), mixed well while the temperature was allowed to rise until the mixture could be scraped off the mortar using a Teflon scraper, and transferred to a centrifuge tube placed on ice. The extracts were centrifuged at 4000 rpm for 10 min (4°C). The supernatant was neutralized with 9 M KOH in D_2O and centrifuged at 4000 rpm for 10 min at 4°C to remove precipitated potassium perchlorate. Thereafter the supernatant was freeze-dried.

Results and Discussion

It has been pointed out previously, using ^{1}H MRS in vivo, that gliomas have little or no PCr (Bruhn et al. 1989). We examined PCA extracts of normal brain, astrocytoma, and glioblastoma. The ^{31}P spectra (results not presented) show a sharp decrease in PCr in astrocytoma compared to normal brain, and in the case of glioblastoma PCr is almost absent in the MR spectrum. The PME concentration shows the opposite trend. The ratio of NTP to nucleoside diphosphate changes in favor of nucleoside diphosphate and diphosphodiesters in astrocytomas and glioblastomas. This is in contrast to in vivo ^{31}P MRS results, in which PCr is present (Hubesch et al. 1990). It therefore appears likely that the

Table 1. Patient data

Patient	Tumor type	Therapy	MRS examinations
PA	Glioblastoma	Irradiation	1 + 3
TO	Anaplastic astrocytoma	Resection and irradiation	1 + 2
MAF	Glioblastoma	Resection and Irradiation	1 + 2
LI	Glioblastoma	Irradiation	1 + 2
AS	Nonspecified astrocytoma	Irradiation	1 + 1
BJ	Glioblastoma	Irradiation	1 + 1
DA	Nonspecified astrocytoma	Irradiation	1 + 1

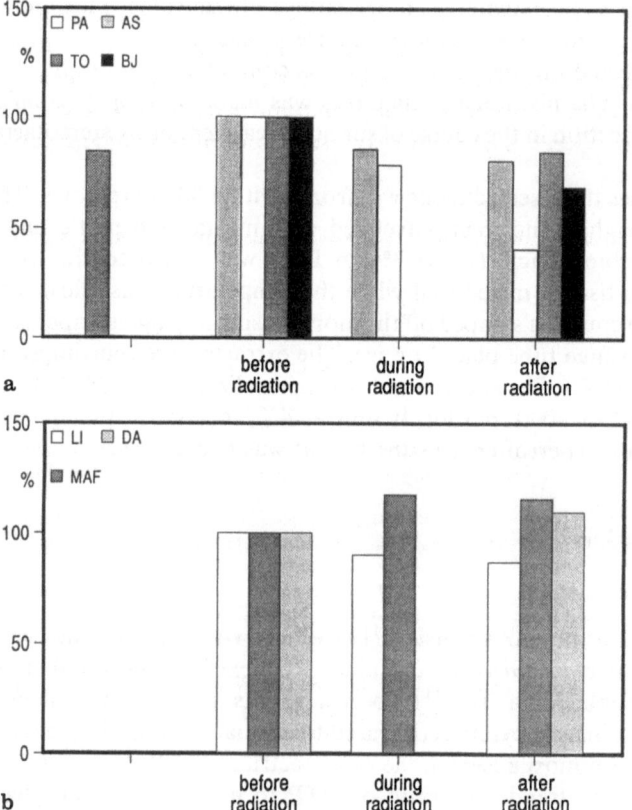

Fig. 1a, b. Total phosphorus signals before, during, and after radiation. **a** Tumor volume responders. **b** Tumor nonresponders. *Abbreviations*, patient initials (see Table 1); *PA*, preliminary examination

metabolites in the tissue surrounding the tumor contribute considerably to the spectrum.

Seven brain tumor patients were monitored before, 2 weeks after, and in some cases several months after total irradiation of the head (see Table 1 for diagnosis). Two groups of patients were defined, responders and nonresponders, taking into account the tumor response seen by MR imaging and other clinical factors. The responders were all surviving after 1 year while the nonresponders did not survive 1 year.

Comparison of PCr/NTP and PME/NTP ratios in the tumor and control volumes did not reveal any trends, and there were also no consistent changes in these ratios during therapy. The type of data analysis that has shown success has been the comparison of the tumor spectra between follow-up examinations. On the whole, intensities tended to decline at least 19% in the four patients who responded (Fig. 1a) as treatment proceeded, although no single metabolite behaved consistently. Two of the nonresponding patients showed an increase in total intensity after treatment and one non-responder showed a decrease in intensity of 11% (Fig. 1b). A tentative interpretation of these results is that responding tumor cells become severely damaged by radiation, which results in a decrease in high-energy phosphates. The nonresponding tumor cells seem to divide rapidly, as indicated by an increase in signal intensity in two cases.

^{31}P MRS thus appears to be a potentially useful tool in monitoring early response to radiotherapy.

Acknowledgments. We gratefully acknowledge the help of Åse Johanne Svarliaunet, Knut Nordlid, and Terje Grønås.

References

Arnold DL, Shoubridge EA, Villemure J-G, Feindel W (1990) Proton and phosphorus magnetic resonance spectroscopy of human astrocytomas in vivo. Preliminary observations on tumor grading. NMR Biomed 3: 184–189

Bruhn H, Frahm J, Gyngell ML (1989) Noninvasive differentiation of tumors with use of localized H-1 MR spectroscopy in vivo: initial experience in patients with cerebral tumors. Radiology 172: 541–548

Chance B, Bond M, Leigh JS Jr, McDonald G (1978) Detection of ^{31}P nuclear magnetic resonance signals in brain by in vivo and freeze-trapped assays. Proc Natl Acad Sci USA 75: 4925–4929

Glickson JD (1989) Clinical NMR spectroscopy of tumors: current status and future directions. Invest Radiol 24: 1011–1016

Hubesch B, Sappey-Marinier D, Roth K, Meyerhoff DJ, Matson GB, Weiner MW (1990) P-31 MR spectroscopy of normal human brain and brain tumors. Radiology 174: 401–409

Segebarth CM, Baleriaux DF, Arnold DL, Luyten PR, den Hollander JA (1987) MR image-guided P-31 MR spectroscopy in the evaluation of brain tumor treatment. Radiology 165: 215–219

Segebarth CM, Baleriaux DF, De Beer R, van Ormondt D, Marien A, Luyten PR, Den Hollander JA (1989) ^{1}H image-guided localized ^{31}P MR spectroscopy of human brain: quantitative analysis of ^{31}P MR spectra measured on volunteers and on intracranial tumor patients. Magn Res Med 11: 349–366

Semmler W, Gademann G, Bachert-Baumann P, Zabel H-J, Lorenz WJ, van Kaick G (1988) Monitoring human tumor response to therapy by means of P-31 MR spectroscopy. Radiology 166: 533–539

Radiotherapy of Pituitary Adenomas: Treatment Technique and Follow-Up

K. Neumann[1], W. Kornmesser[1], R. Ullrich[1], K.-J. Gräf[2], and R. Felix[1]

Introduction

Both postsurgical and primary radiotherapy have proven very effective in the treatment of pituitary adenomas [2, 3, 6, 7]. With the availability of modern accelerators in recent decades, irradiation techniques have been refined to minimize side effects. However, because radiotherapy of pituitary adenomas is infrequent compared to other tumors, there is no generally recommended treatment regime. We report here on the irradiation technique used in our clinic and on outcome of patients treated since 1987.

Patients

A total of 30 patients (19 women, 11 men; aged 18–80 years) with pituitary adenoma were treated by radiotherapy. The tumors included 19 that were non-functioning, 9 growth hormone secreting, and 2 ACTH secreting; there were 28 macroadenomas and 2 microadenomas. In three patients who received primary radiotherapy due to medical inoperability or refusal of surgery, diagnosis of pituitary adenoma was established by magnetic resonance imaging (MRI) or computed tomography (CT). Another patient treated without prior operation had a severe Cushing's disease but showed no tumor on MRI or CT. Twenty-six patients underwent neurosurgery prior to irradiation. The indication for radiotherapy in these patients was remaining postoperative endocrine activity or incomplete resected tumor.

[1] Strahlenklinik und Poliklinik, Universitätsklinikum Rudolf Virchow/Charlottenburg, Freie Universität Berlin, Spandauer Damm 130, 1000 Berlin 19, FRG
[2] Medizinische Klinik und Poliklinik, Universitätsklinikum Rudolf Virchow/Charlottenburg, Freie Universität Berlin, Spandauer Damm 130, 1000 Berlin 19, FRG

Advanced Radiation Therapy Tumor Response Monitoring and Treatment Planning
Breit (Editor-in-Chief)
© Springer-Verlag, Berlin Heidelberg 1992

Treatment Technique

Radiotherapy was performed with 20 MV photons of a Siemens Mevatron KD
linear accelerator. Twenty-six patients received a moving coronar arc field
irradiation. To permit coronal orientation of CT scans for treatment planning
and coronal plane of radiation posterior to the eyes, patients lay in prone
position with maximally reclined head. Reproducible positioning of the patient's
head was achieved by an individually casted Orfit fixation mask attached to a
special device holding the patient's chin. This could be mounted on the
treatment couch or on the CT or simulator couch. Midline and lateral marks
drawn on the fixation mask and aligned with the localizing laser beams in the
simulating and treatment rooms permitted easy and exact repositioning. Treatment fields marked on the mask and radiographs obtained with accelerator
radiation in horizontal gantry position verified correct adjustment.

In 25 patients a 240° arc field was used; one patient received bilateral moving
coronal fields (each 115° arc) with reversing wedge filters to compensate skull
deformity. Isodose curves were generated on basis of coronal CT data in the
tumor plane. The 90% of maximum isodose was adapted to the target volume

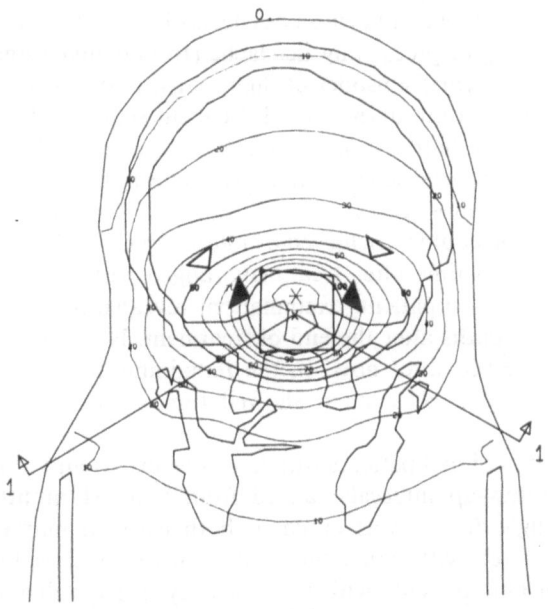

Fig. 1. Isodose curve of a 240° moving coronal arc field irradiation (20 MV photons, linear
accelerator, field size 4 × 4 cm). *Quadrangle*, target volume, for which the 100% isodose is adapted
(*arrowheads*). Difference between each isodose is 10% (*open arrowheads* indicate 50% isodose). Dose
maximum is 111% (*central cross*); dose at the skin is less than 20%, in most of the hairy regions less
than 10%

and then recalibrated as 100% of nominal dose, so that the maximum of absorbed dose was 111% of nominal dose, lying in the center of tumor (Fig. 1).

Because of an extremely large target volume one patient was irradiated with two lateral and one superior field. Three patients were not able to maintain the necessary reclined head position; these were treated with bilateral opposed fields. The total dose was 45–46 Gy in 17 patients, 47–48 Gy in 11, and 49–50 Gy in 2. Single doses were 1.8 Gy in 28 patients and 2 Gy in 2 patients, delivered 5 days per week. The mean field size was 5×5 cm (minimum 3×3 cm, maximum 10×6 cm).

Results

At presentation 13 patients suffered from visual disorders, including decreased visual acuity, visual field deficits, and abducent nerve palsy. Six complained headache; at least three had decreased libido; one had amenorrhea, and another had gustatory and olfactory deterioration. Nine patients were acromegalic; two had Cushing's disease. Hormone analyses revealed hypopituitarism in 15 patients.

Radiotherapy was well tolerated by all patients. Adjuvant corticoid medication was not necessary. The most frequent acute side effects of irradiation were transitory headache or increasing of preexisting headache (15 patients). Other side effects were weariness (13 patients), episodes of slight nausea (9), gustatory deterioration (8), vertigo (4), and mouth dryness (4). Infrequent sequelae (three patients or fewer) were sore throat, hair loss, and transitory visual or auditory deterioration. In no patient is the persistence of these side effects known, but preexisting headache remained in most cases.

Tumor response to irradiation could be achieved by follow-up CT or MRI in a total of 23 patients. Follow-up time after treatment ranged from 6 to 35 months (median 20 months). In seven patients examinations revealed reduction in tumor size, first seen 6–18 months after the end of treatment. No regrowth of these tumors has been observed until now. In the remaining 16 patients tumor extent remained unchanged. No patient showed tumor growth after radiotherapy.

Clinical follow-up was achieved in 8 patients with hormone excess and in 12 with inactive adenomas. Follow-up intervals ranged from 5 to 31 months (median 20 months). Cushing's disease was cured in both cases, a marked decrease in growth hormone levels with time after irradiation was observed in five of six patients. Seven of nine patients with no deficiency in hypophyseal hormones prior to irradiation developed a partial hypopituitarism. Gonadotropin deficiencies were found in six, decreased cortisol and prolactin levels in two, and a fall in thyroid-stimulating hormone in another. In 6 of 11 patients with preexisting hormone deficiencies a further fall was observed. Four patients had unchanged decreased hormone levels or received hormone replacement. In one patient with Cushing's disease the reduced gonadotropin level increased after radiotherapy. Other late side effects than hypopituitarism were not observed within the follow-up time.

Discussion

In radiotherapy of pituitary adenomas, the sparing of surrounding normal tissue is of particular importance because of the benign nature of the tumors and the closeness of sensitive structures (e.g., eyes). Coronal rotating irradiation with a modern linear accelerator provides an optimal dose distribution [4]. Care must be taken in exact and reproducible positioning of the patient's head during preparatory procedures and treatment. This can readily be achieved by the technique described above, which as a great advantage allows CT scan and irradiation in the identical position. Some patients may not be able to recline the head sufficiently; in these cases another field arrangement must be chosen.

Follow-up examinations indicate (albeit rather short-term in some patients) that our treatment technique is very effective in terms of control of tumor growth and fall in hormone levels; our results are similar to those of other studies [2, 3, 6, 7]. No tumor recurrence after treatment was observed, and hormone excesses were markedly improved or cured in seven of eight patients. Side effects during therapy were reversible. The only observable but frequent late sequelae of irradiation were the development of hypopituitarism or the worsening of preexisting hypophyseal hormone deficiencies, as observed by others [5]. Endocrinological examinations in long-term follow-up are mandatory, and hormones must be replaced if necessary. With the administered dosage and fractionation other late complications such as optic nerve injury or brain necrosis are not to be expected [1].

References

1. Aristizabal S, Caldwell WL, Avila J (1977) The relationship of time-dose fractionation factors to complications in the treatment of pituitary tumors by irradiation. Int J Radiat Oncol Biol Phys 2: 667–673
2. Chun M, Masko GB, Hetelekidis S (1988) Radiotherapy in the treatment of pituitary adenomas. Int J Radiat Oncol Biol Phys 15: 305–309
3. Grigsby PW, Simpson JR, Stokes S, Marks JE, Fineberg B (1988) Results of surgery and pituitary irradiation or irradiation alone for pituitary adenomas. J Neurooncol 6: 129–134
4. Halberg FE, Sheline GE (1987) Radiotherapy of pituitary tumors. Clin Endocrinol Metab 16: 667–684
5. Littley MD, Shalet SM, Beardwell CG, Ahmed SR, Applegate G, Sutton ML (1989) Hypopituitarism following external radiotherapy for pituitary tumours in adults. Q J Med 262: 145–160

6. Rauhut F, Clar HE, Bamberg M, Benker G, Grothe W (1986) Diagnostic criteria in pituitary tumour recurrence — combined modality of surgery and radiotherapy. Acta Neurochir (Wien) 80: 73–78
7. Rush SC, Newall J (1989) Pituitary adenoma: the efficacy of radiotherapy as the sole treatment. Int J Radiat Oncol Biol Phys 17: 165–169

A. med Center of Diagnostic Imaging
Neuroendocrine Treatment Planning
Institution de radio(?)
Springer-Verlag Berlin Heidelberg 1992

Tumor Response Monitoring of Posterior Fossa Tumors in Children by Plain and Gd-Enhanced Magnetic Resonance Imaging

P. Baierl and T. Wendt

Introduction

Posterior fossa tumors account for about 50% of pediatric brain tumors. Because magnetic resonance imaging (MRI) has proven an effective method for the examination of this area [1], we decided to perform the follow-up in these patients by MRI whenever feasible [2]. The purpose of this study was to identify the different forms of tumor response and to assess the detectability of local tumor recurrence and metastatic tumor spread.

Materials and Methods

A total of 26 children were included in this study. There were 74 MRI examinations. The length of follow-up varied from 3 months to 6 years. Almost all MRI scans were recorded at 1.0 T. In about half of the MRI examinations Gd-DTPA was given at a dose of 0.1 mmol/kg. The tumors and the therapeutic modalities fall into three main groups. Medulloblastomas ($n = 10$) were treated by surgery and whole brain/spinal cord irradiation. Brain stem tumors ($n = 6$) were treated by local radiation therapy. Therapy of the gliomas ($n = 8$) depended on the type and extent of tumor.

Results

In 17 of 26 patients complete remission was observed. MRI follow-up scans showed either defects ($n = 10$), no residuum ($n = 3$), or high-intensity areas in T2-weighted sequences ($n = 4$). The source of these changes was initially unclear; however, these hyperintense areas did not change in follow-up examinations,

Department of Radiology, University of Munich, Klinikum Großhadern, Marchioninistr. 15, 8000 Munich 70, FRG

Advanced Radiation Therapy Tumor Response Monitoring and Treatment Planning
Breit (Editor-in-Chief)
© Springer-Verlag, Berlin Heidelberg 1992

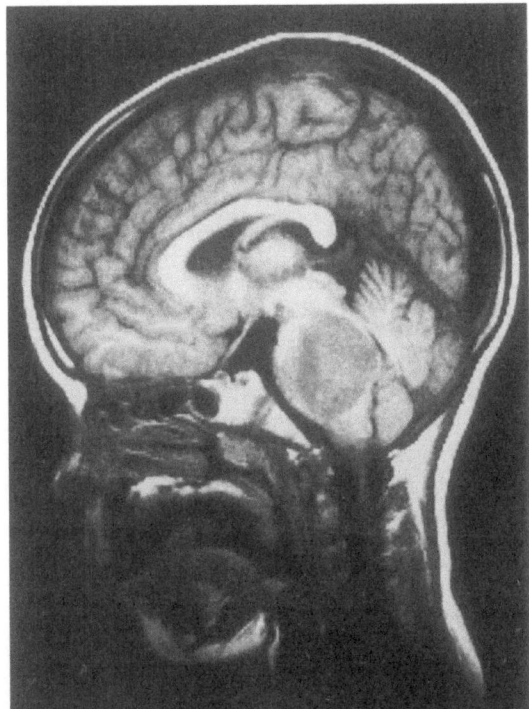

a

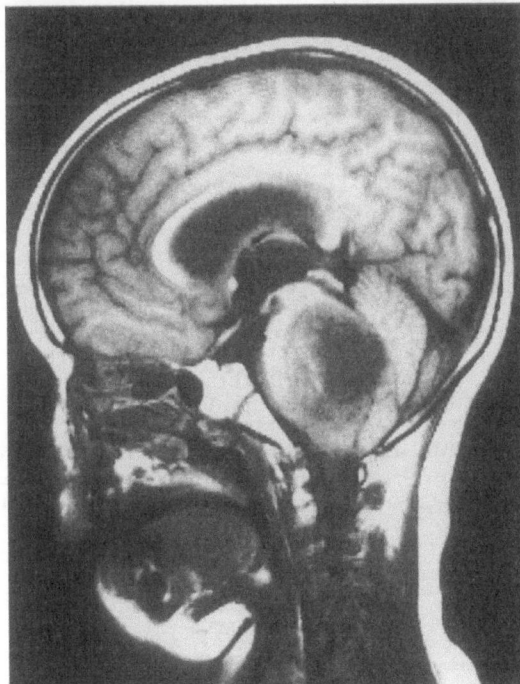

b

Fig. 1a, b. Brain stem tumor in a
4-year-old boy (unknown
histology). **a** Pretherapy MRI
scan (T1-weighted). **b** Posttherapy
scan (T1-weighted). The tumor
has increased in size and
developed a central necrosis

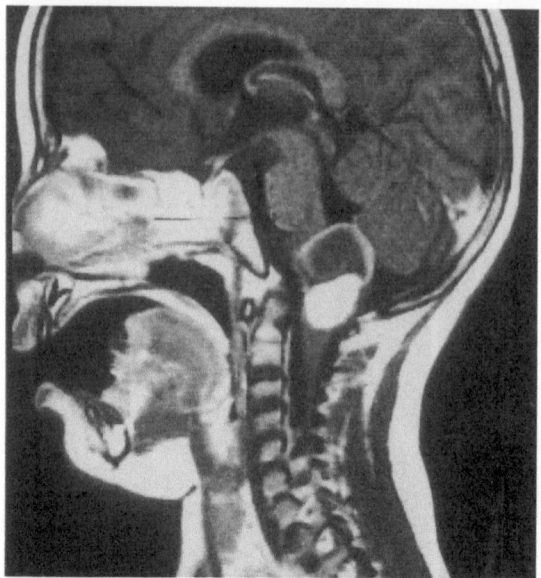

a

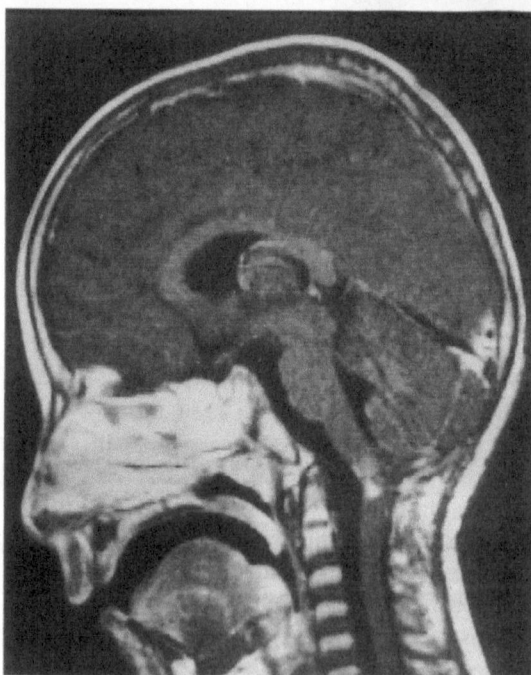

b

Fig. 2a, b. Ependymoma of the fourth ventricle in a 4-year-old boy. **a** Pretherapy MRI scan (T1-weighted) after Gd-DTPA. **b** MRI examination 1 year after therapy; T1-weighted scan after Gd-DTPA. The cyst has disappeared completely, and there is some retraction of the medulla. A small area of enhancement can still be observed

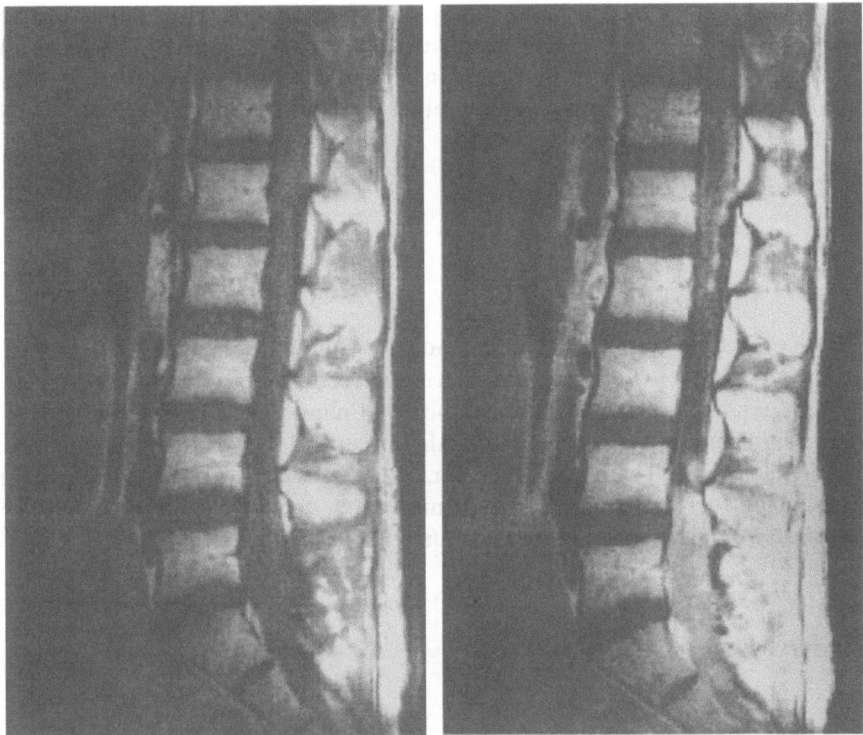

a   b

Fig. 3a, b. Spinal metastases of a medulloblastoma in a 16-year-old boy. **a** Plain MRI (T1-weighted) of the lumbar spine. **b** After Gd-DTPA, the caudal sac can be shown to be filled with tumor. Small drop metastases at L1/L2

sometimes over a period of several years. In addition, there were no signs or symptoms of tumor recurrence. One can therefore conclude that these lesions represent gliotic scarring. In all tumors with contrast enhancement before treatment a lack of enhancement after therapy was a strong indication for a complete remission.

Three children treated only by irradiation showed no remission. An example is presented in Fig. 1. In six patients a partial tumor response was observed. In four of these cases the tumor size had decreased considerably, but more than 1 year after therapy a small focus of contrast enhancement could still be observed (Fig. 2). The source of these lesions is not clear. A residual tumor, a tumor recurrence, and even a sort of enhancing gliosis are possible.

All three local tumor recurrences were gross tumors and were easily detected by plain MRI. Metastatic disease of the spinal cord could also be seen in the precontrast scans when large parts of the cord were involved. However, small drop metastases and meningeal involvement were detected only with Gd-DTPA (Fig. 3).

Brain damage caused by the therapy was found in one patient. A 12-year-old boy with histiocytosis X had been treated with local irradiation and chemotherapy (vinblastine) because of a brain stem tumor. He developed a diffuse toxic leukencephalopathy. In none of the other 25 children were pathologic changes outside the tumor area observed.

Conclusion

MRI proved to be an effective method for follow-up in pediatric brain stem tumors. Complete remission, local tumor recurrence, and metastatic tumor spread could be diagnosed unequivocally. Enhancement with Gd-DTPA was necessary for diagnosis in some of the cases and was of value in almost all patients [3, 4]. There are, however, a few slowly regressing tumors with enhancing foci persisting 1 year or more after therapy. Additional follow-up studies are required to clarify the source of these lesions.

References

1. McGinnis BD, Brady TJ, New PFJ, Buonanno FS, Pykett IL, DelaPaz RL, Kistler JP, Taveras JM (1983) Nuclear magnetic resonance (NMR) imaging of tumors in the posterior fossa. J Comput Assist Tomogr 7: 575–584
2. Baierl P, Wendt T, Bauer WM, Rohloff R, Förster C (1989) Der Wert der Kernspintomographie bei der Strahlentherapie kindlicher Tumoren der hinteren Schädelgrube und der Pinealisregion. Fortschr. Geb Rontgenstr 150: 663–669
3. Powers TA, Partain CL, Kessler RM, Freeman MW, Robertson RH, Wyatt SH, Whelan HT (1988) Central nervous system lesions in pediatric patients: Gd-DTPA-enhanced MR imaging. Radiology 169: 723–726
4. Bird CR, Drayer BP, Medina M, Rekate HL, Flom RA, Hodak JA (1988) Gd-DTPA-enhanced MR imaging in pediatric patients after brain tumor resection. Radiology 109: 123–126

Computed Tomography and Magnetic Resonance Imaging After Brain Tumor Resection: How To Obtain Useful Baseline Scans

M. Forsting[1], F.K. Albert[2], and K. Sartor[1]

Introduction

The overwhelming majority of studies that address the role of surgery in the management of malignant gliomas in adults rely solely on the surgeon's impression of the degree of resection accomplished. Estimations of tumor bulk reduction arising from impressions at the time of surgery continue to form the basis of very recent reports (Newell et al. 1988; Shapiro et al. 1989). Most studies retrospectively review the records of patients operated on by various surgeons. Among the few available studies based computed tomography (CT) there is no consistency in the methods of estimating residual tumor volume or in the timing of postoperative radiographic studies (Ciric et al. 1987; Cairncross et al. 1985; Ammirati et al. 1987). Questions remain concerning the relationship between the timing of postoperative scans and surgically induced as opposed to tumor-induced enhancement, and about the methods for obtaining useful baseline scans. Such scans are absolutely necessary to evaluate the effectiveness of different therapeutic regimens in patients with glioblastoma.

We report here the results of our prospective study on the natural history of postoperative enhancement in patients with glioblastoma. Our long-term results will be analyzed separately.

Methods

In a prospective study, we used contrast-enhanced CT and magnetic resonance imaging (MRI) to monitor 60 patients after resection of a glioblastoma. All CT scans were obtained before and after contrast enhancement with 100 ml iohexol (Omnipaque) on a Picker Vista 1200 SX scanner. MRI was performed on a 1.0-T Picker Vista unit. Pre- and postcontrast (0.1 mmol/kg Gd-DPTA, intravenous) T1-weighted images were obtained with a TR of 600 ms and an echo time (TE) of

[1] Department of Neuroradiology, University of Heidelberg, Im Neuenheimer Feld 400, 6900 Heidelberg, FRG
[2] Department of Neurosurgery, University of Heidelberg, Im Neuenheimer Feld 400, 6900 Heidelberg, FRG

Advanced Radiation Therapy Tumor Response
Monitoring and Treatment Planning
Breit (Editor-in-Chief)
© Springer-Verlag, Berlin Heidelberg 1992

20 ms. With both CT and MRI the slice thickness was 8 mm. The first postoperative scan was obtained as soon as possible after surgery, usually between the 1st and 4th postoperative days. Follow-up scans were obtained 1–2 weeks, 4 weeks, 2 months, and 6 months after surgery.

Results

Residual tumor was shown most reliably and graphically as abnormal enhancement on scans obtained shortly after surgery (Fig. 1a). With CT this was the case in 29 patients (48%), with MRI in 45 (75%). In ten patients we were sure that there was no residual tumor left, while in the remaining five patients findings were equivocal, in two of them due to early reparative enhancement on the 4th day after surgery. The main tissue alteration confounding the interpretation of the early CT scans was hemorrhage along the resection hole and enhancement due to luxury perfusion of the adjacent parenchyma (Fig. 1b). On CT and MRI images obtained 2 weeks after surgery linear enhancement that occurred at the border of the resection hole was difficult to distinguish from tumor. Moreover, increasing protein content and ongoing hemoglobin degradation within the surgical defect made interpretation of the MRI more difficult (Fig. 1c, d). Two months after surgery this benign postoperative enhancement had almost completely resolved.

Discussion

Glioblastoma multiforme and anaplastic astrocytoma account for at least 35% of all primary brain tumors, which translates into 6600 new cases annually in the United States (Liebermann et al. 1982). The current treatment of supratentorial gliomas consists of surgery followed by radiation and/or chemotherapy. The overall survival rate of these patients is far from satisfactory: the 24-month mean survival for patients with glioblastoma is 8%–12%, while the median postoperative survival is 8 months (Andreou et al. 1983). Recent attempts at improving the median survival have focused primarily on the use of new chemotherapeutic regimens or different forms of radiation therapy, with little attention given to the possibility of improving the surgical aspect of the treatment plan (Shapiro et al. 1989). When information on the extent of surgical resection is given, it is based primarily on the surgeon's impression and not on objectively quantifiable neuroradiological criteria. Comparable data in a multimodality treatment plan must necessarily rest on an objective quantification of all therapeutic methods used. Consequently, it is important to quantify the extent of surgical resection of a malignant glioma when assessing the results of treatment.

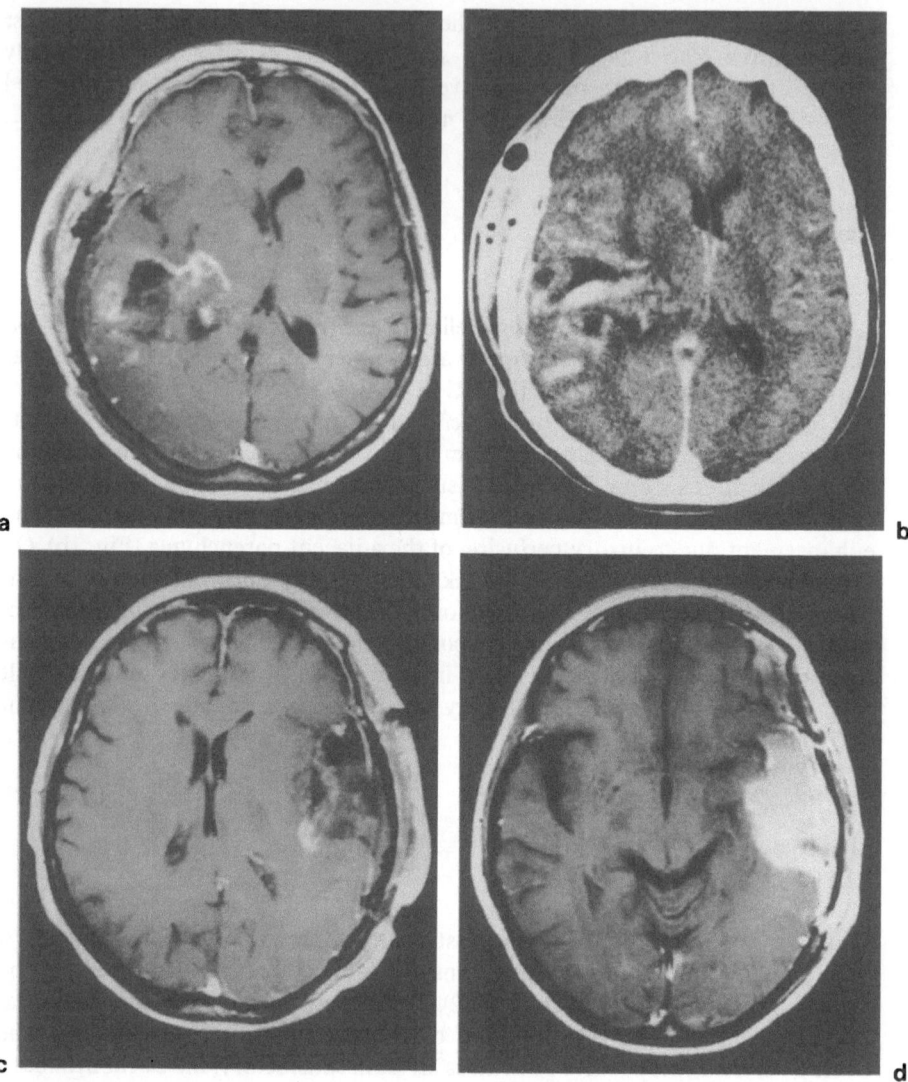

Fig. 1. a MRI obtained 1 day after surgery clearly shows residual enhancing tumor at the medial margin of the resection hole. **b** It is impossible to differentiate between tumor enhancement, blood artifacts, and luxury perfusion. **c** Clear delineation of residual tumor 1 day after surgery. **d** Ten days later there is extensive T1 shortening due to hemoglobin degradation within the resection hole

Despite long-standing availability of CT and now of MRI effectiveness of these methods in the postoperative management of patients is reduced by the difficulty in differentiating tumor enhancement from surgically induced enhancement. The excellent collaboration between the Departments of Neuroradiology and Neurosurgery at our institution made possible this large prospective study to evaluate the natural history of contrast enhancement after glioblastoma resection. Results of animal experiments and of sequential CT scanning after brain tumor resection did show a delay of enhancement along the operative margins up to 5 days after surgery (Cairncross et al. 1985; Jeffries et al. 1981). Despite these results, early CT did not become an accepted method for postoperative imaging.

In our series the main difficulty was differentiating between residual enhancing tumor and enhancement due to luxury perfusion of the adjacent parenchyma or artifacts caused by blood clots within the resection hole. The first postoperative MRI showed contrast enhancement reflecting residual tumor in 75% of the patients. There were no problems with identifying luxury perfusion phenomena in early MRI scans, and although some patients had methemoglobin within the resection hole due to intraoperative use of hydrogen peroxide, we also encountered no major difficulties differentiating blood from enhanced tissue (as may be the case with CT). Another advantage of MRI is that this modality is about 20 times more sensitive in detecting Gd-DPTA than CT is in detecting iodinated media; this means that smaller amounts of enhancing residual tumor are visible on MRI (Runge et al. 1985).

In conclusion, serial MRI should become an essential diagnostic tool for following brain tumor patients under and after therapy. The scan-to-scan status of the residual tumor size may be important for maintaining efficacy and determining the value of treatment (Forsting et al. 1991). The first MRI should be performed soon after operation, preferably during the first 24 or 48 h, at which time the postoperative vascular response is still incomplete, and any demonstrable enhancement can be assumed to be due to residual tumor. Quantitative data from tumor response curves based on the amount of residual tumor are probably more accurate than clinical observation in measuring the efficacy of new therapeutic regimens.

References

Ammirati M, Vick N, Liao Y et al. (1987) Effect of the extent of surgical resection on survival and quality of life in patients with supratentorial glioblastomas and anaplastic astrocytomas. Neurosurgery 21: 201–206

Andreou J, George AE, Wise A et al. (1983) CT prognostic criteria of survival after malignant glioma surgery. AJNR 4: 488–490

Cairncross JG, Pexman JHW, Rathbone MP, DelMaestro RF (1985) Postoperative contrast enhancement in patients with brain tumor. Ann Neurol 17: 570–572

Ciric I, Ammirati M, Vick N, Mikhael M (1987) Supratentorial gliomas: surgical considerations and immediate postoperative results. Neurosurgery 21: 21–26

Forsting M, Albert FK, Sartor K, Kunze S (1991) Early postoperative CT and MRI in glioblastoma. Neuroradiology 33 (Suppl): 25–27

Jeffries BF, Kishore PRS, Kanwalcharan SS et al. (1981) Contrast enhancement in the postoperative brain. Radiology 139: 409–413

Liebermann AN, Ransohoff J (1982) Treatment of primary brain tumors. Neurosurgery 10: 450–453

Newell J, Ransohoff J, Kaplan B (1988) Glioblastoma in the older patient. How long a course of
    radiotherapy is necessary? J Neurooncol 6: 325–327
Runge VM, Clanton JA, Price AC et al. (1985) Evaluation of contrast enhanced MR imaging in a
    brain abscess model. AJNR 6: 137–47
Shapiro WR, Green SB, Burger PC et al. (1989) Randomized trial of three chemotherapeutic
    regimens in postoperative treatment of malignant gliomas. J Neurosurg 71: 1–9

Magnetic Resonance Imaging and Magnetic Resonance Angiography in Treatment Planning and Response Monitoring of Single High-Dose Radiotherapy in Intracerebral Arteriovenous Malformations

H.-U. Kauczor[1], G. Layer[1], B. Kimmig[2], L.R. Schad[1], R. Engenhart[2], M. Müller-Schimpfle[1], B. Wowra[3], W. Semmler[1], and G. van Kaick[1]

Introduction

Arteriovenous malformations (AVM) are regarded as congenital anomalies consisting of a racemose convolution of pathological vessels which predispose to intercerebral bleeding. The bleeding risk is about 4% per year, with a combined rate of major morbidity and mortality of 2.7% per year (Ondra et al. 1990). Cerebral AVM can be graded according to Spetzler et al. (1986). This system is based on the size of the AVM, localization of draining veins, and eloquence of adjacent brain tissue. It is derived from the potential postoperative complications, such as neurological deficits and mortality. AVMs of grade I or II are easily resectable, while those of grade IV or V are correlated with a high risk of major postoperative neurological deficits. This grading allows comparison with other therapeutic approaches: (a) embolization is very helpful preoperatively in preventing excessive bleeding but does not obliterate a large AVM alone (Fox et al. 1990); (b) stereotactic single high-dose radiotherapy, or "radiosurgery," shows good results for complete occlusion of the AVM after a latency of approximately 2 years (Engenhart et al. 1989).

This study evaluated the possible role of magnetic resonance imaging (MRI) and magnetic resonance angiography (MRA) in treatment planning, which is routinely performed by conventional angiography. As radiogenic occlusion of the AVM develops slowly, MRI and MRA were also employed in follow-up every 6 months to observe early reactions and the time course of beginning occlusion and potential side effects.

[1] Department of Radiology and Pathophysiology, German Cancer Research Center, Im Neuenheimer Feld 280, 400, 6900 Heidelberg, FRG
[2] Department of Radiotherapy, University Clinic, University of Heidelberg, Im Neuenheimer Feld 400, 6900 Heidelberg, FRG
[3] Department of Neurosurgery, University Clinic, University of Heidelberg, Im Neuenheimer Feld 400, 6900 Heidelberg, FRG

Advanced Radiation Therapy Tumor Response
Monitoring and Treatment Planning
Breit (Editor-in-Chief)
© Springer-Verlag, Berlin Heidelberg 1992

Patients and Methods

Preradiation MRI and MRA was performed in 25 patients (14 men, 11 women) with an intracerebral AVM; the mean age was 35 years, ranging from 7 to 62 years. Twenty-one of these patients (12 men, 9 women) whose AVM was clearly visualized by preradiation MRA were included in the prospective follow-up study. Treatment planning was based on conventional angiography in all patients. MRI was used for exact identification of adjacent brain structures, and MRA was performed to detect physiologic flow conditions.

MRI was carried out using a Magnetom 1.5 T (Siemens, Erlangen, FRG) superconducting whole-body imager. Imaging included SE 680/15 in coronal plane and SE 2800/20, 90 in transversal plane, slice thickness being 4 mm. A three-dimensional flow-compensated fast-imaging sequence with steady-state free precession (FISP) was used for MRA. Parameters were TR = 40 ms, TE = 7 ms, FA = 15°, matrix 256 × 256, 64 or 128 partitions (depending on the size of the AVM) with an effective slice thickness of 1 mm. The maximum-intensity projection (MIP) technique served for three-dimensional reconstructions of the obtained angiograms.

Single high-dose radiotherapy under stereotactic conditions allows exact definition of the target volume. Using the technique introduced by Hartmann et al. (1985), a steep dose gradient with optimum protection of normal brain tissue is achieved. The mean dose applied to the target margins was 19 Gy (80% isodose). The diameter of the target was about 19 mm.

Our prospective follow-up study consisted of MRI and MRA examinations every 6 months over a period of 2 years. So far, 11 patients have been examined 6 months after radiotherapy. As therapy monitoring by MR techniques is not yet established, the interpretation of alterations requires the evaluation of the following newly defined criteria: (a) in spin-echo images: development of new texture elements within the AVM, alterations in already existing texture elements within the AVM, and new hyperintensities on T2-weighted images in the adjacent brain; (b) in MRA also: decrease in number, size, and intensity of feeding arterial signals, decrease in nidus signals, alteration in nidus signal patterns (e.g., segmentation), and decrease in draining venous signals.

Results

MRA depicted flow signals from the AVM region in 24/25 patients. Feeding arteries were identified on MRA in 20/25 cases. Identification proved to be exact by comparison to conventional angiography. The nidus itself was clearly delineated in 21/25 patients (Fig. 1); a certain differentiation among arterial components, arteriovenous shunts, and venous structures, however, was not

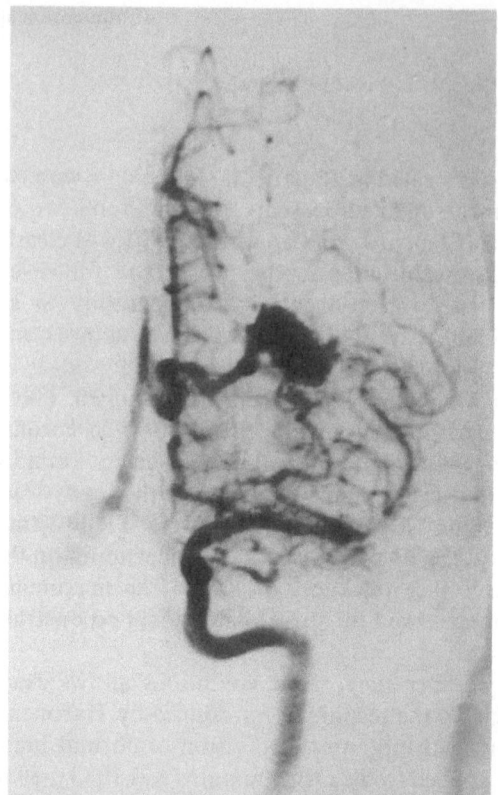

a

Fig. 1. **a** Preradiation angiography of an arteriovenous malformation of the left basal ganglia (courtesy of Prof. Dr. K. Sartor, Department of Neuroradiology, Heidelberg University). **b** Coronal MIP of a transverse three-dimensional angiogram displaying physiologic flow conditions within the AVM

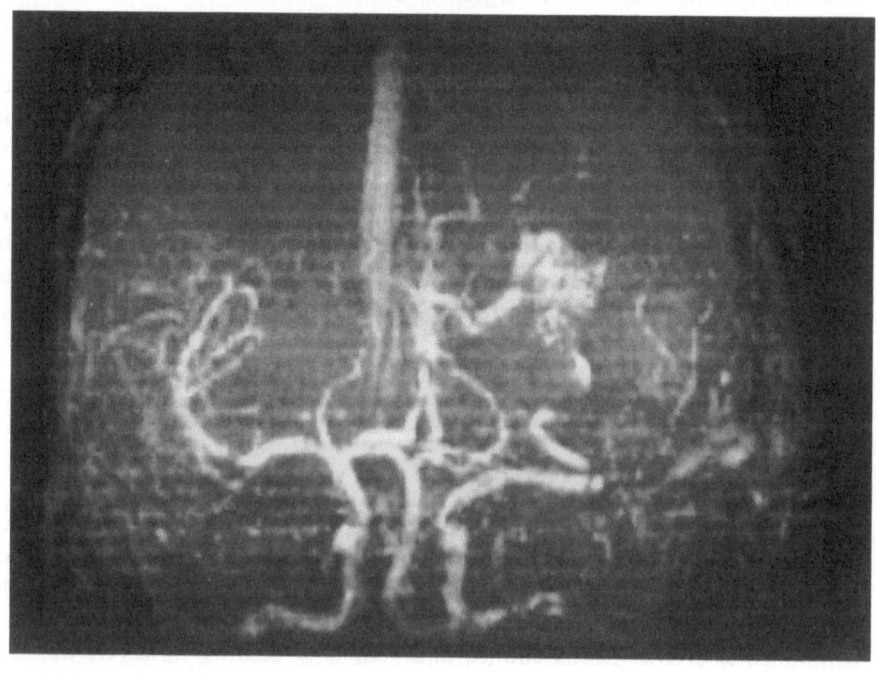

b

possible. Draining veins were frequently visualized (17/25 patients). Exact definition of the target volume by MRA (MIP reconstructions) was impossible due to superimposition in four patients. In these cases the assessment of individual slices with their high spatial resolution (effective slice thickness of 1 mm) provided the basis for the definition of the target volume.

In therapy response monitoring MRA and MRI exhibited changes as early as 6 months after radiotherapy. These alterations were more frequently visualized by MRA (7/11); MRI indicated early reactions in only four patients.

In MRA feeding arteries were almost always visualized; their appearance remained unchanged in 9 of 11 patients. In the other two patients feeding arteries could still be identified, but the coherence of flow signals was lost. Flow signals from the nidus appeared reduced in seven patients 6 months after radiotherapy. We also observed a change to more spotty flow patterns as well as segmentation of signals. The number of veins was reduced in 2 of 11 patients.

Spin-echo imaging revealed an augmentation of texture elements within the AVM in four patients after 6 months. On T2-weighted images small hyperintense regions in the adjacent brain representing edema were visible in 5/11 patients 6 months after radiotherapy. None of these patients, however, exhibited clinical symptoms.

Discussion

Edelman et al. (1989) and Marchal et al. (1990) introduced MRA in the diagnostic work-up of intracerebral AVM. Our sequence protocol (Layer et al. 1991) is based on T1- and T2-weighted spin echo images and the FISP sequence for flow detection. This sequence is sensitive for flow velocities presumed in arteries and arteriovenous AVM shunts. Veins past the AVM are not visualized under low-flow conditions. The whole examination lasts about 35 min and can be routinely included in follow-up studies.

All patients underwent conventional angiography under stereotactic conditions; this is the prerequisite for treatment planning of single high-dose radiotherapy and also serves as the gold standard for MRA, MRA clearly displayed the nidus in 21/25 patients. Superimposition may impair the delineation of the nidus. If MRA itself was not conclusive, the assessment of the individual slices always provided the additional information necessary for definition of the target volume.

A certain differentiation of feeding arteries and draining veins could not be achieved in some cases. This problem may be overcome by the use of a transverse presaturation pulse to eliminate inflowing spins from the carotid and vertebral arteries.

An important advantage of MRA is the potential of three-dimensional reconstructions in any desired viewing angle, ameliorating spatial impression and possibly preventing superimposition. In contrast, additional projections in conventional angiography require longer examinations.

The effect of radiotherapy is thought to be the induction of an inflammatory response in the vessel walls which slowly leads to occlusion by ultimate thrombosis (Steiner 1984). This was shown by Reinhold et al. (1980) in the rat. The exact time course in humans, however, is difficult to demonstrate because of the risks of selective angiography.

Our preliminary results show first indications of beginning occlusion 6 months after radiation. In the detection of these radiogenic alterations MRA was more sensitive than spin-echo imaging. This may be due to earlier visualization of hemodynamic changes in comparison to morphologic alterations of the vessel wall.

MR techniques, including angiographic studies and spin-echo imaging, are an ideal modality to monitor effects and side effects of radiotherapy in AVM patients completely noninvasively.

References

Edelman RR, Wentz KU, Mattle HP, O'Reilly GV, Candia G, Liu C, Zhao B, Kjellberg RN, Davis KR (1989) Intracerebral arteriovenous malformations: evaluation with selective MR angiography and venography. Radiology 173: 831–837

Engenhart R, Kimmig B, Wowra B, Sturm V, Höver KH, Schneider S, Wannenmacher M (1989) Stereotaktische Einzeitbestrahlung cerebraler Angiome. Radiologe 29: 219–223

Fox AJ, Pely DM, Lee DH (1990) Arteriovenous malformations of the brain: recent results of endovascular therapy. Radiology 177: 51–57

Hartmann GH, Schlegel W, Sturm V, Kober B, Pastyr O, Lorenz WJ (1985) Cerebral radiation surgery using moving field irradiation and a linear accelerator facility. Int J Radiat Oncol Biol Phys 11: 1185–1192

Layer G, Semmler W, Schad LR, Wowra B, van Kaick G (1991) MR-Tomographie und MR-Angiographie cerebraler arteriovenöser Malformationen. Fortschr Geb Röntgenstr 154: 438–444

Marchal G, Bosmans H, van Fraeyenhoven L, Wilms G, van Hecke P, Plets C, Baert AL (1990) Intracranial vascular lesions: optimization and clinical evaluation of three-dimensional time-of-flight MR angiography. Radiology 155: 443–448

Ondra SL, Troupp H, George ED, Schwab K (1990) The natural history of symptomatic arteriovenous malformations of the brain: a 24-year follow-up assessment. J Neurosurg 73: 387–391

Reinhold HS, Hopewell JW (1980) Late changes in the architecture of blood vessels of the rat brain after irradiation. Br J Radiol 53: 693–696

Spetzler RF, Martin NA (1986) A proposed grading system for arteriovenous malformations. J Neurosurg 65: 476–483

Steiner L (1984) Radiosurgery in cerebral arteriovenous malformations. In: Fein JM, Flamm ES (eds) Cerebrovascular surgery, vol 4. Springer, Berlin Heidelberg New York, pp 1161–1215

Tumor Response Monitoring: Head and Neck

Introduction

Diagnoses of ... and the planning of therapy is used ... back factors are based on the patient's history and clinical examination with biopsy histology ... and laboratory findings on the one hand and the results of imaging methods ... on the other. However, determination of response rates ... an important characteristic of ... disease ... the regime as part of immunizable therapy is ... at almost points which use objective criteria of clinical response with ... radiant level of size ... (CT) ... Due to their easily made ... survey of gland ... and metabolic parameters and structural changes toward quantitative render literally, imaging methods lend themselves become a cornerstone of effective therapy involvement, as met- and post-therapeutic follow-up. Among these techniques ultrasound ... is noninvasive, inexpensive, easily available, and readily ... By ... the baseline imaging method for the ... guided diagnosis of tumors in this region. Our research shows that ultrasound also provide decisive information at the ... level for optimizing and if necessary adjusting the therapeutic concept to changes ... in tumor volume in and characteristics not only in ... clinical but even for changes ... interventions.

Patients and Methods

Between May 19.. and ... here refer treatment by means of ... regimen of therapy and the ... treated again in an interval of ... There were 30 men and ... women, and the mean age was 58.5 ± ... years (26–78 years). The patients received chemotherapy ... etoposide, with 20 mg cisplatin and 1000 mg ... administered per square meter each day for 5 days. Except in cases of therapy induced fever or thrombocytopenia, the chemotherapy courses were repeated in ...

1 Klinische Radiologie und Poliklinik, Klinikum ..., Universitätsklinik im Neuenheimer Feld 400, ... Heidelberg.
2 Universitätsklinik für ... Hals-Nasen-Ohrenheilkunde, Im Neuenheimer Feld 400, ... Heidelberg.

Ultraschalldiagnostik in ... und ... im Kopf-Hals-Bereich (ed.) ... Springer-Verlag, Berlin Heidelberg 199..

Ultrasound Monitoring of Chemotherapy in Tumors of the Head and Neck Region

U. Mende[1], J. Zöller[2], I.A. Born[3], and M. Loth[1]

Introduction

Diagnosis, staging, and the planning of therapy in head and neck tumors are based on the patient's history and clinical examination with biopsy, histology, and laboratory findings, on the one hand, and the results of imaging methods, on the other. However, determination of response rates in an aggressive antineoplastic chemotherapeutic regime as part of multimodality therapy is based almost exclusively on the subjective criteria of clinical evidence, with a certainty level of merely C1 [1]. Due to their ability, more objectively, to define and measure volumetric and structural changes toward optimizing tumor therapy, imaging methods must therefore become a cornerstone of effective therapy monitoring as intra- and posttherapeutic follow-up. Among these techniques ultrasound — noninvasive, inexpensive, easily available, and effective — has become the first-line imaging method for therapy-guided diagnosis of tumors in this region. Our research shows that ultrasound also provides decisive information at the C2 level for optimizing and if necessary adjusting the therapeutic concept to chemotherapy response, reasonable and mandatory not only for ethical but even for economic considerations.

Patients and Methods

Between May 1986 and July 1990 we treated 65 patients with tumors of the oral cavity and the oropharyngeal region in advanced stages. There were 59 men and 6 women, and the mean age was 54.2 ± 8.6 years (36–78 years). The patients received antineoplastic chemotherapy with 20 mg cisplatin and 1000 mg 5-fluorouracil per square meter each day for 5 days. Except in cases of therapy-induced leuko- or thrombopenia the chemotherapy courses were repeated at

[1] Klinische Radiologie und Poliklinik, Radiologische Universitätsklinik, Im Neuenheimer Feld 400, 6900 Heidelberg, FRG
[2] Universitätsklinik für Mund-Kiefer-Gesichtschirurgie, Im Neuenheimer Feld 400, 6900 Heidelberg, FRG
[3] Pathologisches Institut der Universität, Im Neuenheimer Feld 220, 6900 Heidelberg, FRG

Advanced Radiation Therapy Tumor Response
Monitoring and Treatment Planning
Breit (Editor-in-Chief)
© Springer-Verlag, Berlin Heidelberg 1992

3-week intervals. The standard procedure consisted of three courses; this varied from one to four depending on clinical and ultrasound response, laboratory findings, and the general condition of the patient. All patients underwent accurate ultrasound examinations before and after completion of the chemotherapeutic schedule; 50 patients (76.9%) were also examined in the intervals between the individual courses. All examinations (before, during, and after therapy) were performed under identical conditions in respect to the examiner, equipment (Picker LSC 7000), setting, reproducible ultrasound sections, and documentation, as previously described [2]. Response was analyzed on the basis of measurable volumetric changes of the 65 primary tumors and the 140 lymph nodes (calculated from the measured areas and perpendicular diameters) and the changes in echogenicity, objectified by gray-scale histograms. Clinical and ultrasound data could be compared to histopathological findings in 44 out of the 65 patients (67.7%) who underwent surgery.

Results

The 65 primary tumors showed a reduction in mean pathologic echodifferent volume from 44.3 ± 39.8 ml (range 1.4–180.9 ml) before therapy to 28.1 ± 40.0 ml (1.4–231.3 ml), or $57.7\% \pm 39.8\%$ (14.3%–242%) after therapy. Complete remission (CR) or partial remission of more than 50% (PR) was found in 37 patients (56.9%) and a moderate response of between 25% and 50% (MR) in 16 patients (24.6%). Of these 53 primaries, 33 (62.3%) with a decrease in volume also became more echogenic as a sign of structural tumor response with fibrosis. Unchanged echogenicity was seen in 11 patients (20.7%), and 9 (17.0%) showed less echogenic necrotic area. In the 12 nonresponders (no change, NC; progressive disease, PD) the target volume was more echoic in three tumors (25%), unchanged in three (25%), and markedly less echoic in six (50%).

The mean volume of the 140 analyzed lymph nodes before therapy was 4.1 ± 16.3 ml (range 0.20–187 ml); after therapy this was reduced to 2.8 ± 12.5 ml (0.05–143.2 ml), or $59.1\% \pm 44.7\%$ (6.3%–318%). CR or PR was determined in 69 nodes (49.3%); MR in 28 (20.0%), with 70 of these 97 nodes (72.2%) also showing fibrotic regression with increased echogenicity; and NC or PD in 24 (17.1%), with unchanged or reduced echogenicity in 18 (75%), coincidental with the findings in the primary tumors.

In seven patients (10.8%) ultrasound monitoring revealed initial response of the primary tumor and/or lymph nodes but subsequent progression. Discrepant response between primary tumor and lymph nodes was found in five patients (7.7%).

Clinical (C1) and ultrasound (C2) monitoring were correlated as follows. Of the seven patients with clinical CR six showed excellent PR on ultrasound, Five with elevated echogenicity and one unchanged (the other case, of ultrasound

PD, proved to be a misdiagnosis upon excision biopsy). In 29 of 49 patients clinical PR was confirmed with ultrasound PR; 16 showed MR (27.9%–49.7%), one NC, and three PD. The three patients with NC clinically were PD on ultrasound. In the six patients with clinical PD five also showed ultrasound PD, while one with a relapse after surgery and radiotherapy achieved good PR according to ultrasound.

Discussion

Imaging methods now form an integral part of the diagnostic schedule for primary staging, surgical therapy planning, and posttherapeutic care in head and neck tumors; however, this is not yet the case for the assessment of expensive and aggressive, systemic antineoplastic therapy regimes during the course of therapy. Among these methods, the routine use of computed tomography unfortunately leads to unsatisfactory results, at rates up to 30% in tumors of the oral cavity, because of artifacts and often poor demarcation of the changes, especially in axial slices; it is also restricted by side effects of the contrast medium and by its costs [3]. The still higher costs and the still limited availability of magnetic resonance imaging have prevented it from becoming a standard technique despite its undisputed technical advantages.

We examined the ultrasound monitoring of chemotherapy response based on volumetric changes in the primary tumors and representative lymph nodes and on changes in structure and echogenicity as determined by gray-scale histograms. Such monitoring provides the objective criteria for early and effective assessment of the therapy-induced tumor reduction or the failure of the therapeutic regime. Excellent response (CR or PR) is shown in decreased volume but usually also increased echogenicity, with signs of regression, fibrosis, or recalcification (Fig. 1). Volumetric response and decreased echogenicity due to necrotic areas are rather uncommon. Lack of response (NC or PD) is usually associated with persistently low or decreasing echogenicity.

The ultrasound evaluation of therapy is therefore mandatory in cases of (a) equivocal clinical evidence, (b) insufficient response or progression, (c) initial response with (volumetric and structural) signs of subsequent progression, and (d) discrepant response between primary tumor and lymph nodes. These cases of chemotherapeutic failure can be assessed safely and economically to modify the multimodality therapy concept and perform surgery and/or radiotherapy earlier. Taking into account the cost for inpatient chemotherapeutic treatment, the failure rate with insufficient response, on the one hand, and, on the other, the cost of the imaging modalities (ultrasound versus computed tomography or magnetic resonance imaging), ultrasound is clearly the monitoring technique with definite economic advantage. This monitoring technique thus means a gain in quality of life and possibly in prognosis for the patient as

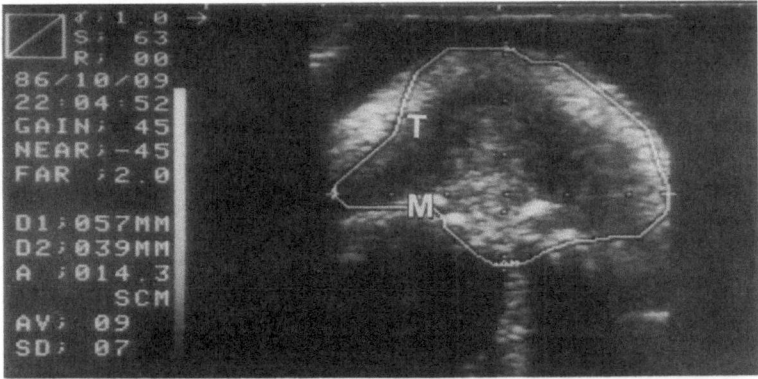

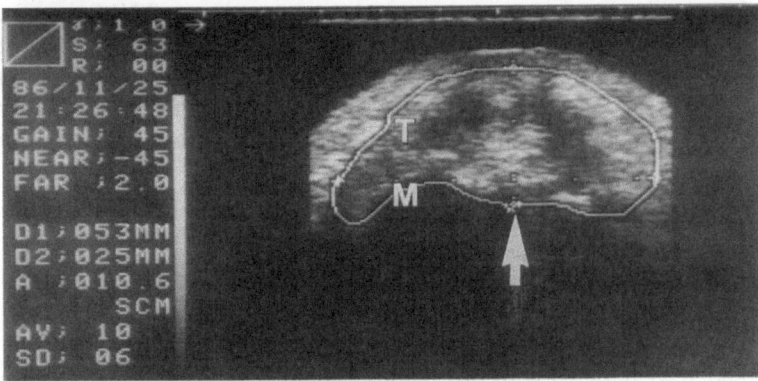

Fig. 1. Ultrasound image (transverse section) of a squamous cell carcinoma of the floor of the mouth and the alveolar process (osteolytic destruction of the mandible; T4 N2C MX) in a 46-year-old man. *T*, Tumor; *M*, mandible. *Above,* before therapy; *below,* after two courses of chemotherapy good volumetric and structural response; tumor smaller and more echogenic. *Arrow*, recalcification

well as a contribution to reducing the costs of treatment due to the excellent cost-benefit relation (1:6).

References

1. Hermanek P, Scheibe, O, Spiessl B, Wagner G (eds) (1987) TNM Klassifikation maligner Tumoren, 4th edn. Springer, Berlin Heidelberg New York
2. Mende U, Flentje M, Weischedel U, Zöller J, Lenarz T (1989) Sonographische Diagnostik von Kopf-Hals-Tumoren im therapeutischen Umfeld. Rontgen B latter 42: 19–23
3. Wolfensberger M, Jecklin A, Franze I, Kikinis R (1987) Der Beitrag der Computertomographie zur präoperativen Klassifizierung von Mundhöhlen- und Oropharynxkarzinomen. Laryngol Rhinol Otol (Stuttg) 66: 324–328

Planimetry Versus Relaxometry as Therapy Monitoring of Head and Neck Tumors

C. Wagner-Manslau[1], U. Gebhardt[1], R. Dorn[1], P. Lukas[2], B. Clasen[3], M. Herzog[4], and H.W. Pabst[1]

Introduction

The use of magnetic resonance imaging (MRI) ensures a better TNM classification. MRI offers the advantage of multiplanar imaging and high resolution with good soft-tissue differentiation. The aim of the study was to compare planimetry to relaxometry for assessing tumor response to radio-chemotherapy (RCT). The determination of T1-times is proposed as a means for staging, therapeutic planning and monitoring.

Materials and Methods

We investigated 41 patients with histologically confirmed squamous cell carcinoma of different malignant head and neck tumors. These included 38 men and 3 women aged 41–76 years (median 54). They had inoperable tumor (T3 or T4) and were examined before therapy for staging and were controlled after the first and second course of combined RCT: mitomycin C and 5 fluorouracil during the first 5 days of both courses of RCT each with 30 Gy for the head and neck region and 10–15 Gy to supraclavicular lymph nodes. Localisation of tumors was as follows: Nasopharynx, 3; palate, 2; tongue, 5; floor of the mouth, 7; tonsils, 6; hypopharynx, 14; larynx, 4. Tumor gradings were: G1, 4; G2, 21; G3, 10; G4, 6. In terms of treatment modalities there were three groups: 24 patients with an inoperable tumor received RCT; 11 patients were operated on primarily; 6 patients were operated after the first course of RCT. Lymph node involvement was confirmed histologically as follows: 11 patients were operated on primarily; and 3 lymph nodes were studied by needle biopsy.

[1] Nuklearmedizinische Klinik und Poliklinik, Technische Universität München, Ismaningerstr. 22, 8000 Munich 80, FRG
[2] Klinik und Poliklinik für Strahlentherapie, Technische Universität München, Ismaningerstr. 22, 8000 Munich 80, FRG
[3] Hals-Nasen-Ohren Klinik und Poliklinik, Technische Universität München, Ismaningerstr. 22, 8000 Munich 80, FRG
[4] Klinik und Poliklinik für Mund-, Kiefer- und Gesichtschirurgie, Technische Universität München, Ismaningerstr. 22, 8000 Munich 80, FRG

Advanced Radiation Therapy Tumor Response
Monitoring and Treatment Planning
Breit (Editor-in-Chief)
© Springer-Verlag, Berlin Heidelberg 1992

MRI parameters were the following:

- Staging
  SE T1, transversal, TR 500–600, TE 20
  SE T2, transversal, TR 2000–3500 ms, TE 30/100 ms
  IE, coronal, TR 1400, TE 30 ms, TI 120 ms
- Control MRI
  SE T2, transversal, TR 2000–3500 ms, TE 30/100 ms
  IE, coronal, TR 1400 ms, TE 30 ms, TI 120 ms
- Relaxometry
  IE, coronal, TR 1400 ms, TE 30 ms, TI 300, 400, 500 ms

All MRI examinations were performed on 1.5 T Philips (Gyroscan S 15), with slice thickness 6 mm, field of view 256 mm.

Results and Discussion

According to reports in literature (Bottomley et al. 1987; Dewes et al. 1986; Dooms et al. 1985), the results of our study showed malignancy to be associated with an elevated T1 relaxation time.

Tumors

The T1 time of tumors was 819 ± 128 ms before therapy and 698 ± 110 ms after the first course RCT (30 Gy); in nonresponders after the second course RCT (total 60 Gy) this was 737 ± 92 ms and after a boost (total 70 Gy) 700 ± 86 ms (Table 1). The determination of T1 values for the tumors shows no specific relation to tumor grading. During therapy the relaxometry is not relevant in cases of complete remission. In cases of partial remission or nonresponse,

Table 1. T1 relaxation times (ms) of tumors and lymph nodes

	Tumors	Lymph nodes with[a] T1 time	Lymph nodes with high[a] T1 time
Before therapy	819 ± 128	648 ± 112	924 ± 119
After RCT course 1 (30 Gy)	698 ± 110	635 ± 145	747·195
After RCT course 2 (60 Gy; nonresponders)	737 ± 92	568 ± 66	624 ± 104
After RCT boost (70 Gy; nonresponders)	700 ± 86	540 ± 63	632 ± 39

[a] At staging examination.

relaxometry cannot differentiate between edema and tumor rest. Fibrous changes can be distinguished from recurrent tumor on T2-weighted SE modes in control MRI about 8 weeks following RCT.

Malignant Lymph Nodes

Lymph nodes in histologically confirmed cases of squamous cell carcinoma showed T1 values before therapy of 924 ± 119 ms (830–1200 ms). RCT reduced T1 time of proposed malignant lymph nodes to 747 ± 195 ms after the first course of RCT, 624 ± 104 ms after the second course RCT and 632 ± 39 ms after the boost (Table 1). Complete remission was defined for this group of proposed malignant lymph nodes as a T1 time on relaxometry of 500–750 ms and no palpable lymph node, partial remission as a T1 time of 750–830 ms and regressive lymph node size, and nonresponding as a T1 value over 830 ms and a size equal to or greater than that prior to treatment. Imaging and planimetry showed a reduction in the size of supposedly malignant lymph nodes after the first course of about 20%. In contrast, we found in 69% of these cases a clear reduction of the T1 time, reaching values of nonmalignant lymph nodes. After the second course there was further size diminution (62%) and T1 time diminution (Table 2, Fig. 1).

Hyperplastic Lymph Nodes

In contrast to the above-mentioned group, lymph nodes with histologically confirmed cases of hyperplasia as well as those according to these data supposed to be nonmalignant showed little change in T1 values during RCT (Table 1).

Table 2. Relaxometry versus planimetry in assessing response to therapy

	After RCT course 1		After RCT course 2		After RCT boost	
	T1 ms	ml	T1 ms	ml	T1 ms	ml
Tumors						
Complete remission	15	3	20	11	21	19
Partial remission	6	15	3	10	1	2
Nonresponders	2	5	0	2	1	2
Malignant lymph nodes						
Complete remission	13	1	18	11	20	10
Partial remission	4	16	1	11	1	11
Nonresponders	7	7	5	2	3	3

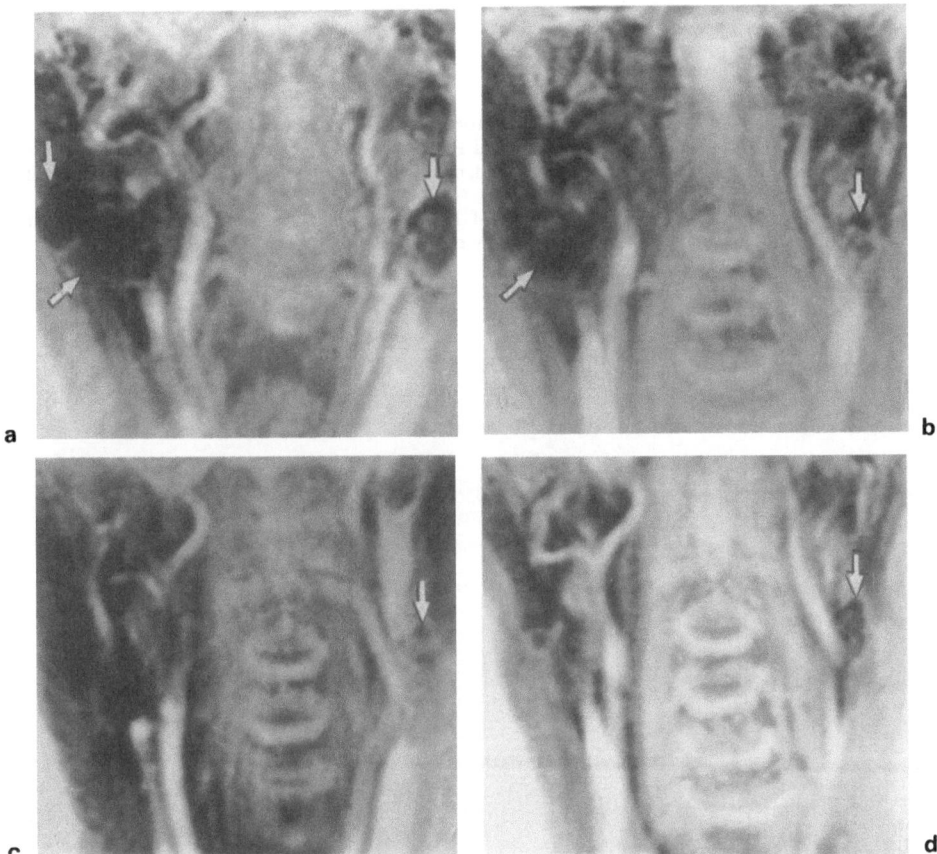

Fig. 1a-d. MR images of two lymph nodes before and after RCT. *Right lymph node*, level III, malignant. **a** Before therapy. T1 1150 ms, 35 ml. **b** After RCT first course. T1 780 ms, 9 ml. **c** After RCT second course. Responder, no remaining lymph node, edema. **d** After RCT boost. Responder, no recurrency, edema and fibrosis (T2-weighted image). *Left lymph node*, level III, hyperplastic. **a** Before therapy. T1 620 ms, 8 ml. **b** After RCT first course. T1 650 ms, 6 ml. **c** After RCT second course. T1 630 ms, 6 ml. **d** After RCT boost. T1 580 ms, 6 ml

Conclusion

Relaxometry measurements based on T1 values are easy to perform and provide a means to aid in the discrimination between malignant and hyperplastic lymph nodes. The information obtained in this way can thus improve the accuracy of TNM classification and therapy monitoring. The differentiation between malignant and hyperplastic lymph nodes is possible, however, only at T1 values below 750 ms or over 850 ms.

References

Bottomley PA, Hardy CJ, Argersinger RE, Mooreb A (1987) A review of H1 NMR relaxation in pathology: are T1 and T2 diagnostic? Med Phys 14: 1–37

Dewes W, Träber F, Gieseke J, Uexküll-Güldenland (1986) Zur Diagnostik von Lymphomen im MRT. ROFO 145: 560–564

Dooms GC, Hriacak H, Moseley M, Fischer M, Higgins C (1985) Characterization of lymphadeno-pathy by MR relaxation times, preliminary results. Radiology 155: 691–697

Monitoring of Therapy in Head and Neck Tumors Using Magnetic Resonance Snap-Shot Imaging

P. Held[1], P. Lukas[2], A. Atzinger[1], S. Braitinger[1], W.-D. Gassel[1], F. Fellner[1], N. Obletter[1], G. Schenk[1], and K. Pfaendner[1]

Introduction

The influence of radiotherapy on vascularization [1, 6–8] has to be established. It was the objective of our study to identify changes in the vascular bed of neoplasms [4, 5, 10–12] during the 1st min after intravenous injection of 20 ml Gd-DTPA to obtain prognostic information about tumor response to therapy. This requires very short acquisition times.

Methods

We performed studies on intensity versus time [2] using a T1-weighted Turbo-FLASH sequence [9]: TR 6.5 ms, TE 3 ms, TI 500 ms, flip angle 8°, slice thickness 1 cm, matrix 128×128, number of measurements 30, number of acquisitions 1 or 2, delay between the measurements 1 s, delayed scan T1-weighted SE. The scans were made before beginning radio-chemotherapy, 2 h after the end of the first irradiation, and on the 3rd, 6th, 10th, and 21st days. Identical slice positioning was obligatory. For contrast enhancement Gd-DTPA (Magnevist) was injected intravenously, 10 ml/5 s, 0.1 ml/kg body weight.

A computer-aided analysis was performed in addition to the visual analysis of signal behavior, especially in evaluating the changes in signal intensity (SI) over a period of 60 s in the individual examinations and the change in signal behavior in the course of radio therapy or radio-chemotherapy. The SI changes were thus objectified to provide a more accurate evaluation of the degree of homogenity of the tumor matrix.

Regions of interest were marked in the tumor area for this purpose. Polygons were defined within the tumor area to calculate standard deviations and SI histograms. A square was defined within the polygon so established to calculate run-length histograms. Only those runs that finished within the square were

[1] Klinikum Passau, Bischof-Piligrim-Str. 1, 8390 Passau, FRG
[2] Klinikum rechts der Isar, Technische Universität München, Ismaninger Str. 22, 8000 Munich 80, FRG

Advanced Radiation Therapy Tumor Response
Monitoring and Treatment Planning
Breit (Editor-in-Chief)
© Springer-Verlag, Berlin Heidelberg 1992

recorded. Thus the area surrounding the square was considered in calculating the run length. The peak values within the polygons with a known range of values were used to calculate the run-length histograms. The degree of homogenity of the tumor texture was established on the basis of standard deviation, SI histograms, and run-length histograms.

The curves and histograms were compared during the course of therapy or at the end of radiotherapy. In addition, studies of intensity versus time were made.

Patients with squamous cell carcinomas and anaplastic carcinomas were examined.

Results and Discussion

Although a number of the originally planned examinations could not be conducted, a certain trend can be observed from the data obtained regarding the influence of radiotherapy on tumor vascularization and the vessels of the host tissue. A marginal area of high SI composed of tumor vessels and new vascularization in the host tissue [12–15] is visible in studies on intensity versus time between the tumor and the surrounding (inflammatory and edematous) tissue. This is best delineated in the first 30–60 s after intravenous injection of Gd-DTPA (Fig. 1). In the course of therapy there was a reduction in contrast between this margin and the tumor area and surrounding tissue. Changes were observed in SI in the intensity-versus-time studies within the (healthy) host tissue and in the tumor only 2 h after the first radiation. We found a stronger and accelerated SI enhancement. This effect was strongest in the surrounding tissue, i.e., in the inflammatory edematous tissue around the tumor and in the normal tissue (especially the tongue). In the tumor matrix there were similar but weaker SI changes [1, 3]. The contrast between the tumor and the marginal area therefore increased.

In the majority of cases the strongest SI enhancement was obtained in the first four scans between the 8th and 10th second after injection of Gd-DTPA. In the fifth and sixth scans the strongest SI enhancement occurred between the 10th and 12th second after injection of Gd-DTPA. The contrast-noise ratio (CNR) between tumor and healthy tissue was very high at the moment of maximum SI enhancement (First to sixth scans), and there was a slight increase at the beginning of the SI plateau (first to fourth scans). The delineation of the tumor nevertheless depends on the tumor/marginal area CNR (rather than on the tumor/healthy tissue CNR). This was highest at the moment of maximum SI enhancement.

During therapy the homogeneity of the signal pattern within the tumor area decreased as a direct result of the change in vascularization and the increase in the number and extent of areas of necrosis. An increase in the standard deviation within the tumor area could be seen beginning in the images of the third scan at

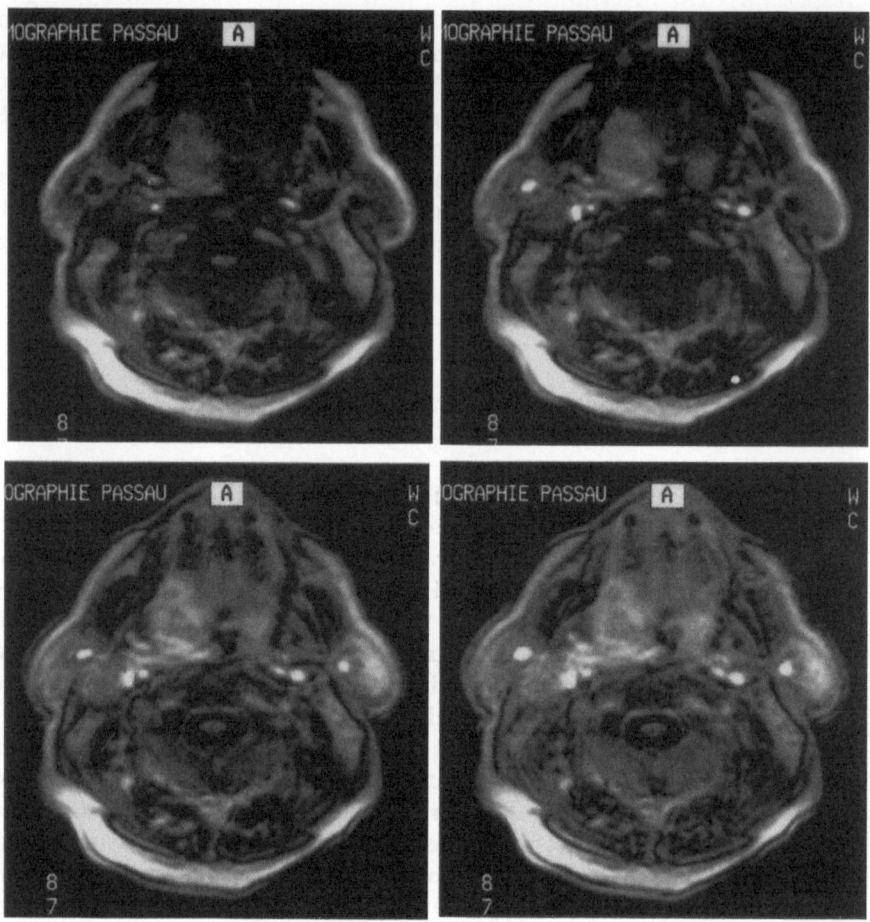

Fig. 1. Squamous cell carcinoma of the oropharynx with cervical lymp node metastasis (*right*). T1-weighted Turbo-FLASH Gd-DTPA scan (intensity-versus-time study) 2 h after the first radiation (second scan). *Upper left*, 8 s after intravenous injection of Gd-DTPA; *upper right*, 10 s after injection; *lower left*, 18 s after injection; *lower right*, 58 s after injection

the moment of the signal plateau. A clear change in standard deviation was perceived in the images obtained at the moment of the maximum SI enhancement of the sixth scan. There was a widening of the curves in the SI histograms (i.e., increase in the number of voxels with different SI), an increase in the number of runs, and a decrease in run length, corresponding to increased inhomogeneity of the texture.

In all cases SI changes occurred before a decrease in tumor volume was visible. These changes in SI appeared earlier on snap-shot Gd-DTPA enhanced scans than on the corresponding spin-echo images (T2-weighted plain scans, T1-weighted contrast scans). It may also be noted that the healthy tissue is affected at an early stage by radiotherapy.

These results must be confirmed by further examinations. However, it is clear that with this method of investigation the influence of radiotherapy on the vascularization of tumor tissue and healthy tissue is identifiable at an early stage, in the first hours after radiation.

References

1. Breit A (1969) Arteriographie vor und nach Tumorbestrahlung. Fortschr Geb Rontgenstr 111: 3–10
2. Claussen C, Lochner B (1983) Dynamische Computertomographie. Springer, Berlin Heidelberg New York
3. Denekamp J (1982) Endothelial cell proliferation as a novel approach to targeting tumour therapy. Br J Cancer 45: 136–139
4. Denekamp J (1984) Vascular endothelium as the vulnerable element in tumours. Acta Radiol Oncol 23/4: 217–225
5. Denekamp J, Hill SA, Hobson B (1983) Vascular occlusion and tumour cell death. Eur J Cancer Clin Oncol 19/2: 271–275
6. Falk P (1978) Patterns of vasculature in two pairs of related fibrosarcomas in the rat and their relation to tumour response to single large doses of radiation. Eur J Cancer 14: 237–250
7. Fike JR, Gillette EL (1978) ^{60}Co gamma and negative PI meson irradiation of microvasculature. J radiat Oncol Biol Phys 4: 825–828
8. Gillette EL, Maurer GD, Severin GA (1975) Endothelial repair of radiation damage following beta irradiation. Radiology 116: 175–177
9. Haase A (1990) Snapshot FLASH MRI application to T1, T2 and chemical-shift-imaging. Magn Res Med 13: 77–89
10. Knierim M, Paweletz N, Finze E-M (1986) Tumor-related constitutive vascularization. An ultrastructural study. Anticancer Res 6: 1305–1316
11. Reinhold HS, Buisman GH (1973) Radiosensitivity of capillary endothelium. Br J Radiol 46: 54–57
12. Schor AM, Schor SL (1983) Tumour angiogenesis. J Pathol 141: 385–413
13. Sholley MM, Gimbrone MA, Ramzi SC (1977) Cellular migration and replication in endothelial regeneration. Lab Invest 36/1: 18–25
14. Sholley MM, Ferguson GP, Seibel HR, Montour JL, Wilson JD (1984) Mechanisms of neovascularization. Lab Invest 51/6: 624–634
15. Shubik P (1982) Vascularization of tumours; a review. J Cancer Res Clin Oncol 103: 211–226

Monitoring of Combined Therapy in Advanced Head and Neck Cancer with Positron Emission Tomography and [18F]fluorodeoxyglucose

U. Haberkorn[1], L.G. Strauss[1], A. Dimitrakopoulou[1], E. Seiffert[3],
C. Reißer[3], F. Oberdorfer[1], and W. Maier-Borst[1]

Introduction

For the evaluation and individual planning of chemotherapy or head and neck tumors it is useful to obtain information about the tumor metabolism and its early changes during chemotherapy. Positron emission tomography (PET) with [18F]fluorodeoxyglucose (FDG) is a specific method that gives information about glucose uptake. These data can be used in follow-up studies to assess the effectiveness of a therapeutic schedule.

Patients and Methods

Twelve patients with histologically confirmed tumors of the head and neck underwent a PET examination prior to the first chemotherapeutical cycle with cisplatin (100 mg/m^2 on day 1) and 5-fluorouracil (1000 mg/m on days 1–4). A second PET examination was performed 1 week after the first chemotherapeutic cycle. All patients had a tumor or lymph node volume larger than 1.5 cm in diameter.

Computed tomography (CT) was performed using a Siemens Somatom DRH. Continuous sections of 8 ml thickness were acquired, and skin markings were made for correct positioning of PET. The volumes were calculated with area and section thickness. For the calculation of tumor growth rate we took an exponential function, $c = \ln(V_0/V_1)/t$ with V_0 and V_1 as the volumes before and after therapy and t as the time interval between V_0 and V_1.

The PET examination used a PC2048-7WB scanner (Scanditronix, Uppsala, Sweden) with two detector rings. Prior to emission scanning, transmission scans were made with more than 10 million counts per section. One hour after

[1] Department of Radiology and Pathophysiology, German Cancer Research Center, Im Neuenheimer Feld 280, 6900 Heidelberg, FRG
[2] Department of Oto-Rhino-Laryngology, University of Heidelberg, Klinikum Mannheim, Theordor-Kutzer-Ufer, 6800 Mannheim, FRG
[3] Department of Oto-Rhino-Laryngology, University of Heidelberg, Im Neuenheimer Feld 400, 6900 Heidelberg, FRG

Advanced Radiation Therapy Tumor Response
Monitoring and Treatment Planning
Breit (Editor-in-Chief)
© Springer-Verlag, Berlin Heidelberg 1992

intravenous administration of 9–12 mCi FDG, PET images were acquired over 10 min. The number of counts per slice in all cases exceeded one million. PET images were generated by an iterative reconstruction program [1] on a VAX 11/750 (Digital equipment, Maynard, Mass., USA) computer system. The image matrix was 128×128; for display an interpolation to 256×256 was made. The spatial resolution was approximately 5.1 mm. The pixel size in all reconstructed images was 2×2 mm. In addition, a correction for attenuation and scattering was included. The quantitative evaluation used a region-of-interest (ROI) technique. The ROIs were defined in tumor and soft tissue with a region size of 32 pixels or more. The PET sections were compared with the CT images to identify anatomical structures. The FDG uptake was then expressed as the standardized uptake value (SUV): SUV = tissue concentration [injected dose (nCi)/body weight (g)].

Results

FDG uptake data were available for six tumors and eight lymph nodes and volumetric data for five tumors and seven lumph nodes. All malignant lesions showed an enhancement in FDG uptake compared to normal soft tissue. We observed differences in FDG uptake in different lymph node metastases of the same patient. The changes in FDG uptake are shown in Fig. 1. Only 50% of the tumors or lymph nodes had a significant decrease in metabolism. The relationship between tumor or lymph node metabolism during chemotherapy and

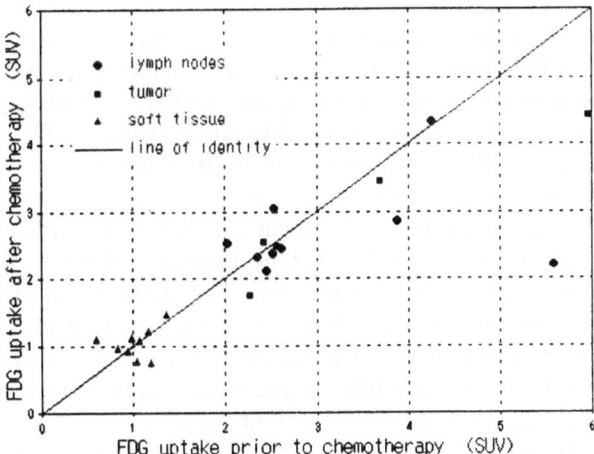

Fig. 1. Change in regional FDG metabolism during chemotherapy in lymph nodes ($n = 9$), tumors ($n = 5$), and soft tissue ($n = 10$)

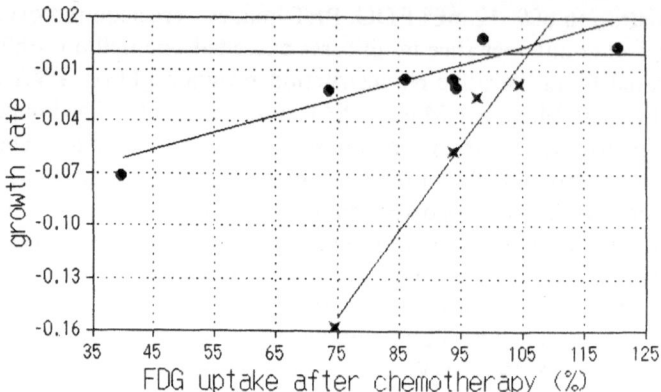

Fig. 2. Relationship between the relative change in FDG metabolism and tumor growth rate

growth rate is shown in Fig. 2. Tumors responded to a greater extent than lymph nodes. The tumor growth rate and the change in FDG uptake were highly correlated in both tumors and lymph nodes ($r = 0.98$ and $e = 0.94$, respectively; $f < 0.01$).

Discussion

FDG, a widely applied tracer in cancer patients, is transported like glucose into the cell and thereafter trapped in its phosphorylated form [2] without further significant metabolism during the examination time. This principle of metabolic trapping has been used for diagnostic procedures as the differential diagnosis of recurrent colorectal cancer [3]. Furthermore, several experimental and clinical studies revealed a reduction in the amount of deoxyglucose after chemotherapy or radiotherapy which was associated with less viable tumor tissue [4–7].

In our study we found that different lymph nodes in the same patient can have different metabolic activity and can also show a different responsiveness to therapy. This may be explained by cell heterogeneity in human tumors. Different metastatic clones lead to metastases with different biologic behavior. We observed a significant decrease in only 43% of cases. This decrease in FDG uptake in only 43% reflects clinical data about the remission rate [8, 9]. Brauneis et al. [10] in a flow cytometric study found no significant difference in tumor reaction to therapy in tumors with different proliferation rates. However there was a higher incidence of regional or distant metastases in tumors exhibiting a high proliferation rate. Minn et al. [11] observed a strong correlation of FDG uptake and the amount of S-phase cells. This supports the thesis that FDG indicates the degree of malignancy and the incidence of metastatic spread. The comparison of tumors and lymph nodes showed a lower response rate for lymph node metastases. A comparable change in FDG uptake was associated with different growth rates in tumors and lymph node metastases. This was also found in the clinical outcome [12].

Therefore, using PET it is possible to obtain absolute and therefore comparable data about tumor metabolism prior to and after chemotherapy. PET is a useful method for the observation and improvement of therapeutic measures in patients undergoing systemic chemotherapy.

References

1. Schmidlin P, Kübler WK, Doll J, Strauss LG, Ostertag H (1987) Image processing in whole body positron emission tomography. In: Schmidt HAE, Csernay L (eds) Nuklearmedizin. Schattauer, Stuttgart, pp 84–87
2. Gallagher BM, Fowler JS, Gutterson NI, MacGregor RR, Wan CN, Wolf AP (1978) Metabolic trapping as a principle of radiopharmaceutical design: some factors responsible for the biodistribution of (18F) 2-deoxy-2-fluoro-D-glucose. J Nucl Med 19: 1154–1161
3. Strauss LG, Clorius JH, Schlag P, Lehner B, Kimmig B, Engenhart R, Marin-Grez M, Helus F, Oberdorfer F, Schmidlin P, van Kaick G (1989) Recurrence of colorectal tumors: PET evaluation. Radiology 170: 329–332
4. Iosilevsky G, Front D, Bettman L, Hardoff R, Ben-Arieh Y (1985) Uptake of gallium-67 citrate and (2-3H)deoxyglucose in the tumor model, following chemotherapy and radiotherapy. J Nucl Med 26: 278–282
5. Abe Y, Matsuzawa T, Fujiwara T, Fukuda H, Itoh M, Yamada K, Yamaguchi K, Sato T, Ido T (1986) Assessment of radiotherapeutic effects on experimental tumors using 18F-2-fluoro-2-deoxy-D-glucose. Eur J Nucl Med 12: 325–328
6. Nagata Y, Yamamoto K, Hiraoka M, Abe M, Takahashi M, Akuta K, Nishimura Y, Jo S, Masunaga S, Kubo S, Konishi J (1990) Monitoring liver tumor therapy with F-18-FDG positron emission tomography. J Comput Assist Tomogr 14: 370–374
7. Minn H, Paul R, Ahonen A (1988) Evaluation of treatment response to radiotherapy in head and neck cancer with fluorine-18 fluorodeoxyglucose. J Nucl Med 29: 1521–1525
8. Rothman H (1985) Changing trends in treatment of advanced head and neck carcinoma: review of the literature and report of a case. Am Osteopath Assoc J: 370–374
9. Schröder M, von Heyden HW, Scherpe A, Nagel GA (1986) Einfluß der Chemotherapie auf die Überlebenszeit von Patienten mit weit fortgeschrittenen Plattenepithel-Karzinomen des Kopf-Hals-Bereiches. Laryngol Rhinol Otol (Stuttg) 65: 11–15
10. Brauneis JW, Laskawi R, Schröder M, Göhde W (1989) Ergebnisse der Impulscytophotometrie bei malignen tumoren des Kopf-Hals-Bereiches. HNO 37: 369–372
11. Minn H, Joensuu H, Ahonen A, Klemi P (1988) Fluorodeoxyglucose imaging: a method to assess the proliferative activity of human cancer in vivo. Comparison with DNA flow cytometry in head and neck tumors. Cancer 61: 1776–1781
12. Deitmer T, Urbanitz D (1986) Zytostatische Primärtherapie von Plattenepithel-Karzinomen des Oro- und Hypopharynx mit Cis-Platin, Bleomycin und Methotrexat. Laryngol Rhinol Otol (Stuttg) 65: 7–10

Lymphoid Lesions of the Eye:
The Role of Magnetic Resonance Imaging

N. Hosten[1], W. Schörner[1], C. Zwicker[1], K. Neumann[1], A. Lietz[1],
S. Serke[2], U. Keske[1], D. Huhn[2], and R. Felix[1]

Introduction

Local radiation therapy is the treatment of choice for both benign (pseudo-) and malignant lymphoma of the ocular adnexa (Kim and Fayos 1976; Jereb et al. 1984; Mittal et al. 1986; Pötter et al. 1989; Dunbar et al. 1990). Various approaches to orbital irradiation have been described by these authors, and selecting one of them requires exact knowledge of the tumor extent and of the relationship between tumor and lens. Magnetic resonance imaging (MRI) of the orbit combines multiplanar imaging capacity and excellent soft tissue contrast. The present study analyzes the ability of MRI to define the extent and anatomic relations of orbital lymphomas toward choosing an optimal radiation protocol.

Patients and Methods

Fifteen patients with a histological diagnosis of orbital lymphoid lesions were studied by MRI and computed tomography (CT). MRI was performed on a 0.5-T Magnetom (Siemens) using a circular surface coil with a diameter of 11 cm that covered both eyes. The in-plane resolution was 0.8 mm/pixel. T1-weighted spin-echo images of both orbits in transverse, sagittal and coronal planes (TR 400 ms, TE 30 ms, 5 mm slice thickness, 4 NEX), and a selected coronal slice of heavier T2 weighting (TR 1600 ms, TE 30, 60 . . . 240 ms, 10 mm slice thickness, 1 NEX) were obtained routinely. MRI was repeated in one slice orientation after administration of 0.1 mmol Gd-DTPA/kg body weight. All CT examinations were performed on a third-generation scanner (Siemens Somatom DR).

Histologically and immunologically the five malignant lymphomas included centroblastoma (one case), centroblastic-centrocytic lymphoma (two cases), and

---

[1] Department of Radiology, Klinikum Rudolf Virchow/Charlottenburg, Free University of Berlin, Spandauer Damm 130, 1000 Berlin 19, FRG
[2] Department of Internal Medicine, Klinikum Rudolf Virchow/Charlottenburg, Free University of Berlin, Spandauer Damm 130, 1000 Berlin 19, FRG

Advanced Radiation Therapy Tumor Response
Monitoring and Treatment Planning
Breit (Editor-in-Chief)
© Springer-Verlag, Berlin Heidelberg 1992

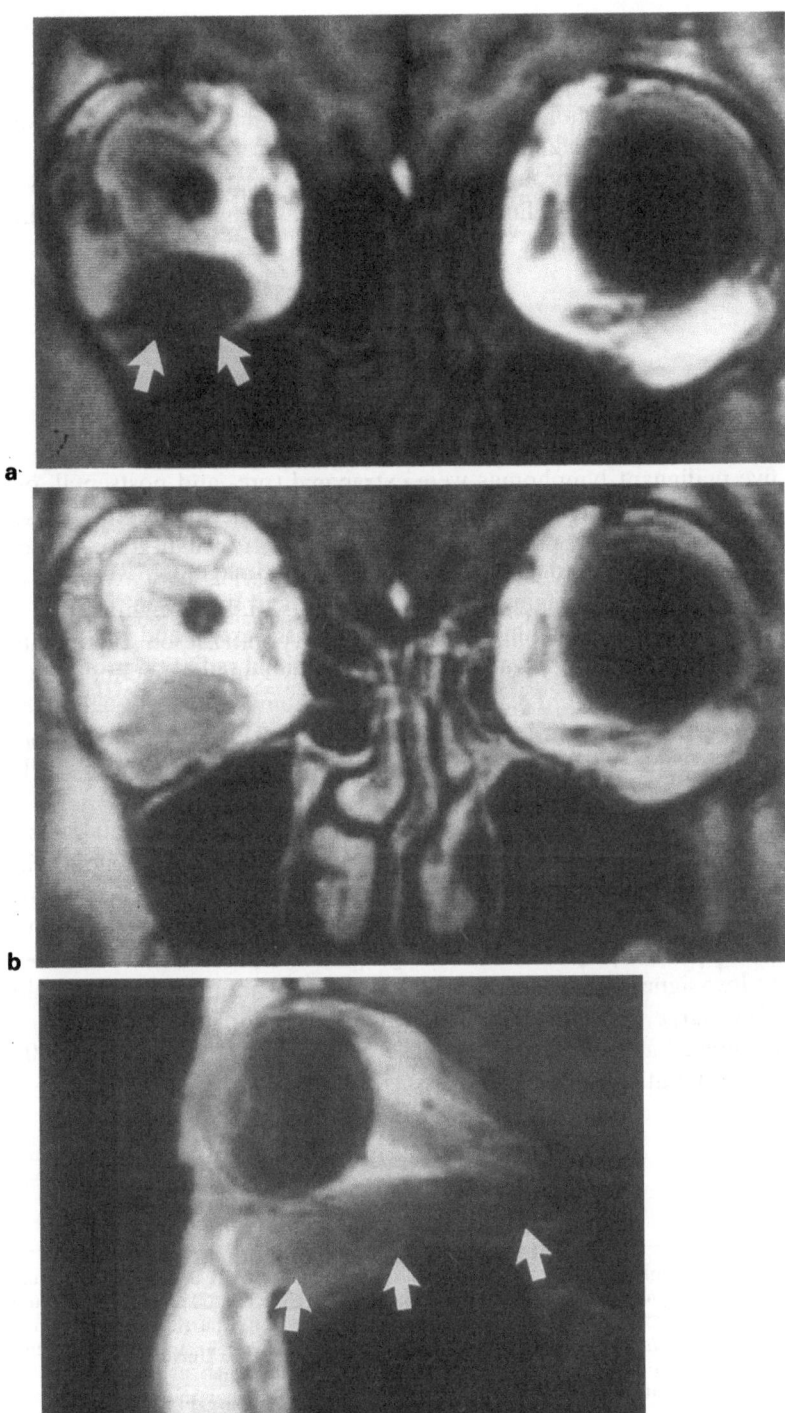

lympo-plasmocytic lymphoma (two cases). Five cases were diagnosed as benign (pseudo-)lymphoma, and five cases of inflammatory pseudotumor were included as this entity is the main differential diagnoses for orbital lymphoma. In three cases of malignant lymphoma follow-up MRI examinations (3 months after radiation therapy) were available.

On MRI, signal intensity, contrast enhancement, location, and morphology of lesions were evaluated. Definition of extension and anatomic relationships were compared to CT findings.

Results

Two of five malignant lymphomas were extraconal (pre- and postseptal, one; postseptal only, one), two were intramuscular (superior rectus muscle and inferior rectus muscle, one each), and one was intraocular. Two pseudolymphomas were intramuscular (superior rectus muscle), two involved the lacrimal gland, and one was extraconal and postseptal. Five inflammatory pseudotumors were all intraconal. Lesions were hypointense on T1-weighted images, slightly hyperintense to muscle on T2-weighted images, and moderately enhanced after Gd-DTPA. On plain CT scans lymphomas were hypodense; they enhanced moderately after intravenous contrast. One intraocular lymphoma presented as a mass with retinal detachment; it was hyperintense on T1-weighted MRI, hyperdense on CT.

Parasagittal MRI defined anteroposterior tumor extension in all cases of malignant lymphoma and in three cases of pseudolymphoma on a single slice (Fig. 1c). Two pseudolymphomas located in the lacrimal gland were best seen on coronal and transverse images. CT did not define anteroposterior extension of lymphomas or pseudolymphomas on a single slice in eight cases. On follow-up MRI only low-signal scars were seen in two cases 3 months after radiation therapy. One large lymphoma with osseous destruction and meningeal involvement showed a significant reduction of tumor mass after radiation (80% were destroyed), but some enhancing tissue remained.

Fig. 1. Appearance of malignant orbital lymphoma on multiplanar MRI in a 46-year-old man; lymphoma of high malignancy. **a** On coronal T1-weighted MRI (SE, TR 400 ms, TE 30 ms, 5 mm, 4 NEX) a low-signal mass is demonstrated inside the right inferior rectus muscle. Contours of mass are irregular (*arrowheads*). **b** T1-weighted MRI after intravenous administration of 0.1 mmol Gd-DTPA/kg b.w. demonstrates moderate enhancement of intramuscular mass. **c** Sagittal T1-weighted MRI demonstrates massive enlargement of infiltrated inferior rectus muscle from the lower lid into the orbital cone (*arrowheads*)

Discussion

Lymphoma of the ocular adnexa is a rare disease constituting approximately 0.03% of all malignant tumors (Dunbar et al. 1990). Local radiation therapy is the most effective treatment (Knowles et al. 1990); doses of 25–40 Gy are recommended for malignant lymphomas (Wannenmacher and Pfannmüller 1976) whereas benign pseudolymphomas are adequately treated with doses as low as 16–20 Gy (Gordon et al. 1986). Various lens-sparing approaches have been described; Dunbar et al. (1990) describe the use of a lead shield mounted on a contact lens. They also give an extensive review of the literature. Immunophenotypic analysis is necessary for differentiating benign and malignant lesions (Knowles et al. 1990), as clinical or radiologic criteria alone are insufficient. Radiologic studies are indicated for defining extension of lesions; additionally, screening for lymphoma of other regions of the body is necessary, as generalization occurs in both benign and malignant orbital lymphoma. CT scans of the orbit are well introduced for preradiation studies of orbital lymphomas; MRI studies are just emerging (Pötter et al. 1989). In our series, T1-weighted MRI defined orbital lymphomas as hypointense structures clearly descernible from orbital fat. The relationship to the lens was clearly depicted, and anteroposterior extension for correct choice of energy was easily determinable on a single sagittal or transverse plane (Fig. 1c). Follow-up examinations demonstrated complete tumor control in two patients; in the remaining patient residual tumor was clearly demonstrated by the persistence of enhancing tissue. In this patient, another control is scheduled presently and may demonstrate the need for further treatment.

Inflammatory pseudotumor was descernible from lymphoma by MRI in our series by location and multifocality; radiation therapy is not primarily indicated in this disease entity, and systemic corticoids are usually helpful.

One case of intraocular lymphoma was not descernible from retinal detachment of other origin by either CT or MRI; knowledge of this extremely rare disease is necessary, however, as involvement of the brain is usually encountered, and this makes further imaging studies and prophylactic or therapeutic radiation of the brain necessary (Margolis et al. 1980).

References

Dunbar SF, Lingwood RM, Doppke KP et al. (1988) Conjunctival lymphoma: results of treatment with a single anterior field. A lens sparing approach. Int J Radiat Oncol Biol Phys 19: 249–257

Gordon PS, Juillard GLF, Selch MT et al. (1986) Orbital lymphomas and pseudolymphomas: treatment with radiation therapy. Radiology 159: 797–799

Jereb B, Lee H, Jakobiec F, Kutcher J (1984) Radiation therapy of conjunctival and orbital lymphoid tumors. Int J Radiat Oncol Biol Phys 10: 1013–1019

Kim YH, Fayos JV (1976) Primary orbital lymphoma: a radiotherapeutic experience. Int J Radiat Oncol Biol Phys 1: 1099–1115

Knowles DM, Jakobiec FA, McNally L, Burke JS (1990) Lymphoid hyperplasia and malignant lymphoma occurring in the ocular adnexa (orbit, conjunctiva, and eyelids) Hum Pathol 21: 959–973

Margolis M, Fraser R, Lichter A, Char DH (1980) The role of radiation therapy in the management of ocular reticulum cell sarcoma. Cancer 45: 688–692

Mittal BB, Deutsch M, Kennerdell J, Johnson B (1986) Paraocular lymphoid tumors. Radiology 159: 793–796

Pötter R, Busse H, Müller RP (1989) Strahlentherapie bei (lokalisierten) Non-Hodgkin-Lymphomen der Orbita. Klin Monatsbl Augenheilkd 413–423

Wannenmacher M, Pfannmüller E (1986) Radiotherapie der Non-Hodgkin-Lymphome. Internist (Berlin) 27: 498–505

Application of Color Doppler Flow Imaging for the Diagnosis of Primary and Secondary Lymph Node Neoplasia and for the Evaluation of Therapy Responsiveness of Malignant Lymphomas

A. Tschammler[1], G. Wittenberg[1], B. Porowski[2], and E. Reinhart[3]

Introduction

Ultrasound is a very sensitive method for detecting superficially located lymph nodes; however, it offers only low specificity in differentiating the alterations between benign and malignant lymph nodes. Color Doppler flow imaging (CDFI) provides the possibility of color-visualizing perfused vessels in real-time sonograms in which flow direction and flow velocity are color coded. Moreover, Doppler spectrum analysis can be performed in individual vessels.

The aim of our study was to examine the possibility of improved differentiation between benign and malignant lymph node alterations by evaluating the perfusion of superficial lymph nodes with the help of CDFI. Additionally, we report our initial results regarding the use of CDFI for therapy control in malignant lymphomas.

Patients and Methods

For primary diagnosis we used CDFI in 220 lymph nodes (76 patients). Among these were 105 benign lymph node alterations, 64 metastases (50 squamous cell carcinomas, 7 bronchial carcinomas, 6 melanomas, 1 carcinoma of the breast), and 51 malignant lymphomas (21 highly malignant non-Hodgkin lymphomas, 30 minor malignant non-Hodgkin lymphomas). The diagnosis was confirmed by histology ($n = 158$) or by clinical follow-up over a period of at least 6 months ($n = 62$). In 21 patients (65 lymph nodes) with malignant lymphomas lymph node perfusion was evaluated during ($n = 33$) and after chemotherapy ($n = 22$) and after radiotherapy ($n = 10$). Six lymph nodes assessed after radiotherapy were additionally treated by chemotherapy.

All lymph nodes were examined in the slow-flow mode with an Angiodynograph (Quantum/Philips) using a 7.5-MHz linear transducer. In large lymph nodes (>3 cm) a 5-MHz transducer was used additionally. To exclude

[1] Institut für Röntgendiagnostik, Universität Würzburg, 8700 Würzburg, FRG
[2] Medizinische Klinik, Universität Würzburg
[3] Klinik und Poliklinik für Zahn-, Mund- und Kiefer-Krankheiten, Universität Würzburg

Advanced Radiation Therapy Tumor Response
Monitoring and Treatment Planning
Breit (Editor-in-Chief)
© Springer-Verlag, Berlin Heidelberg 1992

artifacts, lymph nodes were classified as being perfused only if two-plane, vascular typical Doppler spectra were derived from intranodular color pixels. We evaluated the intranodal flow resistance (quantified by the maximum of the measurable intranodular pulsatility and resistance index, known parameters of Doppler spectral analysis [3]) and lymph node perfusion, which was classified subjectively semiquantitatively in comparison to the surrounding low perfused fat, muscle, and soft tissue.

Results

The median maximum diameter of the benign lymph nodes was 12 (5–32) mm, of the malignant lymphomas 17 (6–55) mm, and of the metastases 18.5 (9–60) mm. With CDFI, perfusion was demonstrated in 171 lymph nodes (78%). In these lymph nodes the increased flow resistance of intranodular vessels (pulsatility index ≥ 1.8 or resistance index ≥ 0.9, norm values determined in the benign lymph nodes [3]) proved to be a highly specific (97%) criterion for differentiating benign lymph nodes from metastases (sensitivity = 53%). This criterion cannot be used to identify malignant lymphomas because its sensitivity is only 18%.

On the basis of the subjective semiquantitative perfusion evaluation, perfusion was found lacking in 49 lymph nodes (17 metastases, 2 malignant lymphomas, 30 benign lymph nodes), low or partial perfusion was found in 45 lymph nodes (26 metastases, 4 malignant lymphomas, 15 benign lymph nodes), and hyperperfusion was demonstrated in 126 lymph nodes (21 metastases, 45 malignant lymphomas, 60 benign lymph nodes). Based on the heperperfusion criterion differentiation between metastases and malignant lymphoma was possible in 77% of lymph nodes. Only by combining CDFI criteria (increased intranodular flow resistance or absent, low, or partial perfusion indicating metastases, and hyperperfusion indicating malignant lymphoma) and B-mode sonomorphologic criteria was it possible to distinguish the benign lymph node alterations. The following parameters of malignancy were examined: maximum diameter over 10 mm [1], minimum diameter at least 8 mm [2], and ratio of maximum diameter to minimum diameter under 2 [4]. In all cases CDFI revealed a higher specificity and accuracy than did B-mode ultrasound. The most sensitive additional criterion (80% in each case) was a maximum lymph node diameter over 10 mm in metastases (Table 1) and malignant lymphomas (Table 2). The highest specificity was achieved in metastases by the additional criterion of minimum diameter of at least 8 mm (95%). In malignant lymphomas the most specific additional criterion (86%) was a pathologic relation in the ratio of maximum/minimum diameter.

Maximum lymph node diameter was chosen as the evaluation criterion during the course of therapy of malignant lymphomas because of its high

Table 1. Differentiation between metastases ($n = 64$) and benign lymph nodes ($n = 105$) by B-mode ultrasound and CDFI

	B-mode ultrasound			CDFI		
	Sensitivity	Specificity	Accuracy	Sensitivity	Specificity	Accuracy
Maximum diameter > 10 mm	95%	38%	60%	80%	76%	78%
Minimum diameter ≥ 8 mm	86%	78%	81%	73%	95%	87%
Maximum/minimum diameter < 2	94%	61%	73%	78%	75%	76%

Table 2. Differentiation between malignant lymphomas ($n = 51$) and benign lymph nodes ($n = 105$) by B-mode ultrasound and CDFI

	B-mode ultrasound			CDFI		
	Sensitivity	Specificity	Accuracy	Sensitivity	Specificity	Accuracy
Maximum diameter > 10 mm	90%	38%	55%	80%	60%	67%
Minimum diameter ≥ 8 mm	69%	78%	75%	65%	82%	76%
Maximum/minimum diameter < 2	63%	61%	62%	57%	86%	76%

sensitivity. A pathologic lymph node size was observed in 12/12 lymph nodes without successful therapy or recurrence. However, a lymph node size over 10 mm was also demonstrated in 17/21 lymph nodes with partial remission and in 14/32 lymph nodes with total remission. Hyperperfusion was identified in 11/12 lymph nodes without remission or recurrence, in 11/21 lymph nodes with partial remission, and in 7/32 lymph nodes with total remission. The criteria used in color Duplex ultrasound — hyperperfusion and pathologic lymph node size — showed the highest correlation to the clinical evaluation of therapy success. These were observed in 11/12 lymph nodes without remission or recurrence, in 10/21 lymph nodes with partial remission, and in 3/32 lymph nodes with total remission.

Discussion

For the detection of superficial lymph node metastases CDFI together with B-mode information offers highly specific additional criteria through the semi-quantitative evaluation of the lymph node perfusion and the Doppler spectrum analysis of intranodular vessels. Also in superficial malignant lymphomas information in addition to the already known sonomorphologic criteria is provided by the semiquantitative evaluation of lymph node perfusion. However, the additional gain in specificity and accuracy is considerably less than in metastases. Initial results obtained during the therapy of malignant lymphomas suggest that CDFI may increase the accuracy of ultrasound evaluation of the therapy success. The degree of reliability of this method, however, has yet to be investigated by means of prospective studies.

References

1. Bruneton JN, Normand F, Balu-Maestro C et al. (1987) Lymphomatous superficial lymph nodes: US detection. Radiology 165: 233–235
2. Gritzman N, Czembirek H, Hajek P et al. (1987) Sonographie bei cervicalen Lymphknoten-metastasen. Radiologe 27: 118–122
3. Tschammler A, Gunzer U, Reinhart E et al. (1991) Dignitätsbeurteilung vergrößerter Lymphknoten durch qualitative und semiquantitative Auswertung der Lymphknotenperfusion mit der farbkodierten Duplexsonografie. Fortschr Geb Rontgenstr 154: 414–418
4. Watzinger F, Weismann C, Doringer E, Schmoller HJ (1989) Größenverhältnisse von Milzen und Lymphknoten bei normalen und krankhaften Zuständen. Ultraschall Med 10: 29–32

Ultrasound: An Effective Imaging Method for the Early Detection of Recurrent Head and Neck Tumors

U. Mende[1], J. Zöller[2], H. Maier[3], M. Flentje[1], and M. Loth[1]

Introduction

Early diagnosis and correct staging of a malignant tumor are the basic requirements for effective primary therapy with the intention of achieving primary control of the locoregional process. Prognosis and quality of life in patients with tumorous diseases in the head and neck region are determined much more by a locoregional recurrence than by distant metastases, which occur infrequently and late at advanced stages. In cases of primary failure the detection of an, if possible, incipient local and/or regional relapse is of major importance for effective secondary therapy [3]. In addition to the often difficult clinical examination — which yields only limited information, especially in cases of fibrotic changes mainly after operation *and* radiotherapy — imaging procedures such as posttherapeutic ultrasound screening help to distinguish recurrent disease from mere therapy-induced residues.

Patients and Methods

The 140 patients included 122 men (87.1%) and 18 women (12.9%) aged between 36 and 85 years. These underwent ultrasound examination on clinical suspicion of a relapse or during posttherapeutic care between February 1985 and May 1990. Each patient underwent between 1 and 24 examinations. In 54 patients (38.6%) the primary therapy consisted of chemotherapy and/or operation without radiotherapy, while the majority of 86 patients (61.4%) received radiation therapy either alone or after chemotherapy and/or operation.

Ultrasound examinations were performed under identical conditions regarding examiner, machine (Picker LSC 7000, with 5-MHz curved and linear array

[1] Klinische Radiologie und Poliklinik, Radiologische Universitätsklinik, Im Neuenheimer Feld 400, 6900 Heidelberg, FRG
[2] Universitätsklinik für Mund-Kiefer-Gesichtschirurgie, Im Neuenheimer Feld 400, 6900 Heidelberg, FRG
[3] Universitäts-Hals-Nasen-Klinik, Im Neuenheimer Feld 400, 6900 Heidelberg, FRG

Advanced Radiation Therapy Tumor Response
Monitoring and Treatment Planning
Breit (Editor-in-Chief)
© Springer-Verlag, Berlin Heidelberg 1992

transducers), setting and calibration, reproducible ultrasound sections, and documentation, as already described [2]. The (least suspected) tumorous processes were analyzed for dimensions and volume (calculated from the measured areas and perpendicular diameters) and the echogenicity objectified by gray-scale histograms. The malignant/benign nature of these (suspected) tumorous changes were confirmed by biopsy or operation and histologic evaluation.

In 55 patients the ultrasound echogenicity of space-occupying processes could be compared to contrast enhancement in computed tomography (CT) examinations performed on the same day or within a short period.

Results

In 136 of the 140 patients the tumorous processes identified by ultrasound were confirmed histologically. Among these were 36 local recurrent tumors without affected lymph nodes (26.5%) and 49 with positive nodes (36.0%), i.e., a total of 85 local recurrences (62.5%). Eleven patients had developed a second primary tumor without metastases in the lymph nodes (8.1%), and 15 (11.0%) also showed positive nodes, resulting in a total of 26 (19.1%) second primaries in the head and neck region. Metastatic recurrences in the lymph nodes were seen in only 25 patients (18.4%). In 28 of the 136 patients (20.6%) clinical examination presented no evidence of a recurrent or second tumor which had been disclosed by ultrasound.

In four patients a tumor relapse was ruled out. One clinically suspected lymph node involvement was correctly regarded as negative on ultrasound because of its echogenicity. The other three were false-positive misdiagnoses by ultrasound. The low echogenicity of one local process in the floor of the mouth and the tongue after operation and radiotherapy (alio loco) was mistaken for tumor relapse. In another patient after repeated operations the swelling of the tongue could not be classified definitely by ultrasound. The low echogenicity of a lymph node in the fourth patient was caused by inflammatory changes and not by tumorous invasion.

The analysis of gray-scale histograms showed significantly higher values of echogenicity (9.94 ± 2.53) for the 85 recurrences and second tumors in which radiotherapy had been part of the primary therapy concept compared to the group of 51 relapses without radiotherapy (7.86 ± 1.92; $p < 0.01$).

The analysis of CT contrast enhancement in 55 relapsed tumors showed a good correlation between hyperdensity (relative to muscle) and lower echogenicity in ultrasound ($p < 0.05$).

Discussion

Whereas the detection and delineation of tumorous processes is usually not problematic for pretherapeutic primary diagnosis and staging, the posttherapeutic clinical examination especially after operation and radiotherapy is often difficult and provides only limited or equivocal information. To differentiate more sensitively and surely between a recurrent tumor and a mere therapy-induced residue imaging techniques must become an integral part of the routine follow-up program.

Especially in posttherapeutic follow-up the standard CT in axial planes yield a high rate of unsatisfactory results for recurrent diseases of the caudal wall of the oral cavity and the oropharynx, in cases of fibrotic, poorly vascularized tumors, and marked asymmetry after reconstructive operation procedures. Also, it is limited principally by artifacts from metal implants and inlays [4]. The main drawbacks of magnetic resonance imaging are the high costs and the still limited availability of this technique despite its technical advantages.

Ultrasound involves low risks and is cheap, sensitive, and effective. It definitely improves the early detection of recurrences or second primary tumors provided that the diagnostic schedule meets a few basic requirements. Together with the clinical evidence only standardized conditions of examination, documentation, and analysis allow the early detection of even tiny structural changes suspected of a relapse. To avoid false-positive results inflammatory processes must be ruled out.

Due to the high rate of second primaries (19.1%) the restriction of ultrasound control examinations to the original local tumor area and the regional lymphatics entails an unjustifiable risk of false-negative results.

Although tumorous processes in the head and neck region usually show irregular borders and lower echogenicity relative to the surrounding tissue, our data clearly demonstrate the unacceptability of the general opinion that tumors (primary, persistent, or recurrent), regardless of primary therapy (mode of operation, chemo-, radiotherapy) are almost always echodeficient [1]. Clinical experience demonstrates that after primary therapy with operation and radiation recurrent tumors are much more fibrotic than without radiotherapy. The detailed analysis of the gray-scale histograms show the significantly higher echogenicity due to stronger fibrosis and generally less expressed vascularization if the region of the relapse had been within the borders of the former radiation field (Fig. 1). Neglecting these facts means reducing the chances for the early detection of the (incipient) recurrence.

In addition, the detailed results of ultrasound screening in the course of posttherapeutic care provide the necessary data for planning and monitoring an adequate relapse therapy.

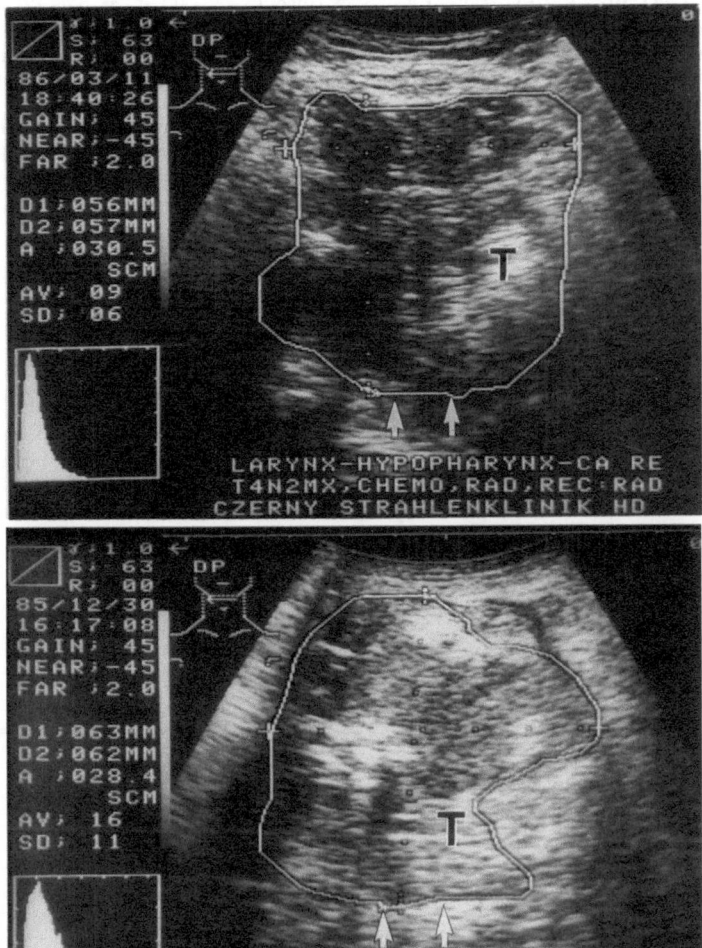

Fig. 1. Echogenicity and radiotherapy. Two ultrasound images (transverse sections). *Above*, carcinoma of the right larynx/hypopharynx (T4 N2c Mx) in a 38-year-old man. Five months after chemo- and radiotherapy, recurrent tumor (oral cavity, oropharynx) mostly beyond the earlier radiation field: lower echogenicity. *Below*, carcinoma of the right alveolar process in a 54-year old man. Sixteen months after operation and radiotherapy, recurrent tumor (oral cavity, oropharynx) within the earlier radiation field: high echogenicity. *Arrows*, surface of the tongue (*T*)

References

1. Frühwald F, Schmid AP, Neuhold A, Schwaighofer B (1986) Real-Time-Sonographie Zur Verlaufskontrolle von Zungenmalignomen während und nach Radiatio. Tumordiagn Ther 7: 150–154

2. Mende U, Flentje M, Weischedel U, Zöller J, Lenarz T (1989) Sonographische Diagnostik von Kopf-Hals-Tumoren im therapeutischen Umfeld. Rontgen-blatter 42: 19–23
3. Wannenmacher M (1987) Mundhöh lentumoren (Mundboden, Zungenkörper und Zungengrund, Ober- und Unterkiefer, Wange). In: Scherer E (ed) Strahlentherapie, 3rd edn. Springer, Berlin Heidelberg New York, pp 447–499
4. Wolfensberger M, Jecklin A, Franze I, Kikinis R (1987) Der Beitrag der Computertomographie zur präoperativen Klassifizierung von Mundhöhlen- und Oropharynxkarzinomen. Laryngol Rhinol Otol (Stuttg) 66: 324–328

Department of Otolaryngology and Pathology, Kidney Central Cancer Research Center, Institute
of ... Prevention and Treatment, ...

Department of ...

Correspondence to: ...

Positron Emission Tomography: A Noninvasive Procedure for the Determination of Tumor Proliferation

U. Haberkorn[1], L.G. Strauss[1], A. Dimitrakopoulou[1], C. Reißer[2], D. Haag[3], S. Ziegler[1], and W.J. Lorenz[1]

Introduction

Morphological parameters such as size are not sufficient for an accurate assessment of biological behavior in tumors. In contrast, the uptake of [18F]fluoro-2-deoxyglucose (FDG) has been found to be correlated with histological malignancy grading in brain tumors [1, 2]. Alavi et al. [3] proposed that these data be used to predict survival rates. Minn and coworkers [4] observed in a mixed tumor population a strong correlation between FDG uptake and the S-phase fraction and suggested FDG imaging as a noninvasive method to assess the proliferative activity of human cancers. We evaluated the relationship between glucose uptake and tumor proliferation rate in patients with squamous cell carcinomas (SCC).

Materials and Methods

Prior to therapy we examined 44 patients with histologically confirmed SCC of the head and neck and four with lymph node metastases of head and neck SCC. In 27 patients specimens were taken by biopsy from the examined region immediately after positron emission tomography (PET) or during surgery 1 day after PET for further flow cytometric analysis.

PET examinations were performed with a two-ring detector system (PC2048-7WB Scanditronix, Sweden). Three PET sections (two primary and one cross-section) with a thickness of 11 mm were acquired. Each detector ring consists of 512 bismuth-germanate-gadolinium-orthosilicate detectors. FDG was used to assess the regional glucose uptake and phosphorylation. One hour

[1] Department of Radiology and Pathophysiology, German Cancer Research Center, Im Neuenheimer Feld 280, 6900 Heidelberg, FRG
[2] Department of Oto-Rhino-Laryngology, University of Heidelberg, Im Neuenheimer Feld 400, 6900 Heidelberg, FRG
[3] Department of Pathology, University of Heidelberg, Im Neuenheimer feld 220, 6900 Heidelberg, FRG

Advanced Radiation Therapy Tumor Response Monitoring and Treatment Planning
Breit (Editor-in-Chief)
© Springer-Verlag, Berlin Heidelberg 1992

after intravenous administration of 9–12 mCi FDG, PET images were acquired to 10 min. Before PET transmission scans were performed with more than 10 million counts per section. The production of FDG followed the method described by Oberdorfer et al. [5], with a radiochemical purity above 98%. PET images were generated by an iterative reconstruction program [6] on a VAX 11/750 computer system. The image matrix was 128×128 and interpolated to 256×256 for display. The pixel size in all reconstructed images was 2×2 mm (spatial resolution 5.1 mm). The images were corrected for attenuation and scatter. For quantitative evaluation, regions of interest were defined in tumor and soft tissue with a region size exceeding 32 pixels in all cases. FDG uptake was then expressed as the standardized uptake value (SUV): SUV = tissue concentration [injected dose (nCi)/body weight (g)].

For flow cytometric analysis, suspensions of single-cell nuclei were prepared with scissors in a solution of 0.5% pepsin in 0.9% saline after acidification with 0.25% hydrochloric acid. Then the homogenate was supplemented with 2 ml pepsin solution and whirled 5 min at room temperature. After sedimentation, 0.1–0.5 ml of the supernatant was injected into 8 ml of a fluorocytochrome solution (0.5 µg 4′6-diamidino-a-phenylindole, DAPI, and 20 µg ribonuclease from bovine prancrease per milliliter in 0.1 M Tris buffer at pH = 7.6), yielding about 10^5 cell nuclei/ml. The nuclear DAPI fluorescence was measured after 30 min with an IPC 22-pulse cytophotometer (Phywe, Göttingen, FRG) using a UG1 and KV550 filter combination. For each probe a total of at least 25 000 pulses were measured. For display and storation a multichannel analyzer (MCA 8100, Canberra Industries, Meriden, CT) was used. We performed the analysis of DNA histograms with a graphic computing system (Tektronix GS 4051 in combination with a 4662 digital plotter) after correction of the superimposed background, according to Haag et al. [7]. Evaluation of the different cell fractions was performed graphically using a trapezoidal model from the increments of the corresponding segments of the plotted curves. The proliferative index (PI) was calculated as: $PI = 100 * (S + G2 + M)/(G0/1 + S + G2 + M)$.

Results

FDG uptake values in the 46 malignant lesions ranged from 1.8 to 6.0 SUV (normal neck muscles 0.8–1.0). The distribution of the 42 primary tumors is shown in Fig. 1. Perfusion values were in the range of 1.5–4.7 SUV (median 3.25). Flow cytometry revealed PI values between 7.5% and 29.4% $S + G2/M$ cells (coefficient of variation between 2.6% and 6.2%; median 3.8%). Two groups were noted when FDG uptake and PI were compared (Fig. 2). Both clusters showed a significant correlation between SUV and PI, with $r = 0.64$ (regression function: $y = 2.11 + 0.024x$) in the lower uptake group and $r = 0.8$ ($y = 3.52 + 0.039x$) in the higher uptake group (both significant at $p < 0.01$).

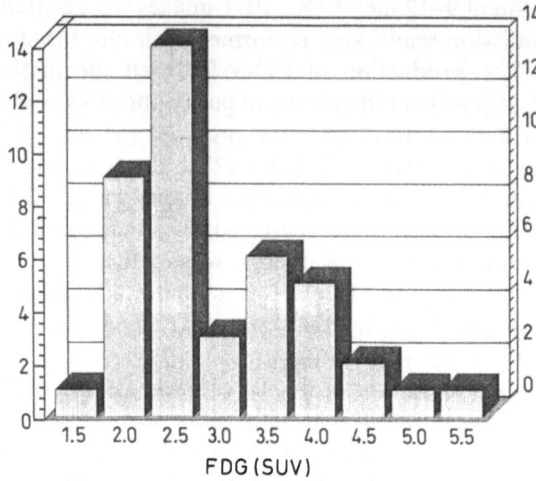

Fig. 1. FDG uptake in 42 squamous cell carcinomas. Height of bars represent the number of carcinomas at each level of SUV (nCi/g)

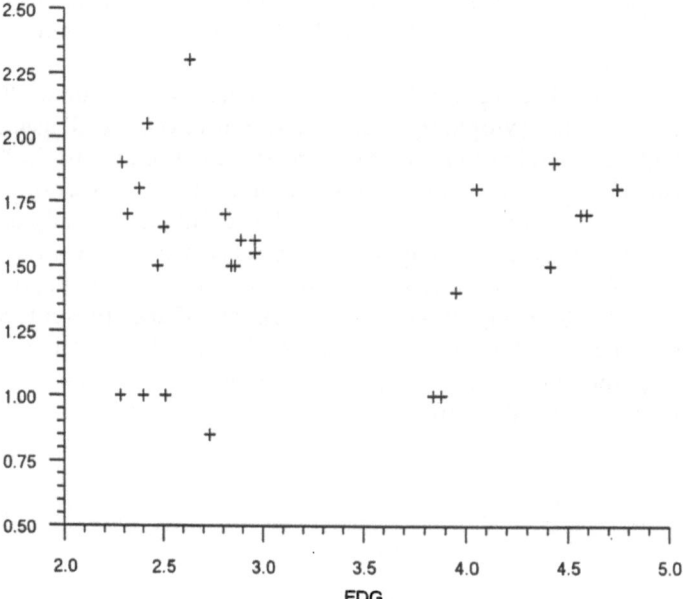

Fig. 2. Correlation of FDG uptake and proliferation index (*PI*) in 27 squamous cell carcinomas reveals two clusters

Discussion

In a study with rat brain tumors Watanabe et al. [8] found a positive correlation between malignancy, as measured by the bromodeoxyuridine labeling index, and local cerebral glucose utilization. From their experiments they suggested that the increase in glucose utilization in these tumors is needed mainly for nucleic acid synthesis. Similar findings are reported by Minn et al. [4], who found a high correlation between FDG uptake and the S-phase fraction. However, the tumor population in their study was inhomogeneous with respect to histology. Furthermore, the use of a gamma camera for data acquisition and the tumor-to-contrast ratios do not permit an accurate quantification of activities in the tumors. Our own results in patients with SCC of the head and neck demonstrate that there are two groups, with different FDG uptake but comparable proliferative activity. The analysis of FDG uptake data from 42 patients with primary tumors gives further evidence that there are two groups with differing glucose uptake pattern. Moreover, in both groups FDG uptake was correlated with the proliferation rate, with flat regression functions, indicating that large differences in tumor cell proliferation may be associated with small changes in FDG uptake.

Some results in the research of tumor physiology and molecular biology may help to explain the observed phenomenon. Barsh et al. [9] observed that the increase in glucose membrane transport and the size of the intracellular glucose pool are dissociated from the increase in DNA synthesis and cell growth. Comparing the uptake of other growth-related substances such as potassium and amino acids with glucose uptake, Weber et al. [10] found that the increase in glucose transport rate exceeds the requirements for growth. Furthermore, cells transformed by Rous sarcoma virus and proliferating at the same rate as normal control cells transported hexoses at a four- to fivefold higher rate than the controls. These data give further evidence that glucose uptake is not directly regulated by the needs for DNA synthesis. Flier et al. [11] demonstrated that elevated glucose transport protein and mRNA levels are found in rat fibroblasts when transfected with src or ras oncogene. Differences in the amount of mRNA for the glucose transporter were also found in hepatoma cells and normal liver cells with an increased rate in the hepatoma cells [12]. In a recent study Yamamoto et al. [13] found elevated amounts of erythrocyte glucose transporter mRNA in a variety of human cancer tissues, including hepatoma, pancreatic cancer, esophageal cancer, and colon cancer. Therefore the underlying molecular mechanism causing a different uptake in our two groups of head and neck tumors may be caused by a different transcription and translation of the glucose carrier gene. Perhaps this difference is due to a varying expression of oncogenes, causing changes in metabolic activity. The results of Flier and others [11, 14–16] with src and ras oncogenes provide evidence for this suggestion. Furthermore, it is known that an elevated expression of multiple oncogenes, including Ha-ras, Ki-ras, and myc, is associated with highly aggressive tumors of the head and neck [17, 18]. PET using FDG may so reflect metabolism regulation or disregulation at the molecular level.

In conclusion, we found that glucose uptake in SCC of the head and neck is correlated with PI. PET with FDG is a noninvasive indicator for the proliferative activity of a tumor. However, the existence of two groups and of flat regression functions indicates that a pure dependence of glucose uptake on the growth rate is too simple as an explanation. These results and the results of a variety of cell experiments suggest that the difference is caused by a difference in glucose carrier expression, perhaps due to oncogenic alterations. This is being explored in an ongoing study at our center.

References

1. DiChiro G, Hatazawa J, Katz DA, Rizzoli HV, DeMichele DJ (1987) Glucose utilization by intracranial meningiomas as an index of tumor aggressivity and probability of recurrence: a PET study. Radiology 164: 521–526
2. Mineura K, Yasuda T, Kowada M, Shishido F, Ogawa T, Uemura K (1986) Positron emission tomographic evaluation of histological malignancy in gliomas using oxygen-15 and fluorine-18-fluorodeoxyglucose. Neurol Res 8: 164–168
3. Alavi JB, Alavi A, Chawluk J, Kushner M, Powe J, Hickey W, Reivich M (1988) Positron emission tomography in patients with glioma. A predictor of prognosis. Cancer 62: 1074–1078
4. Minn H, Joensuu H, Ahonen A, Klemi P (1988) Fluorodeoxyglucose imaging: a method to assess the proliferative activity of human cancer in vivo. Comparison with DNA flow cytometry in head and neck tumors. Cancer 61: 1776–1781
5. Oberdorfer F, Hull WE, Traving BC, Maier-Borst W (1986) Synthesis and purification of 2-deoxy-2-18fluoro-D-glucose and 2-deoxy-2-18fluoro-D-mannose: characterization of products by 1H- and 19F-NMR spectroscopy. Int J Appl Radiat Isot 37: 695–701
6. Schmidlin P, Kübler WK, Doll J, Strauss LG, Ostertag H (1987) Image processing in whole body positron emission tomography. In: Schmidt HAE, Csernay L (eds) Nuklearmedizin. Schattauer, Stuttgart, pp 84–87
7. Haag D, Feichter G, Goerttler K, Kaufmann M (1987) Influence of systematic errors on the evaluation of the S phase portions from DNA distributions of solid tumors as shown for 328 breast carcinomas. Cytometry 8: 377–385
8. Watanabe A, Tanaka R, Takeda N, Washiyama K (1989) DNA synthesis, blood flow, and glucose utilization in experimental rat brain tumors. J Neurosurg 70: 86–91
9. Barsh GS, Cunningham DD (1977) Nutrient uptake and control of animal cell proliferation. J Supramol Struct 7: 61–77
10. Weber MJ, Evans PK, Johnson MA, McNair TF, Nakamura KD, Salter DW (1984) Transport of potassium, amino acids and glucose in cells transformed by Rous sarcoma virus. Fed Proc Fed Am Soc Exp Biol 43: 107–112
11. Flier JS, Mueckler MM, Usher P, Lodish HF (1987) Elevated levels of glucose transport and transporter messenger RNA are induced by *ras* or *src* oncogenes. Science 235: 1492–1495
12. Flier JS, Mueckler M, McCall AC, Lodish HF (1987) Distribution of glucose transporter messenger RNA transcripts in tissues of rat and man. J Clin Invest 79: 657–661
13. Yamamoto T, Seino Y, Fukumoto H, Koh G, Yano H, Inagaki N, Yamada Y, Inoue K, Manabe T, Imura H (1990) Over-expression of facilitative glucose transporter genes in human cancer. Biochem Biophys Res Comm 170: 223–230
14. White MK, Weber MJ (1988) Transformation by the *src* oncogene alters glucose transport into rat and chicken cells by different mechanisms. Mol Cell Biol 8: 138–144
15. Inui KI, Tillotson LG, Isselbacher KJ (1980) Hexose and amino acid transport by chicken embryo fibroblasts infected with temperature-sensitive mutant of Rous sarcoma virus. Biochim Biophys Acta 598: 616–627
16. Weber MJ (1973) Hexose transport in normal and in Rous sarcoma virus-transformed cells. J Biol Chem 218: 2978–2983
17. Field JK, Lamothe A, Spandidos DA (1986) Clinical relevance of oncogene expression in head and neck tumors. Anticancer Res 6: 595–600
18. Field JK, Spandidos DA, Stell PM, Vaughan ED, Evan GI, Moore JP (1989) Elevated expression of the c-*myc* oncoprotein correlates with poor prognosis in head and neck squamous cell carcinoma. Oncogene 4: 1463–1468

Tumor Response Monitoring: Thorax and Breast

Magnetic Resonance Imaging in Mediastinal Hodgkin's Disease During and After Treatment

J.D. Tesoro-Tess, L. Balzarini, E. Ceglia, R. Petrillo, Y. Reyner, and R. Musumeci

Introduction

In Hodgkin's disease (HD), a persistent mediastinal abnormality after clinically successful treatment is common and can simulate persistent disease. Computed tomography (CT) has been used extensively in the follow-up of these patients. It has, however, been repeatedly demonstrated that a residual mass depicted with CT does not necessarily indicate active disease [1]. Gallium-67 imaging has demonstrated a good diagnostic capability for the evaluation of residual disease. The lack of accumulation in fibrotic tissue makes it alternative or adjunctive to CT in the posttreatment diagnostic work-up [2]. Magnetic resonance imaging (MRI) can be very useful in the follow-up of mediastinal HD because it allows differentiation between active tumor and fibrosis, using mainly T2-weighted images [3].

To evaluate the possible role of MRI in the management of patients with treated mediastinal HD we reviewed a number of MRI examinations performed during the follow-up and compared MRI results with those obtained by clinical data and those by gallium-67.

Materials and Methods

The clinical files of 36 histologically confirmed HD patients and the 92 MRI examinations performed during and after therapy were reviewed. All patients had confirmed mediastinal adenopathies at disease presentation and residual mediastinal mass during follow-up. In most patients (61%) a combined modality treatment was provided, but in 28% chemotherapy and in 11% radiotherapy alone were the sole treatments. MRI was performed with a 1.5 T superconductive unit. Single- and double-echo multisection SE sequences were used, and both mainly T1 and T2 ECG-gated images were acquired with TR (repetition time) dependent on heart frequency. As a general rule, low signal intensity in the different pulse sequences was considered compatible with the presence of fibrotic

Diagnostic Radiology E, Istituto Nazionale Tumori, Via Venezian 1, 20133 Milan, Italy

Advanced Radiation Therapy Tumor Response
Monitoring and Treatment Planning
Breit (Editor-in-Chief)
© Springer-Verlag, Berlin Heidelberg 1992

tissue while low intensity on T1 and high intensity on T2-weighted images were considered characteristic of active tumor. Granulation tissue and the occurrence of necrosis, which can exhibit a high signal intensity on T2-weighted images, were also carefully considered. About a half of the examinations (41/92 = 45%) were performed during treatment, one-fourth (23/92 = 25%) within 6 months from the end of therapy, 9% (8/92) after 6–8 months, and 22% (20/92) after more than 8 months.

Results

High signal within the mass was detected in a large number of cases (47/92 = 51%). In only 26 (55%) was this due to active tumor, and 15 (32%) resulted from posttreatment inflammation or cystic degeneration. Six examinations (13%) could not be classified. Finally, in 44/92 (48%) low signal (fibrosis) was found (Table 1).

A correlation between MRI and ^{67}Ga scans was available in 39/92 (42%) examinations (Table 2), and only seven (18%) discordant reports were encountered, due mainly to positive MRI and negative ^{67}Ga findings. The overall accuracy of MRI in comparison with clinical evaluation, ^{67}Ga scan, and other radiological procedures was 92%; sensitivity was 96% and specificity 90%.

Table 1. Correlation between MRI and clinical findings in residual mediastinal masses ($n = 92$)

MRI Finding	Clinical finding	
	Positive	Negative
Positive	26 (28.4%)	6 (6.5%)
Negative	1 (1.1%)	53 (57.5%)[a]

Six cases could not be classified.
[a] Includes 44 (83.1%) fibrosis, 2 (3.7%) necrosis, and 7 (13.2%) inflammation.

Table 2. Correlation between MRI and ^{67}Ga findings in residual mediastinal masses ($n = 39$)

MRI Finding	^{67}Ga finding	
	Positive	Negative
Positive	9 (23.1%)	6 (15.4%)
Negative	1 (2.6%)	23 (58.9%)

Discussion

Achievement of complete remission after initial treatment is one of the most important prognostic factors in Hodgkin's disease. However, partial size regression is often observed, and traditional imaging tests, mainly CT, cannot differentiate viable residual tumor from fibrotic inactive tissue [1, 2].

However, with MRI responding lymphomas in the early posttreatment phase typically exhibit a compound pattern of relatively low, intermediate, and high signals on T2 images, thus representing a mixture of fibrosis, inflammation, and tumor. In fact, unlike a low signal, which correlates well with fibrosis, a high signal on T2-weighted images is not specific for tumor in the first 8–12 weeks after therapy when necrosis, inflammation, and remodeling of tissues is most active. Furthermore, it seems that a lymphomatous mass does not always respond uniformly throughout its volume (Fig. 1). This makes T1-weighted images necessary to ensure that the signal intensity of tumor tissue is not confused with that of fat or other mediastinal structures. Nevertheless, a careful comparison of T1- and T2-weighted images obtained at the same body levels permit differentiation of the superimposition of edema from necrosis on the basis of the pattern and signal intensity and usually allows a correct diagnosis. More than 50% of our case material demonstrated persistently high signal intensity within the mediastinum during follow-up, but only one-half of these were interpreted as residual active tumor. However, in 32% the presence of a pathological inhomogeneous tissue without a well-defined mass was considered compatible with posttreatment inflammatory tissue. Similarly, a residual round mass of homogeneous high signal intensity on T2-weighted images was the result of a necrotic or cystic remnant. It must be emphasized that necrosis usually turns to fibrosis while a cyst usually remains unchanged in size and signal.

Finally in a few cases (6 = 6.5%) the presence of motion artifacts complicated the analysis of signal patterns by the presence of ghost shadows superimposed on mediastinal structures. It must be stressed that the largest number of non-neoplastic conditions which caused inhomogeneous changes in signal intensity were observed during or within the first 6 months from the end of therapy.

Nevertheless, these results strongly support the use of MRI as an indicator of disease activity in the management of Hodgkin's disease. The comparison with ^{67}Ga imaging results (Table 2) demonstrated a good correlation, mostly when active disease was present. Overall, only 2.6% false-negative and 15.4% false-positive results from MRI were encountered. Furthermore, MRI demonstrated 92% accuracy, 96% sensitivity, and 90% specificity.

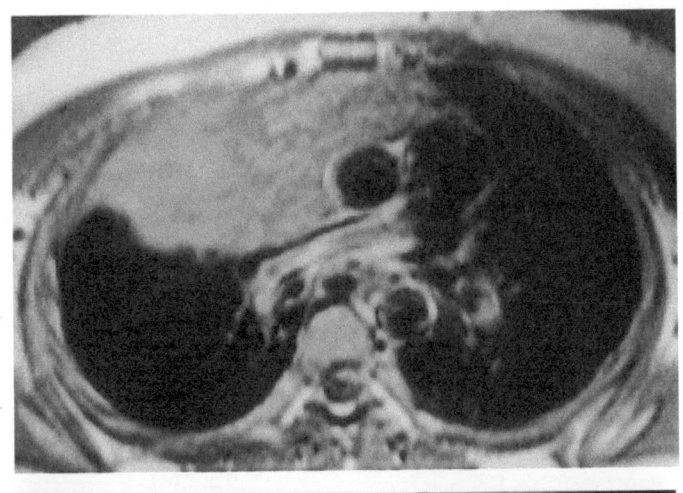

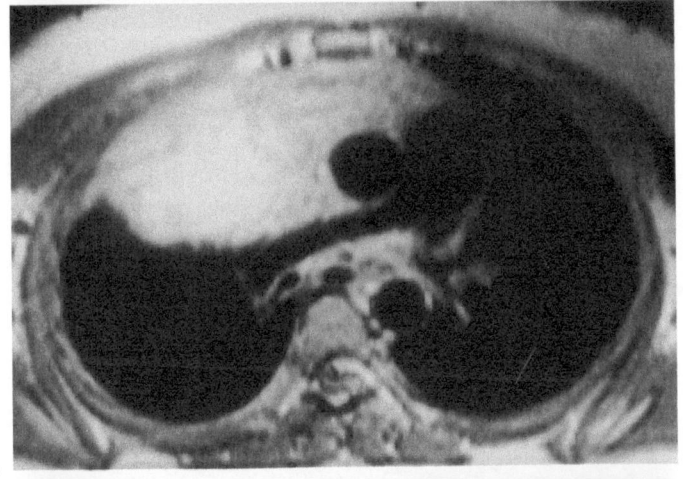

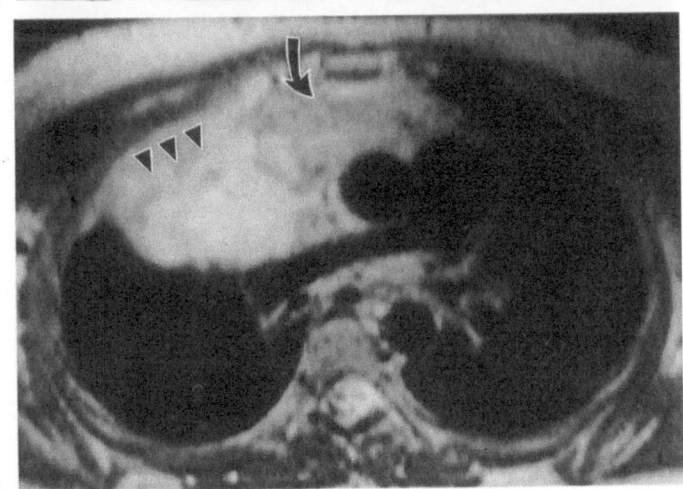

References

1. Lewis E, Bernadino ME, Salvador PG et al. (1982) Post-therapy CT detected mass in lymphoma patients: is it viable tissue? J Comput Assist Tomogr 6: 792–795
2. Drossman SR, Schiff RG, Kronfeld GD et al. (1990) Lymphoma of the mediastinum and neck: evaluation of Ga-67 imaging and CT correlation. Radiology 174: 171–175
3. Nyman RS, Rehn SM, Glimelius BLG et al. (1989) Residual mediastinal masses in Hodgkin disease: prediction of size with MR imaging. Radiology 170: 435–440

Fig. 1a–c. Hodgkin's disease during treatment. Transverse T1 (**a**), proton density (**b**), and T2-weighted (**c**) ECG-gated images. On the T2 image excellent contrast between active tumor (*arrowheads*) and partially fibrotic tissue (*arrow*) is evident

Optimized Therapy Management in Unresectable Bronchogenic Carcinoma by Fluorodeoxyglucose Positron Emission Tomography

M.V. Knopp[1], L.G. Strauss[1], U. Haberkorn[1], A. Dimitrakopoulou[1],
H. Bischoff[2], F. Oberdorfer[1], H. Ostertag[1], F. Helus[1], and G. van Kaick[1]

Introduction

The increasing number of different therapeutic protocols necessitates an early objective evaluation of therapy response. Depending on significant response to the ongoing therapy, the chosen protocol is continued, or alternative protocols are used. Current diagnostic imaging techniques, from conventional radiology to computed tomography and magnetic resonance imaging enable morphologic evaluation of therapy response, limited mainly by the change in tumor volume. Positron emission tomography (PET) with the use of metabolically active substances such as [^{18}F]fluorodeoxyglucose (FDG) enables a direct quantification of the metabolic state with cross-sectional imaging of bronchogenic carcinoma. The technical basis of PET relies, as does that of CT, on computerized reconstruction of cross-sections. Positron-labeled radiopharmaceutical compounds emitted from the body are used as the source for PET images, while the attenuation of X-ray photons from an X-ray tube is used in computed tomography. Despite the fact that PET currently requires very large technical hardware, scanner, and cyclotron, patient studies can be performed in acceptable study times of 25–40 min without inconvenience to the patient due to noise or limited space.

Patients and Methods

A prospective study of 21 selected patients with unresectable bronchogenic carcinoma was performed with FDG PET. There were 16 men and 5 women, aged 35–70 years (mean 57, median 59). Sixteen cases were diagnosed as small-cell carcinoma and five as non-small-cell carcinoma. Seventeen received chemotherapy, one radiation, and three combination therapy. Initial studies prior to therapy and follow-up studies during therapy were performed. At every PET

---

[1] Institute of Radiology and Pathophysiology, German Cancer Research Center, Im Neuenheimer Feld 280, W-6900 Heidelberg, FRG
[2] Thoraxklinik Heidelberg, Amalienstr. 5, 6900 Heidelberg-Rohrbach

Advanced Radiation Therapy Tumor Response
Monitoring and Treatment Planning
Breit (Editor-in-Chief)
© Springer-Verlag, Berlin Heidelberg 1992

study a concurrent CT was performed to enable morphologic correlation. The same field of view was used as for the PET study. In general, one-point studies were performed, in which the patient was injected intravenously with 440 MBq FDG. At the same time the glucose level was determined.

We use a whole-body positron emission scanner manufactured by Scanditronix (WB 2048/7 WB) with a slice thickness of 11 mm and two detector rings. The system enables a concurrent acquisition of three cross-sections. The system resolution is 5.1 mm [1]. At one-point examinations, studies are performed 15 min after injection. Emission scans of 15 min followed by transmission scans of 5 min are acquired. The image reconstruction is performed using an iterative technique with concurrent correction for attenuation and scatter. The calibration of the PET scanner enables a direct quantification of the measured uptake (nCi/cm^3). To enable a quantitative evaluation, regions of interest are placed above the desired area. The measured data allow the determination of a standardized uptake value (SUV) calculated out of the tissue concentration, corrected by the injected dose and the body weight: SUV = tissue concentration (nCi/g)/[intravenous activity (nCi)/weight (g)].

Results

Out of the 21 patients followed, 14 were determined to be responders and 7 nonresponders based on the clinical evaluation by the oncologist at the end of the therapeutic regimen. The first follow-up study of all 21 patients was performed

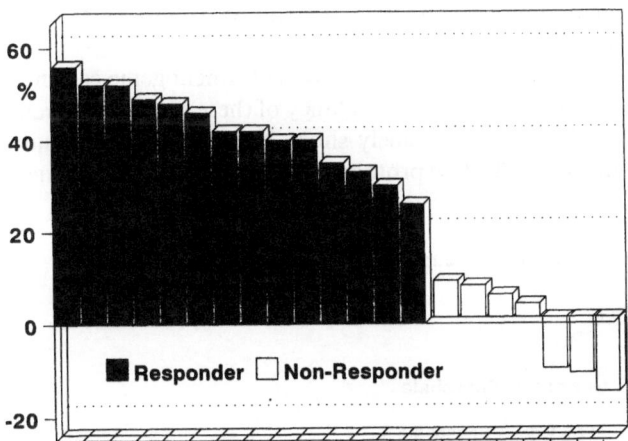

Fig. 1. Change in FDG uptake after second cycle of chemotherapy or 30 Gy radiation, in order of descending response. The first 14 were considered responders (*solid columns*) and the following 7 nonresponders (*open columns*) at the end of the therapeutic protocol

after the second cycle of chemotherapy or 30 Gy of radiation therapy. In all cases PET allowed a reliable detection of response (14/14) or nonresponse to therapy (7/7), as all responders showed unchanged or increased FDG uptake, while all nonresponders showed decreased uptake (see Fig. 1). An evaluation of response with the detection of change in tumor volume as only measure would have been misleading in 7 of the 21 patients, as 3/14 responders showed unchanged or increased tumor volume, while 4/7 nonresponders showed decreased tumor volume.

Discussion

With the introduction of PET, a metabolism-dependent, non-invasive diagnostic imaging technique became available to monitor therapy response [2]. Different radiopharmaceutical compounds can be used to evaluate response. Besides FDG, a direct labeling of chemotherapeutic substances such as 5-fluorouracil is possible. The characteristics of FDG (Fig. 2) as a competitive substrate to glucose in hexokinase-catalyzed phosphorilization is based on the fact that deoxyglucose-6-phosphate remains fairly trapped in tissue during the examination time [3]. Since the glucose metabolism of malignant lesions is significantly increased, a high accumulation of FDG is seen in malignant tissue [4]. An important consideration for imaging is the contrast of a substance compared to its surrounding or normal tissue. We find a very beneficial situation in the thorax due to the fact that lung parenchyma shows only small FDG uptake with a fairly constant value of 0.5 SUV after 60 min. Thereby we have a high contrast relation of the uptake of FDG in tumor, bone marrow, and inflammatory lesions. This unique feature in the thorax facilitates a reliable quantification of FDG uptake [5].

The clinical situation of patients with unresectable bronchogenic carcinoma still remains fairly unsatisfactory. The life expectancy of these patients, especially those with small-cell carcinoma, is extremely short. To improve this situation the clinician must use the most effective protocol at the earliest possible time. As

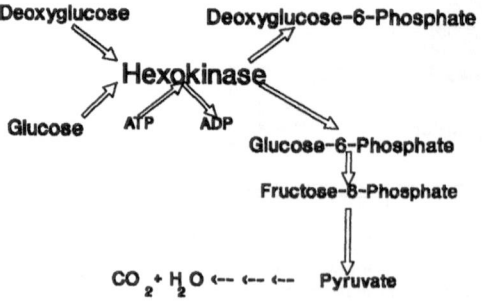

Fig. 2. Biochemical pathway of deoxyglucose

the number of possible therapeutic protocols increase, the current concept of evaluation of response by change in tumor volume may not be sufficient, especially if response must be evaluated after the first or second cycle of chemotherapy. In our selected group of 21 patients, the majority showed decreased tumor volume and were confirmed to be responders. The classification of patients as responders or nonresponders was by our clinical oncologists at the end of the therapeutic regimen. The other observation that the patients classified as nonresponders showed no change in tumor volume (3/7) was also clinically expected. The surprising and clinically important observation is that three of the 14 responders showed no change in tumor volume at the time of initial follow-up. Also, four of the seven nonresponders did show an initial decrease in tumor volume at the initial follow-up. When we compare the change in FDG uptake to the final clinical classification, all 14 responders showed a significant decrease, and none of the seven nonresponders showed a significant decrease or even showed an increase in FDG uptake. This limited study demonstrates that FDG PET can be used to monitor changes in tumor metabolism which can be used to predict the response to the therapeutic regimen.

Conclusion

PET is a new, objective, technique for monitoring of patients receiving therapy for nonresectable bronchogenic carcinoma. It is of special benefit in determining response when the morphologic information from other imaging techniques does not allow a clear and distinct evaluation of response. The clinical oncologist has a new tool for basing his therapeutic decision on objective and individual specific data. The capabilities of PET enable new approaches for comparative evaluation of different therapy protocols in the future. The most important aspect is that PET seems to be able to detect those patients in whom the tumor volume decreases, but at the same time therapy-resistant cell lines are selected which may cause early tumor recurrence.

References

1. Ostertag H, Kuebler WK, Doll J, Schmidlin P, Clorius JH, Strauss LG, Maier-Borst W, Lorenz WJ (1988) A new dual crystal whole-body positron camera. System description, initial results. In: Schmidt HAE (ed) Nuklearmedizin. Schattauer, Stuttgart, pp 7–10
2. Fukuda H, Matsuzawa T, Ito M, Abe Y, Yoshioka S, Yamada K (1984) Experimental and clinical study of cancer diagnosis with (F-18) FDG using positron emission tomography (abstr). J Nucl Med 25: P50

3. Gallagher BM, Fowler JS, Gutterson NI, MacGregor RR, Wan CN, Wolf AP (1978) Metabolic trapping as a principle of radiopharmaceutical design: some factors responsible for the biodistribution of F-18-2-deoxy-2-fluoro-D-glucose. J Nucl Med 19: 1154–1161
4. Som P, Atkins HL, Bandoypadhyay D et al. (1980) A fluorinated glucose analog, 2-fluoro-2-deoxy-D-glucose (F-18): nontoxic tracer for rapid tumor detection. J Nucl Med 21: 670–675
5. Knopp MV, Strauss LG, Haberkorn U, Bischoff H, Wolber G, Vogt-Moykopf I, Kaick G van, Lorenz WJ (1990) PET of the thorax: assessment of its clinical application in tumor staging. Radiology 177:174

Radiotherapy of Lung Cancer: Evaluation of Tumor Response by Computed Tomography

T. Feyerabend[1], R. Schmitt[2], E. Richter[1], and W. Bohndorf[3]

Computed tomography (CT) has proven indispensable in the pretherapeutic staging of bronchogenic carcinoma [1–3]. Conventional X-ray imaging is limited especially in centrally located tumors, atelectasis, and pleural effusion. In most of these cases CT succeeds in delineating exactly the tumor volume pre- and posttherapeutically, thus enabling the evaluation of tumor remission. The goal of our study was to determine the role of CT in the evaluation of tumor remission in irradiated lung cancer patients.

Patients and Methods

We analyzed 434 CT examinations of 133 patients (121 men, 12 women) having histologically confirmed bronchogenic carcinoma (22 with small-cell lung cancer), 96 with centrally located tumors and 37 with peripheral tumors. Of these, 90% were diagnosed in an advanced stage of disease (106 in stage III, 16 in stage IV). All patients received radiotherapy, with a mean dose of 70 Gy isocentrically for non-small-cell lung cancer and 58 Gy for small-cell lung cancer. CT examinations (slice increment: 9 mm; intravenous contrast medium in most cases) were performed before, during, and up to 6 years after radiotherapy.

After irradiation, restaging and remission rates were evaluated in 105 patients. The size of the primary tumor was measured by CT before and after irradiation in 105 patients, and the tumor volume was calculated by the formula for a rotatory ellipsoid. The calculated tumor volumes served to objectify the remission rates. In 37 patients with CT examination 1–3 months and 4–9 months after irradiation the tumor remission was analyzed at the time of reevaluation. The remission of involved lymph nodes was determined in 99 patients with mediastinal or hilar lymph node metastases.

[1] Department of Radiation Oncology and Nuclear Medicine, Lübeck, FRG
[2] Department of Diagnostic Radiology, Ingolstadt, FRG
[3] Department of Radiation Oncology, Würzburg, FRG

Advanced Radiation Therapy Tumor Response
Monitoring and Treatment Planning
Breit (Editor-in-Chief)
© Springer-Verlag, Berlin Heidelberg 1992

Results

In 105 evaluable patients the rate of complete and partial remissions of the tumor disease was 40% and 30%, respectively; no change or progression was observed in 14% and 16%, respectively (Table 1). There were no obvious differences between non-small-cell and small-cell lung cancer.

In patients with non-small-cell lung cancer 36 showed primary tumor volumes of up to 50 cm³, 24 between 50 and 100 cm³, and another 24 greater than 100 cm³ (Fig. 1). After irradiation no tumor was found in 38 patients, 32 had tumor volumes up to 50 cm³ and 14 greater than 50 cm³. Among those with small-cell lung cancer, 11 patients had tumor volumes up to 100 cm³ and 10

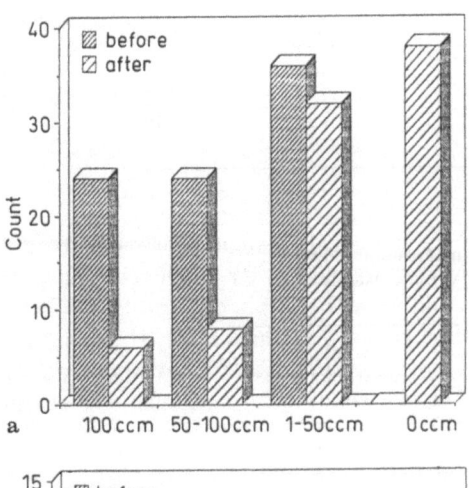

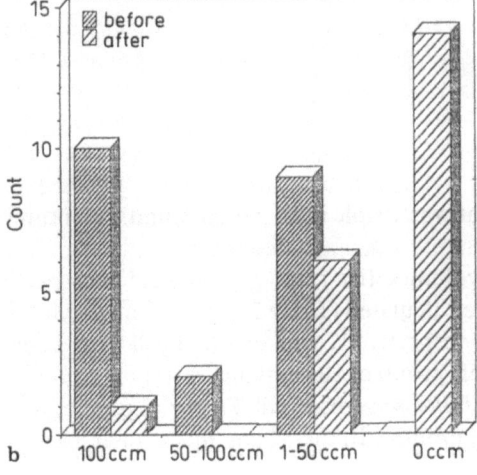

Fig. 1a, b. Tumor volumes in lung cancer patients ($n = 105$) before and after radiotherapy. **a** Non-small-cell lung cancer. **b** Small-cell lung cancer

Table 1. Remission rate in lung cancer treated by radiotherapy

	Non-small-cell lung cancer (n = 84)		Small-cell lung cancer (n = 21)		Total (n = 105)	
	n	%	n	%	n	%
Complete remission	34	40	8	38	42	40
Partial remission	25	30	6	29	31	30
No change	13	15	2	9	15	14
Progressive disease	12	15	5	24	17	16

Table 2. CT-defined remission rate of the primary tumor in lung cancer with pretherapeutically measurable tumor volume

	Non-small-cell lung cancer (n = 84)		Small-cell lung cancer (n = 21)		Total (n = 105)	
	n	%	n	%	n	%
Complete remission	38	45	14	67	52	50
Partial remission	27	32	5	24	32	30
No change	17	20	2	9	19	18
Progressive disease	2	3	–	–	2	2

Table 3. CT-defined remission rate of the primary tumor in lung cancer with pretherapeutically measurable tumor volume examined by CT after irradiation (0–3 and 4–9 months)

	0–3 months after irradiation (n = 37)		4–9 months after irradiation (n = 37)	
	n	%	n	%
Complete remission	7	19	23	62
Partial remission	24	65	8	22
No change	5	14	1	1
Progressive disease	1	2	5	14

even more; after irradiation no tumor was visible in 14 patients, and 6 had tumor volumes up to 50 cm^3.

On the basis of these tumor volumes the rates of complete and partial remission of the primary tumor were calculated (Table 2). In non-small-cell lung cancer these were 45%, and 32%, respectively, and in small-cell lung cancer 67% and 24%. Considering the whole group of 105 patients, a response rate (i.e., complete plus partial remission) of 80% was observed. Tumor regression after irradiation may require more than 3 months. In the 37 patients with at least one

CT examination in the first 3 months and in the 4th–9th months after irradiation (Table 3) the rate of complete remission of the primary tumor increased in this period from 19% to 62% while the rate of partial remission declined from 65% to 22%. The number of those showing no change decreased while those with progression increased.

In another analysis we determined the remission of hilar and mediastinal lymph node metastases in 99 patients. We found complete remission in 59%, partial remission in 7%, and no change in 34%. The response rate (i.e., partial plus complete remission) was far better in small-cell lung cancer than in non-small-cell lung cancer: 83% versus 62%. On the other hand, no change was more frequent in non-small-cell lung cancer: 38% versus 18%.

Discussion

Pre- and posttherapeutical tumor stage evaluation by conventional X-ray diagnostic imaging is often difficult or even impossible in patients with lung cancer if the tumor is centrally located, and if atelectasis, pleural effusion, pneumonitis or fibrosis is present. However, in most cases CT allows exact determination of tumor extent, thus enabling evaluation of remission rates. The method presented here calculates tumor volumes with the help of the formula for rotatory ellipsoids and leads to quantification of remission rates in irradiated bronchogenic carcinomas. This therefore simplifies comparison of therapeutic results since the classification as complete or partial remission, no response, or disease progression relies basically on the quantification of tumor mass.

Our study of 105 irradiated patients shows in 70% a complete or partial remission of the tumor disease while a complete or partial remission of the primary tumor was found in 80% of our patients. This divergent course of disease may be attributed to the radiation-induced regression of the primary tumor, on the one hand, and the development of metastases, on the other. Furthermore, definite evaluation of tumor remission sometimes took 3–9 months after radiotherapy due to slow tumor regression.

We did not correlate histopathologic findings to the remission evaluated by CT. Like Seydel et al. [4], we deem it desirable to control CT findings by bronchoscopy. However, this procedure only an evaluation allows of the endoluminal part of the tumor. Moreover, bronchoscopy often fails to assure the diagnosis histologically due to radiation-induced fibrosis.

In conclusion, our study of 133 patients with lung cancer shows that CT allows the evaluation of tumor remission on the basis of calculated tumor volumes. Consequently, comparison of therapeutic results becomes easier. After radiotherapy we found an overall response rate of 70% in 105 patients. As for the primary tumor, the response rate of 80% was even higher, which expresses the local effectiveness of radiotherapy. According to our results, a definitive evaluation of the remission of lung cancer may not be possible before 3–9 months after irradiation due to slow regression.

References

1. Brion JP, Depauw L, Kuhn G, de Francquen P, Friberg J, Rocmans P, Struyven J (1985) Role of computed tomography in preoperative staging of lung carcinoma. J Comput Assist Tomogr 9: 480–484
2. Frederick HM, Bernardino ME, Baron M, Colvin R, Mansour K, Miller J (1984) Accuracy of chest computerized tomography in detecting malignant hilar and mediastinal involvement by squamous cell carcinoma of the lung. Cancer 54: 2390–2395
3. Khan A, Gersten KC, Garvey J, Khan FA, Steinberg H (1985) Oblique hilar tomography, computed tomography, and mediastinoscopy for prethoracotomy staging of bronchogenic carcinoma. Radiology 156: 295–298
4. Seydel HG, Kutcher GJ, Steiner RM, Mohiuddin M, Goldberg B (1980) Computed tomography in planning radiation therapy for bronchogenic carcinoma. Int J Radiat Oncol Biol Phys 6: 601–606

Restaging of Bronchogenic Carcinoma by Computed Tomography: Diagnostic Signs After Radiotherapy

R. Schmitt, T. Feyerabend, E. Richter, and W. Bohndorf

Introduction

Due to the unfavorable prognosis of bronchogenic carcinomas limiting long-term observations, there are only a few publications about the evaluation of radiotherapeutic results by computed tomography (Bell et al. 1988; Ikezoe et al. 1988; Kono et al. 1981; Libshitz and Shuman 1984; Nabawi et al. 1981; Pagini et al. 1982). However, knowledge about diagnostic signs in CT after irradiation is essential for the determination of remission rates and for the tumor follow-up.

The aim of our study was to clarify whether there are any changes in diagnostic criteria of thoracic CT induced by the irradiation and its side effects on the lung parenchyma.

Patients and Methods

The retrospective analysis included 493 thoracic CT examinations of 150 patients (137 men and 13 women) with advanced stages of bronchogenic carcinoma. In all of the patients CT was performed shortly before and between the 4th and 10th weeks after termination of radiotherapy (short-term analysis). Of these patients 50 were observed later with further 138 CT studies during the follow-up (long-term analysis). During the irradiation interval 55 examinations were performed. Slice thickness and increment were 9 mm; rapid infusion of contrast medium was used in 389 cases.

The standardized evaluation included the following parameters:

Delimitation of the primary tumor. The following score was used: 0, delimitation not possible; 1, possible in less than 50% of the mass contour; 2, possible in 50%–99% of the mass contour; 3, completely possible.

Delimitation of enlarged lymph nodes. Hilar and mediastinal lymph nodes larger than 10 mm were evaluated (same score as above).

Department of Radiotherapy, University of Würzburg, 8700 Würzburg, FRG

Advanced Radiation Therapy Tumor Response
Monitoring and Treatment Planning
Breit (Editor-in-Chief)
© Springer-Verlag, Berlin Heidelberg 1992

Hematogenic metastases of the thorax. The recognizability was compared with the findings in conventional radiography.

Degree of radiation pneumonitis. Using Hounsfield units three degrees were distinguished: 1, homogeneous slight infiltrates with less than -400 HU; 2, patchy infiltrates between -400 and -200 HU; 3, homogeneous dense infiltrates over -200 HU.

Degree of radiation fibrosis. The identification of anatomic structures against fibrotic lung areas was scored: 0, delimitation not possible; 1, vague; 2, possible with restrictions; 3, clear.

Diagnosis of tumor recurrences and progressions. The delimitation of renewed or further growing tumor masses against the surroundings was scored: 0, not possible; 1, possible with restrictions; 2, clear.

Results

Delimitation of the Primary Tumor. Before radiotherapy tumors without atelectasis could be delimited significantly better than tumors with additional atelectasis (score: 2.15 ± 0.73 versus 1.08 ± 0.68). Radiotherapy induced different developments (Table 1 and Fig. 1). In tumors without atelectasis the rate of largely (score 2) or completely (score 3) recognizable tumor margins decreased from 84% (81/97) to 71% (69/97) in early controls and to 29% (10/34) in late controls. Hence, there was a progressive masking of the tumor margins, caused initially by radiation pneumonitis and later by lung fibrosis. In tumors with

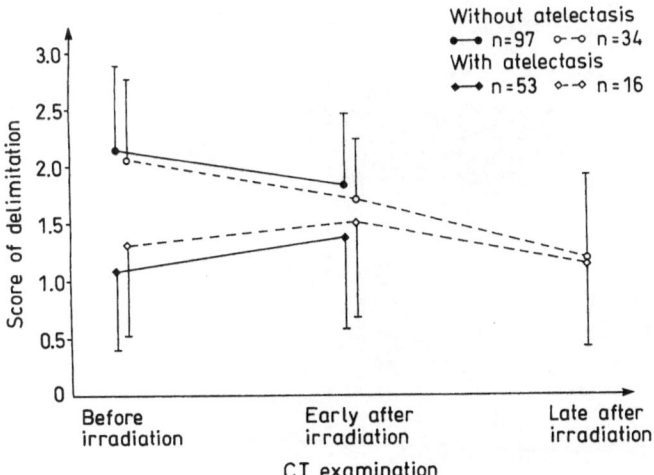

Fig. 1. Delimitation of the primary tumor area (score 0–3) correlated with time of CT examinations (before, early after, and late after radiotherapy)

Table 1. Delimitation of the primary tumor area of bronchogenic carcinomas without and with atelectasis: scores before, early after irradiation (4–10 weeks), and late after irradiation (18–162 weeks)

	Tumors without atelectasis	Tumors with atelectasis
Short-term analysis	$n = 97$	$n = 53$
Before irradiation	2.15 ± 0.73	1.08 ± 0.68
Early control	1.83 ± 0.62	1.37 ± 0.79
Long-term analysis	$n = 34$	$n = 16$
Before irradiation	2.06 ± 0.70	1.31 ± 0.79
Early control	1.70 ± 0.53	1.50 ± 0.82
Late control	1.18 ± 0.73	1.13 ± 0.72

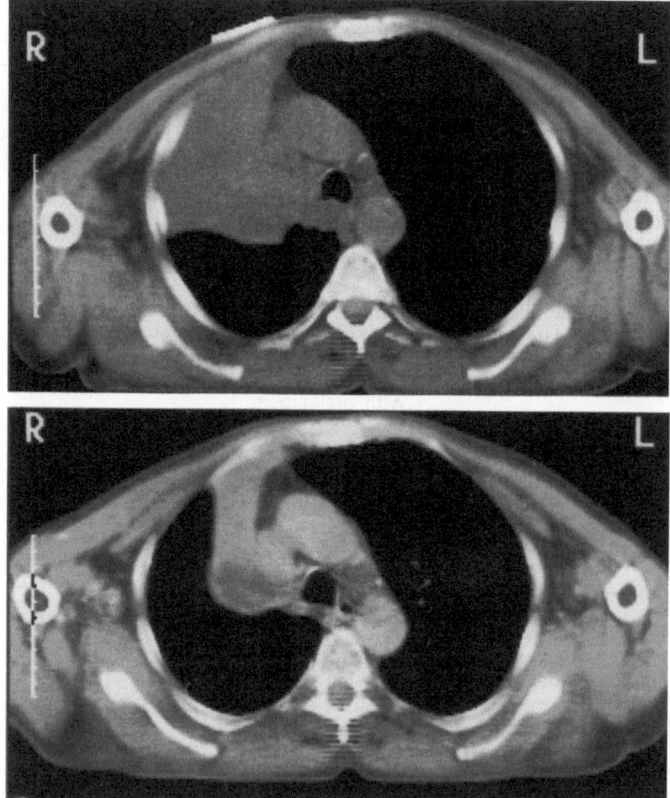

Fig. 2. Central tumor mass of the right lung which is not demarcable from the adjacent atelectasis of the upper lobe (score 0). After the first irradiation interval with 40 Gy the tumor is delimitable over 50% of its border (score 2)

atelectasis the delimitation was temporarily improved (mean score: 1.08 ± 0.68 to 1.37 ± 0.79 in short-term analysis), so that the primary tumor area could be staged adequately (Fig. 2) after complete alleviation of atelectasis in 49% of all cases (26/53). A restricted delimitation of the primary tumor region (score: 1.18 ± 0.73 and 1.13 ± 0.72) resulted after manifestation of lung fibrosis in late controls independently of the existence of an initial atelectasis.

Delimitation of Enlarged Lymph Nodes. A significant change in the contours of the lymph nodes caused by irradiation was not observed (Table 2). The pathologically enlarged hilar and mediastinal lymph nodes were well delimited (scores 2 and 3) in 75% (104/139) before therapy, in 78% (109/139) early after completion of radiotherapy, and in 78% (35/45) of patients in the later tumor follow-up.

Hematogenic Metastases of the Thorax. Thirty-two patients had hematogenic metastases in various thoracic localizations. In comparison to CT, the thoracic M stage was accurately scored in only 66% (21/32) by conventional radiography, with the following distribution: lung metastases 15/20, pleural metastases 2/4, metastases of the chest wall 4/7, and axillary metastases 0/1.

Degree of Radiation Pneumonitis. Of the 150 early CT controls 87 (58%) showed pneumonitic alterations of the lung parenchyma (Table 3). While 43% (23/54) of the homogeneous, slight consolidations (score 1) were visible only by CT, it was possible to confirm 19 patchy infiltrations (score 2) and 14 homogeneous

Table 2. Delimitation of enlarged hilar and mediastinal lymph nodes before, early and late after radiotherapy, scored, 0–3.

Short-term analysis	$n = 139$
Before irradiation	1.77 ± 0.54
Early control	1.79 ± 0.46
Long-term analysis	$n = 45$
Before irradiation	1.87 ± 0.40
Early control	1.82 ± 0.45
Late control	1.80 ± 0.46

Table 3. Degree of radiation pneumonitis during the 4th–8th weeks, after completion of the radiotherapy

Infiltration	CT density (HU)	Patients (n)
Homogeneous, slight	< -400	54
Patchy	-400 to -200	19
Homogeneous, dense	> -200	14
Total		87

consolidations (score 3) by conventional radiography as well. There was a good correlation between the Hounsfield densities of pneumonitis and their delimitations against the surrounding tissues (Table 4).

Degree of Radiation Fibrosis. Of 63 patients 21 developed a focal fibrosis early after radiotherapy (Fig. 3), while all 38 cases with radiation fibrosis in the long-term analysis resulted from former radiation pneumonitis (Table 4). In the four remaining cases CT did not initially reveal pneumonitic signs. There was always a correlation between localization of the fibrotic alterations and the radiation dose. The delimitation to residual tumors and to mediastinal structures was no longer possible in 13% (8/63) and only vague in 70%, (44/63). However, there were always sharp boundaries to the nonaffected lung parenchyma.

Diagnosis of Tumor Recurrences. In the follow-up, 7 tumor recurrences and 13 progressions of residual tumors were confirmed by CT (Table 5). The tumor masses were definitely (score 2) delimited from the surroundings only twice, i.e., in those cases in which the radiation caused no or only small fibrosis. Due to the postradiation changes of the lung parenchyma the other 18 tumors were visible only by indirect signs of a space-occupying process, i.e., by remanifestation of atelectasis, disappearance of traction signs, displacement of central vessels and bronchi, loss of fat septa, or tumorous destruction of the chest wall. Correspondingly, the recurrence tumors could be delimitated 16 times with restrictions (score 1). Only three of the seven true recurrences were seen by conventional radiography.

Table 4. Delimitation of normal anatomic structures within the radiation-induced pneumonitic and fibrotic areas

Delimitation	Pneumonitis (n)	Fibrosis (n)
Not possible	6	8
Vague	26	44
Possible with restrictions	49	10
Clear	6	1
Total	87	63

Table 5. Recognizibility of local tumor recurrences (after complete remission) and of tumor progressions (renewed tumor growth after partial or missing remission)

Delimitation	Tumor recurrences (n)	Tumor progressions (n)
Not possible	0	2
Possible with restrictions	7	9
Clear	0	2
Total	7	13

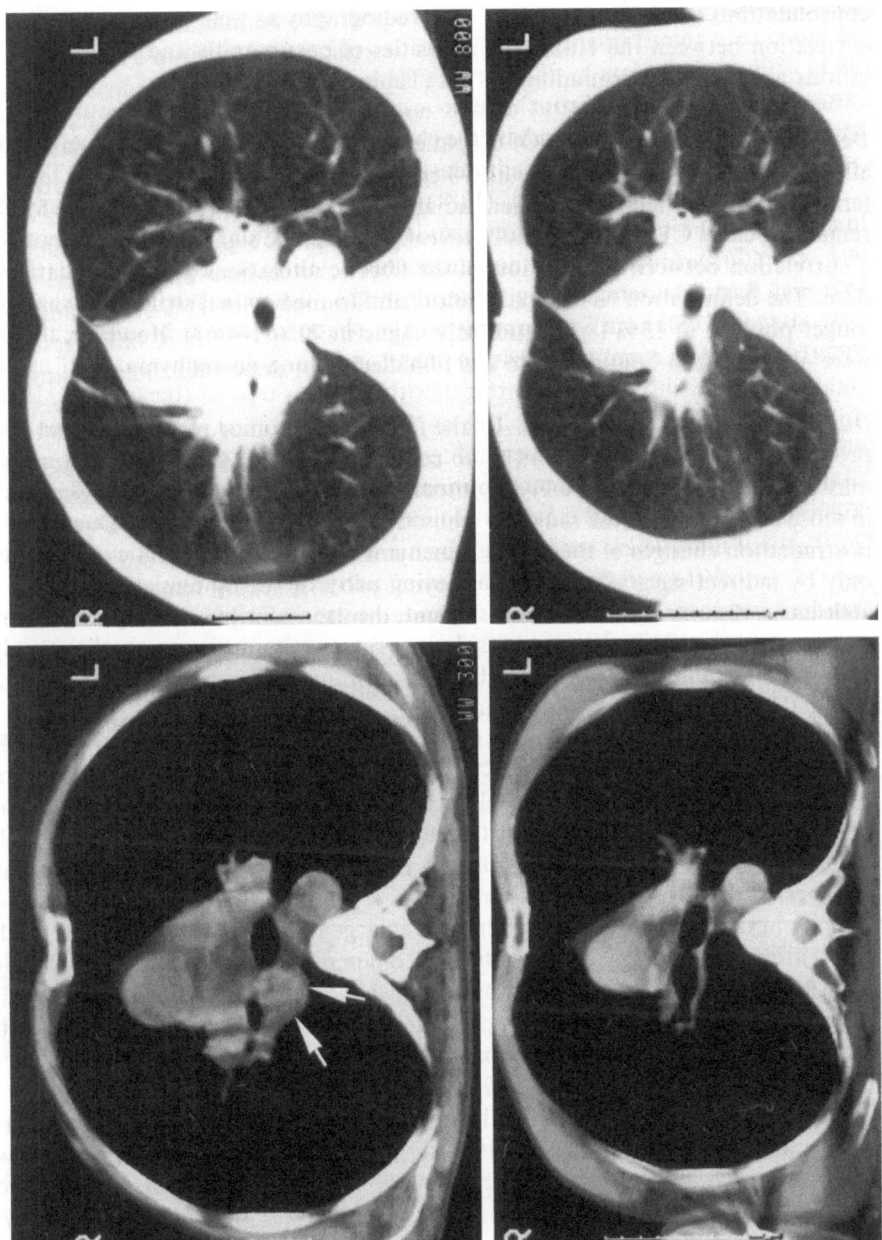

Discussion

After radiotherapy of bronchogenic carcinoma the diagnostic situation is characterized, on the one hand, by the change in tumor size and, on the other, by the reaction of the lung as a radiosensitive organ.

According to Nabawi et al. (1981), the pulmonary radioreaction may be divided into the following phases: exudation, reparation, and development of fibrosis. Concerning the chronological course, Libshitz and Shuman (1984) distinguish the "homogeneous pattern" in the radiation portal, the "patchy consolidation" without conforming to the shape of the radiation field, the "discrete consolidation" as transition phase, and the "solid consolidation" as the analogue of the fibrosis. In accordance with previous reports (Ikezoe et al. 1988; Libshitz and Shuman 1984; Bell et al. 1988, Pagini et al. 1982), our analysis showed that CT confirms the beginning and florid phases of pneumonitis earlier and more extensively than conventional radiography. Also, after the development of fibrosis emphysematous bullae, bronchiectatic changes and paramediastinal and pleura-based lung fibrosis were recognized significantly better by CT. In contrast to conventional radiography the CT shows straight lateral borders between radiation fibrosis and the non-affected lung parenchyma (Pagini et al. 1982). When considering these criteria in an earlier study (Feyerabend et al. 1990) we were able to determine the remission rate in 87% of irradiated bronchogenic carcinomas.

The rate of malignant lymph node involvement is 72% (Brion et al. 1985) for node sizes over 1 cm and 87% (König et al. 1983) for sizes over 1.5 cm. According to our results, the delimitation of enlarged lymph nodes is not influenced by irradiation. The postradiation CT showing a reduction in lymph node size offers even more diagnostic certainty because tumor involvement is then verified retrospectively. Thoracic CT is superior to conventional radiography in determining the persistence of enlarged lymph nodes, as Kono et al. (1981) demonstrated in 29 patients with different thoracic tumors and Lewis et al. (1982) in 13 patients with small-cell bronchogenic carcinomas. However, if enlarged nodes persist, it is not possible to differentiate between malignant, inflammatory, and fibrotic adenopathy.

Whitley et al. (1984) found 9 of 28 tumor residuals or recurrences of chemotherapeutically treated small-cell carcinoma only by CT. In the pneumonectomy study of Glazer et al. (1984), in which conventional radiography was diagnostic in only 5 of 12 tumor recurrences, the recurrent tumor masses were always rounded or oval and had densities of soft tissue. After radiotherapy, however, a differentiation between radiation fibrosis and recurrent neoplasm

Fig. 3. Central squamous cell carcinoma of the right lung (T4 N2 M0). Tumorous mass on the dorsal wall of the right main bronchus occupying the azygoesophageal recess. After radiotherapy complete vanishing of the mass. Now a slight radiation-induced fibrosis in dorsolateral irradiation portal is visible

was difficult in our study, as only two cases out of 20 local recurrences could be diagnosed directly as tumors. The other 18 tumor recurrences were diagnosed only by indirect radiographic findings. In this connection, the subtle comparison with previous CT images was essential. Our study confirms the observation of Pagini et al. (1982) that an expansive change within a radiation-induced fibrosis is suspected to be a tumor recurrence.

References

Bell J, McGivern D, Bullimore J, Hill J, Davies ER, Goddard P (1988) Diagnostic imaging of post-irradiation changes in the chest. Clin Radiol 39: 109–119

Brion JP, Depauw L, Kuhn G, de Francquen, Friberg J, Rocmans P, Struyven (1985) Role of computed tomography and mediastinoscopy in preoperative staging of lung carcinoma. J Comput Assist Tomogr 9: 480–484

Feyerabend T, Schmitt R, Richter E, Bohndorf W (1990) Computertomographische Zielvolumen-bestimmung und Remissionsbeurteilung nach Radiatio beim Bronchialkarzinom. Strahlenther Onkol 166: 405–410

Glazer HS, Aronberg DJ, Sagel SS, Emami B (1984) Utility of CT in detecting postpneumonectomy carcinoma recurrence. Am J Roentgenol 142: 487–494

Ikezoe J, Takashima S, Morimoto S, Kadowaki K, Takeuchi N, Yamamoto T, Nakanishi K, Isaza M (1988) CT appearance of acute radiation-induced injury in the lung. Am J Roentgenol 150: 765–770

König R, van Kaick G, Lüllich G, Vogt-Moykopf I (1983) Computertomographische Beurteilung mediastinaler Lymphknoten beim Bronchialkarzinom. Fortschr Röntgenstr 138: 682–688

Kono M, Hirata Y, Kimura S (1981) The value of computed tomography in the follow-up study of lung cancer and mediastinal tumors. Comput Tomogr 5: 169–189

Lewis E, Bernardino ME, Valdivieso M, Farha P, Barnes PA, Thomas JL (1982) Computed tomography and routine chest radiography in oat cell carcinoma of the lung. J Comput Assist Tomogr 4: 739–745

Libshitz HI, Shuman LS (1984) Radiation-induced pulmonary changes: CT-findings. J Comput Assist Tomogr 8: 15–18

Nabawi P, Mantravadi R, Breyer D, Capek V (1981) Computed tomography of radiation-induced lung injuries. J Comput Assist Tomogr 5: 568–570

Pagini JJ, Libshitz HI (1982) CT manifestations of radiation-induced change in chest tissue. J Comput Assist Tomogr 6: 243–248

Whitley NO, Fuks JZ, Whitacre M, Masler JA, Whitley JE, Aisner J (1984) Computed tomography of the chest in small cell lung cancer: potential new prognostic signs. Am J Roentgenol 141: 885–892

Magnetic Resonance Imaging in the Staging of Hodgkin's Disease and Non-Hodgkin Lymphoma

J.D. Tesoro-Tess, L. Balzarini, E. Ceglia, R. Petrillo, Y. Reyner, and R. Musumeci

Introduction

Treatment and prognosis of patients with Hodgkin's disease (HD) and non-Hodgkin lymphoma (NHL) vary with the extent of the disease at the initial diagnosis. Several authors have reported on the role played by computed tomography (CT) in the staging process [1, 2], and in particular it has been suggested that CT renders chest tomography and even bipedal lymphangiography (LAG) unnecessary [3, 4], mostly for its capability in detecting extranodal involvement or adenopathies not opacified by LAG. Furthermore, the frequently low accuracy rates offered by the various imaging modalities, especially as regards the diagnosis of hepatosplenic or bone marrow involvement, often require invasive staging procedures accurately to detect extranodal disease. The goal of our study was to evaluate the staging possibilities of magnetic resonance imaging (MRI) as well as to assess its value as an alternative tool to the invasive staging procedures.

Materials and Methods

A group of 74 consecutive, previously untreated patients who entered the Istituto Nazionale Tumori in Milan at initial presentation of the disease underwent MRI examination of the chest, abdomen, pelvis, and bone marrow. The diagnosis of HD (39 patients) or NHL (35 patients) was obtained in all cases by nodal or extranodal biopsy and histology. The stage of the disease was established by conventional methods, and MRI results were compared to those obtained by other staging procedures, i.e., chest X-ray, chest and abdominal CT, LAG, laparoscopy and/or laparotomy, hepatic and splenic biopsies, bone marrow aspiration, and histology. MRI was performed with a 1.5 T superconductive magnet. Transverse multislice images were obtained for all patients, and occasionally coronal and sagittal scans were acquired. For chest examination cardiac gating was utilized, and thus TR depended on the heart

Diagnostic Radiology E, Istituto Nazionale Tumori, Via Venezian 1, 20133 Milano, Italyia.

Advanced Radiation Therapy Tumor Response
Monitoring and Treatment Planning
Breit (Editor-in-Chief)
© Springer-Verlag, Berlin Heidelberg 1992

frequency rate (TR = 600–900 ms). Except for liver and spleen, which were studied with both T1 and T2 sequences, all other sites, i.e., abdomen, pelvis, and bone marrow, were evaluated only with mainly T1-weighted images (TR = 450–700, TE = 17). For retroperitoneal lymph node and bone marrow evaluation, further short TI inversion recovery (TR = 1800/TI = 180/TE = 28) combined with a rapid gradient echo sequence (FLASH 30°) were acquired in the coronal plane. The time necessary for a complete examination was 60–90 min.

Results

Chest. Of 32 patients 26 (81.2%) with normal chest radiographs had normal thoracic MRI scans, whereas in about 16% of patients with mediastinal involvement the extent of the disease was unsuspected on chest radiographs. Superior mediastinal nodes were the most frequent sites of disease (Table 1) particularly in HD (100% of patients with demonstrated intrathoracic involvement) rather than in NHL (35%). Except for cardiophrenic nodes (Fig. 1), otherwise involved in a few (5.4%) of all patients, hilar as well as subcarinal or posterior mediastinal nodes were affected much more frequently in HD than in NHL. Pericardial lesions, combined in 60% of cases with pericardial effusion, were encountered in 14.9% of patients.

Abdomen. MRI demonstrated retroperitoneal adenopathies in 22 cases (29.7%), with lower values in HD (9/39 = 23.1%) versus NHL (13/35 = 37.1%). A total of 70 patients underwent both MRI and LAG examinations. The two tests

Table 1. Results of thoracic MRI

	HD (n = 39)		NHL (n = 35)	
	n	%	n	%
High mediastinal adenopathies	31	79.5	6	17.1
Hilar adenopathies	9	23.1	3	8.6
Sub-carinal adenopathies	6	15.4	4	11.4
Posterior mediastinal adenopathies	10	25.6	1	2.9
Cardio-phrenic adenopathies	2	5.1	2	5.7
Lung parenchyma	4	10.3	—	—
Pleural effusion	4	10.3	—	—
Pericardium +/− Pericardial effusion	9	23.1	2	5.7
Chest wall	4	10.3	1	2.9
Other (Axilla)	1	2.6	13	37.1
Total abnormal	31	79.5	17	48.6

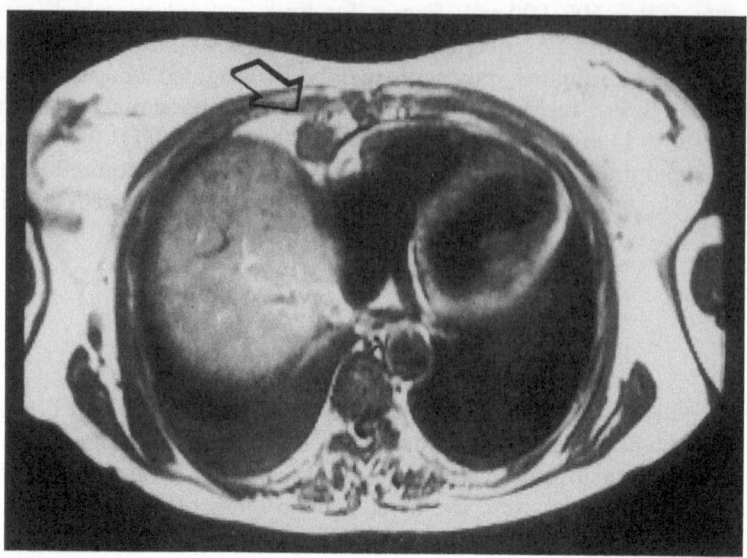

Fig. 1. Non-Hodgkin lymphoma. Transverse T1-weighted (SE 700/17) ECG-gated image. Cardiophrenic angle adenopathy (*arrow*) combined with posterior mild pleural effusion

agreed on the presence (20 patients) or absence (48 patients) of retroperitoneal adenopathies in 68 of 70 cases (97.1%). In both cases in which there was disagreement, LAG showed architecturally abnormal nodes that were normal in size or only slightly enlarged, and thus considered normal with MRI. On the other hand, MRI demonstrated adenopathies at sites not evaluable by LAG (mesenteric, celiac, or splenic hilus) in three patients. However in the same cases LAG findings were positive in the opacified retroperitoneal nodes. Although lymphography is still the single best imaging technique for the evaluation of the retroperitoneal nodes, MRI demonstrated high diagnostic accuracy (97%) and sensitivity (91%) values, considering both retroperitoneal and celiac or mesenteric lymph nodes.

MRI examination of the liver demonstrated a normal pattern in all but one patient (Fig. 2). However, for the spleen in 15% of cases the presence of focal tumor was clearly identified. A correlation of MRI and histological findings was available in 49/74 patients (66.7%; Table 2). For the liver, the values for accuracy and sensitivity cannot be calculated because hepatic involvement was detected in only one patient, and histology was not available in this patient, already assigned to stage IV for diffuse widespread disease. For the spleen, the sensitivity (3/5 patients = 60%) was relatively low, but this value probably is a statistical artifact due to the small number of patients with histologically confirmed splenic involvement. In only 3/13 patients (23.1%) who presented with enlarged spleen was lymphoma detected after biopsy and histology.

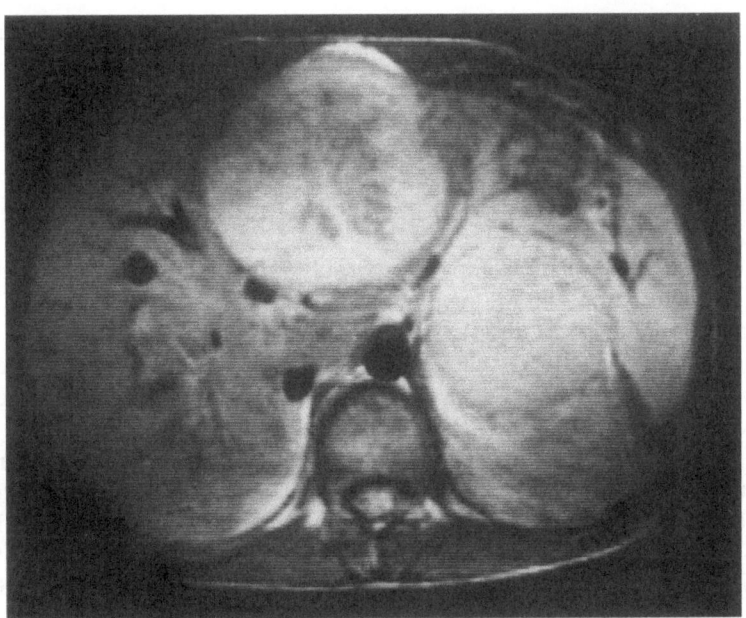

Fig. 2. Non-Hodgkin lymphoma. Proton density (SE 2000/28) image of an 8-year-old child showing inhomogeneous hepatic and left renal masses

Table 2. Infradiaphragmatic involvement: correlation of MRI and histological findings in HD (*n* = 31) and NHL (*n* = 18)

	HD		NHL	
	Histology positive	Histology negative	Histology positive	Histology negative
Liver				
MRI positive	—	—	—	—
MRI negative	—	31	—	18
Spleen				
MRI positive	1	1	2	—
MRI negative	2	27	—	16
Splenomegaly				
MRI positive	2	5	1	5
MRI negative	—	—	—	—

Bone Marrow. In 14/74 patients (18.9%) a bone marrow abnormality was identified by MRI, with larger incidence in HD (28.2%) versus NHL (8.6%). In 72/74 patients (97.3%) bone marrow aspiration from both the iliac crests was performed and MRI/histological correlation was possible. MRI demonstrated a good overall accuracy (83.3%) with similar values for specificity (87.3%) and negative predictive value (93.2%). For sensitivity and positive predictive values rates of 55.6% and 38.5% were obtained, respectively.

Discussion

As a general rule, our data compare favorably with those reported in the literature on the use of CT in the staging of HD and NHL. Castellino et al. [2] reported additional evidence of HD involvement ranging from 0% to 15% at different anatomic sites when chest CT scans were compared with chest radiography. Similarly, Hopper et al. [1] reported that the addition of thoracic CT at the initial examination of these patients changed the clinical stage in 18.7% of cases. Pond et al. [4] published the contribution of LAG and abdominal CT in NHL with influences of 23% for clinical stage and 14% for pathological stage. In our case material the only discordant parameter was the incremental rate of pericardial involvement (23% in HD patients versus 15% reported in the literature) probably due to the increased possibilities of MRI, which can utilize multiplanar and multiecho sequences. Similarly, better values of accuracy and sensitivity in detecting retroperitoneal lymph nodes are encountered when MRI and CT are compared, especially for the capability of MRI to acquire images both in transverse and in coronal planes.

In conclusion, the results of this study suggest that MRI is a valuable method in staging HD and NHL and can be proposed as a competitive method to other diagnostic tests at the initial presentation of the disease.

References

1. Hopper KD, Diehl LF, Lesar M et al. (1988) Hodgkin disease: clinical utility of CT in initial staging and treatment. Radiology 169: 17–22
2. Castellino RA, Blank N, Hoppe RT et al. (1986) Hodgkin disease: contributions of chest CT in the initial staging evaluation. Radiology 160: 603–605
3. Shiels RA, Stone J, Ash DV et al. (1984) Priorities for computed tomography and lymphography in the staging and initial management of Hodgkin's disease. Clin Radiol 35: 447–449
4. Pond GD, Castellino RA, Horning S et al. (1989) Non-Hodgkin lymphoma: influence of lymphography, CT and bone marrow biopsy on staging and management. Radiology 170: 159–164

Biphasic Repair and Prediction of Late Effects Following Lung Irradiation

W. Schmidt and K. Merkle

Introduction

Late effects are essential concomitants in clinical radiotherapy of malignant diseases. Generally these are typical for normal tissues and organs with flexible nonhierarchical structure and a relatively low proliferative activity and consequently consist preferentially of functional cells. In terms of the widely used linear-quadratic (LQ) model, late effects correspond to low α/β ratios, and the incidence and latency times of these effects show a strong dependence on possible changes in the fractionation regime. The α/β ratio of the lung (humans and experimental animals) with respect to the radiation-induced pneumonitis reaction is low and has been determined to be 3–4 Gy. Thus, the lung is a typical late-reacting organ. Indeed, the pneumonitis reaction as one of the most severe side effects of irradiations of the thoracic region appears some months after the end of treatment. Therefore it is highly desirable to have reliable mathematical and statistical methods to analyze clinical and experimental data and to predict the complication rate and mean latency time of the side effects in cases of new schedules. This is an essential precondition for the determination of optimal fractionation schedules in tumor treatment having the lung as dose-limiting organ.

We present a new mathematical model for describing and predicting late effect in terms of the kinetics of the responding target cell loss. The model is a generalization of that proposed by Collis (1982). The model is based on an alternative mathematical conception to describe target cell survival following irradiation; however, it is in good accordance with the LQ model if the parameters are properly chosen. Furthermore, the model describes the repair of the radiation-induced sublethal damage during the interfraction intervals as a biphasic process having a fast and a slow component. This feature is essential especially for the application to accelerated and hyperfractionated irradiation schedules with short interfraction intervals. Presently, the LQ model and its extension to the incomplete-repair (IR) model (Thames 1985) is the most frequently used mathematical framework for analyzing clinical and experimental data from fractionated irradiations. The model has been combined with

Max Delbrück Centre for Molecular Medicine, Dept. Bioinformatics, Robert-Rössle-Str. 10, 0-1115 Berlin, FRG

Advanced Radiation Therapy Tumor Response
Monitoring and Treatment Planning
Breit (Editor-in-Chief)
© Springer-Verlag, Berlin Heidelberg 1992

other statistical ideas and techniques (mixture models, Bentzen et al. 1989; proportional hazards, Taylor et al. 1987) for the different applications.

Nevertheless, the available methods are insufficient with respect to the following two topics. (a) The interfractional repair of radiation-induced target cell damage is an (at least) biphasic process. This became evident from recent experimental results and, indirectly, from the inability of the IR model to describe experimental data consistently (van den Aardweg, personal communication). Indeed, the IR model assumes a simple exponential term to describe the repair. (b) The available mathematical models contain no natural assumptions explaining and describing the latencies in case of late reactions. Therefore, there is a need to formulate such assumptions. In this way it will become possible to use the information content of the observed latency times for the statistical evaluation and to characterize the time course of functional cell loss after the end of irradiation.

Nonmathematical Description of the New Model

To represent cell damage by radiation, the assumption of biphasic repair, and the loss of irreparably damaged target cells in the framework of a unified model, the totality of the irradiated cells is subdivided into a finite number of classes according to the severity of damage: state 0, no damage; state 1, sublethal damage (fast repair); state 2, potentially lethal damage (slow repair); state 3, irreparable damage (limited life time); and state 4, loss of cell function (death). Before irradiation, every cell is assumed to be in state 0, but thereafter a typical distribution of the cells over the states is obtained, depending on the irradiation modalities. The "flow" of the cells between the assumed states is governed and described by a number of parameters. The intensity of irradiation (dose rate) is described by the parameter ρ (Poisson process). The parameters μ_f and μ_s characterize the reflow of cells from states according to the different degrees of damage into state 0, i.e., the two components of the repair process. The probability γ stands for the fraction of cells which are inactivated directly, i.e.,

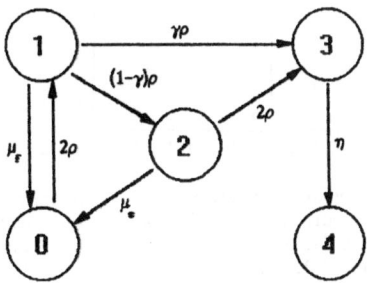

Fig. 1. Schematic representation of the model assumptions. *Numbers (0, ..., 4)* denote the cell damage (for the definitions see text). The transition intensities of the corresponding subpopulations are defined by the parameters (*arrows*) representing this transition

without accumulation of reparable damage (type A damage; Dale 1985). The parameter η describes the time course of functional cell loss. Figure 1 represents these assumptions schematically.

Application: Pneumonitis of the Mice Lung Following Thoracic Irradiation

The model has been applied successfully to a number of fractionation data sets published in the literature concerning reactions of different normal tissues and organs to irradiation. As an example, we present the results of a reanalysis of lung pneumonitis data reported by Vegesna et al. (1986). The details of the experiments are described in the original paper. To give a brief description, 1040 mice were irradiated to the thoracic region with between 1 and 43 fractions with a dose per fraction ranging from 1.15 to 15.5 Gy. There were 90 separate dose groups, each consisting of 10 or 20 mice. The majority of fractions were separated by 3-h intervals, only a few by 12-h intervals. Death was assumed to be due to pneumonitis if it occurred between 56 and 160 days after irradiation. A detailed mathematical analysis of the obtained data was performed by Taylor et al. (1987). The analysis is based on the LQ model combined with the method

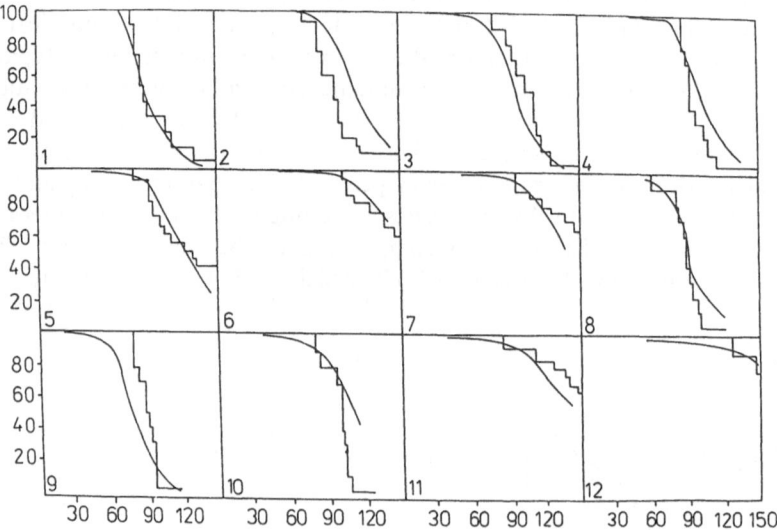

Fig. 2. Lung pneumonitis experiment (Vegesna et al. 1986). Comparison of the experimental survival curves with the model predictions. *Curves 1–7* correspond to single-dose experiments (1:15.5 Gy, 2:14.0 Gy, 3:15.0 Gy, 4:14.5 Gy, 5:13.5 Gy, 6:12.5 Gy, 7:13.0 Gy); *curves 8–12* were obtained from fractionated irradiations (8:11 fractions, 9:12 fractions, 10:10 fractions, 11:9 fractions, 12:8 fractions).

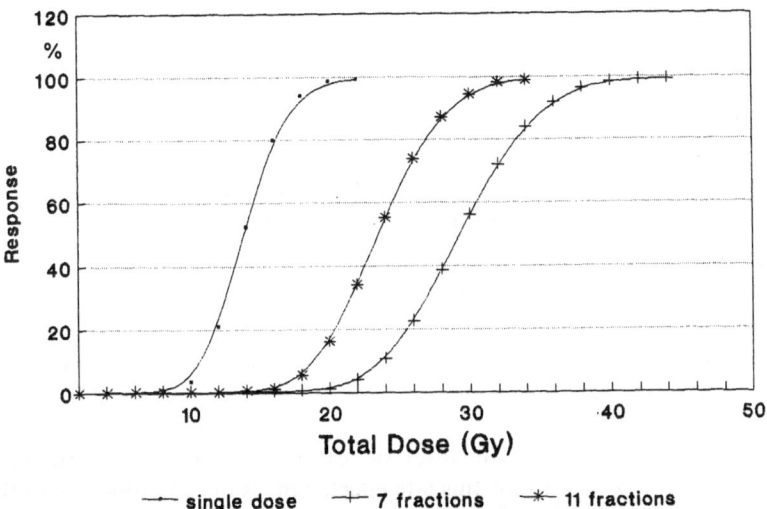

Fig. 3. Model-derived dose-response curves for three different irradiation schedules. The curves are based on the parameters estimated by the maximum-likelihood method from the data of Vegesna et al. (1986)

of proportional hazards (Cox 1972). Figure 2 presents the results from 12 treatment groups. The stairlike curves are the Kaplan–Meier estimates of the survival derived from the experimental data, and the smooth curves are the model predictions based on the maximum-likelihood estimation of the parameters for the model discussed here. These were obtained as follows: $\mu_f = 3.5\,h^{-1}$, $\mu_s = 0.037\,h^{-1}$; $\gamma = 0.346$, $\delta = 0.1084\,Gy^{-1}$, $\pi_0 = 42.5\%$, $\sigma = 2.97\%$, $\eta = 0.1393$ week^{-1}. The parameter π_0 describes the mean critical target cell loss causing death of the animal due to pneumonitis, σ its standard deviation. The constant of the fast repair component is extremely imprecise because shorter interfraction intervals were not tested in the experiments. As can be seen from the Fig. 2, there is a good coincidence between the experimental results and the model prediction for all treatment groups.

The model can be used to predict the outcome of altered fractionation schedules, for example, dose-response curves, ED_{50} values, percentage unrepaired damage for (short) interfraction intervals, and other important entities. Figure 3 demonstrates the predicted dose-response curves for three different fractionation schedules.

Summary and Conclusions

The proposed model permits the simultaneous analysis of incidence and latency times of late injuries following fractionated irradiation of individuals. All data can be used in the analysis, and there is no restriction to isoeffect data.

Estimations of the following radiobiological parameters are obtained:

- μ_f, μ_s: repair constants characterizing the fast and the slow component of the repair process, respectively
- γ, δ: the radiation sensitivity of the responding target cells (equivalent to α and β in the LQ model)
- π_0, σ: mean and standard deviation of the critical target cell loss
- η: the time course of the loss of the irreparably damaged target cells

The model permits the prediction of the incidence of the late injury considered to be expected from altered irradiation schedules (e.g., accelerated, hyperfractionated).

Dose-response curves for given schedules, the fraction of unrepaired damage for short interfraction intervals, and other basic entities can be derived by means of the model.

The parameters γ and δ obtained for the discussed lung pneumonitis data correspond to a low α/β ratio for this late effect. This is in accordance with the findings of other authors. The half-life of the slow repair component, derived from the parameter η, is nearly 26 h. This value is significantly higher than is usually assumed. It follows that for multiple fractions per day in irradiations affecting the lung significant incomplete repair effects must be taken into account.

References

Bentzen SM, Thames HD, Travis EL, Ang KK, van der Schueren E, Dewit L, Dixon DO (1989) Direct estimation of latent time for radiation injury in late-responding normal tissues: gut, lung, and spinal cord. Int J Radiat Biol 55: 27–43

Collis CH (1982) A kinetic model for the pathogenesis of radiation lung damage. Int J Radiat Biol 42: 253–263

Cox DR (1972) Regression models and life-tables. J R Statist Soc [B] 34: 187–220

Dale RG (1985) The application of the linear-quadratic dose-effect equation to fractionated and protracted radiotherapy. Br J Radiol 58: 515–528

Taylor JMG, Withers HR, Vegesna V, Mason K (1987) Fitting the linear-quadratic model using time of occurrence as the endpoint for quantal response experiments. Int J Radiat Biol 52: 459–468

Thames HD (1985) An "incomplete-repair" model for survival after fractionated and continuous irradiations. Int J Radiat Biol 47: 319–339

Vegesna V, Withers HR, Thames HD, Mason KA (1986) Multifraction radiation response of mouse lung. Int J Radiat Biol 47: 413–427

Lung Density Changes Measured by Computed Tomography in Patients Receiving Total Body Irradiation and Bone Marrow Transplantation

P. Feyer, C. Waurick, M. Spengler, C. Größ, O. Titlbach, F.-A. Hoffmann, T. Friedrich, and G. Borte

Introduction

Bone marrow transplantation (BMT) is a well-established therapy for the treatment of various hematological malignancies. The most important indications are acute and chronic forms of leukemia, severe aplastic anemia, severe combined immunodeficiency, and lymphomas. More than 30 000 transplantations have been carried out worldwide, and the frequency is about 4000 transplants per year. The marrow transplant may come from three sources: (a) an identical twin (syngeneic). (b) a histocompatible HLA-identical sibling (allogeneic), or (c) stored marrow from the patient taken in remission (autologous); (Schaefer 1989). The patients must be pretreated with a conditioning therapy by high-dose total body irradiation and/or chemotherapy. An aggressive conditioning regime is necessary to eradicate residual leukemic stem cells, to ensure bone marrow ablation, and to effect complete immunosuppression.

The toxicity of the conditioning therapy may produce problems in the course of BMT. In both autologous and syngeneic BMT treatments failures are due mainly to a leukemia relapse. Allogeneic BMT has introduced a new spectrum of fatal transplantation-related complications limiting success of this treatment. Most prominent among these complications are graft-versus-host disease, interstitial pneumonitis (IP), failures of marrow engraftment, infections, and veno-occlusive disease (Schaefer 1989). The lung is one of the most relevant organs of risk in BMT; complications of the lung are influenced by intensive radiochemotherapy, a following therapy after BMT, individual risk factors, and infections.

One of the major complications after total body irradiation and/or chemotherapy followed by BMT is IP, with an incidence of 10%–84% and associated with a mortality rate of 75%–90% (Barrett 1982; Bortin et al. 1989; Weiner et al. 1986, 1989). IP is a nonspecific response of the pulmonary tissue and belongs to a heterogeneous group of inflammatory disorders affecting predominantly the pulmonary interstitium, resulting in a thickening of the intra-alveolar septa by cellular infiltration (Varecamp 1990). IP may follow an acute or a chronic progressive course. The etiology is often unknown, and the disease must be

Clinic of Radiology, Clinic of Internal Medicine and Institute of Pathology, University of Leipzig, Liebigstr. 20a, 7010 Leipzig, FRG

Advanced Radiation Therapy Tumor Response
Monitoring and Treatment Planning
Breit (Editor-in-Chief)
© Springer-Verlag, Berlin Heidelberg 1992

classified by various clinical-pathological features. The clinical picture is characterized by tachypnea, nonproductive cough, fever, hypoxia. Chest X-rays show
bilaterally diffuse infiltrations from linear to patchy patterns and sometimes
honeycombing (Braunschweig et al. 1986). An increase in density and later
patchy infiltrations are remarkable upon computed tomography (CT; Tellkamp
et al. 1986; Slanina et al. 1988). Functional tests show a diminished lung volume
and compliance. At blood gas analysis hypoxemia and normo- or hypcapnia
have been observed as signs of reduced diffusion capacity. Perfusion scintigraphy demonstrates perfusion disturbances.

With our prospective study we sought to determine subclinical lung changes
after BMT with the help of CT. We also tried to measure sensitivity in order to
detect early prestages of IP and to encourage the use of CT as an accompanying
diagnostic method during the IP therapy.

Materials and Methods

Between January 1989 and March 1990 we examined 38 patients; there were 21
women and 17 men, and ages ranged from 16 to 40 years (average, 24). Of these,
23 patients received allogeneic and 15 autologous transplants. In preparing for
the BMT either a fractionated total body irradiation (FTBI $n = 14$) or a
busulfan conditioning therapy (BU; $n = 24$) was used (Table 1). FTBI was given
with a linear accelerator (9 MV) in latero-lateral beam direction. The patients
received six fractions with a dose of 2.0 Gy on each fraction given on 3
consecutive days (days $- 7, - 6, - 5$ before BMT) followed by cyclophosphamide 60 mg/kg BW per day for 2 days (days $- 4, - 3$). The total
midline dose was 12.0 Gy, and the lung dose was 10.0 Gy with a dose rate of
0.1 Gy/min. BU conditioning consisted of 4 mg/kg BW per day on 4 consecutive

Table 1. Patient diagnoses and conditioning regimes

	Allogeneic transplants ($n = 23$)	Autologous transplants ($n = 15$)
Diagnosis	4 ALL	9 ALL
	4 AML	3 AML
	13 CML	3 NHL/LG
	1 AA	
	1 Plasmocytoma	
Conditioning regime	17 BU + CY	7 BU + CY
	6 FTBI + CY	8 FTBI + CY

ALL, Acute lymphocytic leukemia; AML, acute myeloid leukemia; CML, chronic
myeloid leukemia; AA, aplastic anemia; NHL/LG, non-Hodgkin lymphoma/lympho-
granuloma; BU, busulfan; FTBI, fractionated total body irradiation; CY, cyclophosphamide.

days (days − 8, − 7, − 6, − 5) followed by cyclophosphamide 60 mg/kg BW (days − 4, − 3). Prophylaxis against graft-versus-host disease in allogeneic BMT was carried out with cyclosporin A, metothrexate, and corticosteroids.

To obtain a basic scan patients were examined before BMT and at regular intervals up to 1 year afterwards. A Somatom 2 scanner (Siemens) was used for this CT density study. Six axial 8-mm slices through the lung were obtained. The first slice was placed 1 cm below the sternoclavicular joint; a representative slice was taken at the level of the bifurcation and the last slice above the diaphragma. Each position was taken in full inspiration and expiration. Care was taken to reproduce the same scanning conditions, the positioning, and the breathing status of the patient. The density measurement was according to Rosenblum et al. (1978) and El-Khatib et al. (1989) with peripheral region-of-interest and regional density measurements. Visual evaluation was also carried out.

Results

In the early period of 1–3 months after BMT, 8/26 patients after 1 month and 3/13 patients after 3 months showed an increase in lung density. Eight of these patients had received an allogeneic BMT (seven BU and one FTBI). Two of eight patients developed IP with an early density increase above 7% related to the scan before BMT. Later there were also visual CT changes, such as patchy

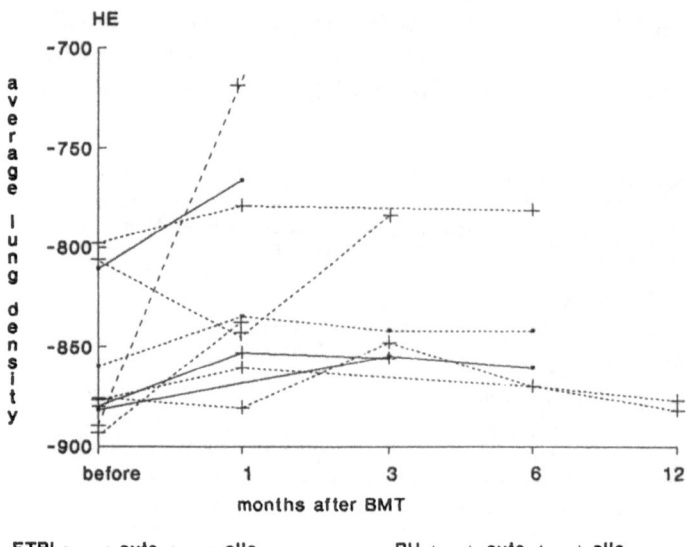

Fig. 1. Average lung density in patients measured before and several months after BMT

infiltrations, in these patients. Lung density increased less than 7%, reversing completely in the follow-up scans (Fig. 1). Figure 2 demonstrates the partial agreement of the reference methods used: chest X-ray, perfusion scintigraphy, and ventilatory tests. Of the patients with a density increase in CT 72% showed changes in chest radiographs. In only 43% were disturbances in lung perfusion scintigraphy evident, and in 43% pathological findings in ventilatory tests were obtained.

Serial measurements of lung density after 6 months showed a nonreversible density increase in 3 of 21 investigated patients (one BU allogeneic, one FTBI autologous, one FTBI allogeneic) and in 3 of 10 investigated patients after 12

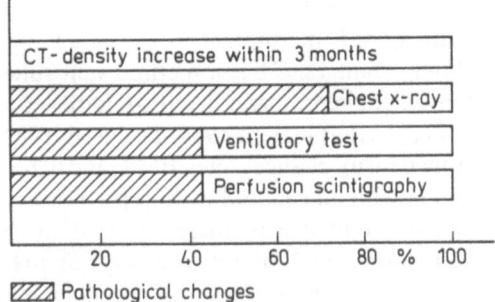

Fig. 2. Comparison of investigation methods to detect pathological changes in patients with CT density increase within 3 months after BMT

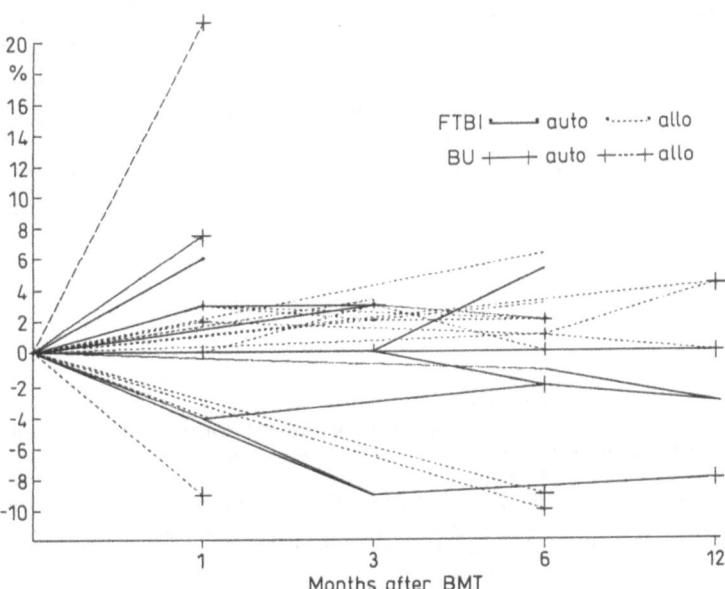

Fig. 3. Changes in average lung density related to the pretransplant values measured on follow-up scans for individual patients up to 1 year after BMT

months (one BU allogeneic, two FTBI allogeneic). In connection with the chest X-ray (83% changes) and functional tests (66% changes), these results suggest a beginning interstitial fibrosis.

We found in our follow-up CT-scans 17 of 38 patients with density increases — 11 in the early period where these changes were reversible and six in the later period as nonreversible changes. Nine of 38 patients showed a lung density decrease not of clinical importance, and 12 of 38 patients had no lung density changes (Fig. 3).

Discussion and Conclusions

In our prospective study of 38 patients CT densitometry was used as a noninvasive test to detect interstitial lung changes. CT is a method well suited for follow-up studies because of its excellent reproducibility (El-Khatib et al. 1989). In agreement with other authors (El-Khatib et al. 1989; Lee et al. 1984), we found three different patterns of lung density changes after BMT. Early lung density increase above 7% was connected with lung complications (two cases of IP, one of cytomegalovirus infection), and a lung density increase less than 7% indicated a reversible lung damage. El-Khatib et al. (1989) and van Dyk and Hill (1983) consider lung density increases to be an indicator of possible lung complications. Therefore CT should be carried out as early as possible in the diagnostic regime of pulmonary reactions following BMT. Some patients showed a decrease in lung density after conditioning therapy (BU or FTBI) and BMT. Thus this does not seem to be a radiation-specific effect, as El-Khatib et al. (1989) conclude from their study. A possible explanation of the density decrease could be changes in ventilation and/or blood flow in the lung after irradiation or after BU and BMT. There are numerous possible influences, such as additional drugs and clinical status. In the later period the lung density changes become irreversible, and we suggest a beginning interstitial fibrosis.

References

Barrett A (1982) Clinical aspects of total body irradiation. J Eur Radiother 3: 159–164

Bortin MM, Ringden O, Horowitz MM, Rozman C, Weiner RS, Rimm AA (1989) Temporal relationships between the major complications of bone marrow transplantation for leukemia. Bone Marrow Transplant 4: 339–344

Braunschweig R, Kubel M, Standke E, Raue I (1986) Röntgenmorphologische Befunde bei 34 Patienten mit akuter myeloischer Leukämie, zytoreduktiver Therapie und Knochenmarktransplantation in Korrelation zu klinischen Daten und Bestrahlungsregime. Radiol Diagn 27: 711–718

El-Khatib EE, Freeman CR, Rybka WB, Lehnert S, Podgorsak EB (1989) The use of CT densitometry to predict lung toxicity in bone marrow transplant patients. Int J Radiat Oncol Biol Phys 16: 85–94

Lee JY, Shank B, Bonfiglio P, Reid A (1984) CT analysis of lung density changes in patients undergoing total body irradiation prior to bone marrow transplantation. J Comput Assist Tomogr 8: 885–891

Rosenblum LJ, Mauceri RA, Wellenstein DE, Bassano DA, Cohen WN, Heitzman ER (1978) Computed tomography of the lung. Radiology 129: 521–524

Schaefer UW, Beelen DW, Neuser J (1989) Knochenmarktransplantation. Karger, Basel

Slanina J, Sigmund G, Hinkelbein W, Wenz W, Wannenmacher M (1988) Die pulmonale Strahlenreaktion nach Mantelfeldbestrahlung. Radiologe 28: 20–28

Tellkamp H, Herrmann T, Voigtmann L, Lorenz J, Rosenkranz G, Köhler K (1986) Computertomographische Untersuchungen zur Erfassung der radiogenen Pneumopathie im Tierexperiment. Digitale Bilddiagn 6: 161–164

Van Dyk J, Hill RP (1983) Post-irradiation lung density changes measured by computerized tomography. Int J Radiat Oncol Biol Phys 9: 847–852

Varekamp AE (1990) Interstitial pneumonitis following bone marrow transplantation. Thesis, University of Leiden. Publication of the Institute of Applied Radiobiology and Immunology TNO, Rijswijk

Weiner RS, Bortin MM, Gale RP, Gluckman E, Kay HEM, Kolb HJ, Hartz AJ, Rimm AA (1986) Interstitial pneumonitis after bone marrow transplantation. Assessment of risk factors. Ann Intern Med 104: 168–175

Weiner RS, Horowitz MM, Gale RP, Dicke KA, van Bekkum DW (1989) Risk factors for interstitial pneumonia following bone marrow transplantation for severe aplastic anaemia. Br J Haematol 71: 535–543

Radiation Therapy Combined with Intraarterial Chemotherapy of Nonoperable Non-Small-Cell Lung Cancer

A. Rieber[1], H.-J. Brambs[1], M. Wannenmacher[2], and P. Drings[3]

Introduction

Radiotherapy is at the moment the standard treatment for nonoperable localized non-small-cell bronchogenic carcinoma. The 5-year survival rate has been reported to be between 6% and 9%. Numerous attempts have been made to improve the response rate and the survival of these patients with various chemo- and radiotherapy schemes. Systemic chemotherapy with cisplatin/vindesine is one of the most active treatments, with a response rate of 40%, but it is limited because of its side effects and toxicity [1, 2, 6, 7, 8]. Central bronchogenic carcinomas are fed by one or two bronchial arteries; it is therefore possible to perfuse the chemotherapeutic agents directly intraarterially [7, 8]. We are now testing the combination of intraarterial chemotherapy and radiotherapy. The aim is to improve the response rate and the survival of patients and to reduce the side effects by intraarterial chemotherapy.

Materials and Methods

Patients carcinomas graded T1–4 N0–3 M0 were included, and they had to be inoperable for internal or technical reasons. A precondition was definite histological diagnosis. The bronchial artery was probed transfemorally in the Seldinger technique. The tumor-feeding artery was demonstrated using digital subtraction angiography. A Tracker 18 catheter was then placed peripherad to avoid chemoperfusion of intercostal arteries and arteries which feed healthy tissue. Angiographic compute tomography (CT) was performed in superselective position of the angiographic catheter to show the perfusion of the tumor. If some parts of the tumor are not contrasted in angiographic CT, there must be a

[1] Abteilung für Radiologische Diagnostik, Radiologische Universitätsklinik, Hoppe-Seyler-Str. 3, 7400 Tübingen, FRG
[2] Abteilung für Klinische Radiologie, Radiologische Universitätsklinik, Im Neuenheimer Feld 400, 6900 Heidelberg, FRG
[3] Abteilung für Onkologie, Thoraxklinik der LVA Baden, Amalienstr. 5, 6900 Heidelberg-Rohrbach, FRG

Advanced Radiation Therapy Tumor Response
Monitoring and Treatment Planning
Breit (Editor-in-Chief)
© Springer-Verlag, Berlin Heidelberg 1992

second tumor-feeding artery which is perfused in the next chemotherapy cycle. Four cycles were planned, one per week. The patients were treated twice with an intraarterial infusion of 3 mg/m² vindesine and 20 mg/m² cisplatin and twice with 20 mg/m² cisplatin only. The patients received a simultaneous radiation, 2 Gy per fraction, 5 days per week and a total dose of 60 Gy.

Results

Eleven patients with squamous and adenomatous cell carcinoma, ten stage IIIa/b and one stage II, were treated. Nine patients had only one tumor-feeding artery. The angiographic CT of two patients suggested a second tumor-feeding artery which was then detected in the next angiography. The intraarterial chemotherapy was well tolerated. No major side effects occurred, and systemic toxicity was insignificant. Nausea and vomiting, which occurred on the evening of chemotherapy, was well treated with antiemetic drugs. Three patients were treated with only two cycles of chemotherapy because a dissection of the bronchial artery led to an irreversible occlusion. One patient died of a pulmonary hemorrhage. Two patients refused continuation of the chemotherapy. In one patient metastases of the liver and the cerebrum were detected, so that the chemotherapy was not continued. The other patients showed a response rate of more than 50% (Fig. 1). Five patients survived the first year; the survival of the four patients still alive is between 15 and 21 months.

Discussion

The first report about the treatment of inoperable lung cell cancer with intraarterial infusion of cytostatic agents was in 1964. Although the tumor response was good, the method was given up because of its high risks and complications [7, 8]. The tumor response of intravenous chemotherapy is between 10% and 40%. The tumor response depends on the choice of cytostatic agent and the combination of the drugs [3, 5, 9, 10, 12]. The most active treatment until now is the combination of vindesine and cisplatin [5, 6]. The standard treatment of inoperable non-small-cell lung cancer is radiotherapy. The average survival of patients treated with chemo- or radiotherpy is between 8 and 12 months [5, 9, 10, 12].

The first results of the EORTC study, which began 1984 in several medical centers, show an average survival of 9.9 months in patients treated only by radiotherapy. Patients treated by a combination of radiotherapy and intravenous infusion of vindesine and cisplatin have an average survival of 15 months. The 2-year survival is 13% by radiotherapy alone and 25% by

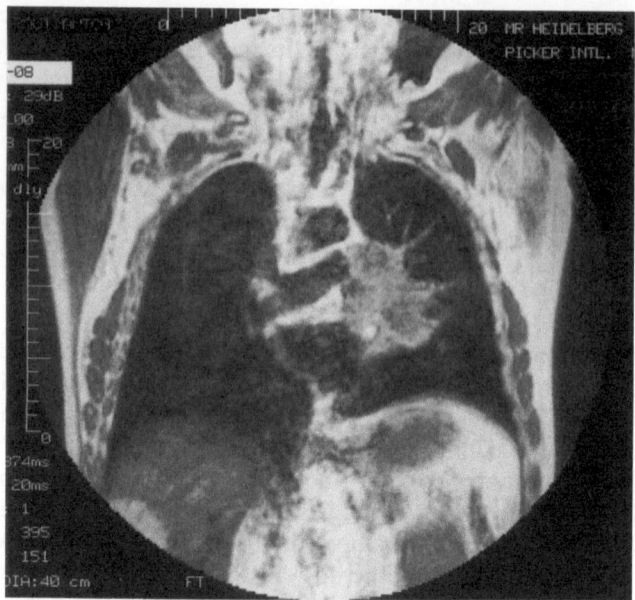

a

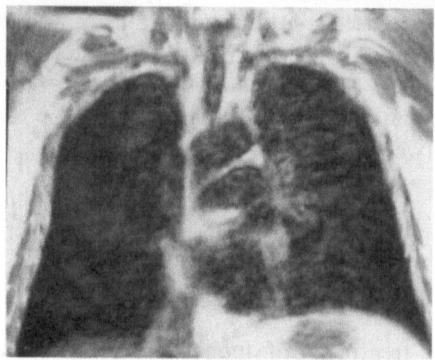

b

Fig. 1a, b. Magnetic resonance images of a central bronchogenic carcinoma (T4 N2) in a 65-year-old patient. **a** Before therapy. **b** After therapy. Therapeutic result shows high tumor regression

combinated therapy [11]. The encouraging results of the EORTC study suggest the development of a similar therapy concept. The side effects can be much reduced by intraarterial chemotherapy. This fact justifies the additional burden of multiple angiographies.

The development of new catheters and the better demonstration of the arteries by digital subtraction angiography allow an intraarterial chemotherapy with which it is possible to spare the intercostal arteries and healthy lung tissue. Angiographic CT allows the demonstration of specific tumor perfusion. The tumor response is higher by this therapy scheme, and survival seems to be longer. The therapy has a principally local effect. Thus, it seems to be convenient to treat patients with locoregional limited tumors only. Finally, it must be emphasized that experience with this scheme is until now limited, and its use is possible only in clinical studies.

References

1. Ekholm S, Albrectsson U, Hellekant C, Jonsson K, Nyman U, Tylen U (1980) Cytostatic infusion into bronchial arteries in bronchogenic carcinoma. Ann Radiol 4: 436–438
2. Ekholm S, Dahlbäck O, Tylen U (1986) Preoperative treatment of squamous cell carcinoma of the lung with mitomycin C in bronchial arteria. Eur J Radiol 6: 9–11
3. Emami B, Perez CA (1987) Carcinoma of the lung. In: Perez CA, Brady LW Jr (eds) Principles and practice of radiation oncology. Lippincott, Philadelphia pp 650–683
4. Georgi M, Vogt-Moykopf I (1988) Stereoangiographie der Bronchialarterien: Technik und Indikation. Fortschr Geb Rontgenstr 149: 158–163
5. Gralla RJ, Casper ES, Kelsen DP, Braun DW Jr, Dukeman ME, Martini N, Yung CW, Golbey RB (1981) Cisplatin and vindesine combination therapy for advanced carcinoma of the lung; a randomized trial investigating two dosage schedules. Ann Intern Med 95: 414–420
6. Helle PA, Planting AST, Yarnold J (1984) Combination chemotherapy + split-dose radiotherapy, a randomized phase II study leading to a phase III study. EORTC Lung Cancer Cooperative Group, EORTC 08842
7. Hellekant C (1979) Branchial angiography and intraarterial chemotherapy with mitomycin C in bronchogenic carcinoma. Acta Radiol Diagn 20: 478–496
8. Hellekant C, Svanberg L (1978) Bronchial artery infusion of mitomycin C in advanced bronchogenic carcinoma. Acta Radiol Oncol 17: 449–462
9. Hesketh PJ, Cooley TP, Finkel HE, Wright J, Hesketh AM (1988) Treatment of advanced non-small cell lung cancer with cisplatin, 5-fluorouracil, and mitomycin C. Cancer 62: 1466–1470
10. Kaasa S, Thorud E, Host H, Lien H, Lund E, Sjolie I (1988) A randomized study evaluating radiotherapy versus chemotherapy in patients with inoperable non-small lung cancer. Radiother Oncol 11: 7–13
11. Karstens JH (1989) Kombinierte Therapie beim nicht-kleinzelligen Bronchialkarzinom. Jahrestagung 1989 der Hessische Gesellschaft für Medizinische Strahlenkunde, Frankfurt
12. Rieber A, Brambs HJ, Kauffmann G, Wannenmacher M, Drings P (1991) Kombinierte intraarterielle Chemo- und Radiotherapie des inoperablen nichtkleinzelligen Bronchialkarzinoms. Strahlenther Onkol 167: 14–18

Positron Emission Tomography with Fluorodeoxyglucose for the Evaluation of Tumor Recurrence of Thoracic Tumors

M.V. Knopp[1], L.G. Strauss[1], U. Haberkorn[1], A. Dimitrakopoulou[1], H. Bischoff[2], D. Branscheid[2], J. Doll[1], S. Delorme[1], W. Maier-Borst[1], W. Lorenz[1], and G. van Kaick[1]

Introduction

The detection of recurrent tumors of thoracic lesions has remained a difficult diagnostic challenge despite the great advances seen in computed tomography (CT) and magnetic resonance imaging (MRI). The common differential diagnostic problem of distinguishing tumor recurrence from scar or inflammatory tissue has increasingly become a difficult clinical problem. Since therapeutic approaches are available in cases of recurrences, a timely and correct diagnosis becomes of increasing importance. The morphologic evaluation of suspect regions of tumor recurrences is quite limited especially if the size of the lesion is still small. Therefore additional information in conjunction with its morphologic information is needed. Positron emission tomography (PET) using metabolically active compounds, such as flour-18 labelled deoxyglucose (FDG) allow imaging of metabolism [1]. As clinical studies to evaluate the potential use of FDG PET imaging for thoracic lesions have shown a great potential benefits [2, 3], this technique is being introduced for the evaluation of recurrent tumors. Two considerations of great importance in the evaluation of recurrent tumors by PET are changes in the metabolic state and function of lesions due to the previous therapy and secondarily due to therapeutic procedures, which may have altered the cross-sectional anatomy. A very careful correlation between the morphologic cross-sectional information obtained by CT and MRI with the functional cross-sectional information available by PET is necessary.

Patients and Methods

A group of 11 patients with previous therapy for malignant thoracic lesions were included in this study. The histologies and modalities of treatment are shown in

[1] Department of Radiology and Pathophysiology, German Cancer Research Center, Im Neuenheimer Feld 280, 6900 Heidelberg, FRG
[2] Thoraxklinik Heidelberg, Amalien str. 5, 6900 Heidelberg-Rohrbach, FRG

Advanced Radiation Therapy Tumor Response
Monitoring and Treatment Planning
Breit (Editor-in-Chief)
© Springer-Verlag, Berlin Heidelberg 1992

Table 1. Patient data

No.	Histology	Inital treatment	Recurrence	FDG (SUV)	Confirmation by
1	Adenocarcinoma	Surgery	Yes	1.9	Surgery
2	Mesothelioma	Surgery	Yes	2.1	Surgery
3	Non-Hodgkin lymphoma	Chemotherapy	Yes	3.0	Surgery
4	Testis tumor	Chemotherapy	Yes	2.2	Surgery
5	Mesothelioma	Surgery	Yes	2.9	Clinical course
6	Squamous cell carcinoma	Surgery	Yes	3.3	Clinical course
7	Adenocarcinoma	Surgery	Yes	3.0	Clinical course
8	Adenocarcinoma	Radiation	Yes	3.0	Clinical course
9	Testis tumor	Chemotherapy	No	0.2	Surgery
10	Hodgkin lymphoma	Chemotherapy	No	1.2	Clinical course
11	Squamous cell carcinoma	Surgery	No	0.1	Clinical course

Table 1. PET studies were performed using whole-body PET scanner manufactured by GE Scanditronix (WB2048/7WB). The whole-body PET scanner consists of a two-ring system with a diameter of 107 cm using 512 BGO/GSO detectors. A field of view of 52 cm is available with slice thickness of 11 mm. With this two-ring system three consecutive cross-sections can be imaged simultaneously [4]. Images were reconstructed with scatter and attenuation correction using an iterative reconstruction technique in a 128 matrix [5]. The spatial resolution was 5.1 mm [6]. A dose of 440 MBq FDG was injected intravenously, and one-point measurements 50 min after injection with an emission scan time of 15 min and a transmission scan time of 5 min were acquired. Tracer uptake concentrations were calculated by a region-of-interest technique and standardized for injected dose and body weight and expressed as a standardized uptake value (SUV). To localize the relevant field of view all patients were scanned by CT prior to the PET study. Anatomical landmarks were evaluated using reconstructed transmission or CT scans of the same level. The inclusion criterion for patients in the study was a finding in CT or MRI studies supportive of tumor recurrence.

Results

PET detected three patients in whom tumor recurrence could be excluded and recurrent tumor in eight patients. These recurrences were confirmed by surgical means in four and by clinical follow-up in the other four. All recurrent tumor lesions showed significant FDG uptake (Table 1) with a range of 1.9–3.3 SUV while the benign lesions showed FDG uptake in the range of only 0.1–1.2.

Discussion

The use of FDG PET in the diagnostic evaluation of indeterminate thoracic lesions has already been established [2, 3]. While the criteria for evaluation of PET studies must be modified for the detection of tumor recurrence, the basic procedure remains the same. Since the overall resolution of the system has been determined at 5.1 mm, lesions smaller than 1 cm in one axis are difficult for quantitative evaluation. Quantitative evaluation, on the other hand, is a necessary tool for objective evaluation since the visual display of uptake of metabolic substance can be influenced by many factors. The differential diagnostic work-up of patients in a postsurgical stage is quite often difficult.

A common and difficult situation in the postsurgical management of patients is presented by small soft-tissue masses, especially considering potential secondary surgical resection which may be scar tissue or recurrent tumor. Figure 1 shows a 63-year-old man who had a surgical resection of two segments of the right lung due to adenocarcinoma. On follow-up studies 1 year after surgical therapy a small soft-tissue mass as seen on the CT scan was observed. Such a situation is of great clinical importance because small recurrent lesions may still be resectable, whereas scar tissue is very frequently the reason. In the evaluation of such small lesions only positive findings, lesions which show significant FDG accumulation, can be used for diagnostic information. In this patient, an intense FDG accumulation was seen despite its small size, and a quantitative evaluation

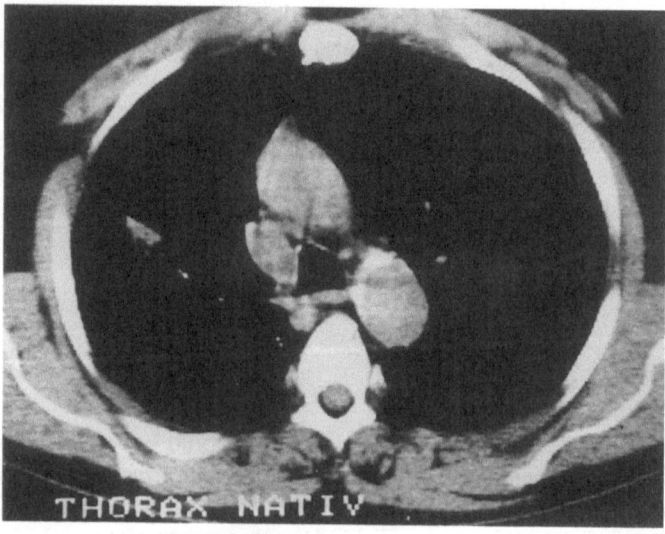

Fig. 1. CT of a 63-year-old man with a soft-tissue mass 1 year after surgical resection of an adenocarcinoma in the right lung

showed FDG accumulation of 1.9 SUV (Fig. 2). This patient was readmitted for a surgical procedure, and the tumor recurrence was confirmed.

A thorough understanding of the metabolic effects of prior treatment is necessary to interpret the findings in PET images. Figure 3 is a PET scan of a

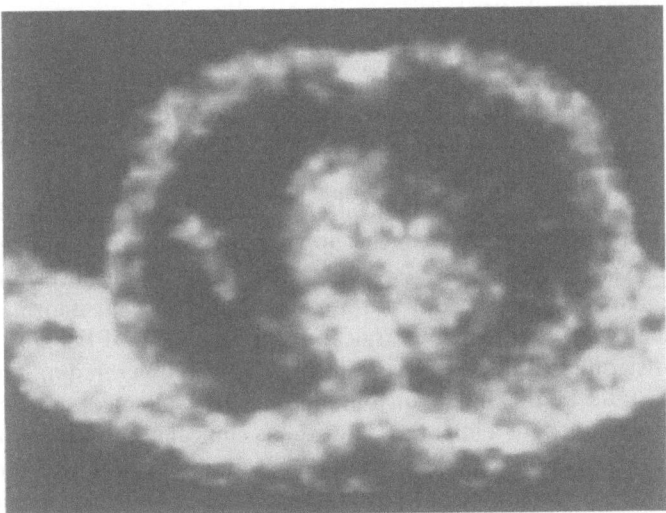

Fig. 2. PET study of the same patient as in Fig. 1 at the same level. The soft tissue mass shows an intense uptake as a sign of metabolic active tissue. The uptake on quantification is above the expected level for scar tissue

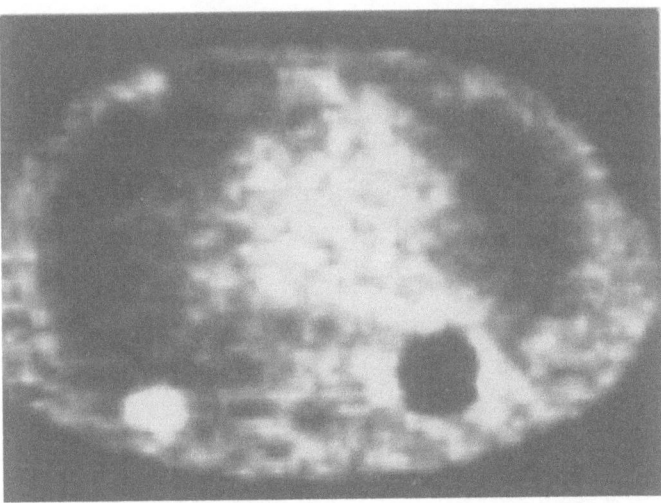

Fig. 3. PET study of a patient with a primary radiated adenocarcinoma of the left lung. The intense accumulation in the mass in the right lung in the PET image is a sign of metastatic lesion. The intense uptake at the edges of the tumor in the left lung are signs of renewed active tumor tissue at the edges of that lesion

45-year-old man with primary unresectable adenocarcinoma of the left lung. The tumor in the left lung was initially treated with radiotherapy. On follow-up studies 6 months after conclusion of the radiotherapeutic protocol a soft-tissue mass was seen in the right lung. A CT scan showed this 1.5-cm round soft tissue mass. The PET scan at the same level showed an intense uptake within this margin; the SUV of 3.0 indicated a malignant lesion. The primary tumor in the left lung showed no significant different areas of soft-tissue masses on CT scan. The PET image gave a quite different perspective of the metabolic state of this region. while no metabolic activity was found within this irradiated lesion, intense uptake was seen at the edges, which is a sign of still active tumor tissue. Clinical follow-up of this patient confirmed the contralateral metastasis as well as an active rest tumor growing at the edges of this treated lesion.

The next patient is a 33-year-old woman with a Hodgkin lymphoma (Fig. 4) who presented with a soft-tissue mass in the upper right lobe. On follow-up studies an increase in size of this mass was seen, leading to the strong suspicion of metastatic malignancy. Bronchoscopy did not reveal any relevant information, and the patient was scheduled for surgical intervention. The PET study (Fig. 5) showed no significant uptake within this region, thereby excluding the possibility of metastatic lesion. Based on our findings, the planned surgical intervention was rescheduled for a later time, awaiting a clinical improvement of these findings. The patient was treated with an intense antibiotic regimen, and follow-up plain film studies revealed a complete disappearance of the soft-tissue mass. This case clearly demonstrates an important application in the exclusion of malignancy.

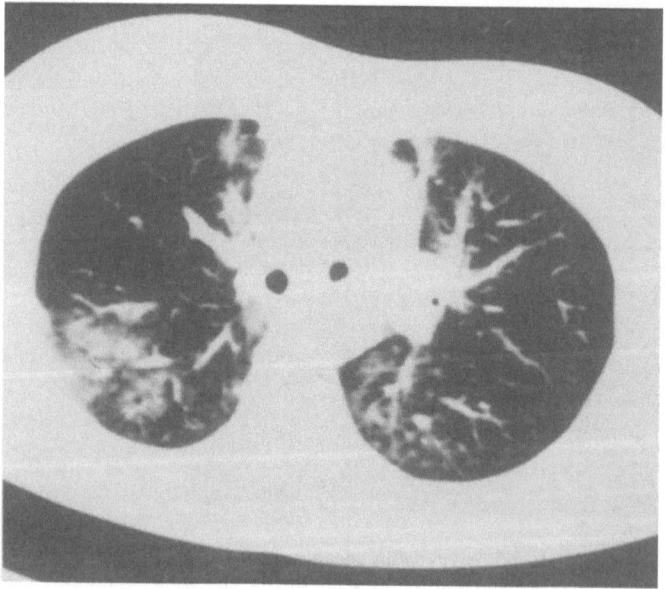

Fig. 4. CT of a patient with Hodgkin lymphoma presenting infiltrative masses in the right lung

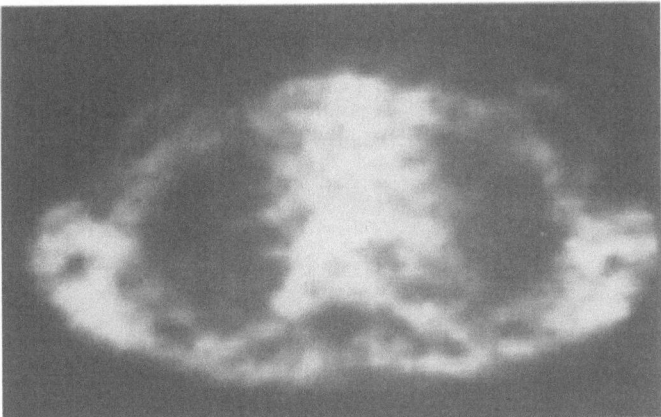

Fig. 5. PET image of the patient in Fig. 4 at the same level shows no increased uptake within the soft-tissue masses in the right lung. Thereby a metastatic process could be excluded

Conclusion

The follow-up of patients after therapy for thoracic lesions either by surgical resection, radiation, or chemotherapy should include plain film, CT, and MRI as necessary. Equivocal findings with these techniques can be evaluated by PET using FDG, thereby enabling the detection of recurrent malignancy. Whereas small lesions can be considered diagnostic only in cases of intense uptake as a sign of malignancy, borderline uptake may be due to malignant lesions with partial volume or motion artifacts as well as benign processes such as scar tissue or inflammatory processes. We conclude that FDG PET is a new diagnostic technique for the detection or exclusion of malignant tumor recurrence.

References

1. Gallagher BM, Fowler JS, Gutterson NI, MacGregor RR, Wan CN, Wolf AP (1978) Metabolic trapping as a principle of radiopharmaceutical design: some factors responsible for the biodistribution of F-18-2-deoxy-2-fluoro-D-glucose. J Nucl Med 19: 1154–1161
2. Knopp MV, Strauss LG, Dimitrakopoulou A, Haberkorn U, Blatter J, van Kaick G (1990) Positron emission tomography for the diagnostic work up in thoracic oncology. In: Schmidt HAE, van der School JB (eds) Nuklearmedizin. HAE Schattauer, Stuttgartt, pp 58–60
3. Kubota K, Matsuzawa T, Fujiwara T, Ito M, Hatazawa J, Ishiwata K, Iwata R, Ido T (1990) Differential diagnosis of lung tumor with positron emission tomography: a prospective study. J Nucl Med 31: 1927–1933
4. Kuebler WK, Ostertag H, Hoverath H, Doll J, Ziegler S, Lorenz WJ (1988) Scatter suppression by using a rotating pin source in PET transmission measurements. IEEE Trans Nucl 35: 749–752

5. Lewitt R, Muehllehner G (1986) Accelerated iterative reconstruction for positron emission tomography based on the EM algorithm for maximum likelihood estimation. IEEE Trans Med Imaging 5: 16–22
6. Ostertag H, Kuebler WK, Doll J, Schmidlin P, Clorius JH, Strauss LG, Maier-Borst W, Lorenz WJ (1988) A new dual crystal whole-body positron camera. System description initial results. In: Schmidt (ed) Nuklearmedizin. Schattauer, Stuttgart, pp 7–10

High-Resolution Computed Tomography for Detecting Lung Tissue Damage After Radiotherapy of Mammary Carcinoma

B. Allgayer, O. Wittmann, A. Heuck, K. Mühlbauer, L. Hölzer-Müller, and K. Brandstetter

Introduction

In the treatment of breast cancer, damage to pulmonary parenchyma is a well-known side effect of chest-wall irradiation. Radiation-induced changes are usually not visible in plain chest radiographs until 1 month after the end of radiation therapy (RT) [1, 3]. Alterations are rarely seen with doses below 20 Gy; as a rule, they appear if more than 60 Gy are administered [3]. Compared with plain films, computed tomography (CT) demonstrates lung tissue damage with higher accuracy [1]. Lung tissue density changes can be quantified [4, 6].

New developments in CT of the lung, such as the high-resolution technique, provide improved visualization of pulmonary structures. The following study was designed to show whether high-resolution CT(HR-CT) detects damage to lung tissue in breast cancer patients earlier than conventional CT. Additionally, the role of densitometric measurements in HR-CT was assessed in comparison to visual quantification of radiation-induced damage.

Materials and Methods

A total of 25 patients with breast cancer (mean age 59.5 years) were evaluated. Of these, 14 patients had undergone mastectomy, and 11 had had conservative surgery (i.e., tumorectomy plus axillary dissection). Adjuvant chemotherapy was performed in three patients. Irradiation to the chest wall was given by opposed portals with a dose of 50 Gy (after mastectomy) or 56 Gy (after conservative surgery). Irradiation to supraclavicular, axillar, and sternal fields was administered additionally, relative to the location of the primary tumor.

CT was performed in maximal inspiration using a Somatom Plus scanner (Siemens, Erlangen, FRG). Scanning was planned with a scout view, starting at the posterior end of the first rib. Ten scans with a slice thickness of 10 mm were acquired and reconstructed with a normal algorithm. In the middle of each

Technische Universität München, Klinikum rechts der Isar, 8000 Munich 80, FRG

Advanced Radiation Therapy Tumor Response
Monitoring and Treatment Planning
Breit (Editor-in-Chief)
© Springer-Verlag, Berlin Heidelberg 1992

10-mm slice, a scan with 1 mm thickness was obtained and reconstructed with a special algorithm [4]. Respiratory gating was not used.

CT-scans before RT, immediately after completion of RT, and 4–6 weeks and 7–12 weeks after completion of RT were compared. CT scans were categorized visually as:

– Grade 0 = no changes
– Grade I = slight changes (such as small pleural nodules)
– Grade II = medium to major pathologic changes

Densitometric measurements were performed in five patients with no visible changes, five patients with grade I or grade II changes were evaluated by means of a semiautomatic algorithm [4]. This algorithm detects the outline of the lung and provides equal area segmentation. Average Hounsfield density is expressed by area.

Results

One week after completion of RT, 20 patients were examined. Ten-millimeter conventional CT scans showed no changes in 19 patients (95%) versus 18 patients (90%) with HR-CT. Subsequently, 4–6 weeks after RT, nine patients were examined. Four patients showed no changes in normal CT (44%) and two in HR-CT. Grade I changes were found in two patients (22%) by normal CT and in four patients (44%) with HR-CT. Grade II changes were demonstrated in three patients (33%) with both normal CT and HR-CT. Then, 7–12 weeks after RT, 11 patients were examined. No changes were found in four patients (36%), grade I changes in five patients (45%) and grade II changes in two patients (18%). There was no difference between normal CT and HR-CT.

An early case (a patient from the group examined 1 week after RT) showed discrete pleural nodules in HR-CT. Plain chest film and normal CT did not reveal these changes (Fig. 1). In the cases with grade II changes, patchy consolidation with linear and streaky densities were found in normal CT and HR-CT. In HR-CT, the irradiated areas in which identification of lobules was possible showed a perilobular, a bronchovascular, and a pleural distribution of changes.

In ten patients, the mean lung density and the standard deviation of the pixel values was determined in the anterior quarter of the irradiated lung in comparison to the contralateral side. This was done in normal CT and HR-CT slices (Fig. 2). In patients with positive radiological findings (CT and HR-CT), the mean lung density of the anterior segments was increased. The difference between the mean lung density in areas with and without radiological findings was statistically significant ($p < 0.001$).

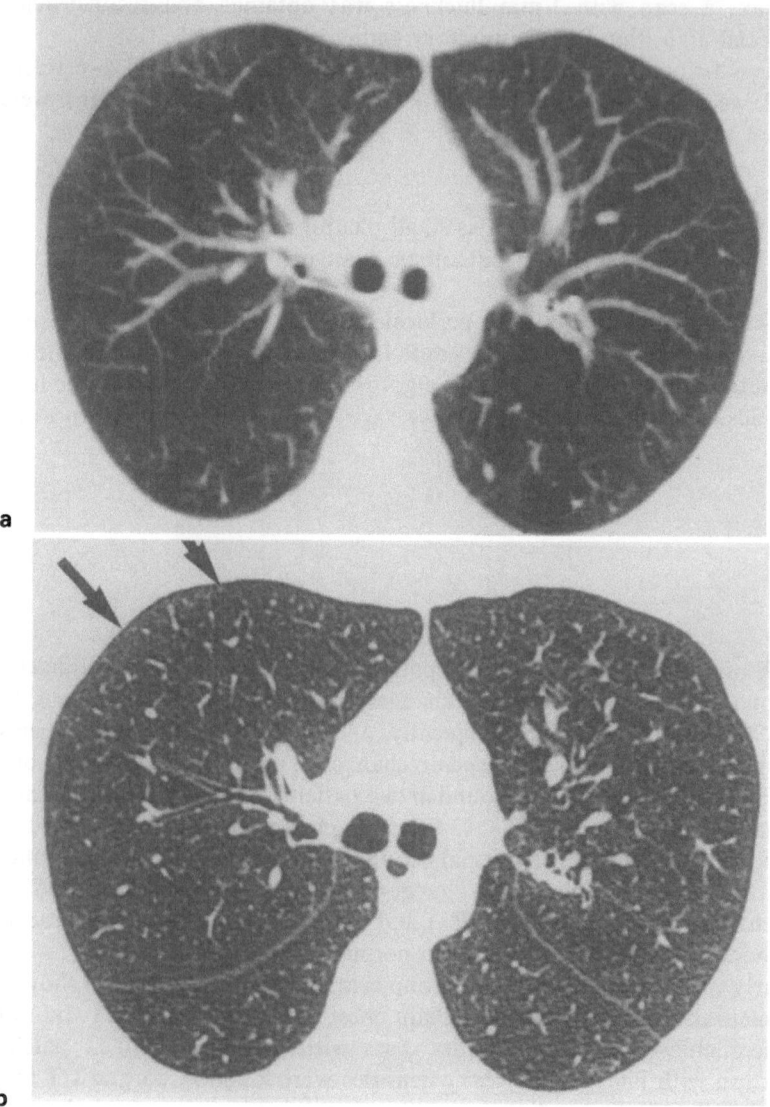

Fig. 1a,b. Examination of a 48-year-old patient (C.G) 1 week after radiotherapy. **a** Normal computed tomography, no pathologic finding. **b** High-resolution computed tomography, small pleural nodules (*arrows*) were found

Discussion

RT in patients for the treatment of breast cancer is usually followed with plain chest radiographs. Recent publications show that CT has a higher sensitivity in the detection of radiation-induced lung damage than conventional X-ray. Lung

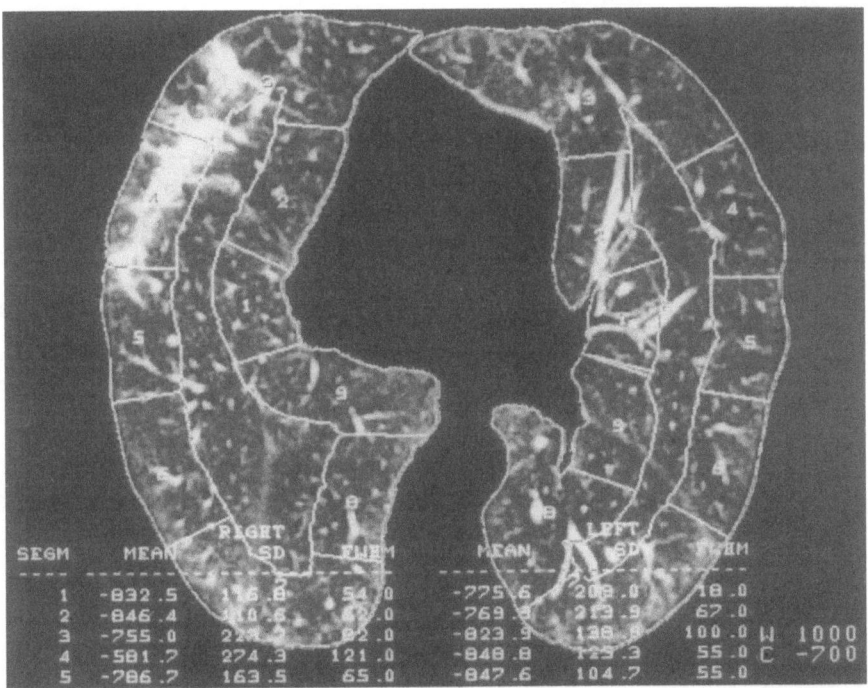

Fig. 2. Regional lung evaluation in a 43-year-old patient (H.F.) 12 weeks after radiotherapy. Central and peripheral regions of interest are defined. Right region 4 shows several areas of damage (HE − 581.7; SD 274.3). Left contralateral region 4 shows no damage (HE − 848.8; SD 129.3)

damage may be present in the absence of radiologically obvious findings. HR-CT slices allow the identification of lung lobules and interlobular septa [5]. The classification of pulmonary parenchymal abnormalities is based on the lobular distribution and categorized in centrilobular, panlobular, and bronchovascular. In our patients with severe lung damage, the identification of the lobular structures was not possible. In lung areas with minor changes, we found a perilobular, a bronchovascular, and a pleural distribution in HR-CT. In one patient, pleural reaction was only detected in HR-CT, while findings were normal in chest films and conventional CT. In all patients with visually demonstrable changes in normal and HR-CT, densitometric differences were found. In our small series, it was not possible to detect densitometric differences when no visible changes were present. HR-CT seems to be the most sensitive method for early detection of lung tissue damage in radiotherapy for breast cancer.

References

1. Ikezoe Y, Takashima S, Shizno M et al. (1988) CT appearance of acute radiation — induced injury in the lung. AJR 150: 765–770
2. Roswit B, White DC (1977) Severe radiation injuries of the lung. AJR 129: 127–136
3. Libshitz HI, Brosof AB, Southard ME (1973) Radiographic appearance of the chest following extended field radiation therapy for Hodgkin's disease. A consideration of time–dose relationships. Cancer 32: 205–215
4. Kalender WA, Fichte H, Bautz W, Skalej M (1991) Semiautomatic evaluation procedures for quantitative CT of the lung, J Comput Assist Tomogr 15(2): 248–255
5. Murata K, Khan A, Herman PG (1989) Pulmonary parenchymal disease. Evaluation with high-resolution CT. Radiology 170: 629–635
6. Rotstein S, Lax I, Svane G (1990) Influence of radiation therapy on the lung-tissue in breast cancer patients: CT-assessed density changes and associated symptoms. J Radiat Oncol Biol Phys 18: 173–180

[18F]fluorodeoxyglucose Uptake
for the Measurement of Metabolic Therapy Effects
in a Mammary Carcinoma Model

U. Haberkorn[1], L.G. Strauss[1], S. Ziegler[1], M. Reinhard[1], M.R. Berger[1], D. Haag[2], V. Rudat[1], A. Dimitrakopoulou[1], and G. van Kaick

Introduction

The advantages of ether lipids are their relatively low systemic toxicity and their suitability for oral application [1]. In a clinical phase I study, hexadecyl-phosphocholine (HPC) was found to be effective in the topical treatment of skin metastases of breast cancer [2]. It is suggested that HPC is metabolized by phospholipase C to its active form [3]. However, the exact mechanism of action is not known. We performed in vivo studies of glucose uptake before and after therapy in a mammary carcinoma model to assess drug-induced changes in the glucose metabolism of these tumors.

Materials and Methods

Female Sprague-Dawley rats were kept under conventional controlled conditions. Mammary carcinomas were induced according to Berger et al. [4] by three intravenous injections of methylnitrosourea (MNU) into the tail vein on days 50, 71, and 92 of life. The rats were weighted and palpated twice weekly beginning 6 weeks after the first injection of MNU to observe tumor manifestation. We used two different doses for the treatment: 100 mg/kg HPC in group 1 ($n = 9$) and 200 mg/kg HPC in group 2 ($n = 3$). The drug was given orally after baseline measurement with FDG.

Only animals with tumor diameters above 2 cm were accepted for examination by positron emission tomography (PET). After premedication with ketamine the animals were kept in an inhalation narcosis comprising halothane, nitrous oxide, and oxygen during the examination. The PET studies were performed with a PC2048-7WB scanner (Scanditronix, Sweden) after administration of 1–2 mCi FDG in a permanent catheter positioned in the jugular vein.

[1] Department of Radiology of Pathophysiology and Institute of Chemotherapy and Experimental Toxicology, German Cancer Research Center, Im Neuenheimer Feld 280, 6900 Heidelberg, FRG
[2] Department of Pathology, University of Heidelberg, Im Neuenheimer Feld 400, 6900 Heidelberg, FRG

Advanced Radiation Therapy Tumor Response
Monitoring and Treatment Planning
Breit (Editor-in-Chief)
© Springer-Verlag, Berlin Heidelberg 1992

Prior to the FDG measurement 10 mCi ^{15}O-labeled water was given to study the tumor perfusion. The perfusion study was done during the first 5 min after bolus injection with seven acquisitions. Thereafter the FDG uptake was measured over 60 min (five 1-min and eight 5-min acquisitions). Prior to PET a transmission scan was performed.

PET images (average slice thickness 11 mm) were generated by use of an iterative reconstruction program [5] on a VAX 11/750 computer system. The image matrix was 256×256. The pixel size in all reconstructed images was 2×2 mm (spatial resolution 5.1 mm). The images were corrected for attenuation and scatter. For quantitative evaluation, regions of interest were defined in the tumors with a region size exceeding 32 pixels in all cases. FDG uptake was then expressed as the standardized uptake value (SUV): SUV = tissue concentration/[injected dose (nCi)/body weight (g)]. The same ROIs were used for the ^{15}O-labeled water and the FDG images. Tumor perfusion was evaluated using the image 5 min after bolus injection of ^{15}O-labeled water, while the 10-min image 60 min after FDG application was used for the evaluation of glucose uptake.

Tumor samples were taken from the six animals in group 1 which had PET follow-up studies and from three tumors in an untreated animal. Thereafter suspensions of cell nuclei were prepared with scissors and 0.5% pepsin in 0.9% saline after acidification with 0.25% hydrochloric acid. The homogenate was supplemented with 2 ml pepsin solution and whirled 5 min at room temperature. After sedimentation, 0.1–0.5 ml of the supernatant was injected into 8 ml of a fluorocytochrome solution (4,6-diamidino-a-phenylinode, DAPI). The nuclear DAPI fluorescence was then measured after 30 min with an IPC 22 pulse cytophotometer (Phywe, Göttingen, FRG) with a UG1 and KV550 filter combination. A total amount of 25 000 pulses was measured for each probe. The display and storation used a multichannel analyzer (MCA 8100, Canberra Industries, Meriden, CT). The analysis of the DNA histograms was performed graphically after correction of the superimposed background [6].

Results

Baseline measurements were carried out in all animals. Follow-up studies were evaluable in seven rats (six of group 1, one of group 2) 24 h and in six rats (group 1) 1 week after therapy. In group 2 two animals died due to side effects. In one animal of this group we observed a decrease in FDG (50%) and in ^{15}O-labeled water (30%) activity 1 day after therapy. Figure 1 shows the time-activity curves of three tumors in the same animal prior to therapy. In one of the tumors (number 1) an increase in FDG accumulation was seen during the examination time, whereas number 2 decreased, and number 3 remained stable. The S-phase fractions in tumor numbers 1 and 2 were identical (2.4%), whereas the amount of S-phase cells was comparatively low in tumor number 3 (1.1%). In Fig. 2 the

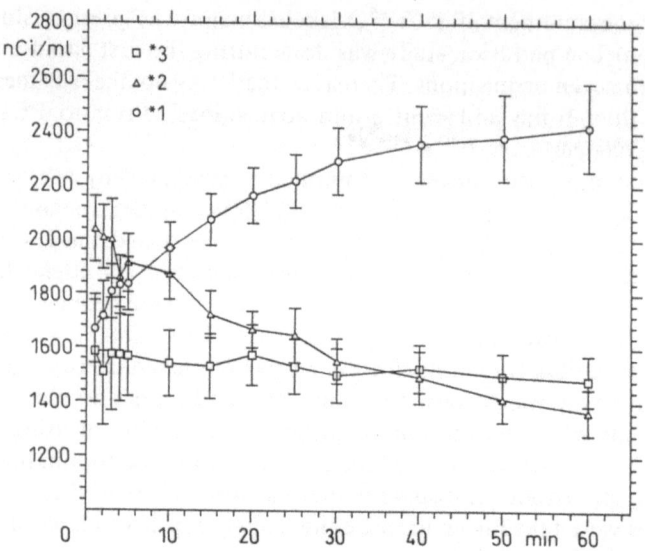

Fig. 1. Time-activity curves for the uptake of FDG (nCi/ml) in three tumors of a single animal before therapy

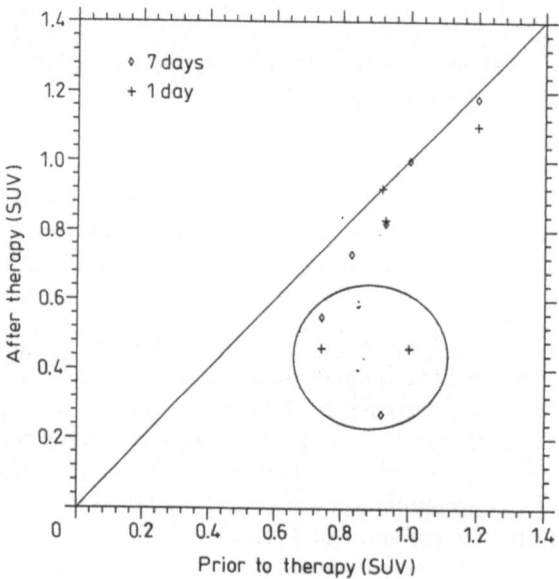

Fig. 2. Changes in the regional FDG uptake (SUV) prior to and 1 day and 1 week after therapy

FDG uptake before and 1 day and 7 days after therapy in group 1 is demonstrated. Only 30% showed a decrease in FDG accumulation. This effect was observed on day 1 and lasted until day 7. The FDG uptake 7 days after therapy was correlated with the proliferative index ($r = 0.77$).

Discussion

HPC is a new drug with a variety of biological properties. Some of the proposed mechanisms are interaction and incorporation in cell membranes and partial restructuring of the chromatin which may contribute to an inhibition of the DNA synthesis [7]. Interaction with the cell membrane and inhibition of DNA replication are likely to influence transport processes such as that of glucose. Therefore we conducted this study to measure early and later effects of HPC on glucose uptake. One interesting finding is that different tumors in the same animal can behave differently with respect to FDG uptake during the examination time. The best explanation for the behavior of tumor number 1 (Fig. 1) is that this tumor differs from the others in its hexokinase activity. Differences are observed not only with respect to metabolism; the tumors may also show a difference in the S-phase fractions. Chemically induced autochthonous mammary carcinomas are also inhomogeneous with respect to morphology and malignancy when appearing at different sites [8]. This may also explain the second finding: a decrease in FDG uptake was found in group 1 in only two cases. This decrease occurred on the 1st day after therapy. Abe et al. made similar observations in a mammary model under radiotherapy [9]; in their study a decrease was found 1–2 days after radiation. Finally, the correlation of FDG uptake with the proliferation rate 7 days after therapy is consistent with the proposed interaction of the drug with the DNA replication.

These preliminary results of our ongoing study show that metabolic changes due to therapy can be measured with PET at a very early stage before morphologic changes occur. In group 2 only one animal could be evaluated 1 day after therapy. However, we observed a marked decrease in FDG accumulation, indicating that the metabolic alterations depend on the dose. Differences in the metabolic behavior prior to and also after therapy may be due to the heterogeneity of these chemically induced tumors. Since 50% of them show alterations in *ras* oncogene expression, oncogene-induced changes may contribute to the observed effects. This is now under research in our institute. Moreover, the animal model allows study of the meaning of resting activity in a treated tumor by histologic examination.

References

1. Fleer EAM (1988) Ether lipids and analogues. J Cancer Res Clin Oncol 114: 655–656
2. Unger C, Eibl H, Breiser A, von Heyden HW, Engel J, Hilgard P, Sindermann H, Peukert M, Nagel GA (1988) Hexadecylphosphocholine (D18506) in the topical treatment of skin metastases: a phase-I trial. Onkologie 11: 295–296
3. Berger MR, Muschiol C, Schmähl D, Eibl HJ (1987) New cytostatics with experimentally different toxic profiles. Cancer Treat Rev 14: 307–317
4. Berger MR, Habs M, Schmähl D (1983) Non-carcinogenic chemotherapy with a combination of vincristine, methotrexate and 5-fluorouracil (VMF) in rats. Int J Cancer 32: 231–236
5. Schmidlin P, Kübler WK, Doll J, Strauss LG, Ostertag H (1987) Image processing in whole body positron emission tomography. In: Schmidt HAE, Csernay L (eds) Nuklearmedizin. Schattauer, Stuttgart, pp 84–87
6. Haag D, Feichter G, Goerttler K, Kaufmann M (1987) Influence of systematic errors on the evaluation of the S phase portions from DNA distributions of solid tumors as shown for 328 breast carcinomas. Cytometry 8: 377–385
7. Hochhuth C, Berkovic D, Eibl H, Unger C, Doenecke D (1987) Effects of antineoplastic phospholipids on parameters of cell differentiation in U937 cells. J Cancer Res Clin Oncol 116: 459–456
8. Scherf HR, Schuler B, Berger MR, Schmähl D (1987) Therapeutic activity of ET-18-OCH3 and hexadecylphosphocholine against mammary tumors in BD-VI rats. Lipids 22: 927–929
9. Abe Y, Matsuzawa T, Fujiwara T, Fukuda H, Itoh M, Yamada K, Yamaguchi K, Sato T, Ido T (1986) Assessment of radiotherapeutic effects on experimental tumors using 18F-2-fluoror-2-deoxy-D-glucose. Eur J Nucl Med 12: 325–328

Intraarterial Dynamic Computed Tomography of Tumor Perfusion Before Regional Chemotherapy Combined with Simultaneous Radiotherapy in Lung and Breast Cancers

A. Rieber[1], H.-J. Brambs[1], M. Wannenmacher[2], and P. Drings[3]

Introduction

Dynamic computed tomographic (CT) scans obtained after an intraarterial bolus of contrast media are used increasingly in the diagnosis of liver metastases because this method has a higher sensitivity than CT after an intravenous bolus of contrast media [2–4]. For this the angiographic catheter is placed in the superior mesenteric, splenic, or proper hepatic artery, and CT scans are performed after an intraarterial bolus of contrast media of several milliliters for each scan [3, 4]. The intraarterial angiographic CT allows an evaluation of the vascularization of the tumor [1].

We performed this method in eight patients with inoperable bronchogenic carcinoma and eight patients with breast cancer. These patients were treated with combined intraarterial chemotherapy and radiotherapy. The aim of the intraarterial angiographic CT was: (a) determination of whether the tumor is perfused completely or only partially by intraarterial chemotherapy, and (b) control of whether healthy tissue is perfused by intraarterial chemotherapy after superselective placement of the angiographic catheter.

Materials and Methods

The angiographies were performed transfemorally in the Seldinger technique in all patients. Eight patients had an inoperable non-small-cell lung carcinoma. The tumor-feeding artery was probed with a 5-F catheter. In coaxial technique a 3-F catheter was placed peripherad to avoid a perfusion of intercostal artery and healthy lung tissue. In the eight patients with breast cancer the internal

[1] Abteilung für Radiologische Diagnostik, Radiologische Universitätsklinik, Hoppe-Seyler-Str. 3, 7400 Tübingen, FRG
[2] Abteilung für Klinische Radiologie, Radiologische Universitätsklinik, Im Neuenheimer Feld 400, 6900 Heidelberg, FRG
[3] Abteilung für Onkologie, Thoraxklinik der LVA Baden, Amalienstr. 5, 6900 Heidelberg-Rohrbach, FRG

Advanced Radiation Therapy Tumor Response
Monitoring and Treatment Planning
Breit (Editor-in-Chief)
© Springer-Verlag, Berlin Heidelberg 1992

mammary artery was probed with a 5-F catheter. The coaxial catheter was placed peripherad to avoid a backward flow in the subclavian artery. To reduce the flow off, the internal mammary artery was occluded distad with particles of Gelfoam in three patients. The intraarterial angiographic CT was of the pathologic region with a slice thickness of 9 mm. There was given 1–3 ml of contrast media through the coaxial catheter for each scan. The chemotherapy was performed after the angiographic CT.

Results

The superselective probing of the tumor-feeding artery was possible in all cases. Two patients with bronchogenic carcinoma had hypovascular tumors, and the others were hypervascular. The hypovascular tumors showed only a sparse contrast enhancement in angiographic CT in correlation with the angiographic findings. The tumor response did not depend on the degree of vascularization. Two patients showed a partial deficiency in angiographic CT, which suggested a second tumor-feeding artery (Fig. 1a). This suspicion was confirmed in a second angiography (Fig. 1b). The second cycle of chemotherapy was therefore infused in this artery.

The perfusion of healthy lung tissue was reduced, that of segments of the esophagus could be avoided. Four patients with breast cancer or recurrence of breast cancer showed very hypervascular tumors in angiography and CT (Fig. 2). Four cancers had poor vascularization and showed a contrast enhancement in CT of 40%.

A punctual embolization distad to the tumor was performed in three patients to reduce the flow off of the cytostatic agents. The cytostatic drug was infused superselectively into a branch of the internal mammary artery in two patients. The tumor response also did not depend on the degree of vascularization in breast cancers. Thus there was no correlation between contrast enhancement in angiographic CT and tumor response.

Discussion

An important hypothesis in oncology is that tumor response depends on the concentration of cytostatic agent in the tumor [6, 7]. Systemic chemotherapy is limited by its toxicity to healthy cells. The aim of regional chemotherapy is to reach a higher concentration and dose of cytostatic agent in the tumor and to reduce the overall dose in the organism. The expectation is to improve the tumor response and reduce systemic side effects [6, 7].

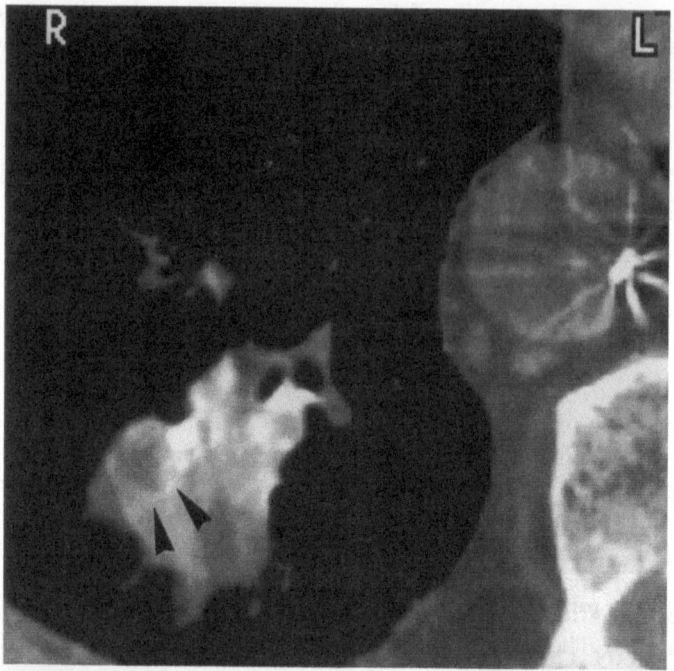

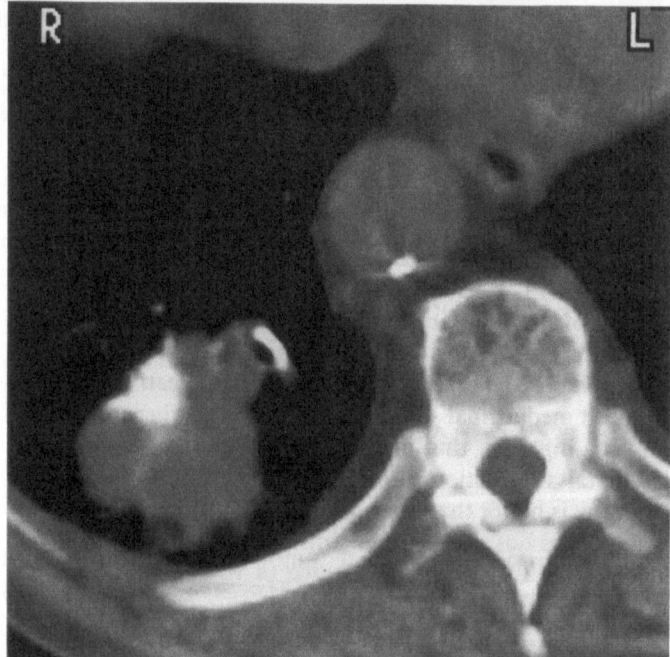

Fig. 1a, b. Angiographic CT of a patient with bronchogenic carcinoma. a The noncontrasted area suggests a second tumor-feeding artery. b A second image verifies the existence of the second tumor-feeding artery

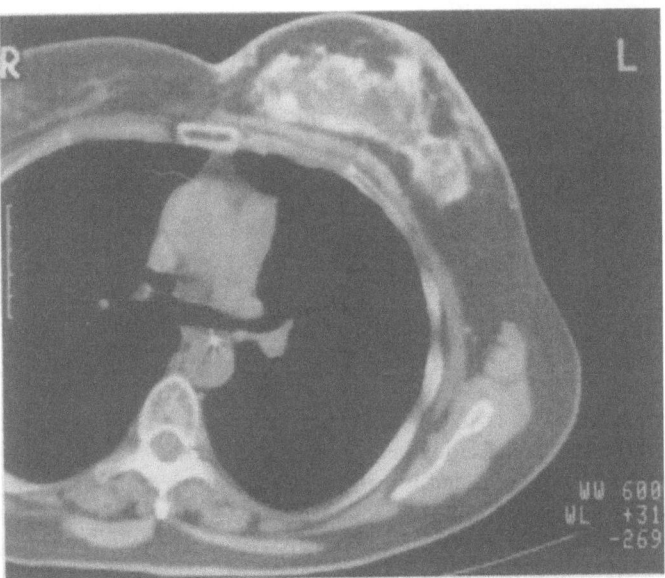

Fig. 2. Angiographic CT of a patient with breast cancer

The development of new catheter techniques allows superselective intra-arterial perfusion. Angiography shows only insufficiently whether the probed artery feeds only the tumor or healthy tissue as well. Breast cancers and recurrences are fed by arteries. Superselective digital subtraction angiography usually demonstrates a high contrast enhancement of the tumor. If it is impossible or inconvenient to probe superselectively a branch of the internal mammary artery, punctual embolization of the artery should be performed distad to the tumor to reduce the flow off of the cytostatic agent. The punctual embolization leads to a collateralization distal to the occlusion.

The following angiography CT demonstrates the extension of the tumor and its perfusion. Metastases of the lung are fed by pulmonary arteries; however, central bronchogenic cancers are fed by one or two bronchial arteries [4, 5]. In this region the angiographic catheter must be placed superselectively because these arteries can also feed mediastinal structures, the intercostal space, and the vertebral canal. There is a high risk that mediastinal or vertebral branches are not noticed even in digital subtraction angiography. The tumor response to intraarterial chemotherapy is better than that to intravenous infusion. But until now the influence on survival has not been established [4, 5].

Intraarterial angiographic CT shows the degree of vascularization of the tumor, but it does not allow a conclusion concerning the intracellular uptake or metabolism of the cytostatic agent [1]. In our experience hypovascular and hypervascular tumors of the lung and the breast show the same tumor response.

The method demonstrates whether all parts of the tumor can be reached potentially by the cytostatic agents. Deficiencies in the contrast CT suggest a second tumor-feeding artery. This must be detected in a second angiography and perfused cytostatically to avoid local recurrences [4]. If there is also healthy tissue contrasted in angiographic CT, the angiographic coaxial catheter is not placed sufficiently superselectively. In this case the angiographic catheter must be corrected before chemotherapy is started. This is very important especially in lung cancers to avoid complications such as paraplegia and perforations of the esophagus.

Conclusions

Intraarterial angiographic CT is performed only as an additional diagnostic method in the detection of liver lesions because it has a higher sensitivity than intravenous contrast CT. In a planned intraarterial chemotherapy this method allows control and correcting of the catheter placement. A second tumor-feeding artery can be detected, and the perfusion of healthy tissue can be avoided. An estimation of the expected effect of the therapy is not possible because the contrast media has a completely different metabolism than the cytostatic agent.

References

1. Flentje M, Hohenberger P, Adolph J, Kober B (1986) Intraarterielle dynamische Computertomographie in der Charakterisierung von Lebermetastasen kolorektaler Karzinome. Fortschr Geb Rontgenstr 145/3: 263–267
2. Köster O, Harder Th, Steudel A, Sommer H-J (1989) CT-Portographie bei malignen Raumforderungen der Leber. Fortschr Geb Rontgenstr 150/2: 156–162
3. Moss AA, Dean PB, Axel L, Goldberg HI, Glazer GM, Friedman MA (1982) Dynamic CT of hepatic masses with intravenous and intraarterial contrast material. AJR 138: 847–852
4. Nelson RC, Chezmar JL, Sugarbaker PH, Bernardino ME (1989) Hepatic tumors: comparison of CT during arterial portography, delayed CT, and MR imaging for preoperative evaluation. Radiology 172: 27–34
5. Müller H, Walther H, Aigner KR (1988) Regional chemotherapy of lung tumors and metastases. Reg Cancer Treat 1: 44–49
6. Schlag P, Hohenberger P (1988) Regionale Chemotherapie von Lebertumoren — eine Situationsanalyse. Chirurg 59: 218–224
7. Stephens FO (1988) Why use regional chemotherapy? Principles and pharmacokinetics. Reg Cancer Treat 1: 4–10.

Tumor Response Monitoring: Abdomen

Evaluation of Regional Processing of Chemotherapy in Patients with Metastatic Colorectal Cancer

A. Desllaugiers, J. Doesallaeg, J. Morderkes, M. V. Ismar, M. Sallies,
J.H. Oosterm, P. Robert and W.J. Mook

Introduction

Materials and methods

Evaluation of Regional Fluorouracil Chemotherapy in Patients with Metastatic Colorectal Cancer

A. Dimitrakopoulou, L.G. Strauss, U. Haberkorn, M.V. Knopp, P. Schlag, H. Ostertag, F. Helus, and W.J. Lorenz

Introduction

The standard chemotherapeutic agent for the treatment of hepatic metastases from colorectal cancer is 5-fluorouracil (FU) [1]. Depending on both the selection process and the response criteria used, the reported response rates have varied from 8% to 82% [1]. Based on a literature survey, Kemeny reported that the average response rate for hepatic metastases is 23%. Therefore, the regional administration of FU has found use for improving the selectivity of the cytostatic drug [2]. Theoretically, regional delivery can potentially increase drug concentrations at tumor sites and lower systemic drug exposure when compared with systemic drug administration. We examined patients with ^{18}F-labeled FU and positron emission tomography (PET) to obtain quantitative data about the distribution pattern of FU and metabolites in metastases, normal liver parenchyma, and aorta as a function of time. Furthermore, ^{15}O-labeled water was used to determine the relative perfusion of the lesions, and we compared the absorption of the non-metabolized tracer with the metabolized cytostatic drug. Our primary goal was to evaluate the tracer concentrations following intravenous and intraarterial infusion of FU. Furthermore, we compared the change in perfusion due to regional administration with the altered FU accumulation.

Materials and Methods

We report on the evaluation of 26 examinations in 13 patients after intravenous and intraarterial tracer administration. All patients had surgically implanted catheters in the gastroduodenal artery. Patients were examined prior to the first chemotherapeutic cycle or at least 1 week following the last FU administration in the drug-free interval of the chemotherapeutic cycle.

Liver metastases were diagnosed prior to referral to the PET examination. Computed tomography (CT; Somatom DRH, Siemens) immediately preceeded

German Cancer Research Center, Im Neuenheimer Feld 280, 6900 Heidelberg, FRG

Advanced Radiation Therapy Tumor Response
Monitoring and Treatment Planning
Breit (Editor-in-Chief)
© Springer-Verlag, Berlin Heidelberg 1992

the PET examination and was used in each patient to identify the region of greatest metastasis diameter. Only patients who had at least one metastasis identified in two contiguous CT slices (8-mm slice thickness) were included in the study, due to the limited resolution of PET. Skin markings were used for proper positioning in PET, after the image level had been determined with CT. We used identical supports for CT and PET.

A PET scanner with two ring detectors (PC2048-7WB, Scanditronix) was used. This system provides for the acquisition of three slices simultaneously (two primary sections, one cross-section). Each of the two rings, 107 cm in diameter, contains 512 BGO/GSO detectors and provides field of view of 52 cm. Transmission scans with more than 15 million counts per section were obtained prior to the radio nuclide administration to obtain data for the attenuation correction of the acquired PET images.

Oxygen-15 was produced using the procedure described by Del Fiore [3]. We obtained ^{15}O-labeled water by bubbling O_2 through sterile physiologic saline. All patients were examined with ^{15}O-labeled water (1110–3700 MBq) prior to the FU infusion. Five 1-min images were acquired after the intravenous administration of ^{15}O-labeled water. A second tracer injection via the intra-arterial route was performed 10 min following the first series, and again five 1-min images were acquired.

$[^{18}F]FU$ was prepared by direct fluorination of uracil in acetic acid using $^{18}F_2$ diluted in neon [4]. Quality control included HPLC. $[^{18}F]$ FU (370–444 MBq) was given together with 500 mg unlabeled FU in a 12-min infusion using an infusion pump (Perfusor secura, Braun Melsungen) following the perfusion studies. Sequential images (typically 22 images) were acquired for 2 h after onset of FU infusion. Intravenous and intraarterial examinations were performed in each patient on different days.

PET cross-sections were generated using an iterative reconstruction program and a 128*128 matrix (interpolated to 256*256 for display, spatial resolution 5.1 mm). The transverse slices were compared to the corresponding CT images to permit certain identification of the lesions using anatomical landmarks. This was followed by a quantitative evaluation of the PET images, using a region-of-interest (ROI) technique. ROIs were placed over the metastases, normal liver parenchyma, and the aorta. Time-activity data were calculated from each image series for further evaluation. The standard uptake value (SUV) [5] was used to express tracer uptake: SUV = concentration (nCi/g) [injected dose (nCi)/body weight (g)].

SUV values for ^{15}O-labeled water were calculated from data obtained from the last of the five 1-min scans. The ^{18}F concentration values 2 h after FU infusion were used to compare the accumulation of the cytostatic agent. Furthermore, time-activity integrals (AUCs) were calculated from the FU data for all ROIs. The values of the aortic region were used as an estimate for the systemic toxicity.

Results

The FU metabolite concentrations 2 h after intravenous and intraarterial FU infusion are shown in Fig. 1. Higher tracer concentrations were obtained after regional application in 55% of the lesions. The change in lesion accessibility was higher than the change in FU accumulation (Fig. 2). We compared the increase in FU metabolite concentrations with the systemic toxicity (Fig. 3).

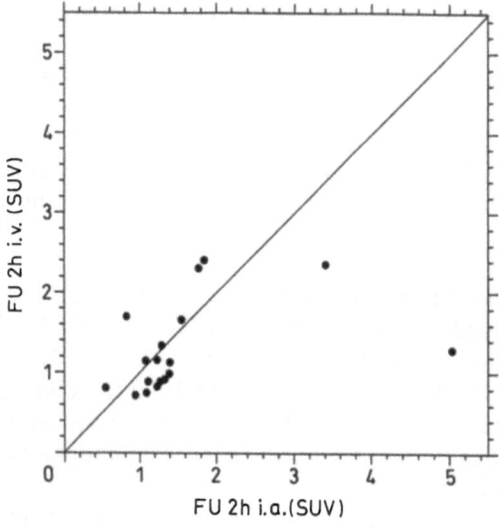

Fig. 1. FU metabolite concentrations 2 h after intravenous or intraarterial FU infusion in 13 patients (26 studies, 18 metastases). The regional administration resulted in enhanced metabolite concentrations in 10 of 18 metastatic lesions (55%)

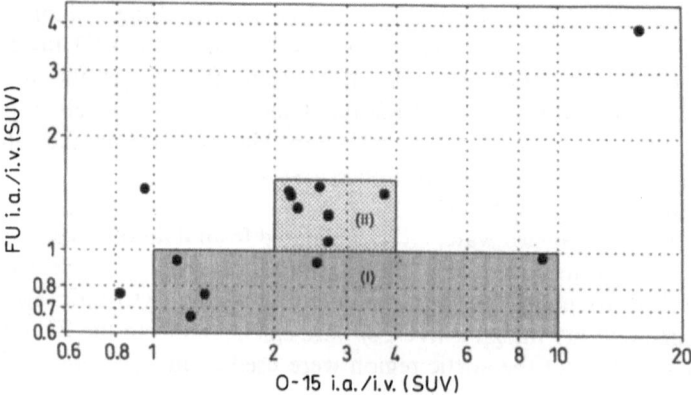

Fig. 2. Lesion accessibility versus FU metabolite concentrations. The improvement in perfusion resulted in a decrease of the FU metabolite concentrations in 5 (28%) of 18 metastases (*field I*), while in 7 lesions (39%) the FU metabolism was enhanced (<50%) by regional administration (*field II*)

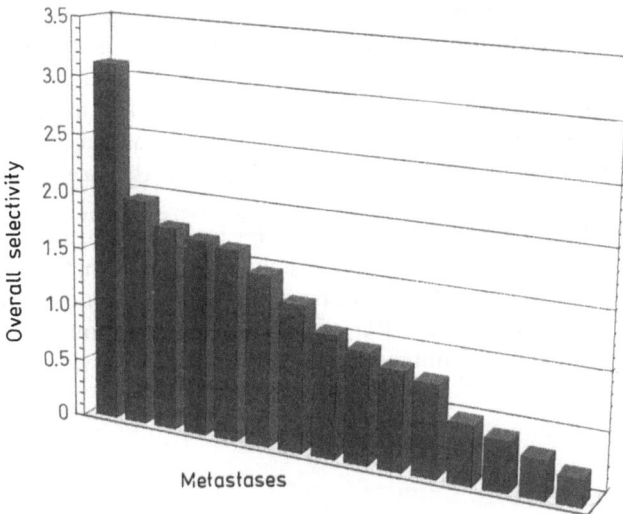

Fig. 3. The change in FU accumulation in the metastases and the change in the systematic toxicity were used to compare the systematic application with the regional infusion: overall selectivity = (^{18}F, metastasis, intraarterial/^{18}F, metastasis, intravenous)/(^{18}F, aorta, intraarterial/^{18}F, aorta, intravenous)

Discussion

Chemotherapy with FU has found extensive use since its introduction more than three decades ago. Since FU uptake in the malignancies is a prerequisite for therapy response, regional administration has found limited use for enhancing the drug exposure of the tumor. The primary goal is to convert some partial responses into complete responses and some minimal responses into at least partial responses [2]. We investigated both systemic and regional infusion of FU in 13 patients. The double examinations with the perfusion tracer ^{15}O-labeled water demonstrated that regional injection improved access to the lesions in 13 of 15 metastases, while the FU metabolite concentrations were enhanced in only nine metastases (Fig. 2). These results show that high tumor perfusion is not the only parameter for increased FU uptake in metastatic lesions. FU transport into the tumor cells, demonstrated by the PET images acquired shortly after the end of the FU infusion, may not be correlated with the perfusion. Furthermore, even a high FU transport into the cells is not necessarily followed by a high FU metabolism (obtained from PET images 2 h after FU infusion). We should emphasize that successful chemotherapy requires a preferential perfusion of a mass, a high FU transport into the tumor cells, and an increased metabolism of FU.

Tumor response to the FU chemotherapy can occur only when high metabolite concentrations are present in the lesions. We were able to demonstrate a significant response to FU chemotherapy in one case. The perfusion, FU transport, and metabolite concentrations were extremely high in this metastasis. The perfusion was enhanced by a factor of 16, while the FU metabolite concentrations were fourfold higher after regional FU infusion. The increased FU metabolite concentrations in the metastasis were associated with a twofold higher systemic toxicity as demonstrated by the AUCs for the aorta and vertebrae.

The PET studies with ^{15}O-labeled water and [^{18}F] FU demonstrate that regional drug administration does not necessarily enhance the FU metabolite concentrations. Since only some patients profit from this approach, individual measurements of tumor perfusion, and FU transport and metabolism are required to evaluate the possible advantage of regional chemotherapy.

References

1. Kemeny N (1983) The systemic chemotherapy of hepatic metastases. Semin Oncol 10: 148–158
2. Collins JM (1984) Pharmacologic rationale for regional drug delivery. J Clin Oncol 2: 498–504
3. Del Fiore F, Depresseux JC, Bartsch P, Quaglia L, Peters JM (1979) Production of oxygen-15, nitrogen-13 and carbon-11 and of their low molecular weight derivatives for biomedical applications. Int J Appl Radiat Isot 30: 543–549
4. Oberdorfer F, Hofmann E, Maier-Borst W (1989) Preparation of ^{18}F-labelled 5-fluorouracil of very high purity. J Labelled Compounds Radiopharmaceuticals 27: 137–145
5. Matsuzawa T, Fukuda H, Abe Y et al. (1985) Current and future aspects of cancer diagnosis with positron emission tomography: biological and clinical aspect. In: Matsuzawa T (ed) Proceedings of the international symposium on current and future aspects of cancer diagnosis with positron emission tomography. Tohuko University, Sendai, pp 1–23

Semiautomatic Tumor Volumetry of Liver Metastases for the Monitoring of Therapy

H. Daschner[1], B. Möller[2], A. Wunderlich[1], K. Lehner[1], and K. Brandstetter[1]

Volumetry of primary or secondary malignomas of the liver is difficult because there is no exact demarcation of the tumor from normal liver tissue. Moreover, there is a risk of superimposed scans due to irregular breathing. These two factors up to now have restricted the reproducibility of volumetry. Nevertheless, clinicians call for a method allowing the objective monitoring of chemo- or radiotherapy. There is a need especially to test the efficacy of new drugs.

We examined nine patients using the Siemens Somatom Plus over 1 year. They suffered from multiple metastases originating from colon or rectum carcinomas. These patients were inoperable and received chemotherapy with an investigative cytostatic agent in a phase II trial. Examinations using computed tomography were conducted every 1–3 months. In each examination two to four liver metastases were measured. First a native CT then a CT with intravenous contrast injection was performed. We injected 200 ml of a nonionic contrast medium over a definite time. The liver was scanned with 1-cm slice thickness and without a gap. The lesions had to have a minimum size of 1×1 cm. The demarcated liver metastases were evaluated by a region-of-interest (ROI) technique, either circle or ellipse, which could be enlarged or reduced. Another possibility was demarcation of the metastases by hand; this allowed best demarcation especially of irregular lesions. The circle was used in small and round metastases; the ellipse was used only seldom. The area of the ROI was calculated by computer and added to the scans above or below. This appeared in the left corner of the scan after a few seconds. To obtain the most objective comparison with the last CT examination it was essential to choose the same window. Besides the volume the number of liver metastases was a criterion.

Native CT scans showed very inaccurate demarcation of the metastases. The volumes calculated for one scan differed up to 100% (Fig. 1). Therefore it seems inappropriate to measure metastases in native CT. We should use the native CT, rather, to look for metastases masked in contrast enhanced CT. On the other hand, volumetry can be performed efficaciously in contrast-enhanced CT. Here we normally find an exact demarcation of the metastases from the surrounding liver tissue. One lesion we demarcated four times by hand; nevertheless we obtained volumes differing from each other by a maximum of only 10% (Fig. 2).

[1] Institut für Röntgendiagnostik, und
[2] Chirurgische Klinik-chirurgische Tumorambulanz des Klinikums rechts der Isar der Technischen Universität München, Ismaninger Strasse 22, 8000 München 80

Advanced Radiation Therapy Tumor Response
Monitoring and Treatment Planning
Breit (Editor-in-Chief)
© Springer-Verlag, Berlin Heidelberg 1992

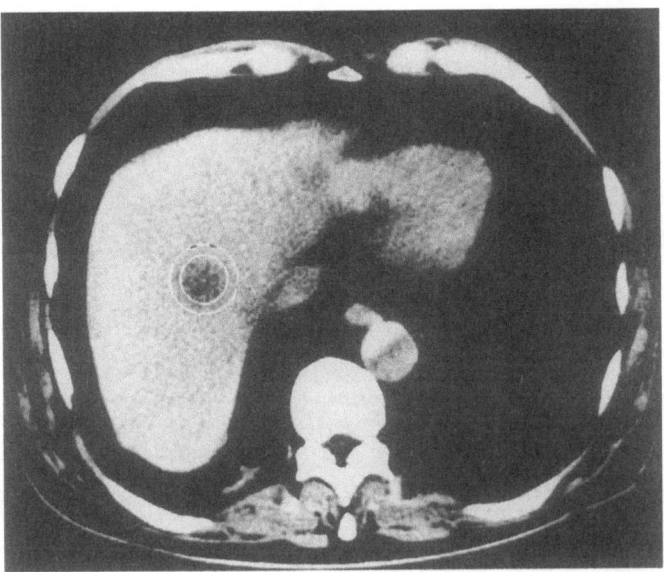

Fig. 1. Native scan of a liver metastasis. There is a poor demarcation of the metastasis so that the measured slice volume differs more than 50%

Especially small metastases can be demarcated exactly. Since they are rather round, they can be put into a circle. If their diameter totals about 1 cm, these lesions lie in one scan. In this case volumetry is no problem.

In each scan a maximum of three metastases can be measured. If there are more, the scan is repeated. In large metastases demarcation from surrounding structures is more difficult, and an inaccuracy of the radius of up to 0.5 cm must be considered. If the demarcation in contrast-enhanced CT is too inaccurate, this lesion should not be measured. In small metastases inaccuracy of the estimated radius can be about 0.1 cm. This means in a scan with 1-cm thickness an increase in volume of 19.3% (Fig. 3a). The volume of the corresponding sphere would increase 29.2%. In larger metastases a radius of 4.3 cm in comparison with a radius of 4 cm results in a growth of the disc of 14.1%; the sphere would increase 24.1%. A radius of 4.5 cm, however, would result in a volume 46% greater than a sphere with a radius of 4 cm (Fig. 3b). This means that there is an increased measuring error in cases of larger metastases. Therefore it seems better to perform a control CT later (after about 3–6 months), especially in cases of low tumor growth.

A disadvantage of the demonstrated method is the inaccurate demarcation of some metastases, although administration of the contrast injection was optimal. Generally it seems justifiable to measure only some of the metastases, which must be considered as reference lesions prospectively. Since in our cases there were always multiple liver metastases, this aspect was unimportant. The

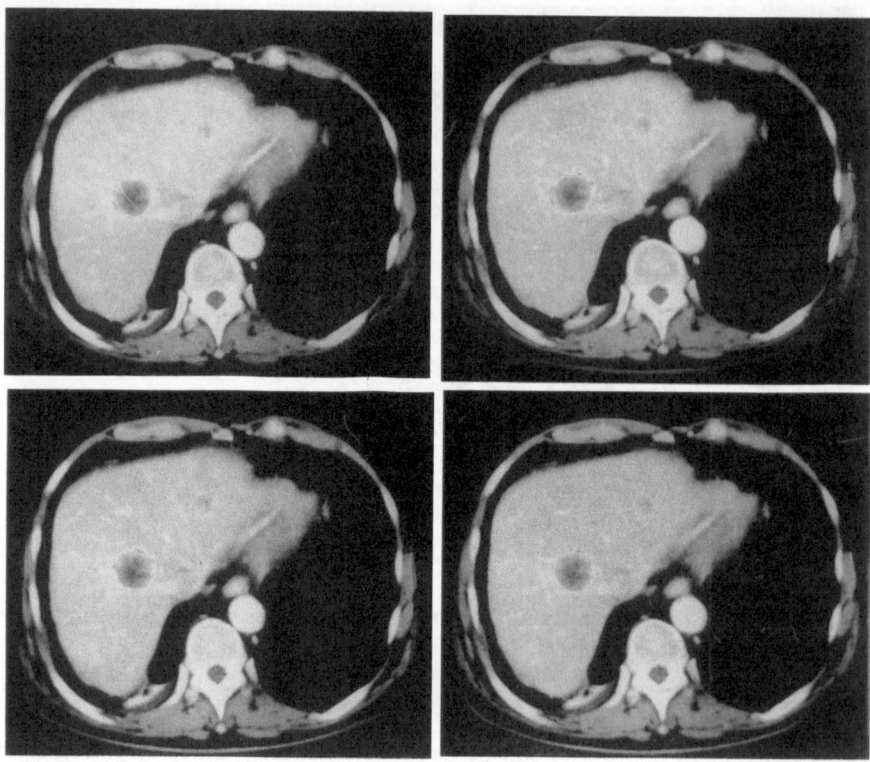

Fig. 2. Using contrast enhancement the measured slice volume of the same liver metastasis can be reproduced adequately

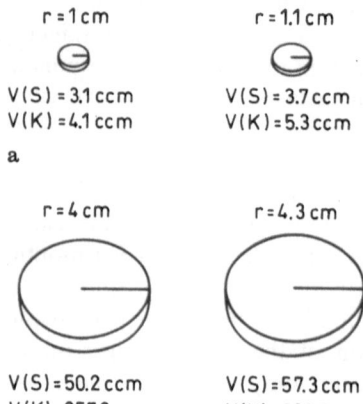

r = 1 cm

V(S) = 3.1 ccm
V(K) = 4.1 ccm

a

r = 1.1 cm

V(S) = 3.7 ccm
V(K) = 5.3 ccm

r = 4 cm

V(S) = 50.2 ccm
V(K) = 257.9 ccm

b

r = 4.3 cm

V(S) = 57.3 ccm
V(K) = 320.3 ccm

Fig. 3a,b. Dependence of volume upon radius (r). **a** Radius of 1 cm versus 1.1 cm. **b** Radius of 4 cm versus 4.3 cm

application of this method in practice will be rather difficult because it is time consuming, taking about 1 h for an examination. To avoid a superimposition in large metastases, it is necessary to compare exactly corresponding scans. If possible, spiral CT should be performed in future. Since scan time is very short, an essential risk of volumetry — the superimposition of slices — can be avoided.

In summary, we believe that the demonstrated method can be reproduced with a good correlation if standardized conditions are used. The introduction of spiral CT would undoubtedly bring essential progress in the tumor volumetry of liver metastases.

[31]P Magnetic Resonance Spectroscopy Follow-Up After Local Chemotherapy and Chemoembolization of Liver Tumors

A. Schilling[1], B. Gewiese[1], G. Berger[2], and K.-J. Wolf[1]

Introduction

[31]P magnetic resonance (MR) spectroscopy is a noninvasive method used to investigate the energy metabolism of an organ or tumor. Changes in tumor metabolism after various types of therapy can be demonstrated by ^{31}P MR spectroscopy [4]. The aim of this study was to examine and quantify the changes in the ^{31}P MR spectra of liver metastases and primary liver tumors during local chemotherapy and chemoembolization. It was also tested whether ^{31}P MR spectroscopy is a suitable method for follow-up, and how soon after the start of therapy the response or non-response of a tumor to a given type of therapy can be reliably evaluated. This early evaluation is of considerable importance for the patients, as ineffective treatment methods straining the patient can be discontinued in the initial phase and substituted by others.

Materials and Methods

We studied ten patients with liver metastases of colorectal carcinomas. There were 5 women and 7 men, with an average age of 54.5 years (range 38–79). Six of these patients underwent local cytostasis and four chemoembolization. We further studied two patients with primary hepatocellular carcinomas submitted to chemoembolization. The diagnoses were confirmed histologically in nine cases. The diameter of the tumors ranged from 8 to 15 cm; the distance from the surface was not over 4 cm.

During local chemotherapy, 5-fluorouracil was infused via a Port-A-Cath system previously implanted in the gastroduodenal artery. Chemoembolization was also performed by means of this system or by use of an angiography catheter placed according to Seldinger. This method comprised supraselective temporary embolization of the tumor vessels using microspheres (Spherex) or

---

[1] Department of Radiology, Steglitz Medical Center, Free University of Berlin, Hindenburg Damm 30, 1000 Berlin 45, FRG
[2] Department of Surgery, Steglitz Medical Center, Free University of Berlin, Hindenburg Damm 30, 1000 Berlin 45, FRG

Advanced Radiation Therapy Tumor Response
Monitoring and Treatment Planning
Breit (Editor-in-Chief)
© Springer-Verlag, Berlin Heidelberg 1992

gelatine particles (Gelfoam). A cytostatic agent (epirubicin or mitomycin C) was applied to the tumor together with the embolic agent.

The examinations were done in a 1.5-T MR imager (Magnetom, Siemens). A doubly tunable surface coil with a diameter of 120 mm was used for transmission and reception. Position control was performed by obtaining MR images with a FLASH sequence in transverse and sagittal layers (TR 70 ms, TE 5 ms, three layers) prior to the spectroscopic examination.

We then performed ^{31}P MR spectroscopy using the FROGS technique. This technique makes it possible to suppress the signals from one specific layer. By positioning the surface coil directly above the tumor and suppressing the signals from the tissue between the tumor and the coil, signal detection can be restricted to the tumor, largely excluding signals from the surrounding healthy liver tissue and superior muscular layer. The spectra were obtained with 256 acquisitions and a repetition time of 3000 ms.

The first ^{31}P MR tumor spectrum was obtained before the initiation of therapy. The second was recorded 2–4 h after chemoembolization or administration of 5-fluorouracil. The third was performed 12–16 h and a fourth 3–4 days after the start of therapy. As far as possible, additional spectroscopic examinations were performed in the further clinical course. All spectroscopic examinations were carried out in a fasting state, as this has been found to be of considerable importance during a previous study [3]. The normal values for ^{31}P MR liver spectra of the 18 healthy, fasting volunteers from this study were compared to the tumor spectra.

The ^{31}P MR spectra were processed using the convolution difference method (line width 400 Hz, subtraction factor 0.85) with subsequent gaussian multiplication (half-time 40 ms). The signal areas were determined with the aid of the Marquardt fit, an iterative method for line fitting. All spectra were later cleared arithmetically of residual signals from the surrounding muscles.

Results

Table 1 shows the mean values and standard deviations for the relative signal portions of the various phosphorous signals before and at various selected time points after the start of therapy. Both chemoembolization and local chemotherapy led to a decrease in phosphomonoester (PME) signals during the first 4 h. However, in the further clinical course the PME signal portion increased up to 10% over the original values. The opposite tendency was observed for the phosphodiester (PDE) portion, which increased by approximately 5% during the first 4 h and then fell to values far below those recorded before therapy. As anticipated, the strongest influence was observed on inorganic phosphate (Pi). The Pi portion, which had been almost identical to that of healthy volunteers before therapy, increased immediately after the initiation of therapy, and clearly

Table 1. relative individual signal areas (in percent) before and after therapy

	PME	Pi	PDE	Gamma-NTP	Alpha-NTP	Beta-NTP	pH
Before therapy	16.7 (±4.4)	5.1 (±2.5)	38.5 (±9.2)	9.2 (±2.4)	19.1 (±3.6)	11.4 (±3.2)	7.2 (±0.1)
After chemoembolization							
Up to 24 h	17.9 (±3.1)	9.9 (±3.2)	37.8 (±7.8)	7.4 (±1.8)	18.6 (±3.6)	10.7 (±3.3)	7.2 (±0.4)
More than 3 days	18.8 (±2.9)	5.2 (±0.9)	31.8 (±2.4)	9.1 (±1.8)	19.5 (±3.7)	11.1 (±2.9)	7.1 (±0.3)
After local chemotherapy							
Up to 24 h	14.4 (±3.6)	7.5 (±4.7)	41.9 (±6.0)	8.2 (±1.8)	16.2 (±2.1)	11.8 (±3.9)	7.2 (±0.1)
More than 3 days	17.3 (±0.8)	7.5 (±0.3)	33.7 (±0.5)	9.8 (±0.4)	18.3 (±0.6)	11.6 (±1.7)	7.1 (±0.1)
Healthy volunteers	12.6 (±2.7)	5.5 (±1.7)	39.6 (±2.8)	11.4 (±1.0)	19.2 (±2.1)	11.5 (±1.6)	7.3 (±0.2)

remained at a high level during the entire follow-up. This effect was much stronger after chemoembolization than after local cytostasis. The relative beta- and gamma-NTP signal portions decreased during the first 24 h and during the further course increased to their original values or above, whereas no significant changes were observed for alpha-NTP during follow-up. We must, however, emphasize that despite the good reproducibility the groups may overlap due to the relatively wide interindividual deviations. Thus, it may not be possible in some cases to assign an individual spectrum to a specific group. This can also be seen from the wide standard deviations.

The effects of therapy on the tumor spectrum are more clearly illustrated by the changes in individual signal portions (Fig. 1, 2) than by the collective

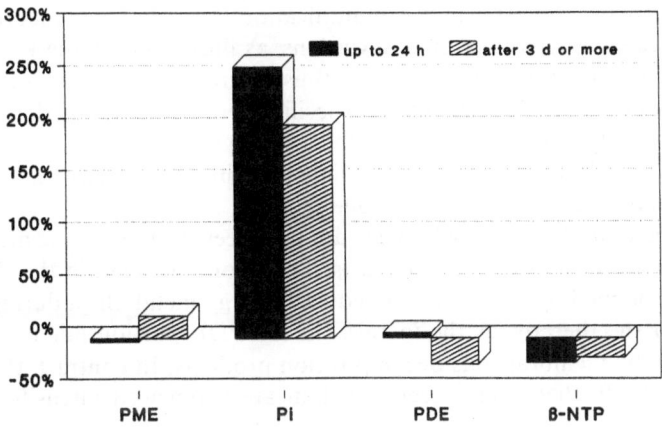

Fig. 1. Intraindividual changes after chemoembolization

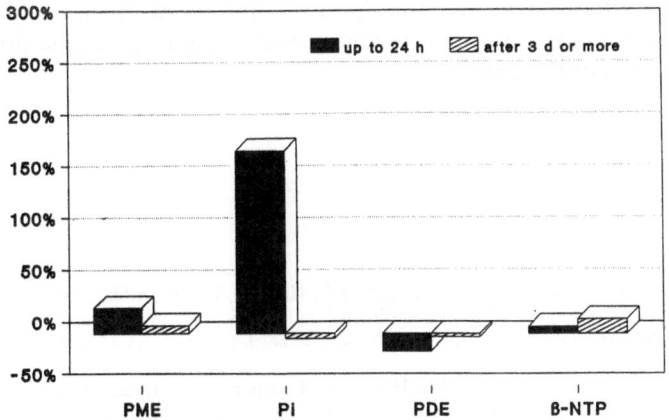

Fig. 2. Intraindividual changes after 5-fluorouracil administration via port-a-cath

changes shown in Table 1. This confirms the effects described above and demonstrates the significance of the changes according to the Wilcoxon's test for paired random samples for Pi, PME, PDE, and beta- and gamma-NTP.

The follow-up ³¹P tumor spectrum of one patient treated with chemoembolization did not show any of the changes described above. In this case, tumor progression was also diagnosed clinically a few weeks later.

Discussion

In accordance with other studies on focal malignant liver lesions [1, 2], we found a marked increase in the PME signal as compared to a series of normal volunteers, but our main interest was the quantification of the posttherapeutic changes. There were wide interindividual deviations, as illustrated by the wide standard deviations. Individual groups may thus overlap, making it very difficult to assign an individual spectrum to a specific group. This means that a single spectrum cannot be considered as sufficient diagnostic evidence. The intraindividual courses, however, are of great diagnostic importance, as similar changes were observed in all spectra under one therapy.

Significant changes in the ³¹P tumor spectrum were seen as early as the first 4 h after chemoembolization or local cytostasis. The strong increase in the Pi signal portion is explained by the markedly reduced energy metabolism during cellular decay after the therapy, as the increase in the PDE portion might be explained probably by membraneous decomposition products. In contrast, the PME increase in the further course seems to indicate a renewed intensified membrane synthesis.

It can be concluded that both chemoembolization and local cytostasis cause significant changes in the ³¹P liver tumor spectrum. Due to the small number of cases and short follow-up, however, these changes do not allow any prognostic conclusions as to the efficacy of the therapy. Spectroscopic follow-up may be the suitable method to distinguish responders and nonresponders within the first 24 h after the initiation of therapy.

References

1. Cox IJ, Bryant DJ, Collins AG, George P, Harmann RP, Hall AS, Hodgson HJF, Khenia S, McArthur P, Spencer DH, Young IR (1988) Four-dimensional chemical shift MR imaging of the phosphorus metabolites of normal and diseased human liver. J Comput Assist tomogr 12: 369–376
2. Oberhaenslli RD, Hilton-Jones D, Bore PJ, Hands L, Rampling RP, Radda GK (1986) Biochemical investigation of human tumors in vivo with phosphorus-31-magnetic resonace spectroscopy. Lancet II 1: 8–11

3. Schilling A, Gewiese B, Stiller D, Römer T, Wolf K-J (1990) Einfluß der Ernährungslage auf das 31P-MR-Spektrum der gesunden Leber. Rofo 153/4: 369–372
4. Semmler W, Gademann G, Bachert-Baumann P, Zabel HJ, Lorenz WJ, van Kaick G (1988) Monitoring human tumor response to therapy by means of P-31 spectroscopy. Radiology 166: 533–539

Clinical ^{19}F Nuclear Magnetic Resonance Spectroscopy in Colorectal Cancer: Monitoring Low-Level 5-Fluorouracil Infusion Therapy and the Metabolic Effects of Additive α-Interferon

M.O. Leach[1], J. Glaholm[1], M. Findlay[2], D. Cunningham[2], J.L. Mansi[2], D.J. Collins[1], G.S. Payne[1], and V.R. McCready[1]

Introduction

^{19}F Magnetic resonance spectroscopy (MRS) has been used to monitor the metabolism of the chemotherapeutic drug 5-fluorouracil (5FU) in patients with hepatic metastatic disease (Wolf et al. 1987; Glaholm et al. 1990; Semmler et al. 1990). Glaholm et al. compared the time course of 5FU metabolism following intravenous and intraperitoneal administration, noting the build-up and decay of 5FU and its major catabolites in the liver. Semmler et al. reported intra-arterial administration of 5FU, observing in one case the presence of fluoronucleotides. In all of these studies 5FU metabolism was observed following bolus administration or rapid infusion of approximately 1 g 5FU.

5FU has been used commonly as a bolus administration to treat patients with metastatic disease from colorectal carcinoma. The response is generally transient and limited to about 20% of patients (Carter 1976). Administration of 5FU by low-dose-rate continuous infusion has recently been reported to improve response rate (Lokich et al. 1989; Hansen et al. 1989). Modulation of treatment by additive α-interferon has also been reported as significantly improving response. In a study by Wadler and Wiernik (1990), in which a 5-day infusion of 5FU was followed by weekly bolus administration of 5FU and α-interferon, an objective response was seen in 20/32 previously untreated patients. Possible synergistic mechanisms include increased formation of fluorodeoxyuridine monophosphate, inhibition of thymidylate synthase and inhibition of cellular thymidine uptake (Gewert et al. 1983; Elias and Sandoval 1989). Clinical ^{19}F MRS studies have not been reported at the low dose rates encountered in continuous infusion therapy, and the objectives of this study were firstly to determine whether signals can be measured at these low dose rates, and secondly to explore the changes in 5FU metabolism that occur during continuous infusion therapy and when this therapy is modulated by α-interferon.

---

[1] CRC Clinical Magnetic Resonance Research Group, Joint Department of Physics, Institute of Cancer Research and Royal Marsden Hospital, Downs Road, Sutton, Surrey SM2 5PT, UK
[2] Section of Medicine and Gastrointestinal Unit, Institute of Cancer Research and Royal Marsden Hospital, Downs Road, Sutton, Surrey SM2 5PT, UK

Advanced Radiation Therapy Tumor Response
Monitoring and Treatment Planning
Breit (Editor-in-Chief)
© Springer-Verlag, Berlin Heidelberg 1992

Methods

Patients admitted to our Gastrointestinal Unit with measurable liver metastases from colorectal carcinoma are being monitored by ^{19}F MRS; a schematic representation of the current trial is shown in Fig. 1. Patients are firstly treated to maximum response by continuous infusion of 5FU at 300 mg m^{-2} per day via a Hickman line using an ambulatory pump. Maximum response is assessed by carcinoembryonic antigen (CEA) and liver ultrasound/computed tomography scans. Additive α-interferon delivered as 5 MU subcutaneously three times per week is then added. These doses may be modified to ameliorate toxicity. At maximum response or progression the therapy is again changed. ^{19}F MRS measurements are taken as indicated in Fig. 1, with the main objectives in this preliminary study being to measure metabolism prior to commencement of α-interferon and then at intervals following treatment with α-interferon.

MRS measurements are performed using a 1.5-T Siemens Magnetom MR system, using a 16-cm surface coil for the spectroscopy measurements. Patients are generally positioned supine with the coil placed over the liver. Measurements commence with an imaging study using the body coil and a FISP sequence, the sequence parameters being set to maximise liver contrast. Shimming is then performed using the surface coil. A susceptibility map may be taken using the body coil. The system is switched to the fluorine frequency, and the signal from a reference sample contained in a fixed position in the surface coil is measured. This sample contains 1 M sodium fluorobenzoate in a deuterated solution and is doped with Gd-DTPA. The frequency of the system is then adjusted to lie between the resonant frequencies of 5FU and the catabolite 1-fluoro-beta-ureido-proprionic acid (FUPA), and acquisitions proceed. Shimming, the reference sample measurement and 5FU measurements are performed

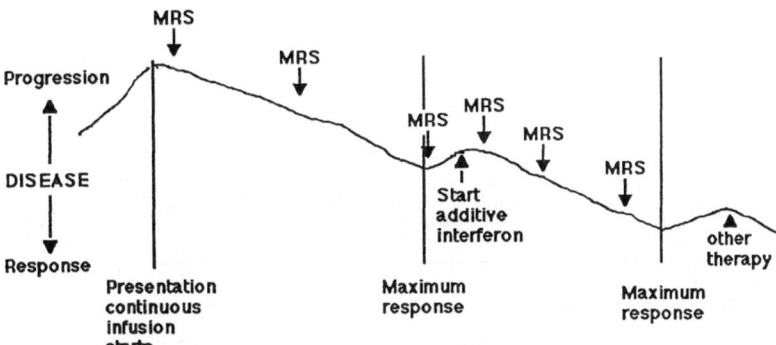

Fig. 1. An idealised schedule for MRS monitoring during the course of the study. Following presentation, continuous infusion therapy commences, and this is continued to maximum response. Once maximum response is achieved, α-interferon is added, and the study continues again until maximum response is achieved

using a half-hyperbolic secant adiabatic half-passage pulse. Spectra are acquired using a pulse and acquire sequence with a repetition time of 2 s, spectra being acquired for 20–40 min. Spectra are acquired in multiples of 128 acquisitions.

Results

In our preliminary results signals have been clearly evident from our measurements. Signal was apparent in one patient receiving a dose of only 50 mg 5FU m^{-2} per day, and catabolites were still present in another patient 5 days after the cessation of infusion therapy. The majority of patients studied have shown a pronounced catabolite peak, identified as principally FUPA but which may also contain an unresolved contribution from 2-fluoro-beta-alanine (FBAL), and which during the course of therapy is seen to reduce in amplitude. Such a result is shown in Fig. 2. In some subjects this reduction in FUPA amplitude is associated with the appearance of a peak at − 4 ppm from FUPA that has not yet been identified. As the FUPA peak decreases, a peak attributed

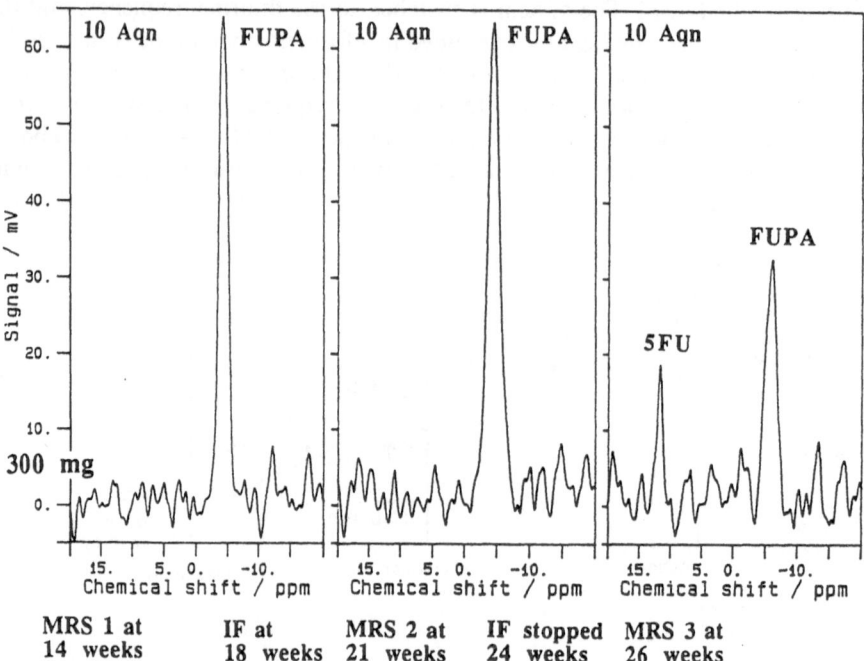

Fig. 2. Measurements performed prior to interferon (*IF*), following interferon and subsequently following the cessation of interferon therapy. The number of acquisitions (*Aqn*) are indicated in units of 128 acquisitions. The measurements are normalised relative to the reference sample

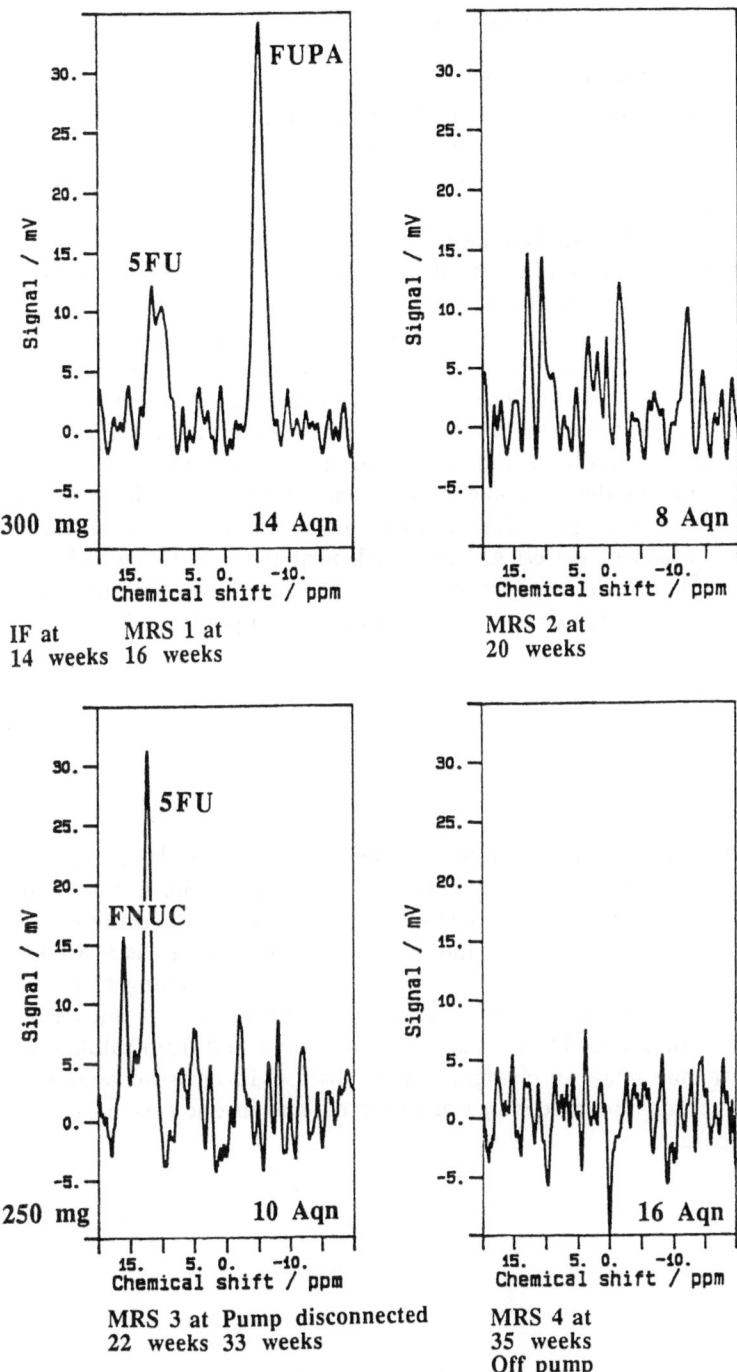

Fig. 3. Measurement 1 following interferon (*IF*). In measurements 2 and 4, significant signal was not acquired. In measurement 2, a relatively short acquisition period was employed, and in measurement 4, 5FU had been discontinued 2 weeks previously, and this measurement therefore serves as a control

to 5FU often becomes apparent. In one patient (Fig. 3), we have also seen a peak attributed to fluoronucleotides. A smaller group of patients initially showed a peak attributed to 5FU with or without accompanying metabolite peaks. An example is shown in Fig. 3. A small number of patients exhibited no signal at first measurement.

In this initial study signal has been localised using only the surface coil, as we anticipated that the metabolite signal would be low due to the low dose rate. There is no internal standard available for fluorine, and thus frequency references must be inferred from the proton frequency and from previous calibration measurements. Although this has been shown to provide an excellent frequency calibration in well-localised studies (Madden et al. 1991), we have observed in this study that there is a significant frequency shift of up to 2 ppm across the liver. This has been confirmed using susceptibility maps. Thus there is some uncertainty in the assignment of individual peaks. We have therefore adopted a conservative procedure in assigning peaks, and a large catabolite peak has been assigned as FUPA, and a single peak in the 5FU region has been assigned as 5FU. During this study additional peaks have been observed in independent measurements at +1.3 ppm and at −5 ppm from 5FU.

Discussion

As this study is currently in progress, we have not yet completed correlation with the response of individual patients. It is clear from the results to date, however, that clear and progressive changes are evident on the serial measurements that we have undertaken, and that the general pattern is a decline in catabolite signal often accompanied by an apparent broadening of the catabolite peak and appearance of 5FU associated with, in at least one case, the presence of an anabolite. These results may indicate a shift from catabolism to anabolism or may relate to changes in bulk disease. In measurements of two isolated masses, catabolic activity was observed, and in one case a 5FU peak was also apparent.

Conclusions

Signal is clearly evident during continuous infusion therapy at dose rates of 50–300 mg 5FU m^{-2} per day. When measurements are normalised to a reference sample a general trend of decreased catabolite signal with treatment duration is seen.

M.O. Leach et al.

References

Carter SK (1976) Large bowel cancer. The current status of treatment. JNCI 56: 3–10

Elias L, Sandoval JM (1989) Interferon effects in 5FU metabolism by HL-60 cells. Biochem Biophys Res Comm 163/2: 867–874

Gewert DR, Moore G, Clemens MJ (1983) Inhibition of mitosis by IFNs. Biochem J 214: 983–990

Glaholm J, Leach MO, Collins D, Al Jehazi B, Sharp JC, Smith TAD, Adach J, Hind A, McCready VR, White H (1990) Comparison of 5-fluorouracil pharmacokinetics following intraperitoneal and intravenous administration using in vivo ^{19}F magnetic resonance spectroscopy. Br J Radiol 63: 547–553

Hansen RM, Quebbeman E, Anderson T (1989) 5-FU by protracted venous infusion: a review of current progress. Oncology 46: 245–250

Lokich JJ, Ahlgren JD, Gullo JJ, Philips JA, Fryer JG (1989) A prospective randomized comparison of continuous infusion fluorouracil with a conventional bolus schedule in metastatic colorectal carcinoma: a mid-Atlantic oncology program study. J clin Oncol 7: 424–432

Madden A, Leach MO, Collins DJ, Payne GS (1991) The water resonance as an alternative pH reference: relevance to 'in vivo' 31-P NMR localised spectroscopy studies. Magn Reson Med 19: 416–421

Semmler WF, Bachert-Baumann P, Guckel F, Ermark F, Schlag P, Lorenz WJ, von Kaick G (1990) Real time follow-up of 5-fluorouracil metabolism in the liver of tumour patients by means of F-19 MR spectroscopy. Radiology 174: 141–145

Wadler S, Wiernik PH (1990) Clinical update on the role of fluorouracil and recombinant interferon alpha-2a in the treatment of colorectal carcinoma. Semin Oncol 17: 16–21

Wolf W, Albright M, Silver M, Weber H, Reichardt U, Sauter R (1987) Fluorine-19 NMR studies of the metabolism of 5 fluorouracil in the liver of patients undergoing chemotherapy. Magn Reson Imaging 5: 165–169

Positron Emission Tomography Measurement of Fluorouracil Uptake Prior to Therapy and Chemotherapy Response

A. Dimitrakopoulou, L.G. Strauss, M.V. Knopp, U. Haberkorn,
P. Hohenberger, G. Wolber, F. Oberdorfer, and G. van Kaick

Introduction

The standard chemotherapeutic agent for the treatment of hepatic metastases from colorectal cancer is 5-fluorouracil (FU) [1]. Depending on both the selection process and the response criteria used, the reported response rates have varied from 8% to 82% [1]. Based on a literature survey, Kemeny reported that the average response rate for liver metastases was 23% [1]. The metabolism of FU has been studied and was recently summarized by Hull et al. [2]. These authors found no significant difference in the metabolite concentrations in plasma between responders and nonresponders to FU chemotherapy. They state that the detection of FU metabolites in tumor tissue is required for an assessment of response to FU. Shani and Wolf showed in an animal study that drug-responsive tumors had a 20:1 tumor-to-blood ratio 12 h after injection, while drug-resistant tumors had only a 4:1 ratio [3]. These data indicate that FU metabolite measurements in tumor tissue may be helpful in predicting response to FU chemotherapy in patients.

We examined patients prior to the first chemotherapeutic cycle with [^{18}F] FU and positron emission tomography (PET) to obtain quantitative data about the distribution pattern of FU and metabolites in metastases as a function of time. Furthermore, studies using computed tomography (CT) were performed before and after FU chemotherapy, and the tumor volume was calculated from the cross-sections. We compared the FU-metabolite concentrations obtained from PET images prior to chemotherapy with the tumor growth rate. Our primary goal was to determine the correlation between these parameters in order to predict therapeutic outcome on the base of noninvasive PET studies.

Materials and Methods

We report on the evaluation of 18 metastases obtained from 12 patients with liver metastases from colorectal carcinoma. All patients were examined prior to the first chemotherapeutic cycle. The standard therapeutic protocol included the

German Cancer Research Center, Im Neuenheimer Feld 280, 6900 Heidelberg, FRG

Advanced Radiation Therapy Tumor Response
Monitoring and Treatment Planning
Breit (Editor-in-Chief)
© Springer-Verlag, Berlin Heidelberg 1992

intravenous or intraarterial infusion of FU (500–1500 mg/m² per day) for 5 days, followed by a 3-week interval without chemotherapy. To exclude potential effects of chemotherapy on PET results the patients were examined with PET prior to the FU therapy. Liver metastases were diagnosed prior to referral to PET. CT (Somatom DRH, Siemens) immediately preceded the PET examination and was used in each patient to identify the region of greatest metastasis diameter. Only patients who had at least one metastasis identified two contiguous CT slices (8-mm slice thickness) were included in the study due to the limited resolution of PET. The volume of each metastasis examined with PET was calculated from the CT slices using a three-axis method [vol = (4/3)π* ·· *a*b*c]. CT studies preceded the first chemotherapeutic cycle and were repeated 3–11 months later. The growth rate was obtained from the volumetric data using the formula: growth rate = ln(Vol₂/Vol₁)/(date of first CT study–date of second CT study), where Vol₁: volume of the metastasis prior to chemotherapy; Vol₂: volume of the metastasis after chemotherapy.

A PET scanner (PC2048-7WB, Scanditronix) with two ring detectors was used. This system provides for the acquisition of three slices simultaneously, two primary sections and one cross-section. [¹⁸F] FU (370–444 MBq) was given together with 500 mg unlabeled FU in a short 12-min infusion using an infusion pump. Images were acquired for 2 h. PET cross-sections were generated using an iterative reconstruction program. The image matrix was 128 * 128 and interpolated to 256 * 256 for display. The spatial resolution in a cross-section was 5.1 mm for the iterative reconstruction. Regions of interest (ROIs) were placed over the metastasis and normal liver parenchyma. Only those metastases visible in at least two consecutive slices were included in the final evaluation.

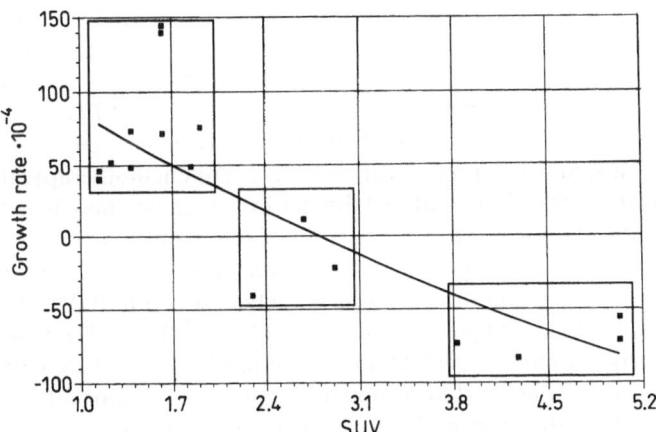

Fig. 1. ¹⁸F concentrations (SUV) in 18 liver metastases 2 h after infusion of [¹⁸F]FU. Three groups were identified by cluster analysis: tumor progression was associated with low tracer uptake (< 2.0 SUV), stable disease was noted in lesions with 2.0–3.5 SUV, while tumor regression was observed only in metastases with high FU metabolite concentrations (> 3.5 SUV). A regression function was calculated with a correlation coefficient of 0.8

The slice showing the largest metastasis diameter was used for the placement of the ROI. The standardized uptake value (SUV) [4] was used to express tracer uptake: SUV = concentration (nCi/g)/injected dose (nCi)/body weight (g). Based on the ROIs, SUV values were calculated for each image of a FU study.

Results

Visual inspection of the late PET image showed the metastasis as a defect, which is indicative for low FU metabolism. The FU uptake in the normal liver tissue was high as compared to the metastases. The data of 18 metastases and the tumor growth rate are summarized in Fig. 1. We noted a high correlation between the FU metabolite concentrations in the metastases and the tumor growth rate.

Discussion

Chemotherapy with FU has found extensive use since its introduction more than three decades ago. Depending on both the selection process and the response criteria used, the reported response rates have varied from 8% to 82% [1]. Based on a literature survey, Kemeny reported that the average response rate for hepatic metastases was 23% [1], with individual response rates low and population response rates highly variable, it is impossible to predict the response rates of individuals or to identify those most likely to respond to therapy. One possible approach for predicting response to FU requires radiolabeling of the chemotherapeutic drug with ^{18}F. PET with [^{18}F] FU gives the oncologist the opportunity to determine the tissue concentration of FU and its ^{18}F-labeled metabolites and to determine their relative tissue concentrations. Since FU uptake by a tumor is a prerequisite for successful chemotherapy, the concentration measurements of FU and metabolites in metastases may help to identify those patients who meet this first criterion of therapeutic success.

The SUV values represent concentration values normalized for the injected dose and the body volume. We noted only 4 of 18 metastases with SUV values exceeding 3.5 (Fig. 1). Late images obtained 2 h after [^{18}F] FU infusion represent total FU metabolite concentrations. It should be remembered that some FU metabolites, such as $\propto$-fluoro-b-alanine, show no significant antitumor activity. Therefore, the measured ^{18}F concentrations may fail to mirror the cytotoxic potency of FU metabolites. It follows that tracer uptake alone, as measured by PET, may not be predictive for the therapeutic success, but therapeutic success cannot occur without uptake of the cytostatic agent. When high ^{18}F concentrations are noted in the tumor, the patient has a high probability of response. While tumor regression occurred only at SUV values exceeding 3.5, no tumor regression was noted for lower concentration values (Fig. 1). The correlation to tumor growth rate was highest for the FU metabolite concentrations 2 h after FU infusion, whereas a significantly lower correlation was obtained for the maximum ^{18}F activity in the metastases. Since the maximum ^{18}F activity reflects the FU transport into the cell, early FU uptake is not representative for the cytostatic effect. A regression function was calculated for the FU metabolite concentration values and the tumor volume. The high correlation of 0.8 demonstrates that this regression function can be used to estimate the tumor growth rate prior to chemotherapy.

References

1. Kemeny N (1983) The systemic chemotherapy of hepatic metastases. Semin Oncol 10: 148–158
2. Hull WE, Port RE, Herrmann R, Britsch B, Kunz W (1988) Metabolites of 5-fluorouracil in plasma and urine, as monitored by ^{19}F nuclear magnetic resonance spectroscopy, for patients receiving chemotherapy with or without methotrexate pretreatment. Cancer Res 48: 1680–1688
3. Shani J, Wolf W (1977) A model for prediction of chemotherapy response to 5-fluorouracil based on the differential distribution of 5-[^{18}F]fluorouracil in sensitive versus resistant lymphocytic leukemia in mice. Cancer Res 37: 2306–2308
4. Matsuzawa T, Fukuda H, Abe Y et al. (1985) Current and future aspects of cancer diagnosis with positron emission tomography: biological and clinical aspect. In: Matsuzawa T (ed) Proceedings of the international symposium on current and future aspects of cancer diagnosis with positron emission tomography, Sendai, pp 1–23
5. Akanuma A (1978) Parameter analysis of Gompertzian function growth model in clinical tumors. Eur J Cancer 44: 681–688

Assessment of Tumor Metabolism in Liver Metastases Using Positron Emission Tomography and [18F]fluorodeoxyglucose

A. Dimitrakopoulou, L.G. Strauss, U. Haberkorn, M. Knopp, W. Kübler, F. Helus, and W. Maier-Borst

Introduction

Metastatic malignant tumors of the liver are common in clinical practice, probably ranking second only to cirrhosis as a cause of fatal liver disease. Hepatic metastases have been reported at autopsies in 30%–50% of patients dying from malignant disease. Patients with metastatic liver involvement usually have imaging studies with ultrasound, computed tomography (CT), or magnetic resonance imaging. All these methods provide morphologic information about the malignant lesions, which are used for therapy management. Besides the morphologic data, functional information about the metabolism of metastases may enhance therapy planning. Therefore, we used positron emission tomography (PET) and [18F]fluorodeoxyglucose (FDG) to assess whether PET gives additional information about the change in tumor metabolism before, during, and after chemotherapy in patients with metastatic colorectal carcinomas.

Materials and Methods

We report our experience obtained in 11 patients with an unresectable, locally recurrent rectosigmoidal malignancy and liver metastases who were directed to chemotherapy. While eight patients received chemotherapy with fluorouracil (FU), three were treated with tumor necrosis factor. Patients were referred to PET to evaluate the potential of using metabolic measurements for therapy planning and follow-up. The study was approved by the appropriate agencies, and informed consent was given by the patients. PET results did not influence the diagnostic or therapeutic modalities which were used in these patients.

Only patients with lesions exceeding 1.5 cm in diameter were included in the study due to the limited resolution of PET. PET studies were performed prior to therapy ($n = 25$) and after therapy ($n = 6$). The results of PET were compared to preexisting clinical data. A PET scanner (PC2048-7WB, Scanditronix) with two ring detectors was used for the examinations. The system provides for the

German Cancer Research Center, Im Neuenheimer Feld 280, 6900 Heidelberg, FRG

Advanced Radiation Therapy Tumor Response
Monitoring and Treatment Planning
Breit (Editor-in-Chief)
© Springer-Verlag, Berlin Heidelberg 1992

acquisition of three slices simultaneously (two primary sections, one cross-section). Each of the two rings, of 107 cm diameter, contains 512 BGO/GSO detectors (crystal size 6 * 20 * 30 mm) and provides a field of view of 52 cm. The data were transferred to a computer system (VAX-11/750, Digital Equipment) for further processing. Transmission scans with more than 10 million counts per section were obtained prior to the radionuclide administration to obtain cross-sections for the attenuation correction of the acquired PET images. Thirty-one examinations were carried out with 126–440 MBq (3–12 mCi) FDG, and 12 sequential images were acquired at 5-min intervals during 1 h following intravenous tracer injection.

PET cross-sections were generated using an iterative reconstruction program. The image matrix was 128 * 128, and interpolated to 256 * 256 for display. The spatial resolution in a cross-section was 5.1 mm for the iterative reconstruction. A 4-mm pixel size was chosen for all reconstructed images. The transverse slices were compared to the corresponding CT images and to the PET transmission images to permit certain identification of the mass using anatomical landmarks. This was followed by a quantitative evaluation of the PET images, using a region-of-interest (ROI) technique. ROIs were placed over the tumor region as well as the gluteal muscles, which served as normal reference tissue. The number of pixels in the tumor region exceeded 32 image elements in all patients. No correction was made for partial volume averaging. Time-activity curves were calculated from each image series for further quantitative evaluation. Tracer uptake was expressed as the standardized uptake value (SUV): SUV = concentration(nCi/g)/injected dose (nci)/body weight (g).

Results

All malignant lesions were visible in the PET FDG images. Furthermore, most metastases showed the highest FDG uptake in the peripheral parts of the lesion, while the central region was hypometabolic, which is indicative for tumor necrosis. This information was not provided by CT. The FDG uptake was more than twofold higher in malignancies as compared to the normal soft tissue (Fig. 1). Follow-up studies demonstrated a decrease in tumor metabolism after FU chemotherapy in two of seven lesions (Fig. 2).

Discussion

FDG is a commonly used radiopharmaceutical for PET brain studies. Di Chiro et al. used FDG to examine patients with tumors of the brain stem and spinal cord. They identified a remarkably close correlation between tumor grade and

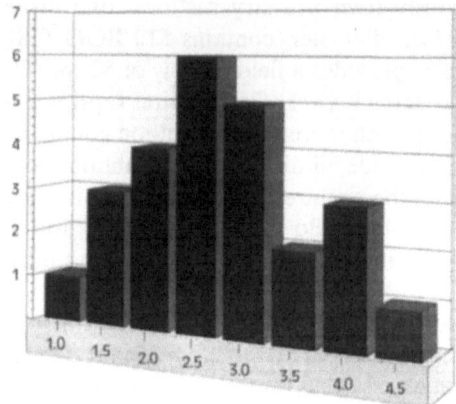

Fig. 1. Histogram of FDG uptake values (SUV) prior to therapy in 25 lesions, *X axis*, FDG uptake (SUV); *Y axis*, number of metastases

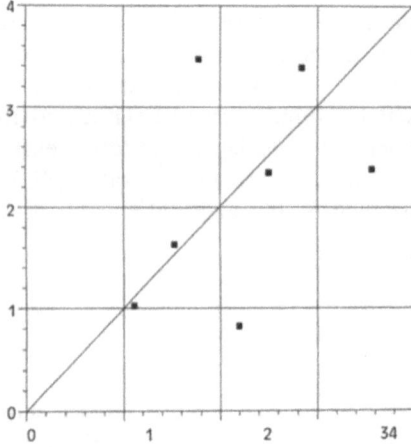

Fig. 2. FDG uptake values prior to and after chemotherapy with fluorouracil. *X axis*, FDG uptake (SUV) prior to chemotherapy; *Y axis*, FDG uptake (SUV) after chemotherapy

glucose utilization. Similar results were reported by Paul et al. [2], who noted consistently high FDG accumulation in both canine osteosarcoma and mammary carcinoma. We demonstrated that PET is helpful in the differentiation of multiple metastases with respect to their metabolism. The results of our study demonstrate that PET with FDG can be used to document the tumor metabolism prior to therapy as well as the change in FDG uptake in metastases due to chemotherapy. The tumor metabolism was different in multiple metastases of the same patients, while CT provided no differences in the lesions. Therefore, the PET information should find use together with morphologic data for therapy management. Different therapeutic protocols may be compared using PET and FDG.

References

Di Chiro G, Oldfield E, Bairamian D et al (1985) In vivo glucose utilization of tumors of the brain stem and spinal cord. In: Breit T, Ingvar DH, Widen L (eds) Positron emission tomography. Raven, New York, pp 351–361

Paul R, Johansson R, Kiures A, et al (1984) Imaging of canine cancers with ^{18}F-Z-fluoro-2-deoxy-D-glucose (FDG) suggests further applications for cancer imaging in man. Nucl Med Commun. 5: 641–646

Evaluation of Modulated Fluorouracil Chemotherapy with Positron Emission Tomography in Patients with Metastatic Colorectal Cancer

A. Dimitrakopoulou, L.G. Strauss, M.V. Knopp, U. Haberkorn, F. Helus, and W. Maier-Borst

Introduction

The standard chemotherapeutic agent for the treatment of hepatic metastases from colorectal cancer is 5-fluorouracil (FU) [1]. Depending on both the selection process and the response criteria used, the reported response rates have varied from 8% to 82% [1]. Based on a literature survey, Kemeny reported that the average response rate for hepatic metastases was 23%. The metabolism of FU has been studied extensively and was recently summarized by Hull et al. [2]. Therefore, modified treatment protocols including d,l-folinic acid have found use for therapy. Trave et al. demonstrated an increased inhibition of thymidilate synthase following pretreatment with d,l-folinic acid [3]. We examined patients with $[^{18}F]FU$ and positron emission tomography (PET) to obtain quantitative data about the distribution pattern of FU and metabolites in metastases, normal liver parenchyma, and aorta as a function of time. Our primary goal was to evaluate the effect of d,l-folinic acid pretreatment on the FU metabolite concentrations.

Materials and Methods

We report on the evaluation of 20 examinations obtained in ten patients with liver metastases from colorectal carcinoma. All patients were examined prior to the first chemotherapeutic cycle. The standard therapeutic protocol included the infusion of d,l-folinic acid (500 mg/m²) and FU (750 mg/m² per day) for 5 days, followed by a 3-week interval without chemotherapy. PET examinations were performed with and without d,l-folinic acid pretreatment in all patients, resulting in a total of 20 PET studies. Computed tomography (CT; Somatom DRH, Siemens) immediately preceded the PET examination and was used in each patient to identify the region of greatest metastasis diameter. Only patients who had at least one metastasis identified in two contiguous CT slices (8-mm slice thickness) were included in the study due to the limited resolution of PET.

German Cancer Research Center, Im Neuenheimer Feld 280, 6900 Heidelberg, FRG

Advanced Radiation Therapy Tumor Response
Monitoring and Treatment Planning
Breit (Editor-in-Chief)
© Springer-Verlag, Berlin Heidelberg 1992

Skin markings were used for proper positioning in PET after the image level had been determined with CT. We used identical positioning supports for CT and PET. A PET system (PC2048-7WB, Scanditronix) with two ring detectors was used for the PET examinations. The system provides for the acquisition of three slices simultaneously. [^{18}F]FU was prepared by direct fluorination of uracil in acetic acid using [^{18}F]F$_2$ diluted in neon [4]. Quality control included HPLC. Typically, 17.5 mg [^{18}F]FU was obtained with purity greater than 99%, and a specific activity of $1.14 * 10^{-5}$ Ci/μM. [^{18}F]FU (370–444 MBq) was given together with 500 mg unlabeled FU in a 12-min infusion using an infusion pump. Images were acquired continuously for 2 h. The second PET examination was performed 1 week later. The pretreatment with d,l-folinic acid (500 mg/m^2, 20–25 min for infusion) preceded the FU application. The same acquisition protocol was used for the second PET study. PET cross-sections were generated using an iterative reconstruction program. The transverse slices were compared to the corresponding CT images to permit certain identification of the mass using anatomical landmarks (e.g., upper pole of the kidney, lower part of the heart, shape of liver, spleen). This was followed by a quantitative evaluation of the PET images, using a region-of-interest (ROI) technique. ROIs were placed over the metastasis and normal liver parenchyma. Time-activity data were calculated from each image series for further evaluation. The standardized uptake value (SUV) [5] was used to express tracer uptake: SUV = concentration(nCi/g)/injected dose (nCi)/body weight (g).

Results

We noted an increase in FU metabolite concentrations in 6 of 14 metastases (Fig. 1). The change in FU metabolite concentrations was compared with the systemic concentrations, which served as an estimate for systemic toxicity (Figs. 2, 3).

Discussion

Chemotherapy with FU has found extensive use since its introduction more than three decades ago. Depending on both the selection process and the response criteria used, the reported response rates have varied from 8% to 82% [1]. Based on a literature survey, Kemeny reported that the average response rate for hepatic metastases was 23% [1]. Two mechanisms of the antitumor effect of FU have been proposed: incorporation into RNA and inhibition of the thymidylate synthase. Therefore, modified treatment protocols including d,l-folinic acid pretreatment have found use for chemotherapy to enhance the

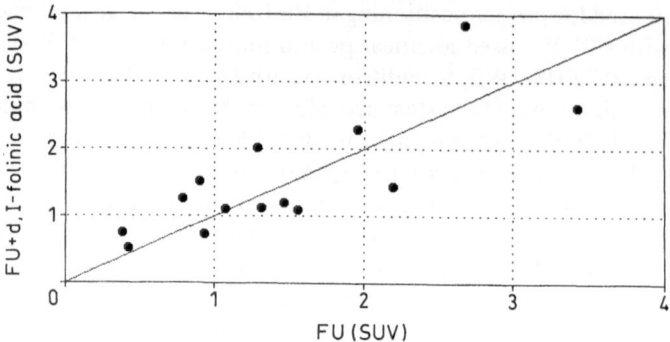

Fig. 1. [18]F concentrations (SUV) 2 h after FU infusion in 14 liver metastases with and without *d,l*-folinic acid pretreatment. Tracer uptake was enhanced (>15%) in 6 of 14 metastases, while decreased FU metabolite concentrations were noted in three lesions following pretreatment with *d, l*-folinic acid

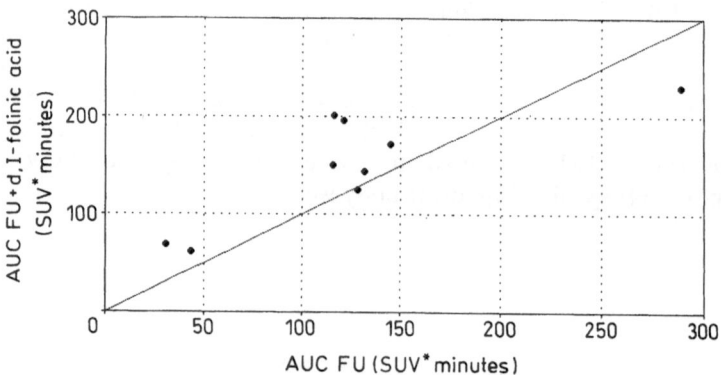

Fig. 2. Standardized time-activity integral values (SUV∗minutes) in the aorta with and without *d,l*-folinic acid pretreatment. Note the increased ^{18}F integral values in most of the patients following pretreatment

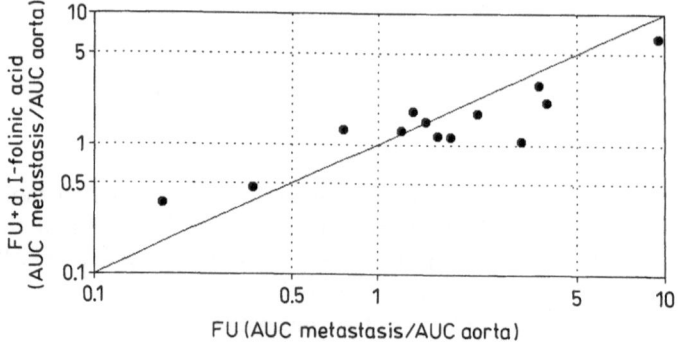

Fig. 3. Ratios calculated from the ^{18}F concentrations in the metastases and the time-activity values of the aorta. The values of the aorta were used as an estimate for systemic toxicity, while the concentration values in the lesions were correlated with therapy outcome

second mechanism. Trave et al. demonstrated an increased inhibition of thymidylate synthase following d,l-folinic acid pretreatment [3]. [^{18}F]FU is biochemically identical to the nonlabeled cytostatic agent FU. Therefore, PET with the ^{18}F-labeled drug gives the oncologist the opportunity to determine the tissue concentration of FU and its ^{18}F-labeled metabolites and to determine their relative tissue concentrations. Since FU uptake by a tumor is a prerequisite for successful chemotherapy, the concentration measurements of [^{18}F]FU and metabolites in metastases may help to identify those patients who meet this first criterion of therapeutic success. Our results demonstrate that the pretreatment with d,l-folinic acid does not necessarily enhance the FU metabolites in all metastases (Fig. 1). In only one of ten patients were the FU metabolite concentrations following pretreatment sufficient to stop tumor growth. Furthermore, the systemic toxicity was increased in most of the patients (Fig. 2). A low FU transport into the tumor cells was noted in the majority of patients (Fig. 1). Therefore, the cytostatic effect of FU was not modified in these patients by pretreatment with d,l-folinic acid. Individual measurements of FU metabolite concentrations are required to select the appropriate therapy.

References

1. Kemeny N (1983) The systemic chemotherapy of hepatic metastases. Semin Oncol 10: 148–158.
2. Hull WE, Port RE, Herrmann R, Britsch B, Kunz W (1988) Metabolites of 5-fluorouracil in plasma and urine, as monitored by ^{19}F nuclear magnetic resonance spectroscopy, for patients receiving chemotherapy with or without methotrexate pretreatment. Cancer Res 48: 1680–1688
3. Trave F, Rustum YM, Petrelli NJ, Herrera L, Mittelman A, Frank C, Creaven PJ (1988) Plasma and tumor tissue pharmacology of high-dose intravenous leucovorin calcium in combination with fluorouracil in patients with advanced colorectal carcinoma. J Clin Oncol 6: 1184–1191
4. Oberdorfer F, Hofmann E, Maier-Borst W (1989) Preparation of ^{18}F-labelled 5-fluorouracil of very high purity. J Label Compds Radiopharm 27: 137–145
5. Matsuzawa T, Fukuda H, Abe Y et al. (1985) Current and future aspects of cancer diagnosis with positron emission tomography: biological and clinical aspect. In: Matsuzawa T (ed) Proceedings of the international symposium on current and future aspects of cancer diagnosis with positron emission tomography, Sendai, pp 1–23

Direct Comparison of two Invasive Computed Tomography Procedures and Correlation with Immunoscintigraphy in the Management of Liver Metastases

N. Rilinger, H. Niemann, H.J. Illinger, and H.J. Halbfaß

Introduction

The number of patients with colorectal carcinoma is growing steadily. In Germany 20 000 new cases are diagnosed each year [5]. At the time of primary tumor diagnosis about 25% of all patients have liver metastases, and on follow-up liver metastases are observed in a further 30%–40%. The average survival rate of untreated patients with liver metastases lies between 6 and 9 months. Using systemic or intraarterial chemotherapy, the average survival rate of the patients rises to about 11–13 months. Only surgery can have a curative effect [1, 8, 11]. The exact topographic localization of the liver metastases and absence of extrahepatic tumor deposits are prerequisites for curative partial hepatectomy.

A variety of imaging tests for the evaluation of the liver are available. Which of these is the most sensitive for detecting focal hepatic lesions continues to be the subject of intense debate among investigators. Several studies have shown computed tomography (CT) to be superior to ultrasound (US) and radionuclide scintigraphy in the detection of liver metastases [2, 14]. Several techniques for the administration of contrast material during CT have been developed in an effort to increase the difference in X-ray attenuation and improve the visual contrast between metastases and normal liver parenchyma [8, 12, 13]. The available data with special regard to the diagnostic value of CT arteriography (CTA) and CT during arterial portography (CTAP) are therefore confusing.

It was the aim of this study to elucidate the diagnostic value of CTA and CTAP in the detection of focal hepatic masses. Furthermore, an attempt was made to evaluate the significance of a ^{99m}Tc labeled monoclonal anti-CEA-antibody (MAb) in the detection of liver metastases.

Methods

We studied a total of 15 patients, nine men and six women, aged between 42 and 72 years. Of these, 13 suffered from colorectal carcinoma and two from other tumors.

Abteilung für Radiologie und Nuklearmedizin, Städtische Kliniken Oldenburg, Dr.-Eden-Str. 10, 2900 Oldenburg, FRG

Advanced Radiation Therapy Tumor Response
Monitoring and Treatment Planning
Breit (Editor-in-Chief)
© Springer-Verlag, Berlin Heidelberg 1992

All CT scans were obtained on a Siemens Somatom DRH system with 4-mm sections at 8-mm intervals throughout the whole liver. Immediately after angiography we performed CTA with injection of contrast material through an angiographic catheter placed in the hepatic artery. Directly after this procedure the patient was transferred to mesenteric arteriography followed by CTAP with contrast material injected into the superior mesenteric artery. Each time we used 60 ml iohexol combined with 30 ml of physiological saline solution so that we obtained a total volume of 90 ml. The liver was examined in fast-scan mode. Contrast material was injected by hand immediately in the case of CTA or — in the case of CTAP — 20 s before scanning and then continued throughout the rapid run. The total amount of contrast material used for angiography and both CT examinations was between 200 and 240 ml. In 13 of the 15 patients immunoscintigraphy (IS) was performed according to the CT procedure. Immediately after CTA and CTAP, 900–1100 MBq of the ^{99m}Tc-labeled MAb was administered in four patients via the hepatic artery and in an additional four patients via the superior mesenteric artery. In five patients the MAb was administered intravenously.

The MAb BW 431/26 that we used is an IgG1 intact molecule and reacts only with a protein epitope on the CEA complex [16]. The labeling procedure with ^{99m}Tc is described by Schwarz and coworkers [16] and allows the direct linkage of ^{99m}Tc to free thiol groups of the activated antibody. After labeling with ^{99m}Tc immunoreactivity is in the range of 90%–95%. The antibody binding to cell membrane integrated CEA is not inhibited by circulating CEA. The MAb does not bind to peripheral blood cells [7]. The labeling kit consists of two components: the antibody and the stannous component, both in lyophilized form and therefore stable for a number of months.

In cases of intraarterial MAb administration we performed sequential scanning during the first 5 min and then planar scans of the thorax, abdomen, and pelvis (gamma camera, Elscint, Apex ECT 256 matrix) 10–20 min after injection. In these and also in the cases of intravenous administration we performed planar scans of the thorax, abdomen, and pelvis 4–8 and 18–30 h after injection. In additional special cases, single photon emission CT studies were carried out (64×64 matrix, 360° rotation, 6°/frame).

Results

Of the 15 patients 13 showed focal hepatic masses. There were 46 lesions detected by CTAP, 43 by CTA, and 20 by IS. The smallest lesion detected by CTAP had a diameter of 0.5 cm. On the basis of the imaging results only three patients were considered candidates for partial hepatectomy, and in these cases our imaging results were completely confirmed by surgery. Table 1 shows the relationship between the size of the hepatic masses and their distribution. The

Table 1. Relationship between size of hepatic masses and their depiction on CT

Liver metastases	CTA	CTAP	Difference
<1 cm	7	10	3
1–2 cm	12	12	—
2–4 cm	19	19	—
>4 cm	5	5	—
Total	43	46	3

most significant result can be seen in those under 1 cm. In three cases CTAP was superior to CTA in the detection of lesions smaller than 1 cm.

Discussion

CTA of the liver shows the hepatic lesions due to their arterial enhancement as hyperattenuated masses compared with the normal hepatic parenchyma. This fact can become a problem in very small lesions (<1 cm) without central necrosis where the distinction between blood vessel and metastasis is almost impossible (Fig. 1). Furthermore, intraarterial administration of contrast material during CT scanning can produce several different types of perfusion abnormalities that may be confused with tumors [9]. To differentiate between perfusion abnormalities and additional tumor masses, accurate interpretation of CTA is required.

On the other hand, CTAP hepatic lesions appear as low attenuation masses because nearly all primary and secondary tumors have a greater arterial than portal venous blood supply. However, normal hepatic parenchyma is supplied predominantly by the portal-venous system. CTAP has several advantages over CTA. In nearly all cases of focal hepatic masses, a better demonstration and localization of the masses was found. Also, because of the anatomic variations of the hepatic artery and the possible failure of superselective catherization, CTA of the entire liver is not always possible. In our study the right liver lobe of one patient was supplied via an arterial branch from the superior mesenteric artery.

Using IS, most of the small liver metastases with a diameter of 1–2 cm showed up as hot spots, whereas almost all the larger metastases (>2 cm) were seen as cold lesions caused by central necrosis and with a hot rim resulting from active tumor tissue (Fig. 2). This is the so-called rim sign. Cold lesions without rim sign were regarded as nonspecific reactions and therefore counted as false-negative findings. In our view the failure to detect 26 liver metastases by IS results from their small size (<1 cm) and perhaps from the lack of CEA production. The poor sensitivity of 43% using the ^{99m}Tc labeled MAb in the detection of liver metastases is confirmed by other groups [3]. However,

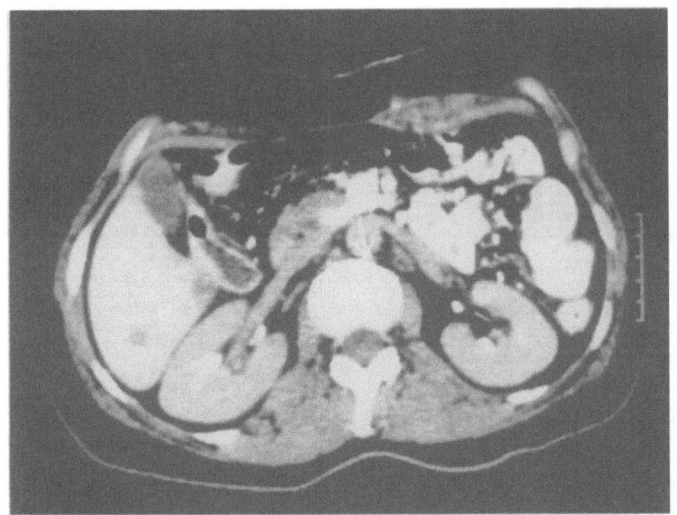

a

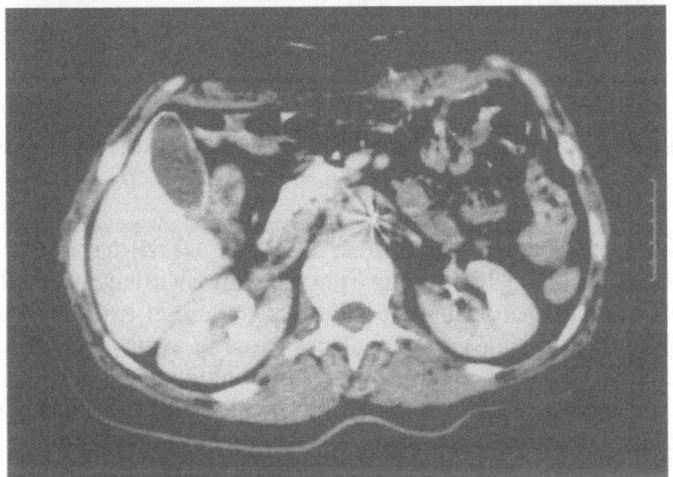

b

Fig. 1a, b. Two liver metastases identified by CTAP. However, one of these lesions was first identified by CTA. **b** as a cross-section of a blood vessel

Bischof-Delaloye and coworkers [6] point out that an increasing sensitivity can be found using iodine-123 antibody fragments for the detection of liver metastases. On the other hand, previous studies show the high sensitivity of IS in excluding extrahepatic deposits [3, 4, 10, 15]. This is, of course, a prerequisite for curative partial hepatectomy. In our hospital IS is therefore performed routinely in patients with liver metastases and planned partial hepatectomy for excluding extrahepatic tumor deposits.

There are at least eight ways of examining the liver for metastatic disease by CT [8, 12, 13, 14]. However, we agree with Miller et al. [13] that the number of

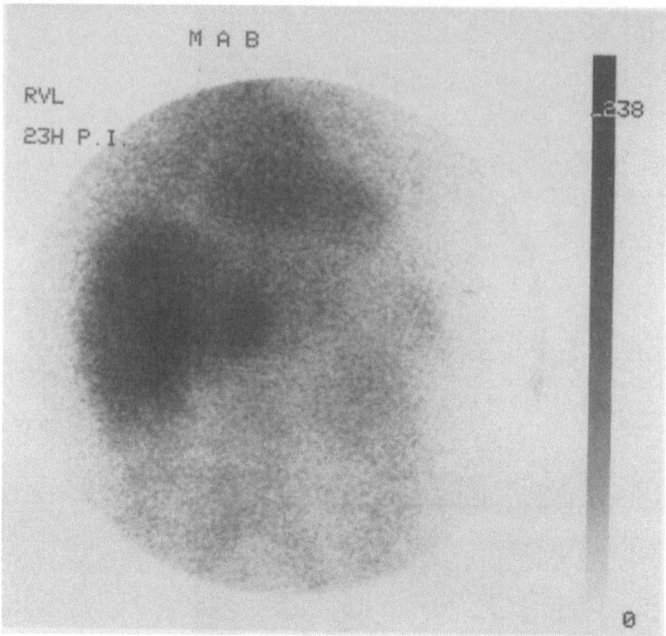

Fig. 2. Detection of three liver metastases partially presented as cold lesion with the rim sign or as hot spot

methods presently in use suggests that neither CTA nor CTAP has proved superior. This is due to the difficulty in comparing these invasive diagnostic CT procedures. A potential criticism of our study is that the use of two different methods for administering the contrast material may cause a mixture of contrast kinetics by recirculating contrast material which may ultimately result in a confused arterial and portal-venous phase. However, in all images from our double invasive study we achieved the typical liver-to-tumor contrast ratio.

Conclusion

The numbers of patients examined and the numbers of lesions evaluated in our study were small. However, the direct comparison of CTA and CTAP shows the advantage of CTAP in the detection of small liver lesions (< 1 cm). Furthermore, because of anatomic variations, CTAP is easier to perform than CTA. On the other hand, IS results with a sensitivity of 43% using intraarterial, portal-venous, or intravenous administration of the ^{99m}Tc-labeled MAb BW 431/26 in the detection of focal hepatic masses are disappointing. Nevertheless, IS is an important additional procedure for excluding extrahepatic tumor deposits in patients who are potential candidates for curative partial hepatectomy.

References

1. Adson MA, van Heerden JA (1980) Major hepatic resections for metastatic colorectal cancer. Ann Surg 191: 576–583
2. Alderson PO, Adams DF, McNeil BJ (1983) Computed tomography, ultrasound, and scintigraphy of the liver in patients with colon or breast carcinoma: a prospective comparison. Radiology 149: 225–230
3. Bares R (1990) Immunszintigraphie kolorektaler Tumoren: Probleme und Grenzen der Methode. Nuklearmediziner 3/13: 173–181
4. Baum RP, Lorenz M, Hottenrott C et al. (1988) The clinical application of immunoscintigraphy: results of a prospective study controlled by surgery, histology, and immunochemistry and compared to CT-scan and sonography. In: Schmidt HAE, Csernay L (eds) Nuklearmedizin, neue Aspekte und Möglichkeiten. Schattauer, Stuttgart, pp 611–615
5. Becker N, Frentzel-Beyme R, Wagner G (1984) Krebsatlas der Bundesrepublik Deutschland, 2nd edn. Springer, Berlin Heidelberg New York
6. Bischof-Delaloye A, Delaloye B, Buchegger F et al. (1989) Clinical value of immunoscintigraphy in colorectal carcinoma patients: a prospective study. J Nucl Med 30: 1646–1656
7. Bosslet K, Lüben G, Schwarz A et al. (1985) Immunohistochemical localization and molecular characteristics of three monoclonal antibody-defined epitopes detectable on carcinoembryonic antigen (CEA). Int J Cancer 36: 75
8. Clark RA, Matsui O (1983) CT of liver tumors. Semin Roentgenol 18: 149–162
9. Freeny PC, Marks WM (1986) Hepatic perfusion abnormalities during CT angiography: detection and interpretation. Radiology 159: 685–691
10. Lind P, Langsteger W, Költringer P et al. (1990) Immunoscintigraphy with Tc99m labeled monoclonal anti-CEA-antibody (BW 431/26) in the follow up of patients with colorectal carcinomas. In: Schmidt HAE, Chambron J (eds) Nuclear medicine — quantitative analysis in imaging and function. Schattauer, Stuttgart, pp 567–569
11. Martin A, Adson MD, van Heerden JA et al (1984) Resection of hepatic metastases from colorectal cancer. Arch Surg 119: 512–516
12. Miller DL (1984) EDE-13 and other contrast agents for computed tomography of the liver. In: van de Velde CJH, Sugarbaker PH (eds) Liver metastases: basic aspects, detection, and management. Nijhoff, Boston, pp 102–117
13. Miller DL, Simmons JT, Chang R et al. (1987) Hepatic metastasis detection: comparison of three CT contrast enhancement methods. Radiology 165: 785–790
14. Rilinger N, Munz DL, Niemann H, Halbfaß HJ, Illiger HJ (1990) I.a./i.v. immunoscintigraphy in comparison with i.a./i.v. contrast-CT using the Tc99m monoclonal antibody BW 431/26 in the detection of liver metastases. In: Schmidt HAE, Chambron J (eds) Nuclear medicine — quantitative analysis in imaging and function. Schattauer, Stuttgart, pp 556–560
15. Rilinger N, Niemann H, Halbfaß HJ (1989) Neue Aspekte in der Immunszintigraphie kolorektaler Tumor-Rezidive mit Hilfe eines 99mTc markierten Anti-CEA-Antikörpers. Rontgenpraxis 7/42: 245–247
16. Schwarz A, Steinsträsser A (1987) A novel approach to Tc 99m labeled monoclonal antibodies. J Nucl Med 28: 721

Monitoring of Tumor Size by Ultrasound: Reproducibility of Measurements

C.F. Hess and M. Bamberg

Introduction

In patients undergoing various treatment modalities for cancer the quantification of tumor size is essential to assess the efficacy of a particular therapeutic protocol [3, 4, 5]. The potential of current imaging modalities to determine progression or regression of malignant disease depends strongly on the interobserver variation of tumor measurements. To determine the reproducibility of ultrasound tumor measurements 57 abdominal tumors were measured by two independent observers, and the resulting differences between corresponding measurements were analyzed.

Materials and Methods

Two independent observers used ultrasound techniques to measure 57 abdominal tumors: 9 cysts of the kidneys, 5 cysts of the liver, 16 liver metastases, 10 lymph nodes, and 17 other tumors. All abdominal tumors were measured in two orthogonal planes defined either by the longitudinal axis of the body (modality A, 176 measurements per observer) or by the longest tumor diameter (modality G, 70 measurements per observer). Measurements A1 (longitudinal diameter) and A2 (anteroposterior diameter) were determined in the sagittal scan and measurements A3 (transverse diameter) and A4 (anteroposterior diameter) in the transverse scan with maximum extension of the lesion. Measurements G1–G4 were defined analogously. All patients were examined initially by observer 1. Observer 2 was informed about the exact location of the lesion, including its photodocumentation for each imaging plane (without measurements). The resulting differences between corresponding measurements underwent detailed statistical analysis [2].

Abteilung für Strahlentherapie, Radiologische Universitätsklinik, Hoppe-Seyler-Str. 3, 7400 Tübingen, FRG

Advanced Radiation Therapy Tumor Response
Monitoring and Treatment Planning
Breit (Editor-in-Chief)
© Springer-Verlag, Berlin Heidelberg 1992

Results

Corresponding measurements of independent ultrasound observers showed excellent agreement ($r = 0.96$ for all measurements; $r = 0.98$ for modality G and $r = 0.94$ for modality A). Differences between corresponding measurements were normally distributed, with a mean of 2 mm and standard deviation of 6 mm. The *absolute* differences between corresponding measurements increased with tumor diameter (Fig. 1); for example, in tumour diameters longer than 5 cm the mean of absolute differences between corresponding measurements was 7 mm, and 16% of absolute differences exceeded 12 mm. Regression analysis revealed a regression line with a slope of 9.5% and a correlation coefficient of 0.58. The statistical distribution of *relative* differences of corresponding measurements is shown in Fig. 2. The probability distribution P ($|\Delta d|/d$) defines the probability of relative differences being less than ($|\Delta d|/d$). Relative differences between corresponding measurements averaged 10% of tumor diameter, but in 5% of the cases they reached 30%. Measurements obtained from a longitudinal plane (A1 and A2) were reproduced better than those from a transverse plane (A3 and A4) or those from planes defined by the longest tumor diameter (G1–G4; Fig. 2). In tumors smaller than 2 cm relative differences of less than 5% were significantly more frequent than in large tumors.

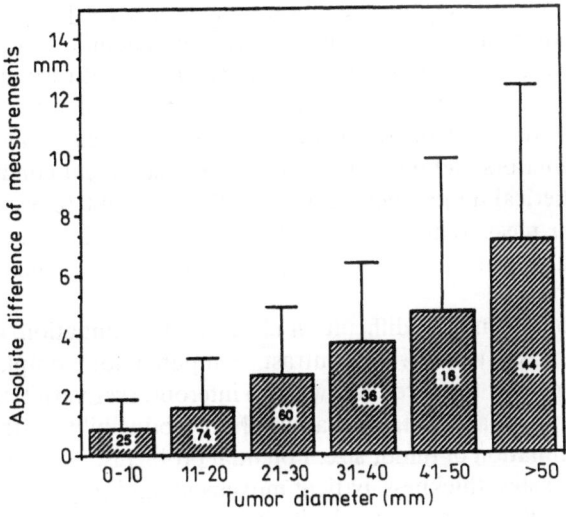

Fig. 1. Absolute differences between corresponding measurements: dependence on actual tumor size

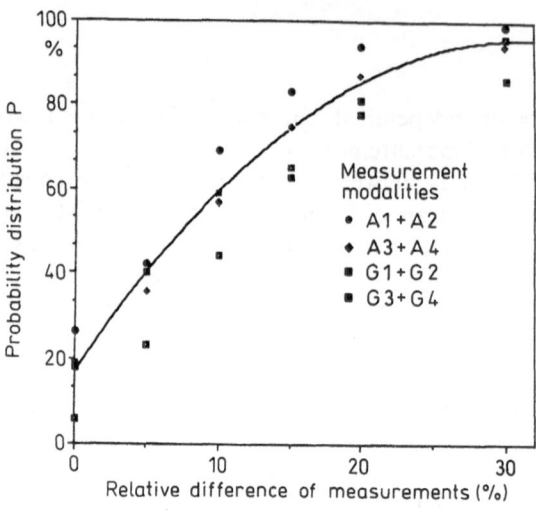

Fig. 2. Probability distributions of relative differences between corresponding measurements

Discussion

Objective assessment of tumor size is mandatory in the follow-up of malignant disease, assessment of sensitivity to therapy, and design of treatment schedules [3, 4, 5]. A number of sources of error must be recognized in the measurement and follow-up of tumors relating to reproducibility of imaging tests, observer error in defining the limits of the lesions, and accuracy in measuring their sizes. However, only few studies deal with the interobserver reproducibility of in vivo determinations of tumor size with current imaging techniques [1, 2, 6].

Our study revealed considerable agreement between corresponding measurements of tumor diameters performed by two independent ultrasound observers. However, relative differences averaged 10%, and 5% of relative differences reached 30% of tumor diameter. Differences may be even greater with less experienced examiners and under less specified measurement conditions. Since increases in spherical tumor *volumes* of 25%, 50%, and 100% result in relative changes in *linear* measurements of 7%, 15%, and 25%, ultrasound measurements of tumor diameters proved to be limited in assessing minor changes of tumor load.

Assessment of tumor volume may be difficult on ultrasound examination, in particular in irregularly shaped tumors. In contrast, computed tomography (CT) volume calculations are easy to reproduce, with an interobserver variation of about 3% [6]. However, no reliable data exist about the reproducibility of the whole process of CT determination of tumor size. Potential problems, including table movement, selection of slice thickness, patient movement, and respiratory motion, may considerably influence the reproducibility of repeated CT examinations [1, 6].

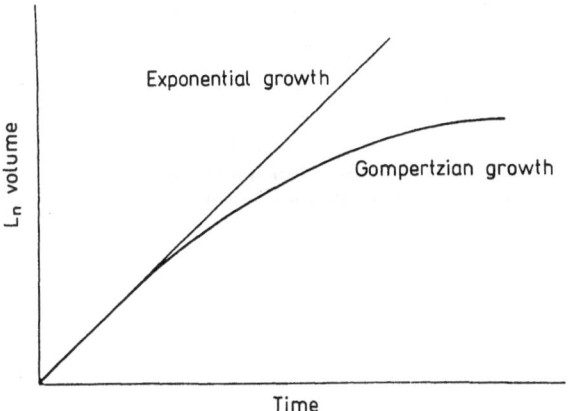

Fig. 3. Exponential and "Gompertzian" tumor growth

It is well accepted in ultrasound routine that tumors should be documented according to some internal landmark, such as vascular anatomy, and that the longest measured diameter should be recorded. However, our data revealed that these assumptions may be inadequate for quantitative tumor follow-up. In our study measurements obtained from a sagittal scan seemed more reproducible than those from other planes, and short diameters could be reproduced better than long linear measurements.

In addition, there is evidence that a constant growth rate (exponential growth) is not valid over the total life of a tumor [3]. Growth seems to be better described by the Gompertz equation (Fig. 3), which describes declining growth rate as the tumor enlarges. Thus, both tumor growth characteristics and reproducibility of measurements suggest that in the case of multiple involvement of malignant disease small tumors should be measured to assess the efficacy of a treatment protocol.

In summary, reproducibility of measurements may considerably influence therapeutic decisions in clinical oncology. Therefore, knowledge of interobserver variation is necessary to read imaging tests adequately, estimate progression or regression of lesions, determine sensitivity to therapy, and choose appropriate intervals between serial imaging examinations. This knowledge may result in a more rational selection of imaging tests and may thus improve the cost-effectiveness of follow-up studies in malignant disease.

References

1. Friedman MA, Resser KJ, Marcus FS (1983) How accurate are computed tomographic scans in assessment of changes in tumor size? Am J Med 75: 193–198
2. Hess CF, Kölbel G, Majer MC (1988) Zur Reproduzierbarkeit der sonographischen

Größenbestimmung intraabdomineller Raumforderungen. Fortschr Geb Rontgenstr Nuklear-med 149: 184–188
3. Norton L, Simon R (1977) Tumor size, sensitivity to therapy and design of treatment schedules. Cancer Treat Rep 61/7: 1307–1317
4. Paling MR, Shawker TH, Dwyer A (1981) Ultrasonic evaluation of therapeutic response in tumors: its value and implications. JCU 9: 281–288
5. Shawker TH (1980) Monitoring response to therapy. In: Brashol DJ, Shawker TH (eds) Abdominal ultrasound in the cancer patient. Wiley, New York, pp 113–134
6. Staron RB, Ford E (1986) Computed tomographic volumetric calculation reproducibility. Invest Radiol 21: 272–274

Magnetic Resonance Imaging in Diagnosis
and Follow-up of Tumors of the Female Breast:
A Comparative Study

Introduction

Patients and Methods

Magnetic Resonance Imaging in Diagnosis and Follow-Up of Testis Cancer Patients: A Comparative Study

O. Klepp[1], G. Myhr[2], O. Smevik[2], Å. Tangerud[3], H. Haarstad[1], A. Nordby[3], and P.A. Rinck[2]

Introduction

Proper staging of the retroperitoneal area is a prerequisite for appropriate treatment of patients with all types and stages of testis cancer. Early detection of any retroperitoneal lymph node metastasis is imperative for the so-called surveillance policy of non-seminomatous germ cell testis tumors in clinical stage 1. Patients with no evidence of metastatic disease are merely surveilled closely after orchiectomy with no other treatment unless a relapse is detected. Computed tomography (CT) has more or less replaced bipedal lymphography as the main radiological imaging method of the retroperitoneal lymph nodes in testis cancer. Both methods have an accuracy of about 70% in early clinical stages. The patient absorbs a midplane X-ray dose of 30–50 m Gy during an abdominal CT examination. As these young male patients also undergo numerous chest X-rays and other radiological procedures and may receive chemotherapy with carcinogenic and mutagenic potential, any alternative imaging method that omits ionizing radiation is of interest if it provides comparable medical information. During the past 4 years we have prospectively compared magnetic resonance imaging (MRI) with CT examination of the retroperitoneal lymph nodes in patients with testis cancer.

Patients and Methods

In the period November 1986 to March 1991 a total of 104 patients with germ cell tumors of the testis underwent primary clinical and radiological staging according to the Royal Marsden Staging System [1] (Table 1) at our hospital. All patients were examined with CT (GE 9800 or Philips Tomoscan 60/TX, both with a spatial resolution of 0.7 mm) of the abdomen and pelvis. The patients received both oral and intravenous contrast to enhance the imaging quality of

[1] Department of Oncology, Trondheim University Hospital, 7006 Trondheim, Norway
[2] Magnetic Resonance Center, Trondheim University Hospital, 7006 Trondheim, Norway
[3] Department of Radiology, Trondheim University Hospital, 7006 Trondheim, Norway

Advanced Radiation Therapy Tumor Response
Monitoring and Treatment Planning
Breit (Editor-in-Chief)
© Springer-Verlag, Berlin Heidelberg 1992

Table 1. The Royal Marsden Hospital Staging of testicular tumors

I		No evidence of metastases
	IMk +	Rising tumor markers with no other evidence of metastases
II		Abdominal node involvement
	A	<2 cm diameter
	B	2–5 cm diameter
	C	<5 cm diameter
III		Supradiaphragmatic node involvement
	M	Mediastinal
	N	Supraclavicular/cervical/axillary
	O	No abdominal lymphadenopathy
	ABC	As above
IV		Extralymphatic metastases
	Lung substage	
	L1	≤3 metastases
	L2	>3 metastases, all ≤2 cm diameter
	L3	>3 metastases, one or more >2 cm diameter
	H+	Liver metastases
	Br+	Brain metastases
	Bo+	Bone metastases
	ABC	As above

the CT. Sections 1 cm thick at 1–2 cm intervals were performed. All patients had a chest X-ray and most of them also a chest CT. During the same time period, 56 (54%) of the 104 patients also underwent abdominal and pelvic MRI examination as part of the primary staging procedures within the same week as the CT examination. The main reason for not performing MRI in the other 48 patients was nonavailability of MRI (due to long waiting lists) during a reasonable time span before start of treatment. Priority was given to patients with non-seminomatous germ cell testis cancer with no evident retroperitoneal metastases on CT. Patients with bulky (>5 cm diameter) metastases on CT had a low priority. Table 2 presents the clinical stage distribution of the patients with and without primary MRI examination (as concluded by the prospective routine overall assessment).

Abdominal MRI examinations were performed with on a Philips S5 (0.5-T) or a Philips S15 (1.5-T) whole-body unit. Transverse, coronal and sagittal T1-weighted (TR 450 ms, TE 20 ms), T2-weighted (TR 2100 ms, TE 100 ms), and intermediate-weighted ("proton density"; TR 2100 ms, TE 29 ms) spin-echo sequences were used. Of the 56 patients 14 (25%) with primary MRI also underwent bipedal lymphography, and 28 (50%) also had ultrasound of the abdomen and pelvis. Any additional 25 patients underwent MRI of the abdomen and pelvis as part of the follow-up after primary treatment. Any positive or equivocal finding was also followed by CT in these patients. Forty-eight of the patients participated in phase II or phase III evaluations of oral superparamagnetic particles as MRI contrast agents for enhancement of the intestines [2]. Most of the patients receiving these had both pre- and postcontrast MRI performed on the same day. If such double MRI examinations are considered as

Table 2. Clinical stage distribution of the 56 patients selected for primary MRI examination of abdomen and pelvis compared to those who underwent only CT scan of the same region

Clinical stage	Primary MRI ($n = 56$)	no primary MRI ($n = 48$)
Seminoma	23 (41%)	27 (56%)
CSI	15	21
CSII	2	1
CSIIB	2	
CSIIC	1	2
CSIIIC	1	
CSIVC	2	3
Non-seminoma	33 (59%)	21 (44%)
CSI	22	10
CSIMk +	2	
CSIIA	2	
CSIIB	5	1
CSIIC		1
CSIIIB		1
CSIIIC		1
CSIV0	1	3
CSIVB		2
CSIVC	1	2

Table 3. Results of the routine prospective evaluations in the 55 evaluable patients who underwent MRI as part of the primary staging procedures

Primary MRI and CT reports	Number of patients	Number of patients with retroperitoneal metastases on final assessment
Both MRI and CT negative	36	4[a]
Both MRI and CT positive	8	8
MRI positive, CT negative	3	3
MRI equivocal, CT negative	1	1
MRI equivocal, CT positive	1	1
MRI negative, CT positive	5	3
MRI negative, CT equivocal	1	0
Total	55	20

[a] One with microscopic metastasis at retroperitoneal lymph node dissection and three with later retroperitoneal relapse during surveillance

single ones, a total of 105 separate MRI examinations of the abdomen and pelvis were performed in 81 different testis cancer patients; 22 had two examinations, and one had three. Five testis cancer patients underwent altogether 13 MRI examinations of the brain (suspect or manifest brain metastases); one patient had five, one had one MRI of the mediastinum, and four had MRI of the lumbar spines. In addition to the prospective (routine) evaluation of the MRI and CT examination, all MRI and CT images with positive or equivocal findings were retrospectively reviewed separately by independent examiners without knowledge of prior conclusions or the follow-up information.

The results of the prospective routine MRI and CT reports and the reviews were compared to the overall clinical information and conclusions obtained by coordinated assessments of serum tumor markers, retroperitoneal lymph node dissection, ultrasound and/or lymphography, reviews of MRI, CT, and the further follow-up of the patients. All the 73 patients who underwent at least one abdominal MRI examination were followed closely until death (two patients) or to March 20, 1991. A questionnaire was sent to 70 patients who had both abdominal CT and MRI to study the patients' preferences regarding one or the other procedure.

Results and Discussion

Of the 56 patients selected for MRI as part of the primary staging procedures 55 were evaluable. The MRI examination had to be discontinued in one patient due to a claustrophobic reaction. The results of the prospective routine evaluations of MRI and CT are presented in Table 3.

If equivocal reports were interpreted as negative findings, MRI detected 11 (55%) out of the 20 regarded as having retroperitoneal metastases. All of the 35 regarded as having normal lymph nodes were described as normal and one as equivocal, indicating an "accuracy" of 84% (46/55) for MRI. The corresponding figures for CT were 60% (12/20), 94% (33/35), and 82% (45/55), respectively. If equivocal reports were interpreted as positive, the "accuracy" of MRI was 85% (47/55) and of CT 80% (44/55). There was no evident false-positive MRI report, but two false-positive CT reports. None of the differences between MRI and CT were statistically significant.

Two of the 55 cases could not be reviewed due to missing CT and/or MRI images. After the review of the 53 evaluable cases we concluded that MRI detected 14 (78%) of 18 cases regarded as having retroperitoneal metastases and CT 11 (61%) of the 18. There were no evident false-positive findings.

There was no significant discrepancy between the 49 MRI examinations performed during follow-up after primary treatment as compared to concomitant or subsequent CT scans. No relapse was detected by routine MRI alone, but three cases with relapse indicated by rising serum tumor markers had both MRI and CT verification of metastases in the retroperitoneal regions and later confirmed by post-chemotherapy normalization. There was no evident case of false-positive or false-negative interpretation of MRI during the follow-up examinations.

As described elsewhere [2], the paramagnetic oral contrast improved the delineation of intra-abdominal and pelvic organs and improved the diagnostic information from postcontrast as compared to precontrast MRI. The ability of MRI to present multiplane (transverse, coronal, and sagittal) images of the retroperitoneal regions seemed particularly useful, especially regarding the assessment of the aortocaval interspace and the retrocrural area.

Repeated MRI examinations proved very useful for one patient with a mature teratoma metastasis remaining in the mediastinum after chemotherapy and reductive surgery. This metastasis was better delineated by a coronal MRI than by CT. Monitoring of this patient gave an early warning both by revealing slight expansion and change of MRI signal as the teratoma started to grow, necessitating further surgery. For this patient with the residual teratoma in the mediastinum, for two cases with negative (normal) CT scans and positive (pathological) MRI of the retroperitoneal region, and for two patients with negative MRI and positive or equivocal CT, the MRI report had a direct and useful influence on the clinical decision making regarding further therapy.

Fifty-six (80%) of the 70 patients answered the questionnaire regarding preference. Six (11%) had no preference regarding MRI or CT. Twenty-eight (50%) of the 56 preferred MRI over CT, and 22 (39%) preferred CT. The main reasons for preferring MRI was the intravenous/oral contrast received as part of the CT examination, concern about irradiation during CT scans, and difficulties due to the need of keeping the arms above the head through the CT gantry. The main reasons for CT preference were the long time spent and tendencies towards claustrophobic fears during the MRI examination.

We conclude that MRI of the retroperitoneal regions in patients with testis cancer provides diagnostic information at least comparable to modern contrast-enhanced CT scans. The information obtained by MRI can be improved by ingestion of oral magnetic particles for delineation of the bowels. The ability of MRI to provide images in the coronal plane of the aortocaval and the retrocrural regions is very useful. The possibility of monitoring residual mature teratoma after chemotherapy is an interesting aspect of MRI, but further experience is needed.

References

1. Horwich A, Brada M, Nicholls J, Jay G, Hendry WF, Dearnalay D, Peckham MJ (1989) Intensive induction chemotherapy for poor risk non-seminomatous germ cell tumors. Eur J Cancer Clin Oncol 25: 177–184
2. Rinck P, Smevik O, Nilsen G, Klepp O, Onsrud M, Øksendal A, Børseth A (1991) Oral magnetic particles in MR imaging of the abdomen and pelvis. Radiology 178: 775–779

Tumor Response to Preoperative Chemotherapy in Nephroblastoma

K. Rieden[1], A. Weirich[2], J. Tröger[1], and R. Ludwig[2]

Introduction

With an incidence of 6.1% of all malignancies in children the nephroblastoma (Wilms' tumor) is the third most common malignant tumor in childhood [2]. This embryonal tumor is typically located unilaterally in one kidney; bilateral nephroblastomas occur in 7%, and an extrarenal localization is seen in 2% [5].

Since January 1989 the Gesellschaft für Pädiatrische Onkologie (GPO) has coordinated a 5-year therapeutic study in the Federal Republic of Germany in association with the International Society of Pediatric Oncology (SIOP). Preoperative chemotherapy for all children aged between 6 months and 16 years is a main part of the therapeutic concept of this study. Preoperative chemotherapy generally starts when the diagnosis is made by diagnostic imaging, including intravenous pyelography, ultrasound, and computed tomography (CT), without preceding biopsy. In trial patients with Wilms' tumors of stages I–III, the tumor response to preoperative chemotherapy is tested by diagnostic imaging (ultrasound and CT) after 4 weeks of treatment. Based on the results of this screening by diagnostic imaging the patients with tumor response undergo randomization. In one group the preoperative chemotherapy is continued for another 4 weeks. In the other groups surgery is performed immediately. The postoperative chemotherapy depends on the stage of the tumor at the time of operation and the histological subtype.

Materials and Methods

Between January 1989 and November 1990, 125 children entered the GPO study. The reference pathologist examined 88% (111/125) of tumors; 69% (86/125) underwent preoperative chemotherapy without preceding biopsy and 92% (79/86) of these preoperatively treated patients had a Wilms' tumor or one

[1] Department of Radiology, Clinic for Radiology, University of Heidelberg, Im Neunheimer Feld 400, 6900 Heidelberg, FRG
[2] Children's Hospital, Im Neuenheimer Feld 150, 6900 Heidelberg, FRG

Advanced Radiation Therapy Tumor Response
Monitoring and Treatment Planning
Breit (Editor-in-Chief)
© Springer-Verlag, Berlin Heidelberg 1992

of its variants. These data correspond to the results of the international findings
of the SIOP 6 study (M.F. Tournade et al. manuscript in preparation). In 15 of
these 79 patients (aged 11 months–10 years) initially diagnosed by intravenous
pyelography, ultrasound, and CT, the tumor response after 4 weeks and in seven
cases after 8 weeks of preoperative chemotherapy was evaluated by follow-up
with ultrasound and CT.

Results

The pretherapeutic volume of the tumors ranged from 90 to 1370 cm^3. The
common volume was 300–600 cm^3. Analysis of the pretherapeutic diagnostic
imaging suggested that only seven patients had a stage I and five stage II. At the
time of operation 11 of these 15 patients had nephroblastoma stage I, one had
stage II, and two had stage III. A bilateral tumor (stage V) was found in
one patient. Other authors [1, 4] have described nephroblastoma of stage I in
22%–28% of primarily operated patients. In our group, which had a much
higher percentage of low-stage nephroblastoma, one effect of the preoperative
chemotherapy must have been a downstaging in some of these tumors.

    The histological findings showed in 13 patients standard malignancy, which
was of the rhabdomyomatous subtype in one case. Two children had an
unfavorable histology with anaplasia, i.e., high malignancy. The ultrasound and
CT follow-up after 4 weeks of preoperative chemotherapy showed in eight
children a significant reduction in tumor size from more than 50% of the
starting volume. Four tumors revealed only a slight reduction of 10%–20%. In
one child the tumor size was not affected. Two tumors showed an increase of

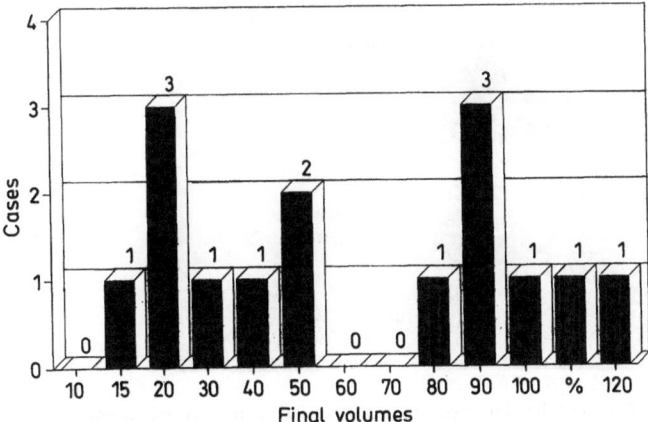

Fig. 1. Tumor volume after 4 weeks of preoperative chemotherapy in relation to the starting volume

10%–20% of the starting volume (Fig. 1). Seven children who underwent preoperative chemotherapy after randomization for 8 weeks showed an additional reduction in tumor size of 10%–50%. The tumor response during the first 4 weeks of preoperative chemotherapy was in accordance with the response

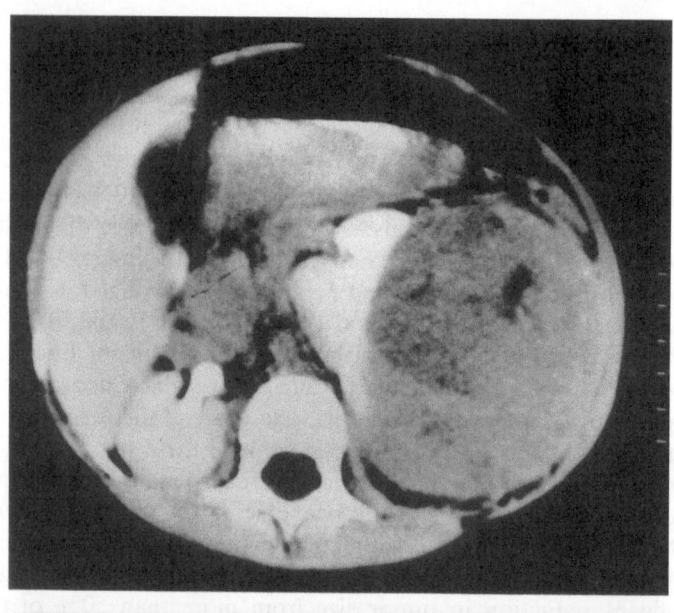

a

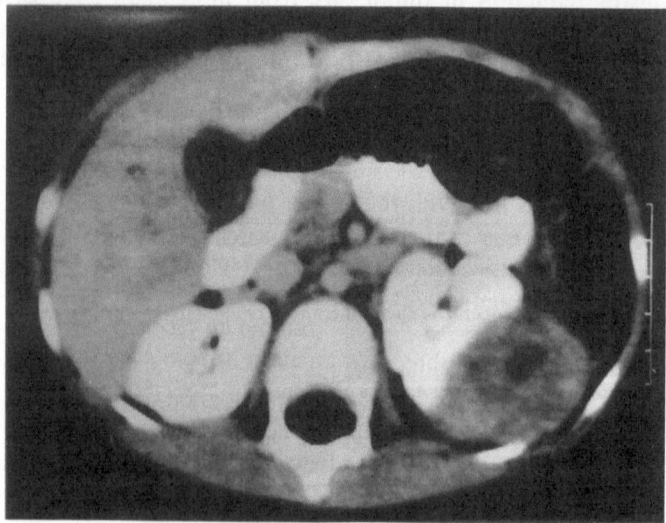

b

Fig. 2. a Admission CT scan of the abdomen shows a large exophytic mass extending from the left kidney. The kidney is flattened. b Postchemotherapy CT scan. Distinct reduction in tumor size with regeneration of the kidney. Multiple areas of low attenuation in the tumor have developed, consistent with necrosis during the 2nd month, i.e., a tumor which showed a small reduction during the 1st month of therapy also revealed only a minor reduction in the 2nd month. Initially good responders showed a further reduction in size of about 50% in the 2nd month of preoperative chemotherapy. In these cases, an impressive regeneration of the affected kidney was seen (Fig. 2).

In our study the tumor response to preoperative chemotherapy did not correlate with the starting volume (Fig. 3). The reduction in initially very small or large tumors was in the range of 10% –60%. The highest reduction occurred in tumors with a volume of 100–600 cm^3. Table 1 shows the analysis of the therapeutic effect in relation to the histological subtype of nephroblastoma. Twelve tumors with standard histology showed a reduction in volume: in eight cases of 50%–85% and in four cases of 10%–20%. In one tumor with standard histology of the rhabdomyomatous type no change in tumor size was detected. Two Wilms' tumors with unfavorable histology revealed a slight increase of 10% to about 20% after 4 weeks of preoperative chemotherapy.

A main part in the analysis of tumor regression is the study of the tumor structure. Nearly all children with standard histology showed significant regres-

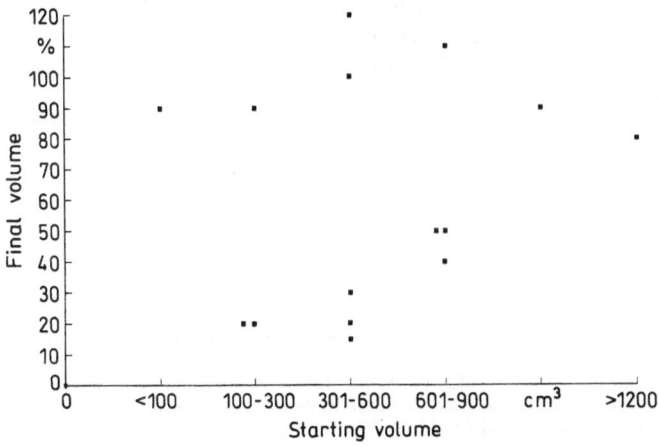

Fig. 3. Tumor volume after 4 weeks of preoperative chemotherapy in relation to the starting volume

Table 1. Tumor volume and tumor structure after 4 weeks of preoperative chemotherapy in relation to the histological type

Histology	Tumor volume	Structure
Standard histology ($n = 12$)	⬇⬇(8) ⬇(4)	Regressive (12)
Standard histology, rhabdomyomatos type ($n = 1$)	No change (1)	Regressive (1)
Unfavorable histology, anaplastic ($n = 2$)	⬆(2)	No change (2)

⬇⬇, Reduction in size of tumor $\geq$ 50%; ⬇, reduction in size of tumor 10–20%; ⬆, increase in size of tumor 10–20%.

sive changes in tumor structure, i.e., anechoic areas in ultrasound and hypo-dense or cystic areas in CT. These changes corresponded to the necrosis of tumor up to 75% as shown by histological analysis. Neither tumor with unfavorable histology revealed any changes in tumor structure in diagnostic imaging under preoperative chemotherapy.

Conclusion

Taken together, the accuracy of diagnostic imaging with 92% true nephroblas-toma in the histological analysis allowed preoperative chemotherapy in Wilms' tumor without preceding biopsy. The majority of patients showed a significant reduction in tumor size during preoperative chemotherapy, facilitating radical oncological surgery [1, 4]. The therapeutic effect can be estimated exactly by the combination of CT and ultrasound. The response can be seen in the reduction in tumor size and in the change in tumor structure. In cases with a slight reduction in tumor size, the occurrence of anechoic or hypodense areas (necrosis or old bleedings) may reveal the tumor response. This effect, mentioned by Shimizu et al. [3], could be seen in all patients with standard histology. The value of the preoperative reduction in tumor size or of the appearance of necrotic areas for the prognosis and long-term survival of the children can be judged only by follow-up data in larger groups.

References

1. Gutjahr P (1990) Bundesweite Wilmstumorstudie 1980 bis 1988. Dtsch Ärztebl 87: 2130–2134
2. Haaf HG, Kaatsch P, Michaelis J (eds) (1990) Jahresbericht 1989 des Kinderkrebsregisters Mainz, Mainz University
3. Shimizu H, Jaffe N, Eftekhari F (1987) Massive Wilms tumor: sonographic demonstration of therapeutic response without alteration in size. Pediatr Radiol 17: 493–494
4. Voute PA, Tournade MF, Delemarre JFM, de Kraker J, Carli M, Burgers JMV Bey P (1987) Preoperative chemotherapy (CT) as first treatment in children with Wilms tumor, results of the SIOP nephroblastoma trials and studies. Proc Annu Meet Am Soc Clin Oncol 6: 880
5. White KS, Grossman H (1991) Wilms' and associated renal tumors in childhood. Pediatr Radiol 21: 81–88

Diagnosis of Suprarenal Metastases in Radiation Treatment Planning Computed Tomography in Patients with Bronchial Carcinoma

K.-R. Wilhelm, K. Rieden, M. Eble, and M. Wannenmacher

Introduction

Many epithelial malignancies have been associated with a predilection for hematogenous spread to the adrenal glands, including those of lung, breast, renal, and gastric regions. Lung cancer represents the primary site from which there is the greatest risk for spread to the adrenals [2]. In staging, adrenal metastases should be evaluated before beginning a radiation therapy [2]. To detect suspected changes of the adrenals and perhaps to integrate them into radiation treatment planning the adrenal gland region was included in computed tomography (CT) scanning for this study.

Patients and Methods

From 1 January to 14 November 1990, CT of the thorax was performed in 240 patients with bronchial carcinomas for radiation treatment planning at the University Clinic for Radiology in Heidelberg. There were 206 men and 34 women; they ranged in age from 36 to 82 years. In these CT examinations the scan region was extended to the suprarenal glands.

Results

The histologic types of the primary tumors of these patients are listed in Table 1. The radiotherapy planning CT scans showed enlarged adrenals suspect for metastases in 15 patients (6.25%), bilateral in three patients. In seven patients no adrenal metastases were known formerly. The known suprarenal metastases of the other eight patients were detected by CT scans in two cases and by

Abteilung für Klinische Radiologie, Radiologische Universitätsklinik, Im Neuenheimer Feld 400, 6900 Heidelberg, FRG

Advanced Radiation Therapy Tumor Response
Monitoring and Treatment Planning
Breit (Editor-in-Chief)
© Springer-Verlag, Berlin Heidelberg 1992

Table 1. Histologic types of bronchial carcinomas

	Average age (years)	Adeno-carcinoma (n) (%)	Squamous cell carcinoma (n) (%)	Small-cell carcinoma (n) (%)	Large-cell carcinoma (n) (%)	Anaplastic carcinoma (n) (%)	"Mixed" tumor (n) (%)	Unclassifiable tumor (n) (%)	Total
Men	58.1	35 17.0	77 37.4	55 26.7	9 4.4	4 1.9	2 0.9	24 11.7	206
Women	60.0	11 32.4	8 23.5	10 29.4	0	0	0	5 14.7	34
Total		46	85	65	9	4	2	29	240

Table 2. Histologic types of adrenal metastases

	Average age (years)	Adeno-carcinoma (n) (%)	Squamous cell carcinoma (n) (%)	Small-cell carcinoma (n) (%)	Large-cell carcinoma (n) (%)	Anaplastic carcinoma (n) (%)	Non-small-cell carcinoma (n)	Total
Men	64.6	5/35 14.3	3/77 3.9	2/55 3.6	1/9 11.1	1/4 25.0	1	13
Women	69.5	1/11 9.1	0/8 0	1/10 10.0	0	0	0	2
Total		6/46	3/85	3/65	1/9	1/4	1	15

ultrasound in six cases. All the adrenal metastases diagnosed by ultrasound had a diameter over 2 cm. The size of the formerly unknown metastases found by our CT scans was less than 2 cm in four patients. The histologic types of the lung cancers of the patients with suprarenal metastases are shown in Table 2. The greatest number of adrenal metastases were diagnosed in patients with adenocarcinoma (6/46, 13.0%); the frequency in small-cell carcinoma was 3/65 (4.6%) and in squamous cell carcinoma 3/85 (3.5%). The adrenal metastases were irradiated with opposite small portals with a total dose of 30–46 Gy and a daily dose of 2 Gy.

Discussion

The routine inclusion of the suprarenal gland region in CT scanning for radiation treatment planning of bronchial carcinomas is valuable, as distant metastases which enlarge the adrenal glands can be evaluated and treated early with a minimum effort of time and material by their simultaneous irradiation with the primary lung cancer. With a 6% incidence in the early stage and with an incidence of up to 52% in the final stage [1], attention should also be paid to this form of metastases in the posttumor care.

References

1. Heilmann HP, Kärcher KH, Seitz W, Schulz U (1987) Tumoren der Thoraxorgane. In: Scherer E (ed) Strahlentherapie, 3rd edn. Springer, Berlin Heidelberg New York, pp 565–593
2. Soffen EM, Solin LJ, Rubenstein JH, Hanks GE (1990) Palliative radiotherapy for symptomatic adrenal metastases. Cancer 65: 1318–1320

Tumor Response Monitoring:
Pelvis

Magnetic Resonance Imaging in Gynecologic Oncology: Role in Pre- and Postradiation Treatment

H. Hricak

Introduction

"The first treatment should be the best possible since it has the greatest chance for curing the patient" [1]. The choice of therapy in cancer patients in general depends on the tumor size, depth of invasion, and stage [2]. Clinical staging is often limited and inaccurate, with the resultant suboptimal therapy [2]. The cross-sectional imaging modalities ultrasound, computed tomography (CT), and magnetic resonance imaging (MRI) have improved the staging of malignant disease [3]. In the pelvis, MRI offers several advantages over the other imaging modalities. In particular, MRI has excellent soft-tissue contrast resolution, allows direct multiplanar imaging, and offers variable imaging parameters (TR/TE), thus facilitating optimal tumor evaluation. However, MRI is not tissue specific, and a histologic diagnosis is required in all cases.

In the postradiotherapy patient, MRI has the ability to demonstrate radiation tissue change and the potential to differentiate radiation fibrosis from recurrent/residual tumor and can therefore be used as a suitable adjunct for assessing treatment response.

Pretreatment Evaluation: Carcinoma of the Cervix

The prognostic factors for carcinoma of the cervix include tumor grade, size, location, depth of stromal invasion, adjacent tumor extension, and lymph node metastases. Except for tumor grade, all other morphologic criteria can be evaluated by MRI.

On the T2-weighted MR image, cervical cancer appears as a high signal intensity mass contrasting against the normal, low signal intensity of cervical stroma [4, 5]. Similar signal intensity changes, however, may be seen with inflammatory disease, postbiopsy changes, and nabothian cyst [3, 6], rendering cervical biopsy essential for the initial diagnosis.

Uroradiology Section, Department of Radiology, University of California, San Francisco, CA 94143-0628, USA

Advanced Radiation Therapy Tumor Response
Monitoring and Treatment Planning
Breit (Editor-in-Chief)
© Springer-Verlag, Berlin Heidelberg 1992

MRI staging parallels the FIGO staging criteria. Stage 0 tumor, i.e., cervical carcinoma in situ, is not identified on MRI. Tumors confined to the cervix (stage I) when larger than 0.5 cm can be demonstrated on T2-weighted MR images as a region of high signal intensity surrounded by the adjacent normal, low signal intensity stroma. When the full thickness of the stroma is invaded, the low intensity stripe is no longer seen, but the symmetric configuration and the signal intensity of the parametrium remain normal. In stage II-A disease, tumor is seen extending into the upper two-thirds of the vagina. In stage II-B tumor, the parametria are invaded. The parametrial invasion is diagnosed when there is eccentric parametrial enlargement, lateral margins are irregular, periparametrial fat planes on T1-weighted images are no longer seen, or on T2-weighted images there is an abnormal high signal intensity present in the involved parametrium. In stage III-A, tumor can be seen extending to the lower third of the vagina. In stage III-B, the normal low signal intensity pelvic wall muscles (levator ani, piriformis, or obturator internus) are disrupted on T2-weighted images. Sagittal images are valuable in the evaluation of stage 1V disease, namely in the demonstration of the bladder or rectal wall invasion. Detection of pelvic lymph node involvement with MRI currently equals that with CT. Both techniques rely on the size of the node, and neither MRI nor CT can distinguish between malignant and hyperplastic nodes.

MRI is not recommended for every patient with cervical cancer. Its value rises in proportion to the volume and stage of the cancer and in the presence of concomitant disease. MRI is indicated in the cervical cancer patient when:

– The tumor size approaches 3 cm on clinical examination (at this point the incidence of lymph node metastases approaches 47%).
– There is a primary endocervical lesion (Fig. 1).
– There is infiltrative tumor growth.
– There are concomitant adnexal or uterine masses.
– It is necessary to exclude extension of tumor to parametrial or adjacent tissue.
– The patient is pregnant.
– Tumor volume assessment is needed for radiation port planning.

Pretreatment Evaluation: Endometrial Carcinoma

On T2-weighted images, the zonal anatomy of the uterus is well visualized, and tumors of the endometrium can be detected [4, 5]. Endometrial carcinoma, however, has nonspecific MRI appearance. It cannot be consistently differentiated from blood clot, benign tumor, or adenomatous hyperplasia, and biopsy to confirm the diagnosis is necessary. However, staging of the disease by MRI is excellent, with 85% accuracy reported by the NCl multicenter study [6]. MRI staging criteria parallels the recommended surgical staging [7]. Stage I tumors are confined to the uterine corpus. If the tumor is small and confined to

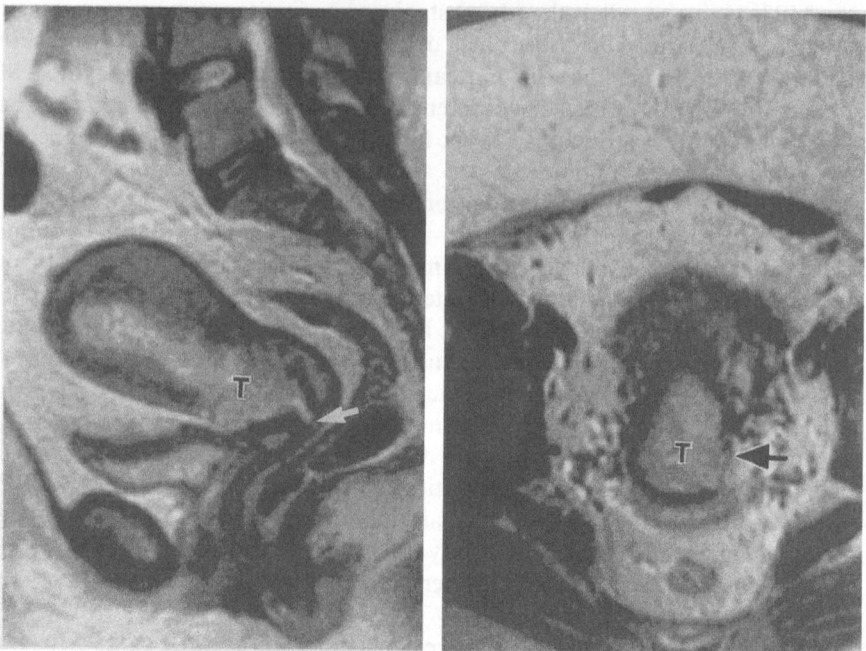

Fig. 1a, b. Endocervical carcinoma (*T*) with full-depth stromal invasion and tumor extension to the left parametria (*solid arrow*). The exocervix (*white arrow*) is free of tumor. T2-weighted images. **a** Sagittal. **b** Transaxial

the endometrium (stage I-A), on T2-weighted images the only abnormality may be increased endometrial width or lobulation of the uterine cavity [4, 5]. The depth of myometrial invasion (inner half stage I-B, and outer half stage I-C) can be assessed with an overall accuracy of 74% [6]. MR stage II disease involves both corpus and cervix. Stage II disease can be further divided into stage II-A (no stromal invasion) and stage II-B (invasion of the cervical stroma, which, when invaded, demonstrates high signal intensity on the T2-weighted image). Stage III disease indicates tumor extension outside the uterus but not outside the true pelvis, and stage IV lesions have extended outside the true pelvis and involve the bladder or rectum.

MRI is indicated in patients with endometrial carcinoma when:

– Physical examination is limited.
– There is a concomitant uterine lesion, for example, leiomyoma, making clinical assessment difficult.
– A histological grade 3 lesion is diagnosed (with the increased likelihood of deep myometrial invasion MRI plays an important role in treatment planning.
– An advanced stage is suspected clinically, warranting initial treatment by radiation therapy rather than surgery.

Evaluation of Postradiation Patients

Radiation-induced tissue changes have been documented in the pelvis [8]. The incidence of MRI-detectable radiation tissue change rises with increasing radiation dose and is significantly higher when the dose exceeds 4500 cGy [8]. In one study, the incidence of bladder and rectal changes rose from 8% and 24%, respectively, when the dose was less than 4500 cGy, to 51% and 48%, respectively, with a dose greater than 4500 cGy [8]. Similarly, radiation changes in the uterus, bone marrow, and pelvic fat occurred with a mean dose greater than 4500 cGy [8].

Radiation change in the premenarchal uterus can be detected. In women of reproductive age, the uterus demonstrates a variety of signal changes [9], mediated by both a direct radiation effect and radiation-induced ovarian hypofunction. As early as 1 month after treatment, the myometrium demonstrates a generalized decrease in signal intensity on T2-weighted images. After approximately 3 months, the uterine zonal anatomy becomes indistinct, and after 6 months, a decrease in the thickness and signal intensity of the endometrium becomes apparent. The uterus also decreases in size after radiation therapy. In the postmenopausal uterus, similar changes occur, but because the postmenopausal uterus is normally small and of low signal intensity, the changes are not as apparent.

The ovaries become smaller after radiation therapy and demonstrate decreased signal intensity on T2-weighted images. These changes reflect atrophy of the ovarian follicles and increased fibrosis with vascular sclerosis.

Immediately following radiation therapy, the wall of the vagina demonstrates increased signal intensity on T2-weighted images, probably caused by edema and hypervascular inflammatory changes. Eventually, fibrotic changes in the vagina cause it to image with low signal intensity on all imaging sequences.

Depending on the severity of postradiation change, a spectrum of findings are seen in the bladder and rectum. Severe radiation change may also lead to fistula formation [10]. Therefore, in the absence of any definite bladder mass lesion, it is important to consider radiation as the cause of high signal intensity change in the postradiation patient, particularly in the first 1–2 years after therapy.

The clinical distinction between residual or recurrent tumor and posttreatment fibrosis may be extremely difficult, and biopsy is often required to resolve the question. Both CT and MRI complement the clinical evaluation, providing information about areas that are clinically inaccessible and allowing better overall evaluation of the patient. Recent reports on MRI indicate that tumor recurrence can usually be differentiated from radiation fibrosis on the basis of signal intensity. Typically, fibrosis images with low signal intensity on both T1- and T2-weighted images. Tumor, however, exhibits a high signal intensity on T2-weighted images. Unfortunately, the inflammation and edema associated with acute radiation change (which may persist for up to 18 months) may also demonstrate high signal intensity on T2-weighted images, sometimes leading to an incorrect diagnosis. Gd-DTPA administration causes enhancement of both tumor and the edematous, inflammatory irradiated tissues and does not contribute to differentiating the two entities.

Conclusion

MRI can demonstrate local tumor stage and identify enlarged pelvic and retroperitoneal nodes. In addition, MRI can be used for the evaluation of the postradiation pelvis in search of suspected persistent or recurrent disease. Knowledge of the MRI appearance of radiation tissue changes is essential for correct image analysis. MRI differentiation between tumor and radiation fibrosis can be achieved in selective cases. However, radiation-induced inflammation and necrosis sometimes precludes the diagnostic ability of MRI, and despite progress in the MRI technology, biopsy and histologic diagnosis have not been superseded.

References

1. Rutledge FN (1962) Cancer of the female genital system. In: Carcinoma of the uterine cervix, endometrium and ovary. Year Book Medical, Chicago, pp 13–18
2. Morrow PC, Townsend DE (1987) Tumors of the endometrium,. In: Morrow PC, Townsend DE (eds) Synopsis of gynecologic oncology, 3rd edn. Churchill Livingstone, New York, pp 159–205
3. Hricak H (1991) The role of imaging in the evaluation of pelvic cancer. In: DeVita VT Jr., Hellmann S, Rosenberg SA (eds) Important advances in oncology. Lippincott, Philadelphia, pp 103–133
4. Togashi K, Nishimura K, Itoh K, Atow (1986): Uterine cervical cancer: assessment with high field MR imaging. Radiology 160: 431
5. Hricak H, Lacey CG, Sandles LG et al. (1988) Invasive cervical carcinoma: comparison of MR imaging and surgical findings. Radiology 166: 623–631
6. Hricak H, Rubinstein LV, Gherman GM, Karstaedt N (1991) MRI in the evaluation of endometrial carcinoma: results of an NCI cooperative study. Radiology 179: 829–832
7. Announcements FIGO stages 1988 revision (1989) Gynecol Oncol 35: 125–127
8. Sugimura K, Carrington BM, Quivey J, Hricak H (1990) postirradiation changes in the pelvis: assessment with MR imaging. Radiology 175: 805–813
9. Tavares NJ, Arrive L, Demas BE, Quivey J, Hricak H (1988) Bladder morphology following radiation therapy: assessment with MR imaging (abstract). RSNA 1988 Scientific Assembly and Annual Meeting
10. Arrive L, Chang YCF , Hricak H, Brescia RJ, Auffermann W, Quivey JM (1989) Radiation induced uterine changes: MR imaging. Radiology 170: 55
11. Ramsey RG, Zacharias CE (1985) MR imaging of the spine after radiation therapy: early recognizable effects. AJR 144: 1131
12. Krestin GP et al. (1988) Recurrent rectal cancer: diagnosis with MR imaging vs. CT. Radiology 169: 307

Clinical Feasibility Determining of the Usefulness of
Magnetic Resonance imaging in the Assessing
of Tumor Response

A. Buchbinder, I. Bank, H. Rosenthal, and Katherine Sena

The purpose of this study was to investigate the usefulness of magnetic resonance imaging (MRI) in the evaluation of tumor response and to monitor the changing signal intensity (SI) and volume of the tumor during and after primary radiation therapy (RT) of coefficient of the uterine cervix.

Patients and Methods

Twenty-four women with histologically confirmed uterine carcinoma were examined by MRI before, during, and following RT. RT-a and to a 12-month follow-up was 3–12 months at present, average 26.1 months. The patients averaged 58.03 years, range 40.5 years. The primary carcinomas were in the FIGO stage IIb or a IIb (Fig. 5.4), IIIb (n = 4-3), IIIb (n = 10) and IVa (n = 3). All patients had a follow-up and a gynecological examination at six-month intervals. The staging was carried out at intervals of biopsy.

The MRI technique included the following features: 1.5-T and 1 MHz (Toroscan Philips) spin-echo pulse sequences TR/TE 550/26 to ms, 2D thickness omit relaxed acquisition of 0.5 scan resolution 256 x 256, two image averaging water fat shift 1.3. Flow compensation presaturation of that scan technique. Immediately before the examination 1 mg glucagon was administered intramuscularly.

In FIGO A the patients received Examined six months after mean 22 by V, 45–48 Gy) and HDR brachytherapy Iridium 192 intracavitary placement, including 2 x 6.5 Gy series.

SI measurements were obtained by evaluating regions of interest within a tumor of least tissue outside the radiation field and within the tumor and least fibrotic tissue. Semiquantitative analysis was performed by evaluation of SI ratios for the SI of the tumor relative to that of muscle and the SI of fibrosis relative to that of muscle (relative signal SI) in the following representation of tumor.

Adapted from ..... Radiation Radiy Report
Radiation on Tumors (Poster)
Springer-Verlag Berlin Heidelberg 1991

Primary Irradiated Carcinomas of the Uterine Cervix: Magnetic Resonance Imaging in the Monitoring of Tumor Response

F. Flueckiger, F. Ebner, H. Poschauko, and K. Arian-Schad

Introduction

The purpose of this study was to investigate the reliability of magnetic resonance imaging (MRI) in the evaluation of tumor response and to monitor the changing signal intensity (SI) and volume of the tumor during and after primary radiotherapy (RTX) of carcinomas of the uterine cervix.

Patients and Methods

Twenty-four women with histologically confirmed cervical carcinoma were examined by MRI before, during, and following RTX and at 6- to 9-month intervals (follow-up 6–48 months at present, average 20.5 months). The patients were aged 34–81 years (mean 60.3 years). The primary carcinomas were in the FIGO stages Ib ($n = 1$), IIb ($n = 9$), IIIa ($n = 3$), IIIb ($n = 10$), and IVa ($n = 1$). All patients had a close clinical follow-up and a gynecological examination at 3-month intervals. The MRI findings were ascertained by transvaginal biopsy.

The MRI technique included the following features: 1.5 T, 64 MHz (Gyroscan, Philips), spin-echo pulse sequences TR/TE 2500/30,90 ms, slice thickness 6 mm, reduced acquisition 70%, scan resolution 256×256, two measurements, water fat shift 1.5, flow compensation (presaturation), half-scan technique. Immediately before the examination 1 mg glucagon was administered intravenously.

For RTX the patients received a combined external beam (photon beams, 23 MeV, 44–48 Gy) and HDR brachytherapy (iridium-192, intracervical placement, afterloading, 2×8.5 Gy).

SI measurements were obtained by determining regions of interest within normal skeletal muscle outside the radiation field and within the tumor and local fibrotic tissue. Semiquantitative analysis was performed by calculation of SI ratios for the SI of the tumor relative to that of muscle and the SI of fibrosis relative to that of muscle (relative SI). In the following presentation SI always

Department of Radiology, University of Graz, Auenbruggerplatz 9, 8036 Graz, Austria

Advanced Radiation Therapy Tumor Response
Monitoring and Treatment Planning
Breit (Editor-in-Chief)
© Springer-Verlag, Berlin Heidelberg 1992

refs to the SI ratios, i.e., relative SI. The tumor volume was measured using a semiautomatic volumetry data program.

Results

Immediate Responders. Sixteen of 24 patients (66.1%) had a total regression in tumor volume 6 months after RTX (Fig. 1). The SI prior to RTX was 5.14 ± 1.16 and dropped to 2.1 ± 0.6 after 3–6 months following RTX (Fig. 2). These changes in SI were statistically highly significant. In all patients total tumor regression was observed in follow-up (follow-up 9–48 months, average 23 months). Figure 2 shows clearly that the decrease in SI in responding tumors was maximal within the first 3 months, and that the decrease was nearly complete 6 months after RTX.

Residual Tumors, Delayed responders, Nonresponders. In 8/24 patients (33.3%) MRI 3–6 months following RTX demonstrated a residual tumor in terms of SI

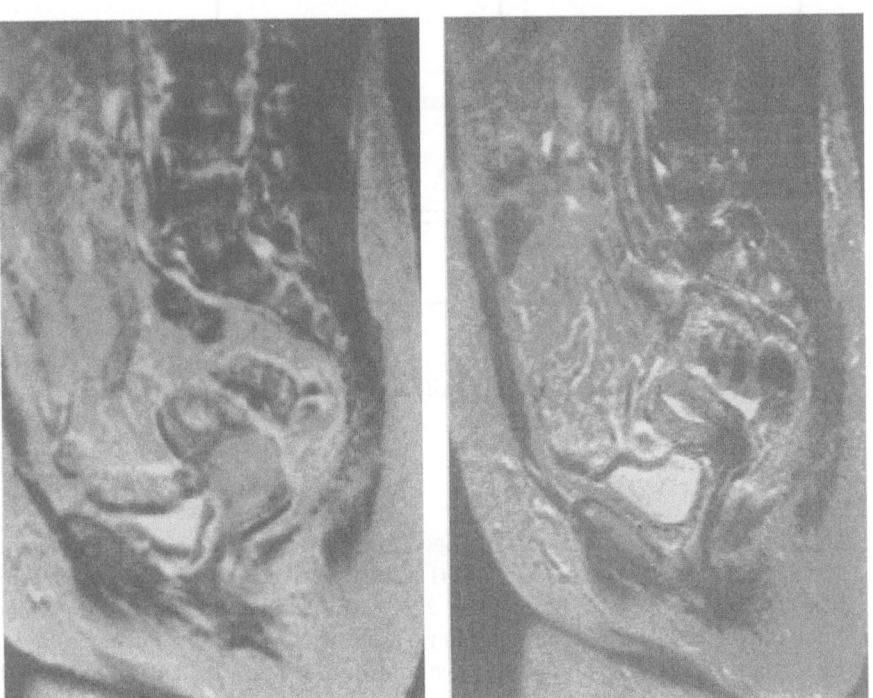

a   b

Fig. 1a, b. Saggital MRI scans in a 60-year-old patient before (**a**) and 5 months after RTX (**b**). Total tumor regression is demonstrable. Radiation fibrosis exhibits low SI

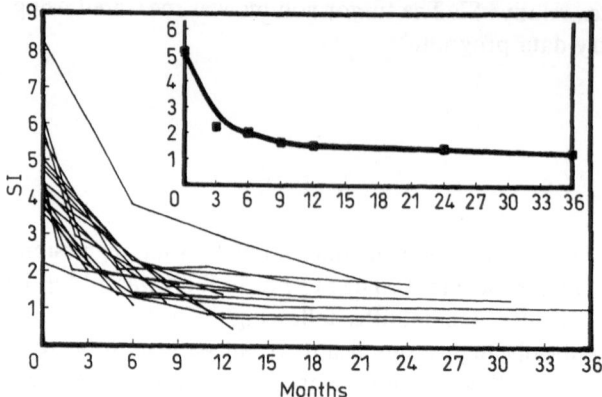

Fig. 2. Changes in relative SI before (0) and following RTX in cases with immediate response ($n = 16$). The SI was measured within the tumor or the cervix after total tumor regression (radiation fibrosis). *Inset,* the averaged SI curve

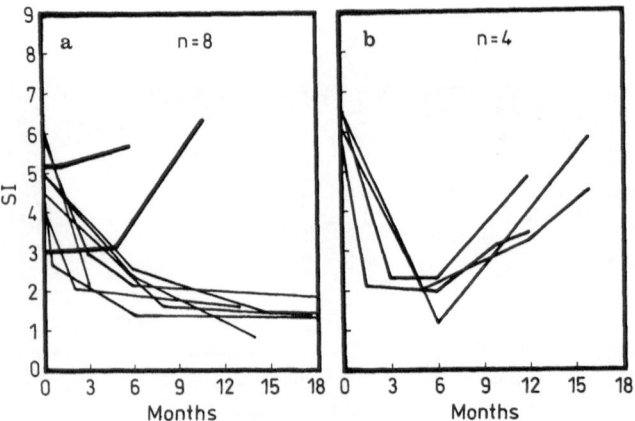

Fig. 3a, b. Changes in relative SI in cases with delayed response (**a,** *thin lines*), no response (**a,** *thick lines*), and with recurrent tumors (**b**)

and volume. Nearly all of these belonged to the group of large tumors, exceeding 50 cm^3. In 6/8 cases a decrease in SI (Fig. 3a) relative to the primary was visible (before RTX, 5.4 ± 0.85; after RTX, 2.58 ± 0.8), similar to that of responders, but a mass lesion was still present after 6 months. Surprisingly, during follow-up these six patients were shown to have total tumor regression 10 months at the latest without additional therapy (delayed response). In 2/24 cases (8.3%) progression of the primary tumor was observed (nonresponders). In these cases no decrease in SI was observed after RTX (Fig. 3a).

Recurrent Tumors. Four of 24 patients (16.7%) developed a recurrent neoplasm after total tumor regression. Two of these patients belonged to the group with immediate and two to the group with delayed response. The recurrent tumors occurred 9–16 months after RTX. All showed high SI, as the primary tumor (Fig. 3b).

Radiation Fibrosis. In the early stage 3–6 months after RTX radiation fibrosis exhibited higher SI (1.9 ± 0.6); 6–9 months after RTX and throughout the observation period of 24–48 months fibrosis showed low SI (1.22 ± 0.15).MRI findings correlated with the clinical courses as well as with gynecologic examination and biopsies in 23/24 patients (95.8%). In one patient MRI findings were suggestive of residual tumor 8 months after RTX. However, transvaginal biopsy showed fibrosis and inflammation but no tumor growth, and follow-up revealed no evidence of residual or recurrent neoplasm.

Discussion

A change in the SI of irradiated tumors has been ascertained by several studies [1, 2, 5]. We found a significant decrease in SI in irradiated tumors with good response to RTX. The decrease in SI corresponded with the progressive replacement of neoplastic tissue by radiation fibrosis. This process was nearly finished 3–6 months after RTX (depending on the size of the primary tumor). High SI in an irradiated tumor does not necessarily reflect vigorous tumor tissue since early fibrosis as well as edema, hemorrhage, hyalinosis, granulation tissue, and inflammation may cause such findings [3, 6]. MRI evaluation of tumor response had reliable results 6 months after RTX in demonstrating significant decrease in SI and tumor volume. Non-responding tumors did not show a decrease in SI.

Recurrent tumors in our study (long TR and long TE spin-echo pulse sequences) showed high SI, as the primary tumor. This was also found in other studies [3, 4, 5]. Since radiation fibrosis showed low SI in such sequences later than 6 months after RTX, recurrences can be well differentiated from fibrosis. MRI is therefore able to detect reliably early recurrent neoplasm during follow-up.

The imaging technique that we used on a high field system achieved optimal contrast to noise, increasing with long TE times, and thus enabled satisfactory differentiation between an irradiated tumor and surrounding tissue. Whether these results are achievable on low or medium field strength systems or with other imaging techniques remains to be established.

Conclusions

We can summarize our findings as follows, (a) In the presented series MRI achieved reliable results in evaluating tumor response to RTX when compared with clinical follow-up in 23/24 patients. (b) A decrease in SI indicated response to RTX. (c) The changes in SI within tumors undergoing RTX were completed within 6 months in the group with immediate response. (d) The most significant decrease in tumor SI occurred within the first 3 months. (e) In cases of large tumor volumes delayed response to RTX was seen (persistence of mass lesion with decreased SI and spontaneous tumor regression later than 6 months). (f) In contrast to previous studies, low SI radiation fibrosis was observed as early as 6 months after RTX.

References

1. Axel L, Kressel HY, Thickmann D et al. (1983) NMR imaging of the chest at 0.12T: initial clinical experience with a resistive magnet. AJR 141: 1157–1162
2. Bies JR, Ellis JA, Kopecky KK, Sutton GP, Klatte EC, Stehmann FB, Ehrlich CE (1984) Assessment of primary gynecologic malignancies. Comparison of 0.15T resistive MRI with CT. AJR 143: 1249–1257
3. Ebner F, Kressel HY, Mintz MC, Carlson JA, Cohen EK, Schiebler M, Gefter W, Axel L (1988) Tumor recurrence versus fibrosis in the female pelvis: differentiation with MR imaging at 1.5T. Radiology 166: 333–340
4. Flückiger F, Ebner F, Poschauko H, Arian-Schad K, Einspieler R, Hausegger K (1991) Stellenwert der Magnetresonanztomographie beim primär bestrahlten karzinom der zervix uteri: Therapie-erfolgsbeurteilung und Nachsorge. Strahlenther Onkol 167: 152–157
5. Glazer HS, Levitt RG, Lee JKT, Emani B, Gronemeyer S, Murphy WA (1984) Differentiation of radiation fibrosis from recurrent pulmonary neoplasm by magnetic resonance imaging. AJR 143: 729–730
6. Glazer HS, Lee JKT, Levitt RG, Heiken JP, Ling D, Totty WG, Balfe DM, Emani B, Wassermann TH, Murphy WA (1985) Radiation fibrosis: differentiation from recurrent tumor by MR imaging. Radiology 156: 721–726

The Use of Magnetic Resonance Imaging in Combined Radio-Chemotherapy of Cervical Carcinoma

H. Junkermann, G. Gademann, H. Schmid, and D.V. Fournier

Since 1987, 25 patients with bulky tumors of the cervix uteri (stage IIb, two; stage III, 20; stage IVa, one; stage IVb, two) have been treated with combined radio-chemotherapy. The first 12 patients were treated with a sequential schedule consisting of two or three cycles of chemotherapy, combined tele- and brachyra-diotherapy, and a further two or three cycles of chemotherapy. Each chemother-apy cycle consisted of cisplatin 20 mg/m^2 and 5-fluorouracil 1000 mg/m^2 for 5 days and was repeated on day 29. Ten patients showed remission under this therapy (Table 1). In eight patients the response was monitored using computed tomography (CT). Despite the good initial response to chemotherapy the intermediate results of this sequentially combined radio-chemotherapy, how-ever, were disappointing (Fig. 1).

Tumor-biological considerations and results of randomized studies using sequential radio-chemotherapy made us change to a simultaneous radio-chemotherapy scheme. One cycle of the chemotherapy described above was given as induction therapy. Concomitant with the second chemotherapy cycle percutaneous whole pelvis radiotherapy was started. A total dose of 45 Gy was given in 5 weeks. During the last week of whole pelvis irradiation the third cycle of chemotherapy was given.

Thirteen patients were treated according to this scheme (in two of these, irradiation was started with the first cycle because of bleeding). In ten women of this group the response of the tumor to the first cycle of chemotherapy was monitored by CT (six patients) and/or magnetic resonance imaging (MRI; six patients). While CT scans in these patients with bulky tumors always showed signs of expansion of the cervix uteri, they did not allow the delineation of tumor against healthy uterine tissues. MRI, however, made this delineation possible. Using MRI, the pretherapeutic extension of the tumor could be visualized exactly. MRI allowed the diagnosis of a viable endocervical tumor residual after combined radio-chemotherapy in cases of a clinically unsuspicious cervix with unsuspicious CT scan. MRI visualized atypical excentric tumor growth which could not be detected on CT. The improved information of tumor extension was important for radiological treatment planning. Using MRI it was possible in every case to evaluate treatment response after only one cycle of chemotherapy. This information might be especially important in therapy schemes with

Department of Gynecological Radiology, Department of Clinical Radiology and Department of General Oncology, University of Heidelberg, FRG

Advanced Radiation Therapy Tumor Response Monitoring and Treatment Planning
Breit (Editor-in-Chief)
© Springer-Verlag, Berlin Heidelberg 1992

Table 1. Local response to chemotherapy in 25 patients with locally advanced squamous cell carcinoma of the cervix uteri

	Complete remission	Partial remission	No change	Progressive disease
Group I (sequential)	2	8	1	1
Group II (simultaneous)	0	8	3	0

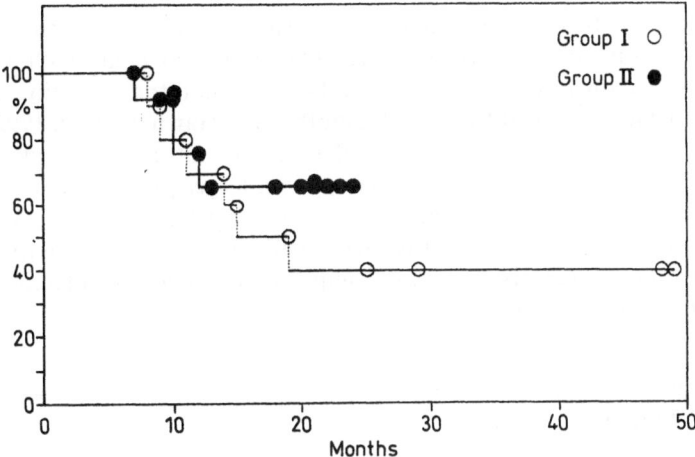

Fig. 1. Survival in ten patients with locally advanced squamous cell carcinoma of the cervix uteri treated with sequential radio-chemotherapy (group I, excluding two patients with primary metastatic disease) and 13 patients treated with concomitant radio-chemotherapy

preoperative down-staging. We see, however, more promise in the concomitant radio-chemotherapy approach. Although radiotherapy had to be interrupted in seven cases because of toxicity (mainly myelotoxicity of the concomitant schedule) the short-term results of this treatment seem to be better than in sequentially treated patients.

MRI is a useful method for pretherapeutic evaluation of large cervix tumors. It is presently the best method for monitoring treatment response under chemotherapy. The information gained by MRI can be used to improve treatment strategy.

Treatment Response in Carcinoma of the Uterine Cervix: Evaluation by Magnetic Resonance Imaging

J.M. Hawnaur, B.M. Carrington, R.D. Hunter, and I. Isherwood

Introduction

The accuracy of magnetic resonance imaging (MRI) in staging surgically treated patients with carcinoma of the cervix is well established (Hricak et al. 1988). We have previously demonstrated the ability of MRI to monitor reduction in tumour size following treatment by radical radiotherapy (Hawnaur et al. 1992). The aim of this study was to assess the ability of MRI to monitor the response of primary carcinoma of the cervix to radiotherapy in a larger group of patients and to detect residual or recurrent tumour at an early preclinical stage. The predictive value of findings on the pretreatment MRI scans and the pattern of response to treatment were also assessed compared with clinical outcome 6 months or more after treatment.

Patients and Methods

Pretreatment MRI scans were obtained in 100 women with stage IB–IV carcinoma of the cervix and repeated routinely 3 and 6 months after completion of radical radiotherapy, comprising one or two intracavitary treatments with or without external pelvic irradiation. Additional scans were obtained if clinically indicated, usually to investigate symptoms and signs suggesting recurrent tumour. Patients were scanned on a 0.26-T superconducting MRI system using conventional spin-echo sequences (SE 740-2000/26-120) in multiple planes. The standard body coil or a corset surface coil were used with a 30- to 45-cm field of view. Section thickness was 7–10 mm with 192–256 views and two signal excitations. Images were analysed prospectively for tumour volume and extent and for lymphadenopathy (enlargement to 1.5 cm or greater), both pre- and posttreatment. Tumour was identified as a hyperintense lesion on T2-weighted MRI scans and its dimensions measured using the electronic cursor on the imaging console. Anteroposterior and craniocaudal diameters were obtained

Department of Diagnostic Radiology, University of Manchester, Oxford Road, Manchester M13 9PT, UK

Advanced Radiation Therapy Tumor Response
Monitoring and Treatment Planning
Breit (Editor-in-Chief)
© Springer-Verlag, Berlin Heidelberg 1992

from sagittal images and the transverse and anteroposterior diameters from oblique scans, passing through the short axis of the cervix. Volume was calculated from the orthogonal measurements using the following formula which assumes an ellipsoid configuration of tumour:

$$V = \frac{4}{3}\pi \cdot \frac{a}{2} \cdot \frac{b}{2} \cdot \frac{c}{2} = 0.52 \, abc$$

where a, b and c are the orthogonal measurements.

MRI findings were correlated with those of pelvic examination under anaesthesia, clinical follow-up of at least 6 months duration and, in some cases, cervical biopsy or hysterectomy.

Results

Complete tumour regression was observed on MRI 3–6 months after completion of radiotherapy in 63% of cases. Regression of the primary tumour was considered satisfactory on MRI when there was complete disappearance of the hyperintense mass demonstrated on pretreatment T2-weighted scans, together with reconstitution of the low signal cervical stroma and no evidence of extracervical spread of tumour or enlarged lymph nodes. There was no consistent relationship between regression rate and tumour size, most patients showing marked reduction in tumour size by 3 months after treatment, despite a wide range of pretreatment tumour volumes. The completeness of tumour regression, however, did appear to have an association with tumour volume: high signal persisting within the cervix on the 3-month MRI scan was observed in 16% of patients, most of whom presented with bulky stage IIB–IV tumours (Fig. 1). To date, seven of these have died or have recurrent or metastatic disease. Biopsy of high signal areas showed only radiation changes in two others. In 16 patients with satisfactory regression of the primary tumour, concomitant development of lymphadenopathy or extracervical recurrence was observed on MRI. A small proportion of patients died of their disease before the MRI study was completed, had a hysterectomy or were otherwise lost to follow-up.

In seven patients, some of whom were being re-scanned for clinically suspected tumour recurrence more than 6 months after treatment, reappearance, persistence or increasing volume of high signal within the cervix was noted on T2-weighted scans, compared with previous MRI scans (Fig. 2). Biopsy or hysterectomy in six of these showed tumour in four, radiation change in one and both radiation change and tumour recurrence in one. There was no consistent difference in morphology or signal intensity, either visually or measured, between radiation change and small volume tumour recurrence. Pelvic sidewall recurrence was demonstrated in three other patients and vaginal recurrence in

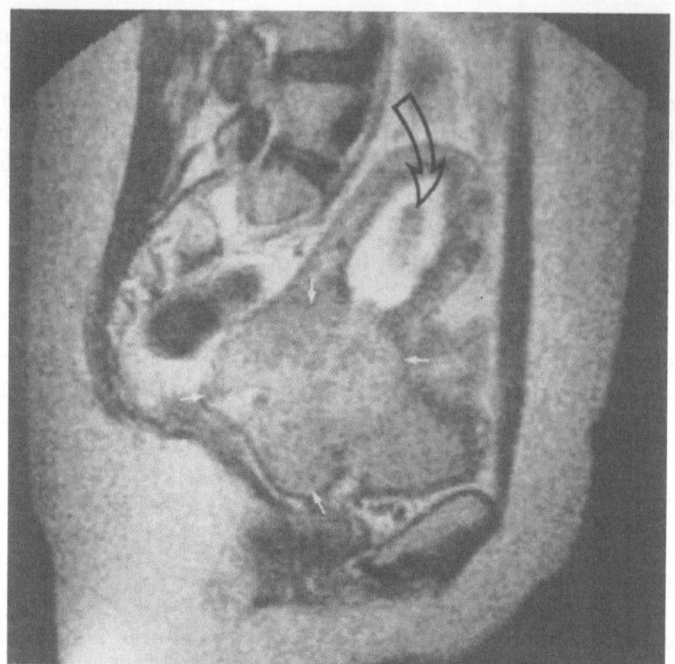

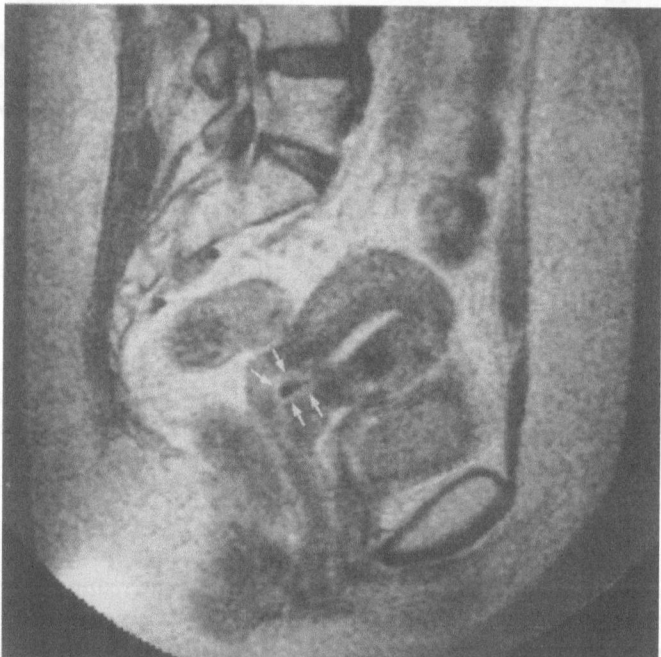

Fig. 1a, b. Sagittal T2-weighted (SE 1500/80) MRI scans of the pelvis in a woman with stage IIB carcinoma of the cervix before (**a**) and 3 months after (**b**) radiotherapy. The untreated tumour is obstructing the uterine cavity, which is distended and contains blood clot (*curved arrow*). There is marked reduction in tumour volume after therapy but with residual signal abnormality probably representing necrotic tumour in the cervix (*arrows*). Note the hyperintense bladder base secondary to radiotherapy

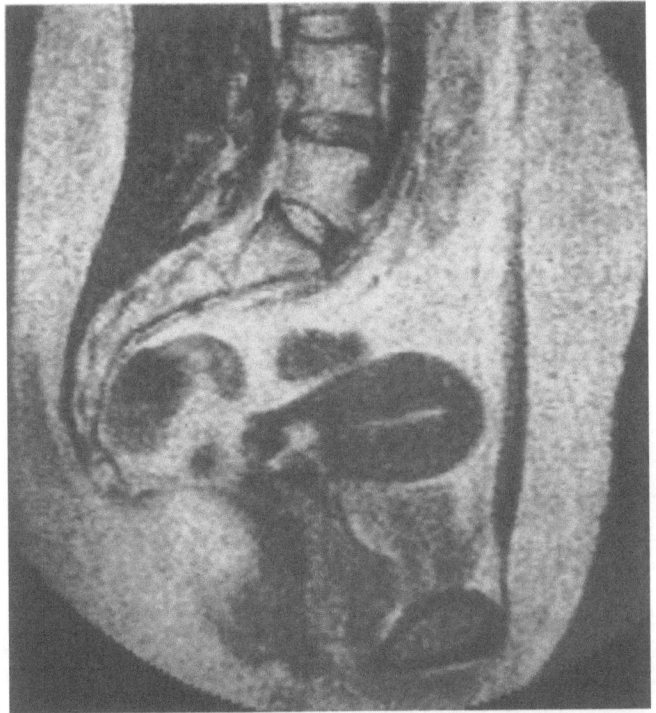

a

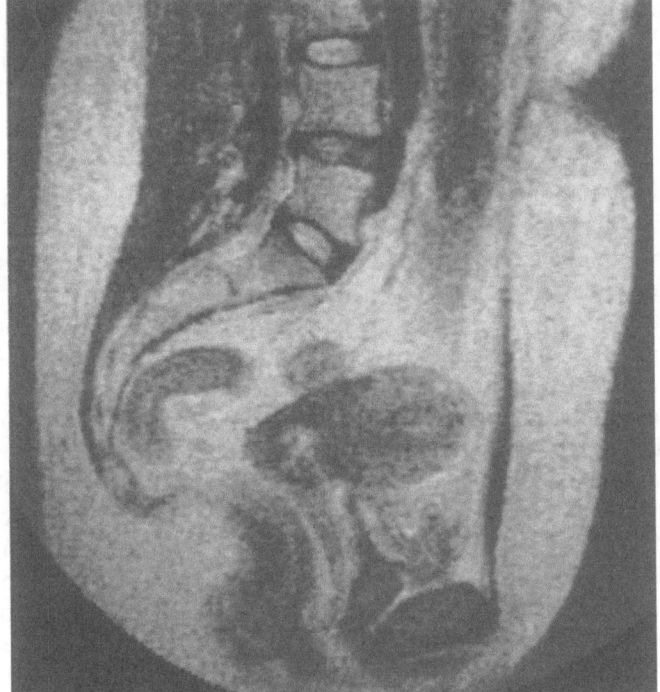

b   Fig. 2a and b

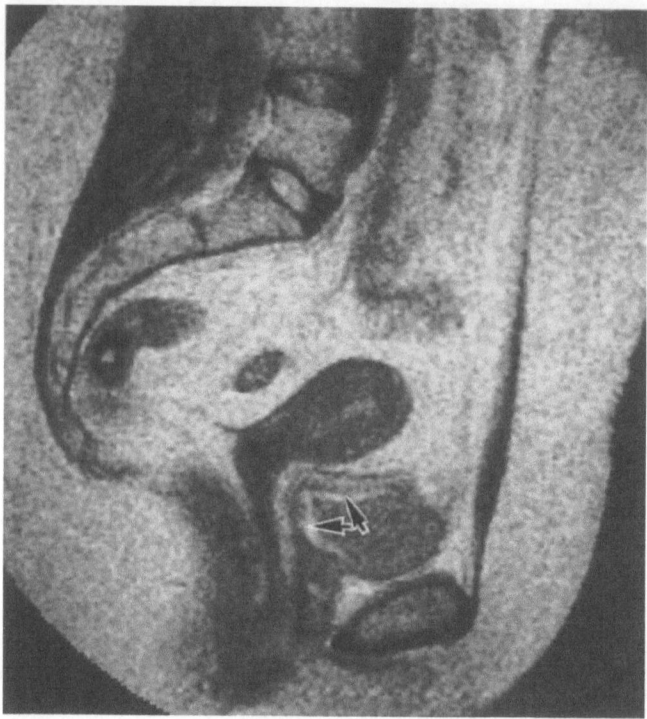

c

Fig. 2a–c. Sagittal T2-weighted (SE 1500/80) MRI scans of the pelvis in a woman with treated carcinoma of the cervix 3 months (**a**), 6 months (**b**) and 2 years (**c**) after radiotherapy. The area of persistent high signal within the cervix was biopsied and consisted of radiation changes only. The patient subsequently presented with symptoms and signs of radiation cystitis, confirmed on MRI

one. In these patients tumour was identified as a mass of low to intermediate signal intensity on T1-weighted sequences and a hyperintense mass on T2-weighted sequences. In one patient given Gd-DTPA, enhancement of recurrent pelvic tumour was observed.

The most useful prognostic factors on pretreatment MRI were tumour volume and the presence and extent of pelvic and/or para-aortic lymphadenopathy. Although an MRI tumour stage of IB had a strong association with a satisfactory outcome and a tumour stage of IIIB or more with a poor outcome, an MRI stage of IIA or IIB was of no predictive value. A tumour volume of less than 40 cm^3 was associated with a good outcome in 84% of patients while only 28% of patients with a tumour volume of more than 40 cm^3 had a good outcome with no evidence of persistent or recurrent disease to date. Most patients with small tumours but a poor outcome had other unfavourable features on MRI. Lymphadenopathy was present on pretreatment MRI in five of seven patients subsequently manifesting metastases, and an incomplete response of the primary tumour on MRI was associated with subsequent central recurrence in three. In 86% of patients with para-aortic lymphadenopathy there was a poor outcome while absence of lymphadenopathy on MRI was associated with a good outcome in 78% of patients. Unilateral or bilateral lymphadenopathy on MRI was of less obvious prognostic value since patients usually received effective treatment in the form of additional radiotherapy or chemotherapy. The presence of a measurable volume of high signal at the site of the previous carcinoma on the 3-month MRI scan was associated with later tumour recurrence or radiation damage.

Discussion

The value of measurement by MRI of tumour volume in carcinoma of the cervix has been previously reported (Hawnaur et al. 1992). Tumour stage, tumour volume and the presence of lymphadenopathy are each important factors influencing the 5-year survival rate of patients with carcinoma of the cervix treated by radiotherapy. MRI is the only imaging technique capable of non-invasively assessing these factors without the use of contrast medium. In addition, monitoring response of tumour to radiotherapy by MRI may provide useful additional prognostic information, identifying patients with significant residual signal abnormality after radiotherapy. Although the ability of MRI to differentiate residual or recurrent tumour from radiation changes in the cervix is limited, it can be used to identify a subgroup of patients in whom cervical biopsy is justified. In addition, MRI is a useful adjunct to clinical examination for early detection of pelvic recurrence and can detect lymphadenopathy or pelvic side wall spread of tumour not readily appreciated on pelvic examination.

References

Hawnaur JM, Johnson RJ, Hunter RD, Jenkins JPR, Isherwood I (1992) The value of magnetic resonance imaging in assessment of carcinoma of the cervix and its response to radiotherapy. Clin Oncol 4: 11–17

Hricak H, Lacey CG, Sandles LG, Chang YCF, Winkler ML, Stern JL (1988) Invasive cervical carcinoma: comparison of MR imaging and surgical findings. Radiology 166: 623–631

Assessment of Bladder Carcinoma and its Response to Treatment by Magnetic Resonance Imaging with Gd-DTPA

J.M. Hawnaur, R.J. Johnson, J.P.R. Jenkins, and I. Isherwood

Introduction

Conventional magnetic resonance imaging (MRI) has been shown to be an accurate method of staging bladder carcinoma (Amendola et al. 1986; Bryan et al. 1987; Rholl et al. 1987; Buy et al. 1988; Johnson et al. 1990). The ability of MRI to differentiate between invasion of the superficial and deep muscle layers of the bladder wall is, however, questionable (Johnson et al. 1990). Such information is vital for the urologist considering endoscopic surgery. The aim of this study was to assess the ability of Gd-DTPA-enhanced MRI sequences to improve definition of the extent of bladder carcinoma compared with conventional MRI. The response of bladder carcinoma to radiotherapy was also assessed, and a subgroup of patients with suspected recurrent tumour after treatment were studied to investigate the ability of MRI with Gd-DTPA to differentiate between recurrent tumour and post-treatment changes.

Patients and Methods

A total of 45 patients (39 men and 6 women, aged 47–78 years) with primary bladder carcinoma or suspected tumour recurrence after treatment were studied. Pretreatment MRI was performed in 34 of these patients with primary tumours and repeated 3–4 months after radiotherapy or chemotherapy in 30. Three patients in this group died before repeat MRI could be obtained, and one was lost to follow-up. Radical radiotherapy was given to 25, consisting of approximately 50 Gy given in 20 fractions over 4 weeks. Two patients received palliative radiotherapy, and three underwent chemotherapy. Eleven patients with suspected recurrence after treatment (previous transurethral tumour resection, radical radiotherapy or chemotherapy) were also examined. MRI findings in all patients were correlated with clinical follow-up, cystoscopy, examination under anaesthesia (EUA) and biopsy and with findings at cystectomy in three patients.

Department of Diagnostic Radiology, University of Manchester, Oxford Road, Manchester, M13 9PT, UK

Advanced Radiation Therapy Tumor Response
Monitoring and Treatment Planning
Breit (Editor-in-Chief)
© Springer-Verlag, Berlin Heidelberg 1992

Scans were performed on a 0.26-T superconducting magnet system using either the conventional body coil or a corset surface coil. Multiplanar T1- and T2-weighted spin-echo sequences (SE 740-2000/26-120) were obtained of the pelvis and abdomen. Following 0.1 mmol/kg Gd-DTPA, T1-weighted sequences were repeated in multiple planes. The field of view was 30–45 cm and slice thickness 7–10 mm.

Results

Bladder carcinoma was shown on MRI as focal thickening or a discrete mass in the bladder wall, iso- or slightly hyperintense on T1-weighted sequences and hyperintense on T2-weighted sequences. Moderate enhancement occurred after Gd-DTPA. No enhancement was shown in two patients following transurethral resection of bladder carcinoma with residual mural thickening at EUA. Tumour necrosis and blood clot did not enhance, helping to differentiate such areas from viable tumour. Enhancement after Gd-DTPA assisted identification of small tumours within the bladder wall and increased contrast between tumour and uninvolved muscle. The latter was demonstrated as a low-signal band between the hyperintense tumour and high-signal perivesical fat on T2- or enhanced T1-weighted images (Fig. 1). No demarcation between superficial and deep muscle layers was demonstrated, preventing differentiation of advanced T2 from early T3a tumours. Tumours were staged T3a when there was poor definition of the low-signal outer bladder wall but an intact interface between bladder and perivesical fat. T3b tumours showed complete loss of integrity of the muscular bladder wall and infiltration of perivesical fat. Gd-DTPA was rarely helpful in tumours more advanced than stage T3a since the conspicuity of perivesical tumour infiltration was reduced on enhanced T1-weighted sequences (Fig. 2). MRI demonstrated lymph node or bone metastases in six patients. These were best shown on unenhanced T1-weighted sequences since contrast with pelvic fat or bone marrow was reduced after Gd-DTPA.

Three to 4 months after radical radiotherapy, all patients showed regression of the primary tumour together with changes in the previously normal bladder wall. Hyperintensity of the mucosal surface of the bladder, particularly postero-basally, was the most frequent abnormality detected and was often associated with moderate bladder wall thickening. An increased signal of the bladder wall was also identified on both T1- and T2-weighted sequences in some patients, with enhancement after Gd-DTPA, most intense on the mucosal surface (Fig. 3). Particularly marked radiation changes were observed in patients receiving intravesical chemotherapy prior to radiotherapy or with evidence of a bladder outflow obstruction due to benign prostatic hypertrophy on pretreatment MRI. Severely affected bladders showed marked circumferential thickening, reduced

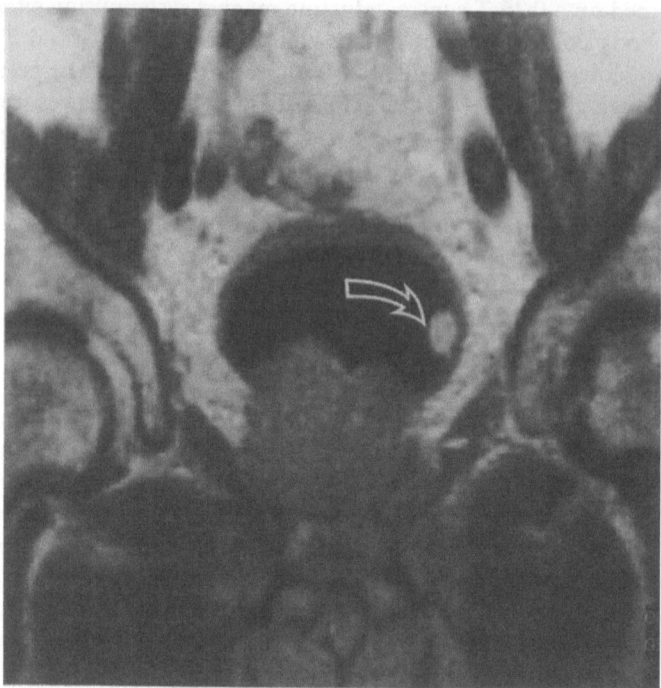

Fig. 1. Coronal T1-weighted (SE 700/40) MRI scan of the bladder showing tumour confined to the bladder wall (stage T2/early T3a) enhanced after Gd-DTPA (*arrow*). Uninvolved bladder wall deep to the tumour remains low signal, but differentiation between superficial and deep muscle layers cannot be made. The low-signal urine, due either to a low concentration of Gd-DTPA or a very high concentration producing super-paramagnetic T2 shortening optimises assessment of the luminal surface of the tumour

volume and poor distensibility with, in some cases, an irregular spiculated interface with surrounding perivesical fat (Fig. 3). Mural thickening, abnormal signal and enhancement after Gd-DTPA were also observed in pelvic organs such as the rectum, seminal vesicles and prostate.

Eleven patients were referred with suspected recurrent tumour on the basis of symptoms such as haematuria or a palpable mass at EUA. In two previously treated by surgery, MRI demonstrated a focal enhancing mass of recurrent tumour within an otherwise normal bladder. Seven patients had received previous radical radiotherapy up to 4 years earlier. In five, MRI demonstrated mural thickening, enhancement and mucosal hyperintensity consistent with radiation injury, but no evidence of tumour recurrence. The MRI diagnosis was confirmed by multiple check cytoscopies and biopsy in four patients and by cystectomy in one, although the latter also had foci of pre-invasive carcinoma in addition to florid radiation change. In two other patients with histological evidence of recurrent tumour MRI demonstrated a focal mass in addition to

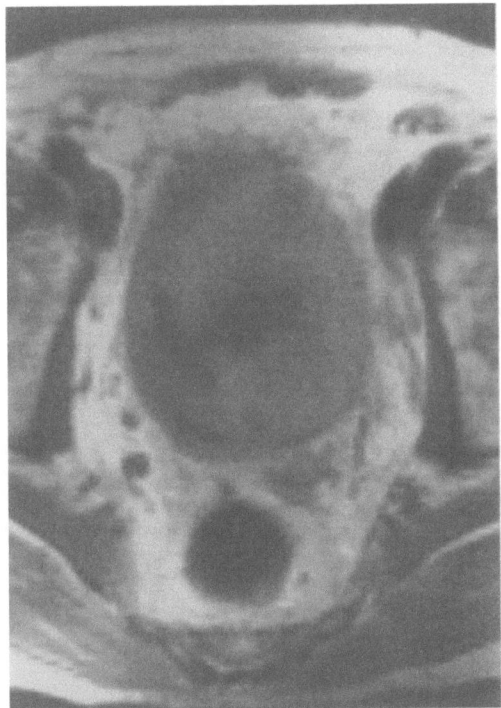

a

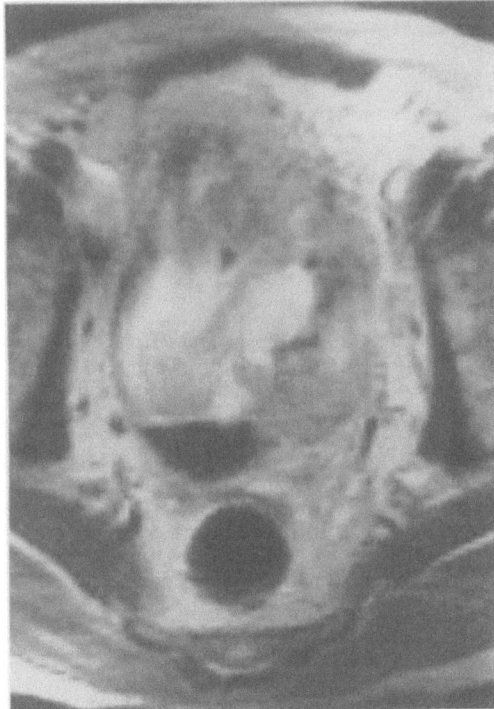

b

Fig. 2a, b. Transverse T1-weighted
(SE 740/40) MRI scans of a patient
with a T3b bladder carcinoma of the
bladder before (**a**) and after (**b**) Gd-
DTPA. Contrast between tumour and
paravesical fat is reduced after
enhancement, and there is a variable
signal intensity of urine

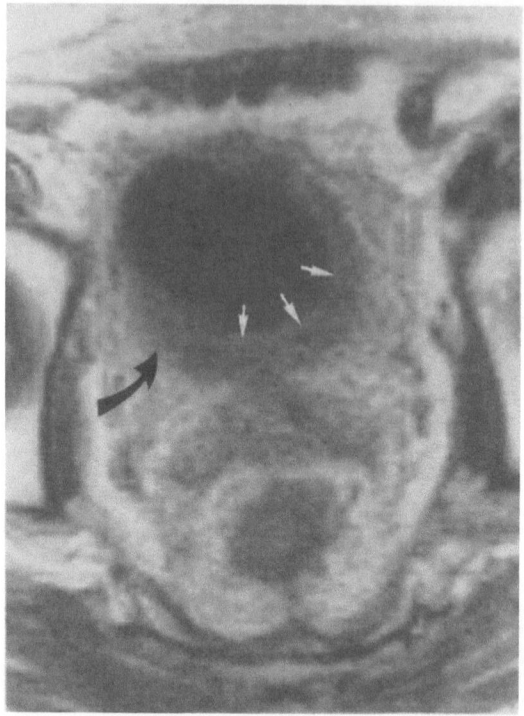

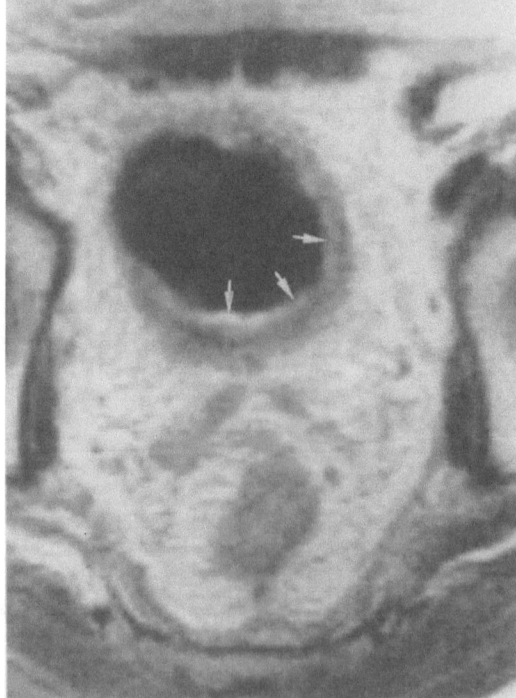

Fig. 3a, b. Transverse T1-weighted (SE 740/40) MRI scans of the bladder before (**a**) and after (**b**) Gd-DTPA 3 months after radiotherapy for bladder carcinoma. There is thickening and irregularity of the bladder wall, with mucosal hyperintensity (*short arrows*) and enhancement, particularly of the mucosal surface posterolaterally. The interface between the outer bladder wall and the pelvic fat is ill-defined (*curved arrow*). Note also enhancement of adjacent pelvic viscera and soft tissues

radiotherapy changes. Two patients that were previously treated by chemotherapy showed no evidence of tumour recurrence.

Discussion

Several technical problems were encountered during this study. Changes in
bladder volume and shape during the examination affected the morphology and
position of tumour within the bladder at the same anatomical level before and
after Gd-DTPA. Urine signal intensity varied according to Gd-DTPA concentration and the degree of mixing. Low signal intensity urine from a low
concentration of Gd-DTPA or a very high concentration producing T2 shortening effects optimised contrast between tumour, bladder wall and urine. High
signal intensity urine due to the T1 shortening effect of Gd-DTPA reduced the
visibility of papillomatous tumours and of superficial plaques of tumour. Inflow
of dilute urine, poor mixing or turbulence of urine could produce apparent
filling defects mimicking tumour on scans after Gd-DTPA.

Although Gd-DTPA improved contrast between tumour and bladder wall,
is rarely added to the information available from conventional T1- and T2-
weighted spin-echo sequences. Contrast of tumour with fat and high-signal urine
containing moderate amounts of Gd-DTPA was reduced after enhancement so
that perivesical and intraluminal extent of tumour were best shown on unenhanced T1-weighted scans. A fat suppression sequence could improve the
conspicuity of tumour extension into fat on post Gd-DTPA scans. Similarly the
demonstration of lymph node or bony metastases was not improved by Gd-
DTPA administration.

Following radical radiotherapy, mucosal changes were observed in the
previously normal bladder wall in the majority of patients. The mucosal
hyperintensity and enhancement after Gd-DTPA suggest underlying hyperaemia. Cystoscopic findings in acute radiation reaction include hyperaemia,
telangiectasia, oedema and ulceration with an inflammatory cell infiltrate
histologically. Several of the patients with suspected recurrence of bladder
carcinoma after treatment showed a small volume thick-walled bladder with
diffuse mucosal and intramural signal abnormalities on MRI. These changes
were subsequently proven to be due to radiation damage. Chronic radiation
bladder injury may produce bladder wall thickening due to mucosal and
submucosal oedema and/or fibrosis resulting in reduced bladder capacity. At
cystoscopy, telangiectasia, mucosal and muscular fibrosis together with ulceration and necrosis may be demonstrated. The pathological process underlying
most of the chronic changes is small vessel disease producing eventual occlusion
of small arteries. The observation that abnormal enhancement also occurs in
other pelvic organs has implications for detecting infiltrating recurrent tumour
after pelvic radiotherapy (Hawnaur et al. 1990).

References

Amendola MA, Glazer GM, Grossman HB, Aisen AM, Francis IR (1986) Staging of bladder carcinoma: MRI-CT surgical correlation. Am J Roentgenol 146: 1179–1183

Bryan PJ, Butler HE, LiPuma JP, Resnick MI, Kursh ED (1987) CT and MR imaging in staging bladder neoplasms. J Comput Assist Tomogr 11/1: 96–101

Buy J-N, Moss AA, Guinet C, Ghossain MA, Malbec L, Arrive L, Vadrot D (1988) Mr staging of bladder carcinoma: correlation with pathological findings. Radiology 169: 695–700

Johnson RJ, Carrington BM, Jenkins JPR, Barnard RJ, Read G, Isherwood I (1990) Accuracy in staging carcinoma of the bladder by magnetic resonance imaging. Clin Radiol 41: 258–263

Hawnaur JM, Johnson RJ, Isherwood I, Jenkins JPR (1990) Gd-DTPA in MRI of bladder carcinoma. In: Contrast media in MRI. Proceedings of the international workshop, Berlin, February 1990. Medicom, pp 357–363

Rholl KS, Lee JKT, Hciken JP, Ling D, Glazer HS (1987) Primary bladder carcinoma: evaluation with MR imaging. Radiology 163: 117–121

Response to Definite Radiotherapy in Patients with Invasive Bladder Carcinoma Evaluated by Contrast-Enhanced Computed Tomography of the Primary Tumor

E.M. Sager[1], S.D. Fosså[2], and S. Ous[3]

Introduction

Definite radiotherapy has been used for many years in the treatment of bladder carcinomas and retains an important place in the management of bladder cancer (Eschwege et al. 1989). Complete response to irradiation as evaluated clinically 3–4 months after treatment is an indicator for beneficial long-term survival (Jacobsen et al. 1989). However, a major problem after definite radiotherapy is the inaccuracy of clinical evaluation of the primary tumor, reported to entail an error as high as 60% (Osborne et al. 1982). Computed tomography (CT) has been used in evaluation of treatment response of the primary tumor in urinary bladder carcinomas after definite radiotherapy (Husband 1990; Yu et al. 1979). Radiotherapy produces bladder wall thickening, reduction in bladder capacity, and generalized increase in density of the perivesical fat (Husband 1990). These findings make interpretation of postradiotherapy CT more difficult than in the untreated patient.

   The aim of the present study was to evaluate the ability of contrast-enhanced CT to demonstrate response of the primary bladder tumor after definite irradiation.

Patients and Methods

We examined 39 patients — 29 men and 10 women, aged 55–81 years (mean 67) — with T2–T4 bladder cancer by means of cystoscopy and bimanual palpation under anesthesia before and 3 months after definite irradiation. Five patients had a T2 tumor, 22 had a T3 tumor, and 12 had a T4 tumor. Fifteen patients had undergone combination chemotherapy before the start of radiotherapy. In only

[1] Department of Diagnostic Radiology, Norwegian Radium Hospital, Montebello, 0310 Oslo 3, Norway
[2] Department of Oncology and Radiation Therapy, Norwegian Radium Hospital, Montebello, 0310 Oslo 3, Norway
[3] Department of Surgery, Norwegian Radium Hospital, Montebello, 0310 Oslo 3, Norway

Advanced Radiation Therapy Tumor Response
Monitoring and Treatment Planning
Breit (Editor-in-Chief)
© Springer-Verlag, Berlin Heidelberg 1992

14 cases was a diagnostic transurethral resection performed 3 months after treatment. As biopsies were not performed in all patients, we compared the CT evaluation with the clinical evaluation. The observation time was at least 12 months in all patients. Based on the clinical examination, the series was divided into a group of completely responding patients and a group with residual tumors.

The irradiation was given to the bladder as the target volume with 2-cm safety margins. A four-field technique was used (anteroposterior/posteroanterior and two lateral portals) after CT-based planning. The patients received a target dose of 60 Gy over 6 weeks with daily fractions of 2 Gy 5 days per week. This regimen gave a cumulative radiation effect (Kirk 1971) of approximately 1750 reu.

CT of the bladder was carried out in all patients immediately before (CT1) and 3 months after radiotherapy (CT2). A GE 9800 Quick body scanner was used. Important aspects of the technique were: a full bladder, either filled with urine or a fat emulsion (Lipofundine; produced for intravenous nutrition for Kabi), the use of 5-mm slice thickness, and a displayed field of view of 30 cm giving a pixel size of approximately 0.6 mm. Both a pre- and postcontrast series were taken: the precontrast series to identify the tumor area, the postcontrast series to evaluate the contrast enhancement in the tumor (Sager et al. 1987a, b). The criterion for the diagnosis of a malignant tumor observed on the CT scans was: a mass in the bladder wall with a significant contrast enhancement relative to the normal bladder wall (Sager et al. 1991).

The size of the tumor was measured in the CT slice where the tumor had its greatest extension. The area was encircled and measured accurately by the use of the region-of-interest function. Based on the World Health Organization criteria for response (Miller et al. 1981), patients were allocated to one of the four response categories as assessed by CT.

Results

Twenty-one patients had no tumor by clinical examination after radiotherapy, but in six of these CT diagnosed a residual tumor (Table 1). In 18 of the 39 patients both clinical examination and CT indicated residual tumor. Taking the size measured by CT into account, 9 of the 18 were categorized as showing no change and 9 as partial response.

The median size of all tumors before treatment was 7.1 cm^2 (range 1.0–23.0 cm^2). The median size of the residual tumors after treatment was 4.3 cm^2 (range 1.3–16.2 cm^2). Only 4 of the 24 residual tumors were larger than 10 cm^2. There was a significant difference in response of the tumors with pretreatment size over 10 cm^2 and those with smaller size ($p < 0.05$, Mann-Whitney test). Of the 15 completely responding patients as assessed by CT, 14

Table 1. Patients with inconsistency between clinical complete response and CT response evaluation after definite radiotherapy

Patient no.	Area CT1 (cm²)	CT2 (cm²)	Comment
1	12.0	4.0	Bowel loop adjacent to the residual tumor.[a] Biopsy was not taken. No sign of recurrence after 8 months.
2	3.3	1.3	Recurrence in the bladder after 6 months.
3	4.7	1.9	Scar tissue adjacent to the tumor.[a]
4	11.2	4.3	Fig. 1. Tumor in the bladder base.[a] Biopsy: radiation induced changes. Recurrent tumor at the same site 10 months later.
5	12.0	9.0	Biopsy: irradiation changes. Residual tumor in the dome.[a] Non-invasive tumor found 12 months later.
6	8.0	4.8	Multiple tumor locations. Biopsy: radiation induced changes. No recurrence after 5 months.

CT1, CT before treatment; CT2: CT three months after definite irradiation.
[a] Discrepancy possibly partly due to location of tumor.

Table 2. CT-based pretreatment tumor size correlated to response category obtained by CT

Tumor size	Complete response	Residual tumor	Total
< 10 cm²	14	14	28
> 10 cm²	1	10	11
Total	15	24	39

Table 3. Comparison of CT-based response category after chemotherapy and definite radiotherapy

Patient no.	After chemotherapy	After definite radiotherapy
1	PR	CR
2	PR	CR
3	PR	CR
4	NC	PR
5	NC	PR
6	NC	PR
7	NC	PR
8	PR	PR
9	NC	NC
10	NC	NC
11	NC	NC
12	NC	NC
13	NC	NC
14	NC	NC
15	PR	NC

CR, Complete response; PR, partial response; NC, no change

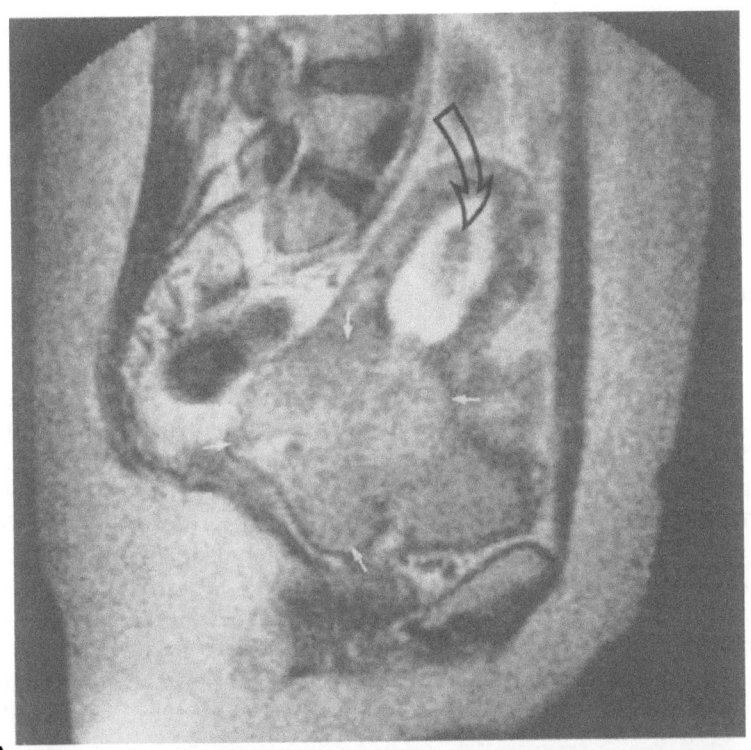

a

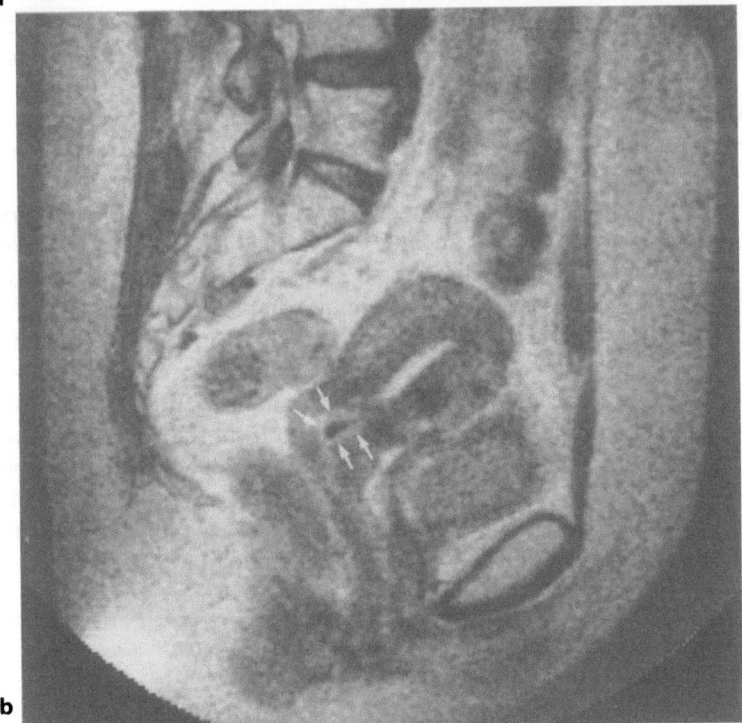

b

(90%) had a pretreatment tumor size less than 10 cm^2. However, in 24 patients with residual tumor, only 14 (58%) had a pretreatment tumor size less than 10 cm^2 (Table 2).

The CT-based response categories of the 15 patients previously treated with chemotherapy, are shown in Table 3. Seven of 15 showed improved response category after radiotherapy.

Discussion

Due to the known irradiation changes, there is a high degree of uncertainity about the clinical response evaluation in bladder cancer patients after definite pelvic radiotherapy. Especially small tumors may be impossible to palpate in the irradiated pelvis.

To increase discrimination of benign from malignant processes, the use of intravenous contrast medium is recommended (Dean et al. 1980). Intravenous contrast medium injection is used both to delineate the structures more accurately and to discriminate between different soft tissues on the basis of the degree of contrast enhancement. In the urinary bladder, the degree of enhancement can be used to discriminate between residual masses without and those with malignant histology after irradiation (Sager et al. 1989; Sager et al. 1991).

It is known that preradiotherapy tumor size influences on the result of treatment (Bloom et al. 1982; Shipley and Rose 1985). Bloom et al. (1982) found that 46% of patients with initial tumor size less than 5 cm were alive 3 years after treatment, whereas only 20% of the patients with tumor size greater than 5 cm survived 3 years. In this study, the patients categorized as complete responders both by clinical examination and CT had small pretreatment tumor sizes. Half of these patient had a tumor size less than 4.0 cm^2, and only one of the tumors was more than 10 cm^2 in size. Pretreatment CT of the bladder and assessment of the tumor size may thus help the clinician to select those patients for radiotherapy who have the greatest chance of attaining complete response.

Three of the six patients with a CT detected residual tumor but complete response by clinical examination underwent a diagnostic transurethral reaction 3 months after radiotherapy, and only inflammatory changes and necrosis were found. The biopsy may, however, not have been taken from the location where CT showed tumor. Baker (1986) found that there was a tendency to understage invasive bladder carcinomas after treatment although transurethral resection biopsies were performed. In the future, a discrepancy between clinical complete response and tumor positive CT should lead to CT-guided biopsies.

Fig. 1. Tumor (*T*) in the bladder base, left side, before (**a**) and after (**b**) treatment (*between curved arrows*). *SV*, Seminal vesicles; *R*, rectum

294

E.M. Sager et al.

References

Baker R (1986) The discrepancy of clinical vs. surgical staging. JAMA 206: 1170
Bloom HJG, Hendry WF, Wallace DM, Skeet RG (1982) Treatment of T3 bladder cancer. Controlled trial of pre-operative radiotherapy and radical cystectomy versus radical radiotherapy. Br J Urol 54: 136
Dean PB (1980) Contrast media in body computed tomography. Experimental and theoretical background, present limitations and proposals for improved diagnostic efficiacy. Invest Radiol 15: 164
Eschwege F, Raoul Y, Wibault P, Droz JP, Court B, Perrin JL (1989) Does radiotherapy still have a place in the treatment of bladder tumors? In: Murphy GP, Khoury S (eds) Therapeutic progress in urologic cancers. Liss, New York, pp 605–611
Husband J (1990) Staging of bladder and prostate cancer In: Husband J (ed) CT review. Churchill Livingstone, London, pp 203–215
Jacobsen A-B, Lunde S, Ous S, Melvik JE, Pettersen EO, Kaalhus O, Fosså SD (1989) T2/T4 bladder carcinomas treated with definitive radiotherapy with emphasis on flow cytometric DNA ploidy values. Int J Rad Oncol Biol Phys 17: 923
Kirk J (1971) Cumulative radiation effect: I. Fractionated treatment regimes. Clin Radiol 22: 145
Miller AB, Hoogstraten B, Staquet M, Winkler A (1981) Reporting results of cancer treatment. Cancer 47: 207
Osborne DE, Honan RP, Palmer MK, Barnard RJ, McIntyre D, Pointon RS (1982) Factors influencing salvage cystectomy results. Br J Urol 54: 122
Sager EM, Talle K, Fosså SD, Ous S, Stenwig, AE (1987a) Contrast-enhanced computed tomography to show perivesical extension in bladder carcinoma. Acta Radiol Diagn 28: 307
Sager EM, Fosså SD, Kaalhus O, Talle K (1987b) Contrast-enhanced computed tomography in carcinoma of the urinary bladder. The use of different injection methods. Acta Radiol Diagn 28: 67
Sager EM, Kaalhus O (1991) Features of irradiated urinary bladder tumors and their correlation with malignancy observed on computed tomography. Acta Radiol Diagn 1: 57
Shipley WU, Rose MA (1985) Bladder cancer. The selection of patients for treatment by full dose irradiation. Cancer 55: 2278
Yu WS, Sagerman RH, King GA, Chung CT, Yu WY (1979) The value of computed tomography in the management of bladder cancer. Int J Rad Oncol Biol Phys 5: 135

Efficiency of Computed Tomography in Calculating Tumor Response After Radiotherapy of Presacral Recurrences

R. Engenhart[1], C. Seyfried[2], J. Romahn[1], and G. van Kaick[2]

Introduction

Locally recurrent rectal cancer following radical surgery is a difficult problem. Pain is frequently present and is usually associated with a mass of recurrent tumor in the presacral space. The most effective therapy for symptomatic local recurrences is radiation therapy. Previous studies with photons have reported an improvement of pain in 60%–80%; however, the palliative effect lasts only about 6 months [1, 5, 8, 9]. Based on clinical and biological observations it has been suggested that patients with recurrent disease may benefit from high linear energy transfer therapy (LET) [3, 4, 6, 7].

A particular problem in the follow-up of patients with colorectal recurrences are residual masses after irradiation. Imaging methods are helpful if the tumor shows significant changes. Radiological reduction in tumor size in 20%–60% of patients are reported, but complete remission is rarely seen [2, 9]. Therefore, there is considerable controversy about the different methods for verifying response rate and duration. Radiotherapists are frequently confronted with the fact that the patient shows good clinical response in spite of the remaining large tumor mass in the pelvis. Tumor volume may have prognostic value; however, methods to determine tumor remission posttherapeutically by volumetric analysis with computed tomography (CT) are seldom used.

This report quantifies the changes, in tumor size in 41 patients with presacral recurrences using a volumetric analysis utilizing CT scans.

Materials and Methods

Patients in this study were referred to radiotherapy because of symptoms caused by recurrent rectal cancer in the pelvis. From 1986 to 1989, 41 patients with presacral recurrences were treated with a combined modality approach of 40 Gy

---

[1] Department of Radiotherapy, University Clinic of Radiology, Im Neuemheimer Feld 400, 6900 Heidelberg, FRG
[2] Department of Radiology and Pathophysiology, German Cancer Research Center, Im Neuenheimer Feld 280, 6900 Heidelberg, FRG

Advanced Radiation Therapy Tumor Response
Monitoring and Treatment Planning
Breit (Editor-in-Chief)
© Springer-Verlag, Berlin Heidelberg 1992

photons followed immediately by a boost of 6.6 or 10 Gy neutrons. All 41 patients underwent baseline CT scans. These were needed for documentation of the pretreatment status and for radiotherapy planning. All were controlled at approximately 3, 6, 9, and 12 months following radiotherapy. The CT scans were performed with a whole-body scanner (Somatom DRH, Siemens). Contiguous sections were obtained with a slice thickness of 8 mm from the pelvic iliac crests to the level of the perineal region after opacifying the small bowel by 5% Gastrografin.

Tumor volume was defined as the product of three diameters, the transverse, the anteroposterior, and the superoinferior. Tumor response was evaluated by CT scan digitized tumor volumetric analysis. For each CT section, the individual margin of the tumor mass was indicated by manually drawing a region of interest (ROI; Fig. 1). The total volume was determined by the number of pixels within the ROI multiplied by the pixel size and slice thickness of 8 mm. Results of this technique were reproducible within ± 15%. In addition the density (Hounsfield units) of the tumor mass was measured from a representative number of CT slices. The volumes were determined during a follow-up of 12 months. The measured tumor volumes were used to determine the stage of remission. Stable disease was defined as less than 50% reduction and less than 25% increase in volume, progressive disease as an increase in tumor size by 25% or more, and partial response as more than 50% decrease in tumor volume.

Pain symptoms were assessed clinically at the initiation of irradiation and at the first follow-up, according to the EORTC/RTOG pain score. To obtain an objective measurement of pain the scoring system takes into account the intensity of pain and the frequency of pain using a nine-point scale [10].

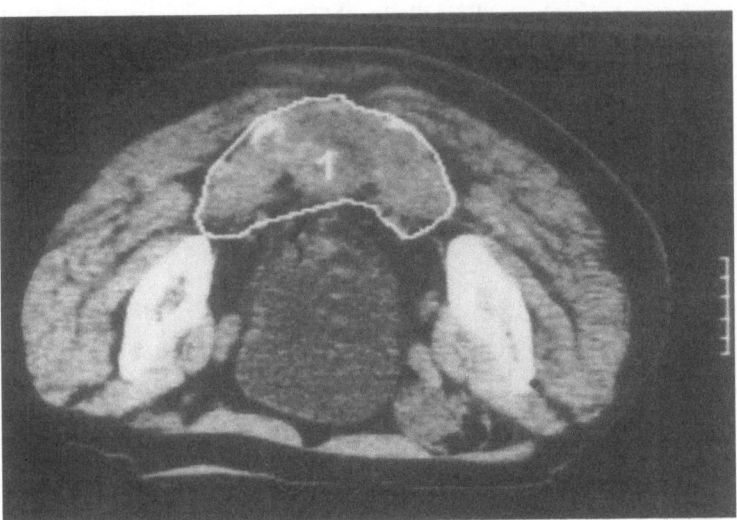

Fig. 1. Quantitative determination of recurrence volume by CT-assisted volumetric analysis. CT scan with a region of interest drawn around the tumor mass

Results

A total of 133 CT examinations of 41 patients were evaluated, and the tumor remission was defined by an exact determination of the tumor volume. Pelvic CT investigations included 37 at 3 months, 30 at 6 months, and 26 at 12 months. All scans were analyzed with respect to presacral tumor mass and response to therapy and were correlated with the results of pain relief. The pretreatment tumor volumes determinated from volumetrical analysis is shown in Fig. 2.

There was a definite presacral mass with a mean tumor volume of 283 cm^3, ranging from 68 to 1200 cm^3, in the 41 patients. The mean tumor volume before radiotherapy as measured by the three diameters was 371 cm^3. The recurrence involved presacral bone with destruction of os sacrum was seen in 15 patients.

Serial CT scans demonstrated the reduction in tumor size over the first 6 months after irradiation. A decrease of more than 10% of tumor mass was shown by CT scans in 23 patients. The regression was 10%–19% in seven patients, 20%–29% in six, 30%–39% in four, and 40%–49% in three. No recurrence treated with irradiation disappeared completely during follow-up; 23 patients (56%) achieved a complete losts of symptoms. A partial response with a 50%–60% reduction in tumor volume was noted in only three patients. Clinical response in terms of relief of severe and progressive pain symptoms was achieved in all but one patient. In 16 patients, follow-up CT scans showed no change at all (± 10% difference of volume) during the first 6 months. Figure 3 illustrates the relative distribution in volume change 3 or 6 months after radiotherapy. Six months after irradiation CT demonstrated no change in size or configuration of the mass. A change in tumor density was not obtained in follow-up investigations. In three patients in whom clinically local failure was suspected, two had a

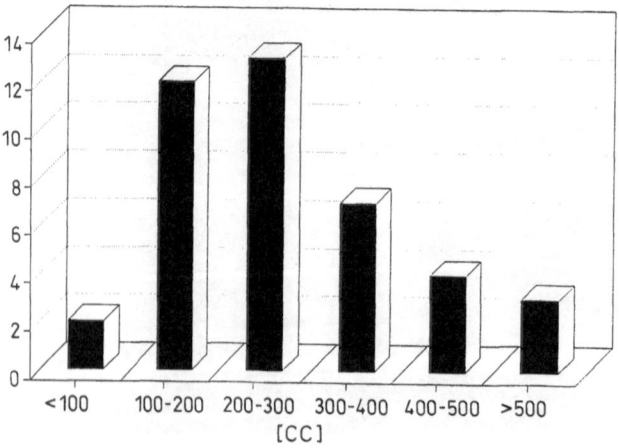

Fig. 2. Histogram of the pretreatment tumor volume distribution for 41 patients with unresectable recurrent carcinoma

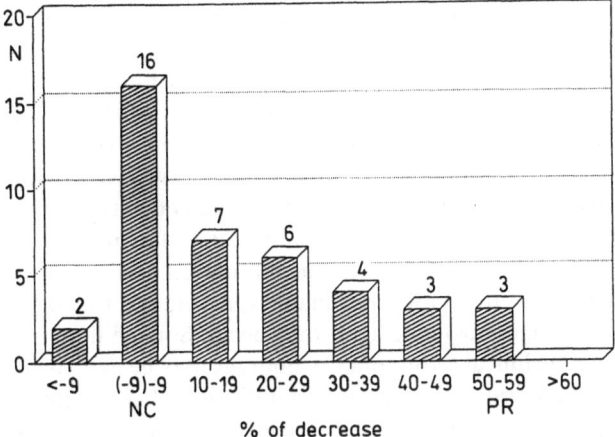

Fig. 3. Percentage change in tumor volume 3–6 months after radiotherapy

positive CT scan, defining the tumor volume as a product of diameter and by volumetric analysis. These two patients had a peritoneal carcinosis already at time of treatment. One showed an increase in volume of 10% at 6 months, and only 12 months after irradiation was a clear progression determined. All patients were nonresponders; the initial mean volume of the patients relapsing within 12 months after therapy was 157 cm^3, with a range of 102–231 cm^3.

Discussion

CT has assumed a main position in tumor staging of rectal carcinoma; it shows metastatic disease in the para-aortic nodes and liver as well as urinary obstruction. It is also valuable in detecting early recurrent rectal carcinoma after surgical excision. It allows decisions about surgery or radiotherapy and helps define the exact target volume for irradiation. However, changes in CT response after irradiation appears to be a less sensitive indicator of effects of treatment than the clinical data determined from pain remission [2, 7, 8]. Although 88% of patients showed excellent clinical remission, changes in CT between 10% and 56% in pre- and posttreatment volume were detected in only 23 patients 6 months after irradiation. In our study a reduction in tumor size of more than 50% was noted in five patients by diameter measurement and in three by exact CT volumetric analysis. In general, primary tumor mass as determined by CT analysis was 30% smaller than estimated by visual diameter examination. An explanation for the differences between the two measurements is that the diameter is a relative measurement. The main advantage of the CT-determined volumetric technique is that it provides an accurate quantification of pelvic mass following treatment.

The volume of recurrent tumor and the response rate may have prognostic significance. Due to the small number of patients included it is difficult to draw definite conclusions. No correlation was found between tumor volume and response or relapse within 12 months after therapy. No patient with reduction in size of more than 10% relapsed during the 1st year. Only exact determination of pre- and postoperative tumor volume enables a quantitative statement concerning tumor remission. Normally only visual volume estimation based on length, width and height were carried out. With large changes in volumes this may be sufficient, but with small changes misjudgements may occur. Some differences in the rate of response between clinical strips and CT findings may be explained by this phenomena. The volumetric technique is generally useful in monitoring responders and nonresponders so that an alternative treatment option can be considered.

References

1. Arnott SJ (1982) Radiotherapy. In: Duncan W (ed) Colorectal cancer. Recent Results Cancer Res 83: 113
2. Aydin H, Richter E, Feyerabend T. Bohndorf W (1990) Die In-vivo-Bestimmung des tumor-volumens: was leistet die CT-unterstützte Berechnung beim Rektumkarzinomerzidiv? Strahlenther Onkol 166: 204–206
3. Battermann JJ (1982) Results of dT fast neutron irradiation of advanced tumors of bladder and rectum. Int J Radiat Oncol Biol Phys 8: 2150
4. Breteau N, Destembert B, Sabattier R, Schlienger ;M (1985) An interim assessment of the experience of fast neutron boost in glioblastomas, rectal and bronchus carcinomas in Orleans. Strahlentherapie 161: 787
5. Ciatto S, Pacini P (1982) Radiation therapy of recurrence of carcinoma of the rectum and sigmoid after surgery. Acta Radiol Oncol 21: 105
6. Eising E, Pötter R, Haverkamp U, Schnepper E (1990) Neutron therapy for recurrence of rectal cancer: interim analysis from Münster. Strahlenther Onkol 166: 90–94
7. Engenhart R, Kimmig B, Höver KH, Strauss LG, Lorenz WJ, Wannenmacher M (1990) Photon-neutron therapy for recurrent colorectal cancer–follow up and preliminary results. Strahlenther Onkol 166: 95–98
8. Flentje M, Frey M, Kuttig H, Kimmig B (1988) Strahlentherapie bei Lokalrezidiven kolorek-taler Tumoren. Prognostische Faktoren, Verlaufsdiagnostik und Ergebnisse. Strahlenther Onkol 164: 404–407
9. Schultz U (1987) Kolorektale Tumoren. In: Scherer E (ed) Strahlentherapie: Radiologische Onkologie, 3rd edn. Springer, Berlin, Heidelberg, New York, pp 632–651
10. Tong D, Gillick L, Hendrickson FR (1982) The palliation of symptomatic osseous metastases. Cancer 50: 893–899

Therapy Monitoring of Rectal Carcinoma by Pharmacokinetic Analysis of Magnetic Resonance Imaging Data

G. Layer[1], G. Brix[1], M. Müller-Schimpfle[1], R. Engenhart[2], P. Schlag[3], W. Semmler[1], and G. van Kaick[1]

Introduction

Colorectal carcinoma is the second most common cause of cancer-related death [1]. Its incidence is about 25/100 000 in Europe, and the American Cancer Society estimates that over 100 000 new cases occur each year in the United States. The malignant tumor recurs in 30%–50% of patients undergoing resection in curative intention, and up to 50% of all patients suffering from rectal cancer die of local recurrence and its complications [2, 3]. Keeping in mind these data, it is easy to understand that early diagnosis of recurrent tumor is a major problem for the oncologist working with this patient group.

The routine follow-up of rectal cancer patients includes the repetition of the history, the physical examination and rectal palpation, chest X-rays, abdominal ultrasound, liver function tests, tumor marker examination (CEA, CA 19-9), and computed tomography (CT) of the pelvis for locoregional reevaluation. However, there are cases in which CT findings are not unambiguous, showing presacral soft tissue areas of varying size and density without infiltration of neighbouring structures. The purpose of this study was to determine whether magnetic resonance imaging (MRI) can help in differentiating tumor recurrence and unspecific scar in these cases.

Materials and Methods

Nineteen MRI examinations of 16 patients were included in this ongoing study. All patients had a history of curatively treated colorectal carcinoma and were now suspect for tumor recurrence. They showed a pelvic mass in prior CT, rising

[1] Institute of Radiology and Pathophysiology, German Cancer Research Center, Im Neuenheimer Feld 280, 6900 Heidelberg, FRG
[2] Department of Radiology/Radiotherapy, University Clinic, University of Heidelberg, Im Neuenheimer Feld 400, 6900 Heidelberg, FRG
[3] Department of Surgery, Division of Surgical Oncology, University Clinic, University of Heidelberg, Im Neuenheimer Feld 400, 6900 Heidelberg, FRG

Advanced Radiation Therapy Tumor Response
Monitoring and Treatment Planning
Breit (Editor-in-Chief)
© Springer-Verlag, Berlin Heidelberg 1992

Table 1. Patient referral and confirmation of diagnosis

Reason for referral	Lesions finally diagnosed by		
	Follow-up	Needle biopsy	Operation
pelvic mass in CT[a]	10	4	1
CEA	2	1	—
Locoregional complaints	1	—	—

[a] Within this group two patients were examined before and after radiotherapy and one patient twice after radiotherapy showing two different lesions.

CEA level, and/or locoregional symptoms suspect for recurrence in the follow-up (Table 1). Six patients had undergone combined photon/neutron radiation therapy 7 months–3 years prior to MRI examination (mean 16 months); two patients were examined before and 3 months after radiotherapy, one patient twice after radiotherapy. Surgical treatment in nonirradiated patients had been performed 4–81 months prior to the MRI examination (mean 28 months).

MRI was performed using a 1.5-T superconducting equipment (Magnetom SP, Siemens). The sequence protocol included T1-weighted and T2-weighted spin-echo images (SE 500/15, SE 2800/22, 90) in axial and sagittal plane sections. Slice thickness was 8 mm, with matrix size 256×256 and two averages each. In a selected slice showing the suspect mass in maximum extension 64 rapid SE images were acquired before (4 images), during (12 images), and after (48 images) perfusor-controlled Gd-DTPA infusion (0.1 mmol/kg body weight). The spin-echo sequence had a repetition time of 100 ms, an echo time of 10 ms, and matrix size of 128×128. The acquisition time was 13 s per scan, and an interscan interval of 11 s was chosen.

The theoretical approach used in this study is complex and has been described in detail previously [4]. The fast SE sequence yielded a linear relationship between the measured MRI signal and Gd-DTPA tissue concentration. Due to this fact, the measured dynamic MRI data set can be analyzed on the basis of a suitable pharmacokinetic model. In our study the complete tissue-specific information contained in a signal-time curve (Fig. 1) is condensed to two parameters: an amplitude A reflecting the degree of MRI signal enhancement and a distribution time t_{21} characterizing perfusion and vascular permeability. Doing the analysis pixel-by-pixel reveals the kinetic tissue properties without losing the spatial information of the MR image.

For quantitative data evaluation regions of interest (ROIs) were placed by a physician in 19 suspect regions and 15 gluteal muscle tissue areas as an internal reference. The 19 suspect lesions included eight recurrent tumors, five irradiated recurrent malignancies, and six benign lesions. The diagnosis was confirmed for six lesions by histology (two recurrences, four benign histologies) and for 12 lesions by clinical follow-up including CT examinations for at least 9 months (Table 1). In one patient a lesion was diagnosed as a recurrence only 4 months

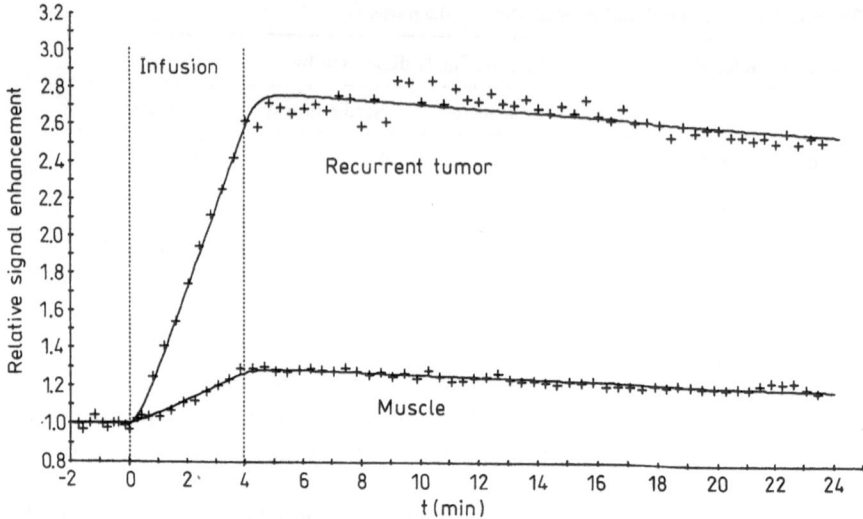

Fig. 1. Signal-time curve in recurrent tumor and muscle

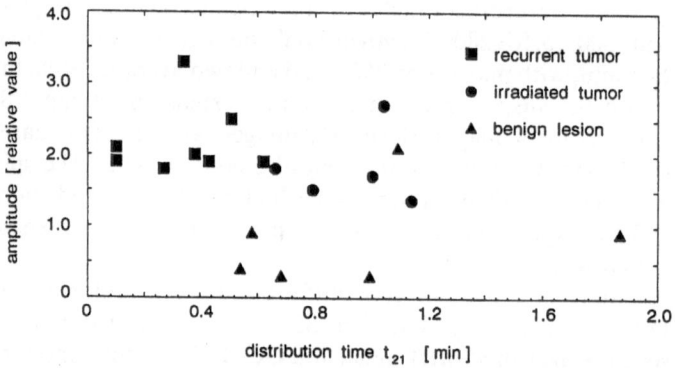

Fig. 2. Distribution of the estimated parameters A and t_{21} in benign and malignant lesions. Note the clustering of malignant nonirradiated lesions within an area of high amplitude A and short distribution time t_{21}

after initial surgery by CT and MRI examinations revealing a large pelvic mass ($10 \times 9 \times 6$ cm). The patient received radiotherapy shortly thereafter.

Results

MRI revealed pelvic masses in all cases. No lesion seen by CT was missed by MRI. Signal intensity on T1-weighted images was equal to or slightly lower than that of muscle tissue. On T2-weighted images the lesions showed as a rule inhomogeneously higher signal intensity compared to muscle tissue. All lesions also contained areas of relatively low signal. Significant differences in signal pattern were not identified between the different lesions.

Using both estimated parameters (A and t_{21}) a discrimination between recurrent tumor, irradiated tumor, and benign tissues was possible with high accuracy (Fig. 2). Malignant lesions showed a high amplitude A after administration of contrast medium. Regarding the amplitude A, with a contrast enhancement of more than 100% chosen as cut-off, benign and malignant lesions were discriminated with only one misclassification. Distribution time t_{21} does not play a major role for this diagnostic decision. After irradiation, the values of t_{21} shifted to longer distribution times.

Discussion

The standard method for local follow-up of surgically treated rectal cancers is pelvic CT. The CT problems concerning the differentiation between recurrent tumor and postoperative or postradiation scar have been discussed in the past [5, 6]. Only the invasion of surrounding structures such as the sacrum or the bladder is a definite criterion to diagnose a recurrent tumor. MRI is considered to have advantages compared to CT by differing signal intensities in the T2-weighted images [7]. However, differentiation is impaired by areas of edema and inflammation within scars or desmoplastic reaction within tumors [8]. According to our results, T2-weighted images are of little benefit.

Diagnostic procedures considering the functional aspect of the suspect tissue have the highest accuracy in the characterization of the lesion. Positron emission tomography studies evaluating the turnover of fluorodeoxyglucose demonstrated a nearly 100% differentiation between unspecific scar tissue and recurrent malignancy [9]. Nevertheless, this method is rarely available and is expensive. Therefore the attempt to map a tissue region by its Gd-DTPA enhancement characteristics in MRI seems a very attractive functional access. It should be emphasized that the proposed model gives a pixel-by-pixel linear relationship between signal intensity and contrast medium tissue concentration. The pharmacokinetic data do not depend on subjective decisions of the observer.

The obtained results with differences between benign and malignant lesions and even between irradiated and nonirradiated tissue components encourage further examinations to obtain sufficient data for statistically assured diagnostic statements.

References

1. Silverberg E, Lubera J (1986) Cancer statistics. CA 36 11
2. Rich T, Gunderson LL, Lew R, Galdibini JJ, Cohen AM, Donaldson G (1983) Patterns of recurrence of rectal cancer after potentially curative surgery. Cancer 52: 1317–1329
3. Olson RM, Perenchevich NP, Malcolm AW, Chaffey JT, Wilson RE (1980) patterns of recurrence following curative resection of adenocarcinoma of the colon and rectum. Cancer 45: 2969–2974
4. Brix G, Semmler W, Port R, Schad LR, Layer G, Lorenz WJ (1991) In vivo mapping of pharmacokinetic parameters in CNS Gd-DTPA enhanced MR imaging. J Comput Assist Tomogr 15(4): 621–628
5. Lee JKT, Stanley RJ, Sagel SS, Leitt RG, McClennan BL (1981) CT appearence of the pelvis after abdoni-perineal resection for rectal carcinoma. Radiology 141: 737–741
6. Reznek RH, White FE, Young JWR, Kelsey FI, Nicholls RJ (1983) The appearences on computed tomography after abdominoperineal resection for carcinoma of the rectum: a comparison between the normal appearences and those of recurrence. Br J Radiol 56: 237–240
7. Krestin GP, Steinbrich W, Friedmann G (1988) Recurrent rectal cancer: diagnosis with MR imaging versus CT. Radiology 168: 307–311
8. de Lange EE, Fechner RE, Wanebo HJ (1989) Suspected recurrent rectosigmoid carcinoma after abdominoperineal resection: MR imaging and histopathologic findings. Radiology 170: 323–328
9. Strauß LG, Clorius JH, Schlag P, Lehner B, Kimmig B, Engenhart R, Marin-Grez M, Helus F, Oberdorfer F, Schmidlin P, van Kaick G (1989) Recurrence of colorectal tumors: PET evaluation. Radiology 170: 329–332

Anti-CEA Immunoscintigraphy in the Detection of Recurrences and Metastases of Colorectal Carcinoma

N. Rilinger[1], D.L. Munz[2], H.J. Illiger[1], H.J. Halbfaß[1], and H. Niemann[1]

Introduction

The number of patients with colorectal carcinoma is growing steadily. With 20 000 new cases each year colorectal carcinoma has become the second most common form of cancer in Germany. Rising trends can also be found in many other European countries [4]. The prognosis is poor especially for those patients with local lymph node metastases at the time of surgery of the primary tumor (Dukes stage C), with a 5-year survival rate of about 40% [12]. Diagnosis of the primary tumor is seldom difficult; however, the detection of recurrences or metastases sometimes presents a great problem.

It was the aim of this study to elucidate the value of immunoscintigraphy (IS) in the detection of recurrences and metastases of colorectal cancer using a ^{99m}Tc-labeled monoclonal antibody (MAb) against carcinoembryonic antigen (CEA; BW 431/26).

Methods

In 41 patients aged between 27 and 80 and with case histories of colorectal carcinoma IS, was performed using the ^{99m}Tc-labeled anti-CEA MAb BW 431/26. The clinical indication for IS was in most of the cases a significantly increased serum CEA level with suspected local recurrence or liver metastases. The MAb used was an IgG1 intact molecule which reacts exclusively with a protein epitope on the CEA complex [6]. Labeling procedure with ^{99m}Tc has been described by Schwarz and coworkers [11]; this allows the direct linkage of ^{99m}Tc to free thiol groups of the activated antibody. After labeling with ^{99m}Tc immunoreactivity ranges from 90% to 95%. The antibody binding to cell membrane integrated CEA is not inhibited by circulating CEA. The MAb does not bind to peripheral blood cells. The labeling kit of Schwarz and coworkers

[1] Abteilung für Radiologie und Nuklearmedizin Städtische Kliniken Oldenburg, Dr. -Eden-Str. 10 2900 Oldenburg, FRG
[2] Abtielung für Nuklearmedizin, Universität Göttingen, Robert-Koch-Str., 3400 Göttingen, FRG

Advanced Radiation Therapy Tumor Response
Monitoring and Treatment Planning
Breit (Editor-in-Chief)
© Springer-Verlag, Berlin Heidelberg 1992

[11] consists of two components: the antibody and the stannous component, both in lyophilized form and therefore stable for a number of months.

In cases of intraarterial MAb administration (suspected liver metastases), sequential scanning was carried out during the first 5 min followed by planar scans of the thorax, abdomen, and pelvis 10–20 min after injection (Elscint gamma camera APEX 409 ECT, 256 matrix, all-purpose collimator). Otherwise planar scans of the thorax and abdomen took place 4–8 and 18–30 h after injection supplemented in special cases by emission computed tomography.

Results and Discussion

The detection of recurrent local disease is based on clinical examination, a rise in serum tumor markers such as CEA, and local imaging. Ultrasound is limited by bowel gas, and X-ray and computed tomography cannot be used reliably to distinguish bowel thickening, local post-surgical scarring or inflammation, and truly recurrent disease. IS examinations for diagnosing local recurrence or metastases of colorectal carcinoma were performed in the early and middle 1980s mainly by the use of ^{111}In- or ^{131}I-labeled antibodies or their fragments. The development of the ^{99}mTc-labeled MAb represented a major step forward in routine (IS).

In 32/41 patients IS was positive, detecting 39/69 liver metastases, 3/3 lymph node metastases, 0/1 lung metastases, and 8/8 local recurrences.

Table 1 shows our results grouped in true- or false-positive and -negative findings. Seven of eight local recurrences detected by IS (Fig. 1) were also seen by CT; however, in one case, IS was the only diagnostic procedure showing the recurrence, confirmed by surgery. These good results in the detection of local recurrences were also found by other authors [1, 3, 5, 9, 10] who report sensitivities in the detection of recurrences between 67% and 92%. Two lymph node metastases were detected only by IS (Fig. 2) and confirmed by surgery, whereas other procedures such as computed tomography and ultrasound produced negative results.

Whereas in our study no false-positive lymph node was found, immuno-histochemical results of other investigators [1] show that positive scans of

Table 1. Immunoscintigraphic results ($n = 41$)

	Liver metastases	Lymph node metastases	Others	Local recurrences
True positive	39	3	—	8
True negative	3	—	—	6
False negative	30	—	1	—
False positive	—	—	—	1

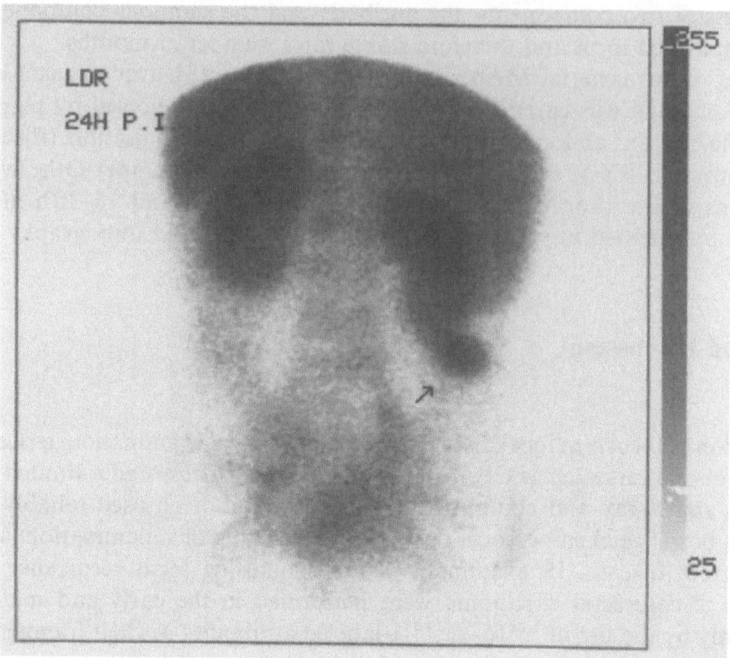

Fig. 1. Recurrence of colon ascendens carcinoma, confirmed by surgery

lymph nodes without any tumor can be due to free CEA. Therefore the sensitivity of IS in the detection of lymph node metastases differs from author to author and drops, according to Bares et al. [2], to 24%.

Most of the small liver metastases with a diameter of 1–2 cm showed up ;as hot spots, whereas almost all larger metastases were seen as cold lesions caused by central necrosis and with a hot rim resulting from active tumor tissue. This is the so-called rim sign. All liver metastases that only showed up as defects without the rim sign were taken as nonspecific reactions and considered to be negative scans. In our view, the failure to detect 30 liver metastases by IS results from their small size (< 1 cm) and perhaps the lack of CEA production. The poor sensitivity of 56% using the ^{99m}Tc-labeled MAb BW 431/26 in the detection of liver metastases is confirmed by other groups [1]. However, Bischof-Delaloye and coworkers [5] pointed out that an increasing sensitivity can be found using ^{123}I antibody fragments for the detection of liver metastases.

We found one false-positive scan in the case of nonspecific colitis. This may be due to a cross-reactivity with NCA 95 [2, 7] expressed at the cellular membrane of granulocytes and their preliminary stage. False-positive results seen by other groups [2] may also be caused by retention of radioactivity in the feces and by bilious excretion of the MAb metabolized in the liver. These false-positive results can be avoided by giving a laxative before MAb administration and by repeated scanning to detect the movement of radioactivity in the bowel.

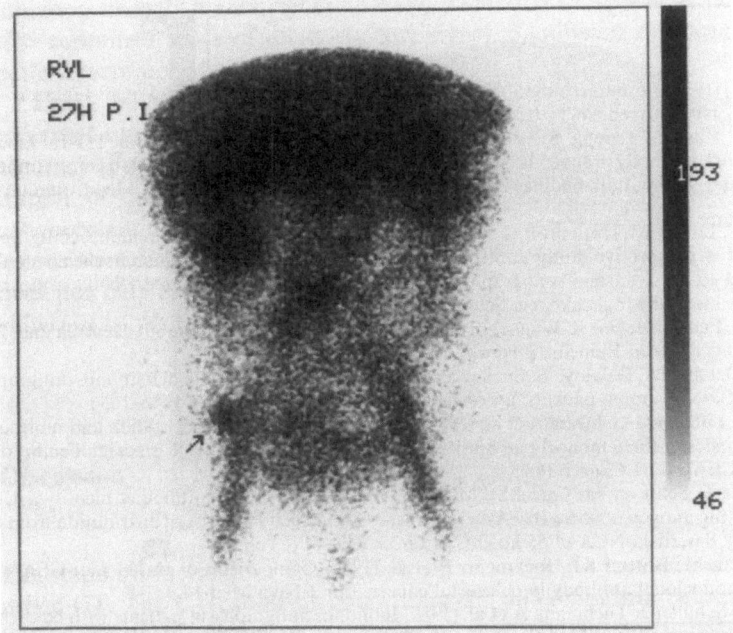

Fig. 2. Focal tracer accumulation in a lymph node metastasis. This finding was negative in computed tomography and ultrasound but was confirmed by surgery

Another, but very unusual, reason for false-positive immunoscans described by Granowska and Britton [8] is the presence of the target antigen in benign soft-tissue tumor without malignancy.

Conclusion

IS with the ^{99m}Tc-labeled MAb BW 431/26 is a very promising approach in the detection of local recurrences of colorectal cancer. It is an important additional procedure for other imaging modalities such as computed tomography to distinguish between local postsurgical scarring and truly recurrent disease. In our study the IS results in cases of liver metastases with a sensitivity of 56% are poor. The detection of lymph node metastases also remains a problem because false-positive scans can be obtained by free CEA in tumor-draining lymph nodes without real malignancy. However, in our study IS was the decisive approach in the detection of two occult lymph node metastases which were later confirmed by surgery.

References

1. Bares R (1990) Immunszintigraphie kolorektaler Tumoren: Probleme und Grenzen der Methode. Nuklearmediziner 3/13: 173–181
2. Bares R, Fass J, Truong S et al. (1989) Radioimmunoscintigraphy with 111-In labeled monoclonal antibody fragments (F(ab)$_2$ BW 431/31) against CEA: radiolabeling, antibody kinetics and distribution, findings in tumour and nontumour patients. Nucl Med Commun 10: 627–641
3. Baum RP, Lorenz M, Hottenrott C et al. (1988) The clinical application of immunoscintigraphy: results of a prospective study controlled by surgery, histology and immunochemistry and compared to CT-scan and sonography. In: Schmidt HAE, Csernay L (eds) Nuklearmedizin, neue Aspekte und Möglichkeiten. Schattauer, Stuttgart, pp 611–615
4. Becker N, Fentzel-Beyme R, Wagner G (1984) Krebsatlas der Bundesrepublik Deutschland, 2nd edn. Springer, Berlin Heidelberg New York
5. Bischof-Delaloye A, Delaloye B, Buchegger F et al. (1989) Clinical value of immunoscintigraphy in colorectal carcinoma patients: a prospective study. J Nucl Med 30: 1646–1656
6. Bosslet J, Lübben G, Schwarz A et al. (1985) Immunohistochemical localization and molecular characteristics of three monoclonal antibody-defined epitopes detectable on carcinoembryonic antigen (CEA). Int J Cancer 36:75
7. Buchegger F, Schreyer M, Carrel St, Mach JP (1984) Monoclonal antibodies identify a CEA crossreacting antigen of 95 kd (NCA-95) distinct in antigenicity and tissue distribution from the previously described NCA of 55 kd. J Cancer 33: 643–49
8. Granowska M, Britton KE, Richmann P et al. (1988) Comparison of In-111 anti-CEA-with PR1A3 monoclonal antibody in colorectal cancer. Eur J Nucl Med 14: C3–8
9. Kroiss A, Schüller J, Tuchmann A et al. (1989) Immunoscintigraphy in patients with colorectal cancer recurrences. Nucl Med Commun 10:222
10. Lind P, Langsteger W, Költringer P et al. (1990) Immunoscintigraphy with Tc99m labeled monoclonal anti-CEA-antibody (BW 431/26) in the follow up of patients with colorectal carcinomas. In: Schmidt HAE, Chambron J (eds) Nuclear medicine, quantitative analysis in imaging and function. Schattauer, Stuttgart, pp 567–569
11. Schwarz A, Steinsträsser A (1987) A novel approach to Tc99m labeled monoclonal antibodies. J Nucl Med 28:721
12. Skindo K (1974) Recurrence of carcinoma in the large intestine. A statistical review. Am J Proctol 25:80

Positron Emission Tomography Studies of Tumor Metabolism: A Prognostic Factor in High-Dose Radiotherapy of Recurrent Rectal Cancer?

J. Romahn[1], R. Engenhart[1], L.G. Strauss[2], U. Haberkorn[2], W.J. Lorenz[2], and M. Wannenmacher[1]

Introduction

Rectal recurrence following a complete resection of a rectal carcinoma accounts for about 50% of all tumor-related deaths in this tumor [12, 13]. These occur with an incidence of 20%–50%, depending on tumor stage, grade, and therapy procedure [9, 19]. About 70%–80% occur within the first 2 years following primary surgery. Radiotherapy is known to be the most effective treatment modality for rectal recurrence, with symptomatic response rates of 50%–90%, but the palliative effect lasts only about 6 months. Because rectal recurrence seems to be relatively radioresistant compared with the primary disease, high linear energy transfer (LET) radiation should bring better results. Based on clinical and radiobiological observations, it has been suggested that patients with macroscopic recurrence may benefit from neutron therapy. An improvement in symptomatic response compared with photon therapy has been reported [2, 3, 4, 5].

[18F]Fluorodeoxyglucose (FDG) is a marker of metabolic tumor activity because it follows the normal glucose pathway into the cell and is trapped there by intracellular phosphorylation. By positron emission tomography (PET) techniques it is possible to achieve images of the metabolic activity of viable tissue in vivo.

Materials and Methods

Out of a total of 52 patients treated with a mixed-beam schedule of 40 Gy photons followed by a neutron boost of 6.6–10 Gy, we performed a study of tumor metabolic activity in 21 patients. All of these patients received a PET

---

[1] Department of Radiotherapy, University Clinic of Radiology, University of Heidelberg, Im Neuenheimer Feld 400, 6900 Heidelberg, FRG
[2] Department of Radiology and Pathophysiology, German Cancer Research Center, Im Neuenheimer Feld 280, 6900 Heidelberg, FRG

Advanced Radiation Therapy Tumor Response
Monitoring and Treatment Planning
Breit (Editor-in-Chief)
© Springer-Verlag, Berlin Heidelberg 1992

study with FDG prior to radiotherapy. After completion of radiation they were followed-up by further PET investigations.

The photon therapy was carried out in the Radiotherapy Center of the University of Heidelberg. The radiation was delivered in a weighted-box technique favoring the AP/PA fields. Target volume was the whole pelvis. We administered 40 Gy in 20 fractions over 4 weeks using 23 or 42 MeV photons. This treatment was followed immediately by a boost of 14 MeV neutrons. The neutrons were delivered by the 14-MeV DT generator of the German Cancer Research Center in Heidelberg. Fractions of 1 or 1.1 Gy were administered three times per week. Patients suffering from distant metastasis at the beginning of radiotherapy received a total dose of 6.6 Gy. Those without distant metastasis were treated with a curative intention to a dose of 10 Gy. The target volume for the neutron boost was the macroscopic tumor with a craniocaudal safety margin of 1.5 cm. The os sacrum in the whole tumor length was included in the target volume. Irradiation with fast neutrons was carried out in an arc therapy technique. The inconstant dose output was controlled and compensated by a computer-assisted system developed at the German Cancer Research Center [6, 7]. This technique results in an optimal and homogeneous dose distribution in the target volume and a good reduction in dose to normal tissues of the risk organs (i. e., small bowel and bladder).

All patients underwent computed tomography (CT) examinations prior to radiotherapy (Siemens whole-body scanner Somatom DRH). These data were used for treatment planning and for identification of regions of glucose accumulation in the PET scans by means of anatomic landmarks. The CT examinations were performed in contiguous sections including the iliac crest, perineal region, and inguinal lymph nodes. A whole-body PET scanner (PC 2048-7WB, Scanditronics, Uppsala, Sweden) with two ring detectors was used for the metabolic studies. The patients received an intravenous bolus injection of 9–12 mCi FDG. Data acquisition began 1 h after injection and lasted about 10 min. FDG was produced and its radiochemical purity determined using the method described by Oberdorfer et al. [10]. The PET images were analyzed using a conventional region-of-interest technique (ROI). ROIs were chosen in the tumor and in the gluteal muscle, the latter serving as reference tissue. FDG concentrations were normalized to the injected dose and body volume to obtain standardized uptake values (SUV). During radiotherapy and in follow-up we used the tumor markers CEA and CA 19-9 for documentation of tumor response and for indication of distant metastasis.

Severe pain is a predominant and most sensitive symptom of rectal recurrence that often leads to the final diagnosis. We used the EORTC/RTOG scoring system for palliation of osseous metastasis to quantify intensity of pain and to objectify the intensity and duration of pain relief after therapy. This nine-point scoring system takes into account the intensity of pain as well as the administration of analgetic drugs (frequency and types of analgetics) [18].

Results

Our series of 21 patients with PET metabolic investigation up to now has a mean follow-up of 14.1 months (4–38). Thirteen patients have died. Seven of the remaining eight patients are currently without evidence of disease. The time to local failure was measured from radiotherapy to objective evidence of local progression or death. Five patients were considered to have local progression at the time of death. Progression-free survival ranges from 6 to 28 months, with a mean of 12.7 months.

Relief of pain was achieved in all but one of our patients: complete relief in 13 and partial relief in 7. Duration of pain relief was 6 months in 81% and 12 months in 76%, and in 53% of our patients we found relief of pain for longer than 18 months. Twelve of our patients could stop administration of analgetics.

Of our 21 patients 18 showed pathological and increasing CEA serum levels when admitted to radiotherapy. The serum level remained in the upper normal range in three patients. Medium pretherapeutic CEA was 15 ng/ml with a range of 3–156 ng/ml. A significant decrease was seen in all but one patient after radiation treatment; the mean CEA level at that time was 4.2 ng/ml (1–74 ng/ml). Normalization of CEA levels correlated with the clinical course in 14 patients. In five no decrease was achieved due to development of simultaneous distant metastasis. Sensitivity and specificity values are presented in Table 1.

We performed 72 PET studies in the 21 patients. FDG uptake was increased in all but one patient prior to radiotherapy. The average FDG concentration was more than twice as high as that seen in scar or normal soft tissue. An increased uptake due to infiltration of the os sacrum was noted in two patients, while CT revealed no signs of sacral destruction. The intensity of FDG accumulation showed a wide range of 1.8–5.0, with a mean SUV of 2.3. With the exception of two patients, we saw a decrease in tumor activity of 30%–60% within 2 months after radiotherapy. However, in only six patients did SUV reach the range of normal soft tissue. Six months after irradiation we found a mean FDG uptake of 1.6 (0.8–2.9). In eight patients we obtained PET data 12 months after radiotherapy. At that time mean SUV was 1.5 (1.1–3.3), but in three

Table 1. Results of FDG, CEA, and pain score in follow-up of colorectal recurrence

	FDG ($n = 14$)	Pain score ($n = 21$)	CEA ($n = 21$)
True positive	5	5	4
True negative	2	13	8
False positive	7	3	8
False negative	0	0	1
Sensitivity	1	1	0.8
Specificity	0.2	0.8	0.5
Accuracy	0.5	0.9	0.6

patients we already noted an increase in metabolic tumor activity. However, in one patient 18 months after an SUV comparable to normal soft tissue was found. Two other patients at that time had a slight increase in FDG accumulation, first noted 6 months after therapy. However, this increase was associated with an increase in CEA levels at the same time, followed by an increase of pain 2 and 6 months later. In four patients we obtained PET examinations more than 18 months after radiotherapy; two showed increased FDG accumulation due to a second tumor relapse, and one showed no clinical sign of progression as the tumor marker level did not leave the normal range. The figures for PET FDG uptake and CEA level and complains of pain are presented in Table 1.

Discussion

A variety of factors influence the prognosis of patients with rectal cancer, such as tumor stage, grade, and therapy procedure [2, 3, 9, 19]. Furthermore, as Welin has pointed out, there is great variability in individual tumor growth rate [20]. James et al. reported that early response to radiotherapy seems to be an indicator for further prognosis of the patient because those with a good early response to radiotherapy show a significantly higher survival rate compared to those without or with moderate improvement of symptoms [8]. Local failure is the usual reason for limited pain relief, caused either by dose inhomogeneity in the target volume or by radioresistance of the tumor cells or cell line. In both cases the administration of a curative tumor dose fails. As usual, the possible dose is limited by the complication rates of normal tissues in the neighborhood of the tumor, in our case bladder and small intestine. The irradiation technique that we used in our series allows the safe delivery of high doses to the target volume, with a good dose gradient outside the tumor [6]. CT and/or magnetic resonance imaging is absolutely necessary in computer-assisted treatment planning to define the correct target volume.

Several studies have demonstrated that CEA is a useful prognostic factor for patients suffering from primary colorectal carcinoma [11, 15]. In follow-up studies several authors have demonstrated a sensitivity of 90% for diagnoses of local recurrences or distant metastasis [17]. Staab reported that it is possible to diagnose a local recurrence about 6 months earlier by observing serum CEA levels than is possible by clinical methods [14]. Arnott observed that pretherapeutic serum CEA levels may be a predictor of treatment response [1]. In our study we found no correlation between decreased serum CEA and patient prognosis. After irradiation all CEA levels were the upper normal region, and in analogy to postsurgical follow-up [17] CEA was a valid parameter to indicate a second relapse or the development of distant metastasis.

FDG uptake is an indicator of tumor metabolism and activity. Strauss et al. [16] demonstrated that it is possible to differentiate recurrent rectal tumor from scar tissue with PET. SUV measurement provides quantitative data to evaluate the treatment response of radiotherapy. The initial decrease in SUV, similarly to that in serum CEA level, is not influenced by existing distant metastasis. However, a complete normalization of SUV after radiotherapy was seen in only 6/14 of our patients, while two of these six patients who had complete normalization 3 and 4 months after radiotherapy developed a second relapse after 6 and 22 months. Our small patient numbers do not allow a conclusion as to whether a normalization of SUV predicts long-term benefit. On the other hand, three patients were misclassified because of increasing SUV values 3, 5, and 12 months after therapy. All three showed worsening of clinical signs, but CEA levels remained unchanged. In all three a small-bowel complication was verified by the surgeon after laparotomy. Final pathology denied the evidence of residual disease. The increased glucose metabolism was caused by the increased glycolytic activity of inflammation.

The earliest indication of a local tumor relapse was given by FDG uptake. We found a concomitantly rising serum CEA level. According to the literature, the clinical symptoms become manifest months later [24]. Because of the problem that enhanced glycolytic activity is related not only to malignant cells, FDG PET studies cannot distinguish between inflammation, proliferation, repair, and residual viable tumor. Necrotic areas in the center of the tumor after radiotherapy may lead to normal SUV values even when the tumor wall consists of viable tumor cells. This could be responsible for the two patients that developed recurrence after a complete normalization of SUV. At the moment it is not possible for technical reasons to obtain contiguous cross-sections of the whole tumor volume. Therefore the investigation is limited to two sections in the position where the tumor diameter is greatest. The tumor metabolism may be normal there, but recurrences may also develop at the cranial or caudal edge.

We can conclude that PET imaging using FDG is a sensitive method for distinguishing scar tissue and viable tumor. The use of PET as a predictor of patient prognosis after radiotherapy is as yet not possible, but the findings of our study warrant further exploration.

References

1. Arnott SJ (1983) Plasma embryonic antigen (CEA) as an indicator for radical or palliative radiotherapy in patients with rectal cancer. Cancer Detect Prev 66: 155–159
2. Breteau N, Destembert B, Favre A, Sabattier R (1986) Neutron boost in inoperable rectal carcinomas in Orleans. Bull Cancer (Paris) 73: 591–595
3. Duncan W, Arnott SJ, Jack WJL, Orr JA, Kerr GR, Williams JR (1990) Results of two randomized clinical trials of neutron therapy in rectal adenocarcinoma. Radiother Oncol 166: 90–94
4. Eising E, Pötter U, Haverkamp E, Schnepper E (1990) Neutron therapy (d > T. 14MeV) for recurrence of rectal cancer: interim analysis from Münster. Strahlenther Onkol 166: 90–94
5. Engenhart R, Kimmig B, Höver KH, Strauss LG, Lorenz WJ, Wannenmacher M (1990)

Photonneutron therapy for recurrent rectal cancer — follow up and preliminary results. Strahlenther Onkol 166: 95–98

6. Engenhart R, Kimmig B, Wannenmacher M, Höver KH, Hesse BM, Lorenz JW (1989) Experience with the computer controlled weighted moving beam therapy (WMBT) in routine clinical use. In: Blattmann H (ed) Proceedings of the international heavy particle therapy workshop (PTCOG/EORTC/ECNEU), 18th–20th September, 1989, Villingen, FRG

7. Höver KH (1987) Neutron isodose distribution obtained by weighted moving beam therapy. Br J Radiol 60: 313

8. James RD, Johnson RJ, Eddleston B, Zheng GI, Jones JM (1983) Prognostic factors in locally recurrent rectal carcinoma treated by radiotherapy. Br J Surg 70: 469–472

9. McDermott FT, Hughes ESR, Pihl E, Johnson WR, Price AB (1985) Local recurrence after potentially curative resection for rectal cancer in a series of 1008 patients. Br J Surg 72: 34–37 (1985)

10. Oberdorfer F, Hull WE, Traving BC, Maier-Borst W (1986) Synthesis and purification of 2-deoxy-2-^{18}F-D-glucose and 2-deoxy-2-^{18}F-D-mannose: characterization of products by ^{1}H and ^{19}F NMR spectroscopy. Int Rad Appl Instrum 37(8): 695–707

11. Persijn JP, Hart AAM (1981) Prognostic significance of CEA in colorectal cancer: a statistical study. J Clin Chem Clin Biochem 19: 1117–1123

12. Rich T, Gunderson LL, Lew R, Galdibini JJ, Cohen AL, Donaldson G (1983) Patterns of recurrence of rectal cancer after potentially curative surgery. Cancer 52: 1317–1329

13. Schulz U (1987) Kolorektale Tumoren In: Scherer E (ed) Strahlentherapie: radiologische Onkologie, 3rd edn. Springer, Berlin Heidelberg New York, pp 632–651

14. Staab HJ (1984) Medizinisch-biologische Bedeutung des Carcinoembryonalen Antigens (CEA): klinische Studien und experimentelle Modelle. Roche, Basel

15. Staab JJ, Anderer FA, Brümmendorf T, Stumpf E, Fischer R (1981) Prognostic value of preoperative serum CEA level compared to clinical staging. Br J Cancer 44: 652–662

16. Strauss LG, Clorius JH, Schlag P, Lehnert B, Kimmig B, Engenhart R, Marin-Grez M, Helus F, Oberdorfer F, Schmidlin P, van Kaick G (1989) Recurrence of colorectal tumors: PET evaluation. Radiology 170: 329–332

17. Sugarbaker PH, Zamcheck N, Moore FD (1976) Assessment of serial carcinoembryonic antigen (CEA) assays in postoperative detection of recurrent colorectal cancer. Cancer 38: 2310–2315

18. Tong D, Gillick L, Hendrickson FR (1982) The palliation of symptomatic osseous metastases. Cancer 50: 893–899

19. Welch JP, Donaldson CA (1979) The clinical correlation of an autopsy study of recurrent colorectal cancer. Ann Surg 189: 496–502

20. Welin S, Youler J, Spratt JS (1963) The rates and patterns of growth of 375 tumors of the large intestine and rectum observed serially by double contrast enema study. Am J Roentgenol 90: 673–685

Treatment Planning and Tumor Response Monitoring: Bone and Soft-Tissue

Magnetic Resonance Imaging of Skeletal Metastases: Evaluation of Therapeutic Consequences

P. Lukas, R. Stepan, R. Bauer, B. Kolb, A. Heuck, and A. Breit

Radiotherapy is an effective treatment modality in the palliation of skeletal metastases. Toward sparing patients with poor prognosis from unnecessarily long treatment periods or hospitalization, we evaluated the therapeutic value of magnetic resonance imaging (MRI) in the treatment of patients with skeletal metastases who are to undergo radiation therapy. Due to its superior soft-tissue contrast, MRI is considered the most sensitive method for differentiating between normal bone marrow and tumorous tissue.

Methods and Materials

To determine the exact tumor extension in patients with skeletal metastases prior to radiotherapeutic treatment we performed 100 MRI examinations of the spine and pelvis. The patients were examined in our two MRI units with 0.5 and 1.5 T (Gyroscan S5 and S15, Philips). The following sequences were used: T_1-weighted SE, $T_R = 500-550$ ms, $T_E = 30-50$ ms; T_2*-weighted FFE, flip angle 20°, TE = 27/54 ms; T_2-weighted SE, $T_R = 1800-2000$ ms, $T_E = 50/100$ ms.

From 100 patients 92 were selected for the study; the examinations of eight patients had to be neglected due to motion artifacts or early breaks caused by patients' pain. There were 42 men and 50 women; mean age was 58 years (range 22–81). The primary tumor sites were: breast, 26; genitourinary, 77; lung, 14; gastrointestinal, 10; thyroid, 5; other, 14; unknown, 6. The most frequently examined regions were the spine with 58% and the pelvis with 22%. A pilot study included MRI examination of 60 patients — 25 men and 35 women, with a mean age of 59 (range 32–79). Both studies were retrospective. Table 1 lists the examinations that were carried out within a 3-week period in each patient. It is interesting that in comparison to our pilot study the number of computed tomography (CT) examinations decreased markedly. This means that in cases of pathological bone scintigraphic findings, the clinicians decided to perform MRI alone as additional screening method, whereas X-ray and CT were, already at an early stage, considered to be less specific.

Institut für Strahlentherapie und Radiologische Onkologie, Technische Universität München, Klinikum rechts der Isar, Ismaninger Str. 15, W-8000, Munich 80, FRG

Advanced Radiation Therapy Tumor Response
Monitoring and Treatment Planning
Breit (Editor-in-Chief)
© Springer-Verlag, Berlin Heidelberg 1992

Table 1. Examinations carried out in patients with bone metastases

	Major study ($n = 92$) n (%)	Pilot study ($n = 60$) n (%)
Bone scan + X-ray + CT	39 (43)	36 (60)
Bone scan + X-ray	28 (30)	17 (28)
Bone scan + CT	6 (7)	3 (5)
X-ray + CT	2 (2)	2 (3)
X-ray only	3 (3)	—
Bone scan only	14 (15)	2 (3)

Table 2. Further results obtained by the MRI examination

	Major study ($n = 92$)	Pilot study ($n = 60$)
No additional information	37%	31%
Additional information		
Without consequence	16%	23%
With consequence	47%	46%
Consequences		
Verification of diagnosis (metastases yes/no)	9%	10%
Change in field size	23%	20%
Change in therapeutic modality	15%	16%
Total	47%	46%

Results

In terms of the accuracy of tumor localization (not the extent of tumor) the comparison between bone scintigraphy and MRI in the region of the axial skeleton, showed equality of the methods in 58% of cases, MRI as superior in 40%, and bone scintigraphy superior in 2%. Even disregarding unspecific scans, there remained 20 of 92 patients (22% of cases, and a much higher number of metastases) in which MRI showed metastatic changes in tissue which could not be seen in bone scintigraphy. Further results of the inclusion of MRI examination are presented in Table 2; the category "metastases yes/no" refers to any kind of therapy (yes or no), change in field size to the size of the portals or addition of a second field, and change in therapeutic modality to chemotherapy or operation instead of radiotherapy.

Discussion

Our results show the obtaining of additional information by MRI which is of therapeutic consequence in 47% of the examined cases. As a result of this, no radiation therapy of skeletal metastases is carried out at our institution without

MRI examination of the axial skeleton. The reason for the superiority of MRI to bone scintigraphy in the detection of skeletal metastases lies in the mechanism of tumor spread in our group of patients. The primary tumors in our group were generally hematogenously spreading tumors. As recent studies of hematogenous tumor spread have shown, tumor cells grow significantly better in bone marrow well supplied with blood than in cortical structures. Due to the excellent contrast between fatty bone marrow and solid tumor tissue, metastases can be found early by MRI while they can be detected by bone scan only if cortical structures are destructed.

Conclusion

1. MRI is superior in the detection of metastases and skeletal structures with a predominance of bone marrow.
2. Bone scan is superior in the detection of metastases in skeletal structures with a predominance of cortical bone.
3. MRI is the most sensitive method for detecting the extension of metastases in the axial skeleton and is therefore of significant therapeutic value.

Magnetic Resonance Imaging of Skeletal Metastases

K. Neumann, N. Hosten, W. Schörner, H. Steinkamp, and R. Felix

Introduction

In patients with malignant disease, the presence of skeletal metastases is very important for treatment and prognosis. Particularly the number and site of metastases influence the choice of field size in radiotherapy. Radionuclide scans carried out for screening or conventional radiographs depict alterations of the bone matrix but do not reflect tumor involvement of the bone marrow, which normally occurs first. Magnetic resonance imaging (MRI) has proven very sensitive in the detection of bone marrow changes [6] and may possibly depict bone metastases before they became apparant scintigraphically or roentgenologically [2–4].

This report examines the use of plain and gadolinium-DTPA (Gd-DTPA) enhanced MRI as a screening method to disclose metastatic invasion of the bone marrow. In addition to a conventional T1-weighted gradient echo (GE) sequence an opposed-phase GE sequence was used, in which red bone marrow shows little or no signal intensity.

Patients and Methods

We studied 20 patients (15 women and 5 men, 41–76 years of age) with known metastases of the spine or pelvis. Primary malignancies included breast cancer ($n = 10$), lung cancer ($n = 2$), colorectal cancer ($n = 2$), hypernephroma ($n = 2$), prostatic cancer ($n = 2$), malignant melanoma ($n = 1$), and malignant neuroectodermal tumor ($n = 1$). All patients had a bone scan prior to MRI. Metastatic bone destruction was confirmed by conventional radiographs or computed tomography scans.

MRI was performed on a 0.5-T Siemens system with a 50 cm field of view body coil. T1-weighted sagittal or coronal images of the spine and pelvis were

Strahlenklinik mit Poliklinik, Universitätsklinikum Rudolf Virchow/Charlottenburg, Freie Universität Berlin, Spandauer Damm 130, 1000 berlin 19, FRG

Advanced Radiation Therapy Tumor Response
Monitoring and Treatment Planning
Breit (Editor-in-Chief)
© Springer-Verlag, Berlin Heidelberg 1992

obtained using an in-phase GE sequence with TR = 400 ms and TE = 14 ms. Opposed-phase images were then generated using a GE sequence with TR = 400 ms and TE = 22 ms, in which magnetic moments of fat and water protons have a phase difference of 180°. Both sequences were repeated after intravenous administration of 0.1 mmol/kg Gd-DTPA. In each sequence 14 slices of 5-mm thickness were obtained in 6.9-min acquisition time. In coronal orientation, a 1.25-mm interslice gap was used. Number, localization, and delineation of lesions detected by MRI were compared with those shown by scintigraphy. Areas of different signal intensity (SI) in MRI were assumed to be metastatic only if they showed contrast enhancement.

Results

In MRI patients were positioned so that in coronal slice orientation lower thoracal and lumbar spine, pelvis, and proximal femura were shown. Using sagittal orientation, thoracal and lumbar vertebrae and lower cervical vertebrae were imaged. On T1-weighted in-phase MR images red bone marrow had a SI comparable to that of muscle. Opposed-phase images depicted red marrow with low SI close to background. Analyzed visually, red marrow showed no increase in SI after administration of Gd-DTPA.

Bone scans depicted 28 metastatic lesions within the vertebrae and 9 lesions of the pelvis. In-phase T1-weighted images showed 23 solitary lesions of the spine and 14 lesions of the pelvis, being slightly or moderately less intense than normal bone marrow. In MRI margination of lesions and spatial resolution were superior to radionuclide scans. Unlike bone scans, MRI allowed certain determination of involved vertebrae. After administration of contrast five more lesions were detected, but increasing intensity obscured depiction of 21 metastases which were seen on plain images.

Opposed-phase images showed metastases with moderately or markedly higher SI than normal red bone marrow (Fig. 1). Thirty-five solitary lesions of the vertebrae and 18 lesions of the pelvis and proximal femurs were detected. All metastases shown on the bone scans were imaged and showed Gd-DTPA enhancement. Increasing SI after administration of Gd-DTPA improved visualization in all lesions. Delineation of lesions on plain and contrast-enhanced images was superior to in-phase T1-weighted images and was distinctly better than on bone scans. In two patients, opposed-phase MR images revealed diffuse metastatic infiltration in nearly all parts of the imaged spine, which was less visible on in-phase images and could not be detected on bone scans.

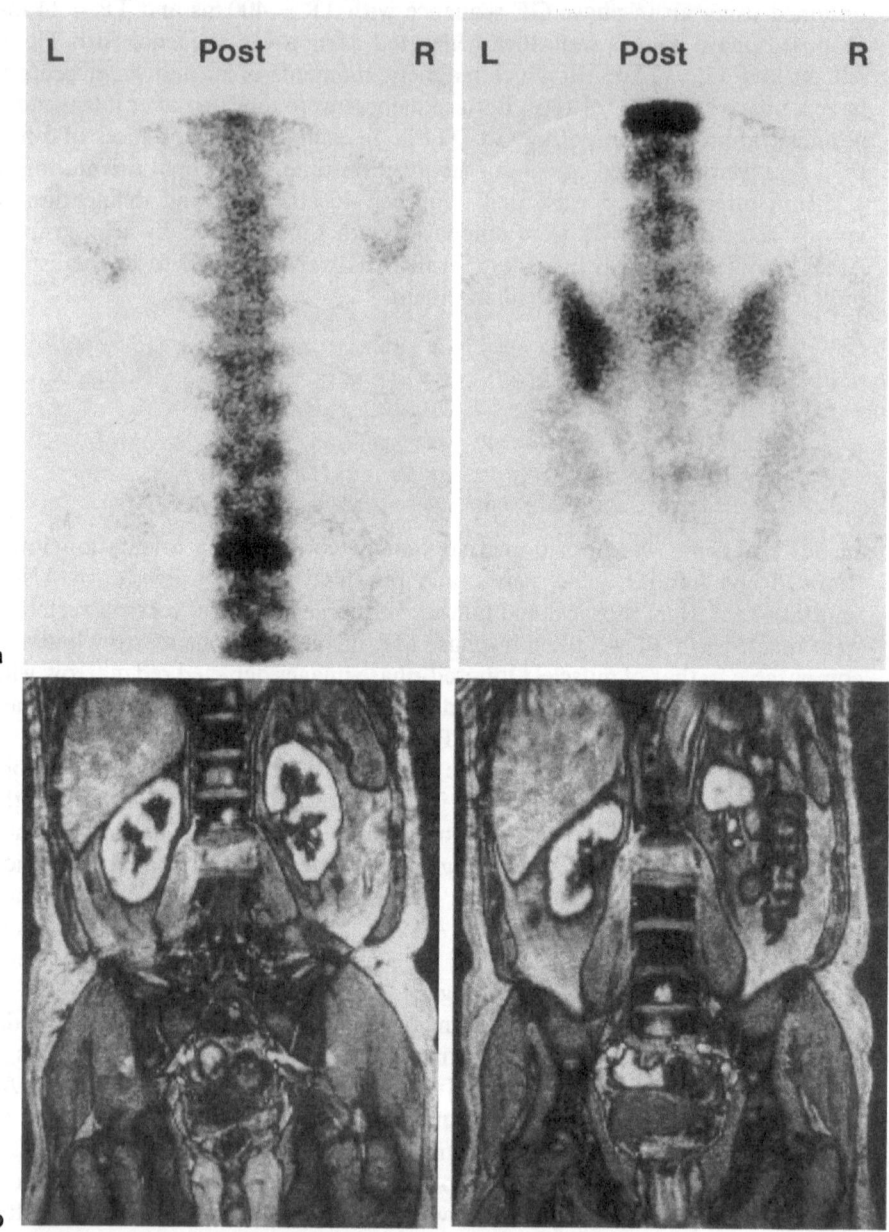

Fig. 1a, b. Bone scan and opposed-phase MR images of a 53-year-old patient with lung cancer. **a** [99mTc] DPD scintigraphy. Enhancement of the radionuclide in the vertebral body L2 indicates metastasis. No other enhancement in thoracal or lumbar spine. **b** Coronal opposed-phase MR images (GE, TR = 400 ms, TE = 22 ms) after intravenous administration of Gd-DTPA. Corresponding to the bone scan, L2 shows high signal intensity. Additionally, markedly hyperintense lesions in the vertebrae T 10, T 12, L1, L5, and S1 are demonstrated

Discussion

Imaging the bone marrow permits sensitive detection of skeletal metastases by MRI [4]. Surface coils provide high spatial resolution [5] but are not suitable for screening because of the small field of view [2]. Use of body coils with a larger field of view but poorer image quality requires a high contrast between metastases and red bone marrow to give appropriate information. Increase in SI differences between normal and abnormal bone marrow may be obtained by short inversion-time inversion-recovery (STIR) images or other chemical shift techniques [1]. SI in the opposed-phase images used in this study depends particularly on the ratio between fat and water protons because their magnetic moments are "subtracted" at time of signal acquisition. Echo-time TE was set to a value at which SI of red marrow was minimal. Lesions having different amounts of fat and water showed higher SI. This resulted in higher lesion to bone marrow contrast and, unlike on in-phase images, improved visualization after Gd-DTPA enhancement.

Compared with bone scans, the number of detected metastases on in-phase T1-weighted images was less in the spine and higher in the pelvis, overall being approximately the same. However, delineation of the lesions was superior. Gd-DTPA enhancement, which was used as a criterion for malignancy, did not improve imaging. Opposed-phase images depicted more metastases both in the spine and in the pelvis. Some lesions in the proximal femura not seen on bone scans or T1-weighted MR images could be detected. Although all metastases detectable on bone scans showed increased SI after Gd-DTPA administration differentiation between benign and malignant lesions by contrast enhancement remains to be confirmed.

In conclusion, sensitivity of opposed-phase images to bone metastases is high and may exceed sensitivity of bone scans. Contrast enhancement improves visualization of lesions in this sequence. Using a body coil, this technique may provide a fast screening method for vertebral and pelvic metastases with good delineation of lesions. Specifity of Gd-DTPA enhanced MRI should be the objective of further investigation.

References

1. Baker LL, Goodman SB, Perkash I, Lane B, Enzmann DR (1990) Benign versus pathologic compression fractures of vertebral bodies: assessment with conventional spin-echo, chemical shift, and STIR MR imaging. Radiology 174: 495–502
2. Decho T, Horstmann G, Randzio G (1990) Vergleichende Untersuchung zwischen Knochenmarkszintigraphie und Magnetresonanztomographie bei onkologischen Patienten. Fortschr Geb Rontgenstr 154: 300–305
3. Kattapuram SV, Khurana JS, Scott JA, el Khoury GY (1990) Negative scintigraphy with positive magnetic resonance imaging in bone metastases. Skeletal Radiol 19: 113–116

4. Stephan R, Lukas P, Kolb B, Breit A (1990) Die therapeutische Relevanz der Kernspintomographie für die strahlentherapeutische Behandlung von Skelettmetastasen. In: Lissner J, Doppman JL, Margulis AR (eds) MR '89. 3. Internationales Kernspintomograhie Symposium, Garmisch-Partenkirchen, 25–29. Januar 1989. Deutscher Ärzte, Köln, pp 52–56
5. Sze G (1990) Magnetic resonance imaging of the spine in oncology. In: Breit A (ed) Magnetic resonance in oncology. Springer, Berlin Heidelberg New York, pp 41–54
6. Vogler JB, Murphy WA (1988) Bone marrow imaging. Radiology 168: 679–693

Advances in Screening and Staging of Malignant Diseases Using Immunoscintigraphy for the Detection of Bone Marrow Involvement

N. Rilinger[1], M.Z.S. Halabi[1], D.L. Munz[2], H. Niemann[1], and H.J. Illiger[1]

Introduction

Although bone marrow scintigraphy has been used since the end of the 1950s, it has not yet achieved prominence as a valid procedure in nuclear medicine. Initially this resulted from the relatively high radioactivity of the isotopes used and from the low level of imaging. The introduction of ^{99m}Tc-labeled microspheres and nanocolloids led to the availability of substances absorbed by the reticuloendothelial system (RES) of the liver, spleen, and bone marrow. Because of their physical and biochemical characteristics these were widely used to achieve relatively good imaging of bone marrow. However, the uptake of these colloids in the RES of liver and spleen unfortunately results in poor or lacking visualization of the middle and lower thoracic and the upper lumbar column. Recently a new and very promising approach has been tried, using immunoscintigraphy (IS) for the detection of bone marrow infiltration. In a first study Reske et al. [3] showed that the monoclonal antibody (MAb) BW 250/183, developed initially for the detection of inflammatory foci [1], is an excellent substance for the detection of bone marrow infiltration.

It was the aim of this study to elucidate the value of IS using this MAb in comparison to colloid scanning in the detection of bone marrow infiltration in patients with solid tumors or systemic disorders.

Materials and Methods

We studied 33 patients aged between 21 and 73 years. Six patients suffered from breast cancer, three from bronchial cancer, one from sarcoma, and 23 from Hodgkin or non-Hodgkin lymphoma (stages I–IV). All patients examined were informed of the procedure and gave their consent.

The MAb 250/183 is a murine monoclonal IgG1 antibody which is directed against carcinoembryonic antigen (CEA) and nonspecific cross-reacting antigen

[1] Abteilung für Radiologie und Nuklearmedizin, Städtische Kliniken Oldenburg, Dr.-Eden-Str. 10, 2900 Oldenburg, FRG
[2] Abteilung für Nuklearmedizin, Universität Göttingen, Robert-Koch-Str., 3400 Göttingen, FRG

Advanced Radiation Therapy Tumor Response
Monitoring and Treatment Planning
Breit (Editor-in-Chief)
© Springer-Verlag, Berlin Heidelberg 1992

(NCA-95) exposed at the cellular membrane of peripheral granuclocytes and myelocytes [1] in bone marrow. About 80% of this cell population is located in bone marrow.

The labeling procedure with ^{99m}Tc is very simple and was carried out according to Schwarz and Steinträßer [4]. The incorporation rate is higher than 95%. Colloid scanning used a commercially available colloid kit with a particle size smaller than 50 nm. Labeling with ^{99m}Tc was carried out according to the manufacturers' instructions. Both diagnostic procedures were conducted over 3 days. Three hours after injection of 400 MBq of the ^{99m}Tc-labeled MAb and 1.5 h after the ^{99m}Tc-labeled colloid (400 MBq), planar scans of the thorax and the pelvic bone in dorsal and ventral views were performed, followed by dorsal views of the lumbar column, humeri and femori, and anterior and lateral views of the skull.

Skeletal scintigraphy, plane radiographs, computed tomography (CT), magnetic resonance imaging (MRI), and bone marrow biopsies were performed to confirm the skeletal lesions.

Results and Discussion

IS showed homogeneous bone marrow and moderate liver/spleen uptake with excellent visualization of all parts of the vertebral column. Table 1 shows the results of our study. All 40 bone marrow lesions detected by colloid scan were also seen by IS. However, IS showed 17 additional lesions which were all confirmed by the diagnostic methods mentioned above. Conventional bone scanning revealed only 37 lesions. Figure 1 shows a typical example of the qualitative as well as quantitative superiority of bone marrow IS in the detection of bone marrow infiltration. Due to the high liver/spleen uptake, colloid scanning was not able to detect many lesions in the lower thoracic or upper lumbar column. However, as Zollinger [5] pointed out, the vertebral column is one of the most essential areas where metastases of different solid tumors can be found.

Table 1 shows the correlation between IS and colloid scanning and between IS and conventional bone scanning. In 28 patients we found a complete and in five patients only a partial correlation comparing IS and colloid scanning. On

Table 1. Correlation between IS and colloid scanning and between IS and conventional scanning ($n = 33$)

Correlation	IS/colloid scanning	IS/conventional scanning
Complete	28	27
Partial	5	4
None	—	2

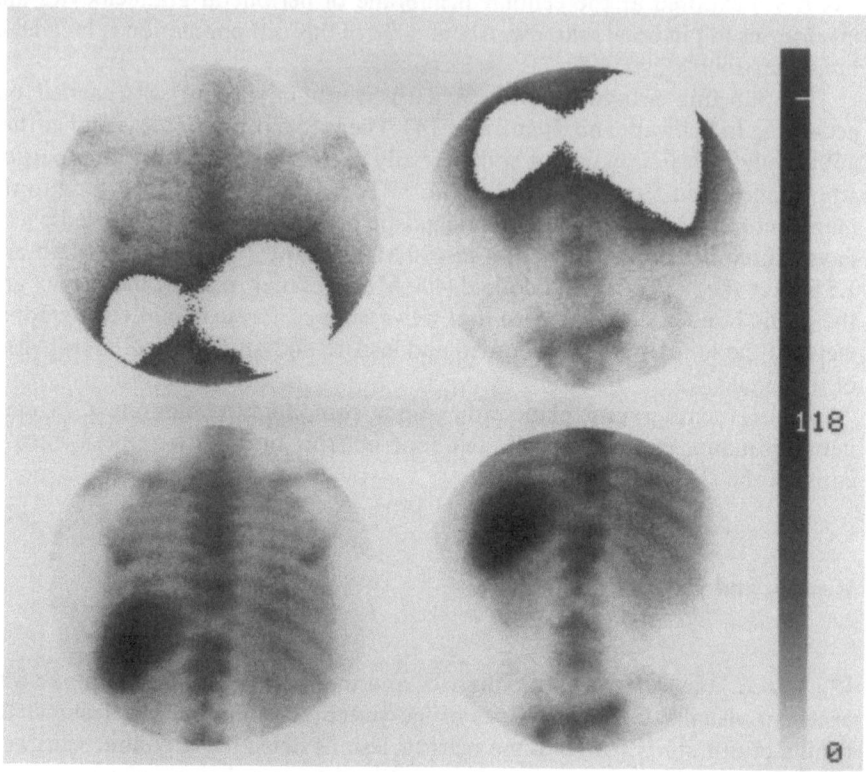

Fig. 1. Patient with known Hodgkin disease. Immunoscintigraphy (*below*) shows several lesions of the vertebral column and is superior to colloid scanning (*above*) especially in the region of the lower thoracic and upper lumbar column

the other hand, correlating our findings using IS and bone scanning we found in 27 cases a complete, in 4 a partial, and in 2 no correlation. Whereas bone scan shows a local increase in osteoblastic activity bone marrow scanning indirectly visualizes the suppression of hematopoietic tissue in the bone marrow cavity. Thus both diagnostic procedures are important complementary methods for correct tumor staging. In three patients with recurrences of Hodgkin lymphoma and with case histories of radiation therapy, 12 bone marrow lesions seen by IS and/or colloid scanning were identified as fatty or fibrotic bone marrow degenerations. These 12 false-positive lesions underline the fact that both diagnostic procedures are nonspecific methods which must be verified by specific procedures such as CT or MRI.

The skeletal system is one of the most important regions where metastases of different solid tumors and systemic disorders can be found. Besides the well-established bone scan, bone marrow scintigraphy is an important procedure for correct clinical staging of these patients [2]. Standard staging procedures such as plane radiographs and bone scans detect indirect signs of neoplasm in cases of 30%–40% demineralization or osteoblastic response to metastatic infiltration. CT and MRI are very sensitive procedures for the detection of bone marrow infiltration; however, whole-body examinations are impractical. This means that in using CT or MRI we must know which region is to be examined.

Conclusion

IS with the NCA-95 monoclonal antibody BW 250/183 is an excellent method for detection of bone marrow infiltration and is superior to colloid scanning. However, IS and colloid scanning are nonspecific examination methods which must be supplemented by other specific diagnostic procedures.

References

1. Bosslet K, Lüben G, Schwarz A, Hundt E, Harthus HP, Seiler FR, Muhrer C, Kloeppel G, Kayser K, Sedlacek HH (1985) Immunohistochemical localization and molecular characteristics of three monoclonal antibody-defined epitopes detectable on carcinoembryonic antigen (CEA). Int J Cancer 36: 75
2. Munz DL, Kötter R, Kornemann I, Brandhorst, Hör, G (1984) Bone marrow involvement of the skeletal system. In: Schmidt HAE, Adam WE (eds) Nuklearmedizin: Darstellung von Metabolismen und Organfunktionen. Schattauer, Stuttgart, p 644
3. Reske SN, Karstens JH, Glöckner, W, Buell U (1989) Sekundäre Knochentumoren Skelett- und Knochenmarksszintigraphie. In: Feine U, Müller-Schauenburg W (eds) Skelettszintigraphie, Knochendiagnostik mit neuen Verfahren. Wacholz, Nürnberg, pp 29–40
4. Schwarz A, Steinsträßer A (1987) A novel approach to Tc99m labeled monoclonal antibodies. Nucl Med 28: 721
5. Zollinger H (1971) Pathologische Anatomie: 1. Allgemeine Pathologie. Thieme. Stuttgart

Improved Radiotherapy Planning and Follow-Up of Bone Metastases by Skeletal Ultrasound

U. Mende, K. Rieden, U. Weischedel, and M. Wannenmacher

Introduction

In oncology ultrasound has become an established imaging method for the diagnosis, follow-up, and posttherapeutic care of most parenchymal organs and has gained growing importance; its application to tumors of the skeletal system, on the other hand, is still very uncommon. Kratochwil's outstanding report on the prospect for ultrasound diagnosis in primary bone tumors [1] unfortunately remained widely unnoticed and without consequences for the diagnostic routine schedule in primary or metastatic malignant diseases of the locomotor system. However, the general opinion that ultrasound analysis of skeletal lesions is impossible due to the high attenuation of ultrasound by the bone matrix ignores the fact that tumorous changes may concern not only the cortical layer and spongiosa (visible in conventional X-ray) but also the periosteum and surrounding tissue. Based on data from a large number of patients, we seek to demonstrate that such reservations toward ultrasound in the evaluation of bone metastases are not justified.

Patients and Methods

We examined 293 patients (140 women and 153 men, aged 24–87 years) with malignant diseases and who underwent radiotherapy between December 1984 and August 1990. A total of 500 bone metastases were examined up to ten times by skeletal ultrasound and by conventional X-rays for diagnosis, therapy planning, and intra-/posttherapeutic follow-up. The most frequent primary tumors were cancer of the breast (29.4%), lung (27.3%), kidney (17.1%), prostate (4.4%), and plasmocytoma (4.1%). The ultrasound examinations were performed on an LSC7000 machine (Picker International, Munich) under standardized conditions with frequencies of 3.5, 5, and 7.5 MHz, preferring the linear 5-MHz transducer as the best compromise between spatial resolution and

Department of Radiology, University Clinic for Radiology, University of Heidelberg, Im Neuenheimer Feld 400, 6900 Heidelberg, FRG

Advanced Radiation Therapy Tumor Response
Monitoring and Treatment Planning
Breit (Editor-in-Chief)
© Springer-Verlag. Berlin Heidelberg 1992

penetration [3]. In addition to the representation in at least two perpendicular planes and their relation to risk organs and field margins (set according to the therapy simulator), the tumorous lesions were analyzed for dimensions, volume, and echogenicity by gray-scale histograms and the extent of an accompanying soft-tissue tumor exceeding the roentgenologically visible structures of the cortical layer. Efficient monitoring and follow-up was based on the comparability in terms of identical examiner, set-up, and documentation.

Results

Depending on the primary tumor and the affected skeletal region the ultrasound analysis of the metastatic appearance showed marked differences less in respect to the intraosseous tumor compartment than to the extent and structure of periosteal and soft-tissue infiltrations. In 241 of the 500 lesions (48.2%) this accompanying soft-tissue tumor was either absent or small, exceeding the roentgenologically visible contours of the compact bone by less than 10 mm. It was larger, however, in 259 cases (51.8%), in 135 instances (27.0%) between 10 and 20 mm and in 124, in fact, (24.8%) above 20 mm. Large processes (> 10 mm) were frequently found with carcinoma of the lung (76.9%), kidney (68.8%), and plasmocytoma (70%) as well as in the flat bones of the thoracic skeleton (67.7%)

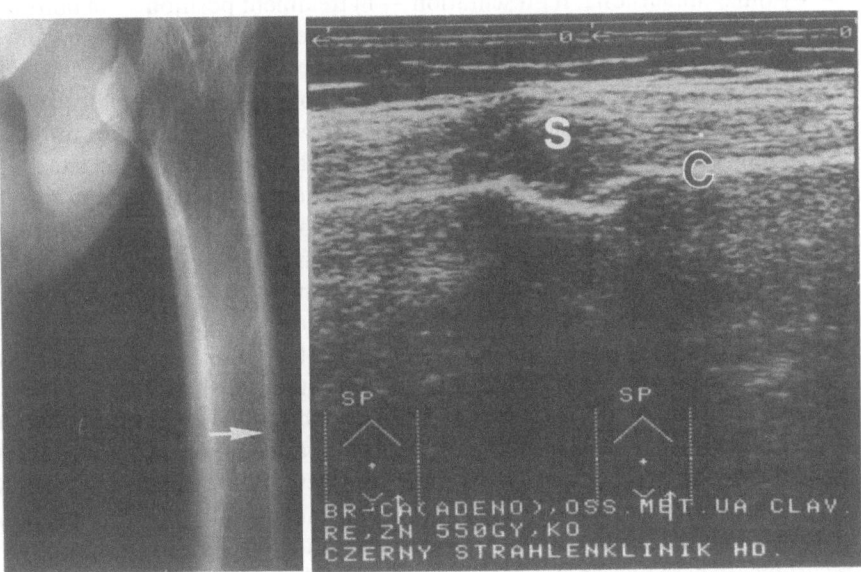

Fig. 1. Adenocarcinoma of the lung in a 58-year-old man. Painful metastasis of the left femur (*arrow*). *Left*, X-ray; *right*, ultrasound (longitudinal section). *C*, Cortical layer; *S*, soft-tissue tumor

and the pelvis (86.7%); these were relatively rare, however, with breast cancer (19.4%) and in the proximal extremities of femur (18.8%) and humerus (19.2%). Dynamic real-time ultrasound also revealed almost pathognomonic differences in vascularization, very good in metastases of thyroid cancer but extreme in those of hypernephroma, which often (90%) showed pulsatile masses with few echoes. Another noteworthy result of these investigations was the morphologic explanation for the local pain of the bone lesions, which was correlated with periosteal reactions and soft-tissue tumors by more than 97% (Fig. 1) [2].

Discussion

Our results clearly indicate that ultrasound is a valuable adjunct to conventional X-ray and can well improve the diagnosis and therapy planning of bone metastases. Although ultrasound tends to underestimate tumorous changes of the medullary space and the spongious bone, it is equal to X-ray in the assessment of the cortical layer but by far superior in the detection of periosteal or soft-tissue processes. This is especially important for radiotherapy planning, which requires reliable data on the dimensions of the tumor as a whole to ensure the correct field size. The radiation field must cover not only the roentgenologically visible lesions of compact and spongious bone but also these sometimes extensive soft-tissue infiltrations.

By three-dimensional representation — in treatment position — of bony *and* soft tissue tumorous structures as well as their neighboring risk organs, ultrasound will become not only the ideal adjunct to the therapy simulator but even a must with negative or equivocal X-rays and in those cases in which localization of primary tumor or metastatic lesion make a larger soft-tissue tumor probable (carcinoma of the lung, kidney, and plasmocytoma as well as affected sites such as thoracic skeleton, pelvis, and skull). The determination or adaptation of radiation method, field size, and beam energy especially with electron therapy becomes easier and safer, therefore reducing the number of more costly examinations using computed tomography or magnetic resonance imaging for therapy planning in particular for low-lying processes (Fig. 2).

Easily, feasible standardized controls to monitor volumetric *and* structural changes such as necrosis, fibrosis, and recalcification, of the tumorous lesions allow objectification of the therapeutic results and modification of the therapy concept very early if necessary. By the change in attenuation and echogenicity ultrasound makes the incipient recalcification detectable earlier than does X-ray, which requires an enhancement in calcium content of about 30%. The same criteria apply to the posttherapeutic care with the detection or exclusion of a recurrency, where ultrasound is almost unlimited by osteosynthetic/endoprothetic metal implants, in contrast to computed tomography and partly to magnetic resonance imaging.

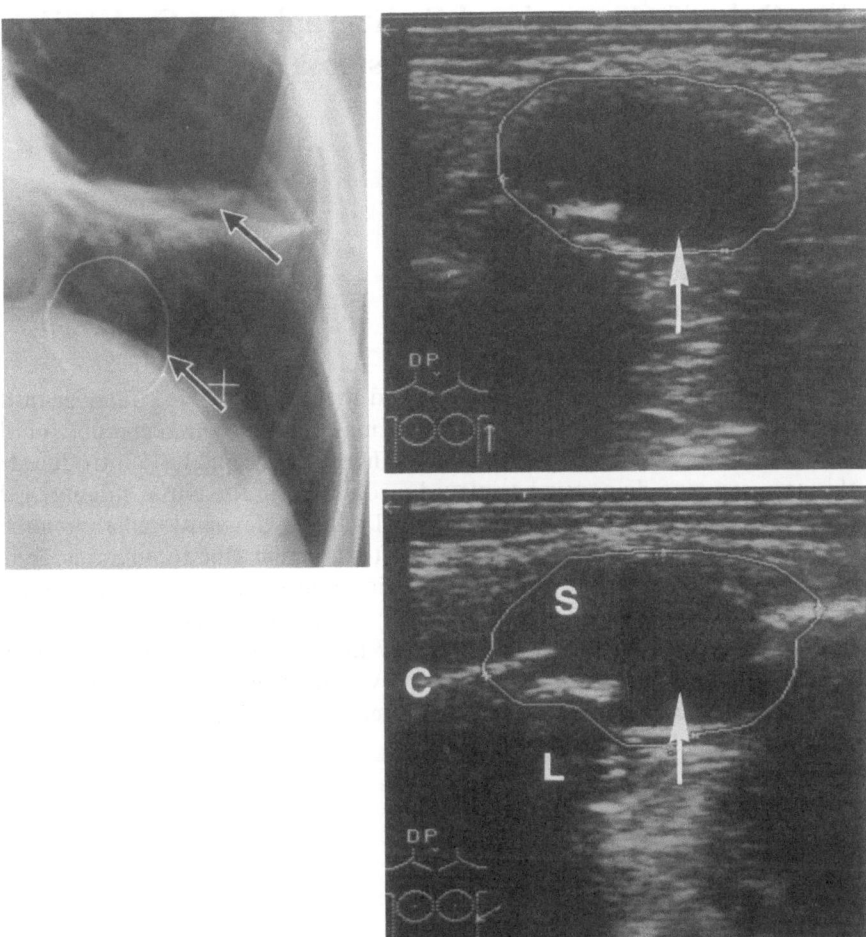

Fig. 2. Large-cell anaplastic carcinoma of the lung in a 65-year-old man. Painful metastasis of the rib (*arrow*). *Left*, X-ray; *right*, ultrasound for therapy planning (field size, electron energy, risk organ), *C*, Cortical layer; *S*, soft-tissue tumor; *L*, lung

References

1. Kratochwil A, Ramach W (1976) Die Ultraschalldiagnostik bei primär malignen Knochentumoren. Z Orthop 116: 503–507
2. Mende U, Rieden K, Braun, A, Weischedel U, zum Winkel K (1986) Die Realtime-Sonographie. Ein wichtiges bildgebendes Verfahren bei Diagnostik und Therapieplanung von Skelettmetastasen. Fortschr Rontgenstr 145: 373–378
3. Mende U, Rieden K, Weischedel U, Braun A, Ewerbeck V, Zöller J (1989) Sonographische Diagnostik von Tumoren des Stütz- and Bindegewebes. Picker aktuell 13: 3–13

The Role of Conventional Radiography for Evaluation of Preoperative Response in Osteosarcoma

T. Riebel

Introduction

The nature of the surgical intervention and the postoperative strategies in the treatment of osteosarcoma depend to a major extent on regression of the primary tumor. Since preoperative chemotherapy concepts were introduced in this area, imaging diagnosis has played a role both in the initial staging of the disease and in the assessment of the local course. Conventional radiological techniques (plain radiography including soft-tissue films and tomograms, angiography) were the first modalities to provide important and fundamental information. These have lost none of their importance even today [3, 4, 13], and they should not be overshadowed by nuclear medical and in particular cross-sectional imaging techniques. Our own positive experience in assessing the course of osteosarcomas of the extremities by means of conventional radiography underscores this view.

Materials and Methods

The initial radiographs of the primary tumor in 61 osteosarcomas were evaluated and compared with the findings during preoperative chemotherapy and with the degree of histological regression, according to Salzer-Kuntschik et al. [16]. In addition to the plain radiographs, initial angiograms were available in 44 patients and preoperative angiograms in 24. This allowed analysis of the behavior of a large number of radiological criteria from the initial finding up to the operation for responding tumors (regression grades I–III = none or less than 10% vital tumor tissue) and for less or nonresponding tumors (grades IV–VI = 10%–100% vital tumor). On the basis of whether their extent and distribution preoperatively were the same or different, the individual criteria were assigned a different indicator status as regards tumor regression. Finally, the response of the tumor responder versus non-responder was assessed globally

Universitätsklinikum Rudolf Virchow-Wedding, Pädiatrische Radiologie, Reinickendorfer Str. 61, 1000 Berlin 65, FRG

Advanced Radiation Therapy Tumor Response
Monitoring and Treatment Planning
Breit (Editor-in-Chief)
© Springer-Verlag, Berlin Heidelberg 1992

on the basis of the radiographs alone. The accuracy of these results was checked by comparing them with the histological findings.

Results

The following features were found to be particularly important for assessing the course of osteosarcomas from conventional radiographs and angiograms: (a) periostal formations (Codman's triangle, spicules); (b) soft-tissue swelling; (c) extraosseous calcifications/ossifications (reactive/tumorous); (d) osseous destruction (substantial increase); (e) tumor length (substantial change); and (f) pathological vascularization.

Changes displaying a major preoperative difference in distribution between tumors with good and unsatisfactory response were considered to be of great value in assessing the response to the treatment. The diagnostic criteria were: (a) Codman's triangle (intensity, characteristics); (b) soft-tissue swelling (intensity); (c) extraosseous ossifications (proximity to and contact with the bone surface, density, delineation); and (d) pathological vascularization (intensity intra- and extraosseous). Although the differences in distribution between osteosarcomas with good and unsatisfactory regression as indicated by other diagnostic features after chemotherapy were not huge, they were still important for the interpretation: (a) osseous destruction (increase of the intensity and spread of nonresponding tumors); (b) osseous sclerosis (arrangement and density); (c) spicules (number, length, characteristics); and (d) extraosseous ossifications (intensity, "periostal shell").

On the basis of these analyses, the final set of findings indicate "good response" of an osteosarcoma (Fig. 1): (a) periostal reactions: disappearance of typical formations or loss of their characteristics due to reactive regeneration of bone (Codman's triangle, spicules; (b) soft-tissue swelling: intensive or complete regression; (c) extraosseous calcifications/ossifications: condensation, increase of density and sharp delineation of tumorous or reactive compactions—accumulation on the bone surface and formation of a cup-shaped "periostal shell;" (d) spread: intraosseous changes constant, constancy or regression of the size of the extraosseous tumor (particularly compared to the spread in the initial angiogram); and (e) pathological vascularization: little or none in the preoperative angiogram.

Osteosarcomas with "poor response" typically show the following characteristics (Figs. 2, 3): (a) periostal reactions: persistence or new development of typical formations (Codman's triangle, spicules); (b) soft-tissue swelling: little or no regression or increase; (c) extraosseous calcifications/ossifications: poor delineation with persistent wide distribution and little contact with the bone surface, no "periostal shell;" (d) spread: increase intra- and extraosseous; and

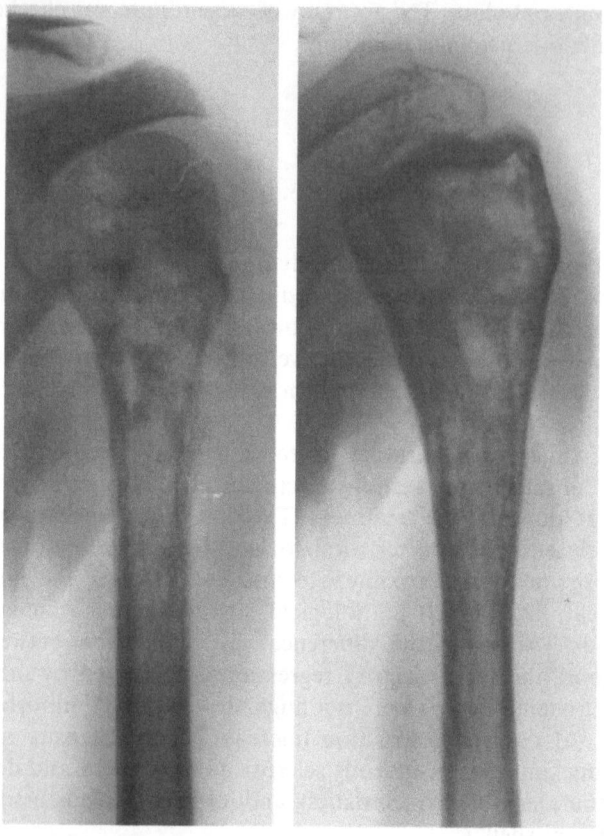

a   b

Fig. 1a, b. Classical osteosarcoma of the proximal humerus with good response to preoperative chemotherapy (histological grade I). **a** Initial plain survey. **b** After chemotherapy. No typical spicules of Codman's triangle left, compact connection of sharp and "shell-like" demarcated extraosseous new bone formations to the surface of humerus; no soft-tissue swelling left; intraosseous destructions still within the initial area

(e) pathological vascularization: moderate to intensive in the preoperative angiogram.

The category "circumscribed vital tumor remains" is recognized by the following findings: (a) periostal reactions: maintained locally and characteristically (Codman's triangle, spicules); (b) soft-tissue swelling: continues in individual sections of the outer tumor border; (c) extraosseous calcifications/ossifications: in some cases still arranged relatively broadly and irregularly around the bone and without good delineation; and (d) pathological vascularization: circumscribed areas with a varying number of tumor vessels (in the preoperative angiogram).

An average accuracy rate of 87% (responders 88%, nonresponders 85%) in comparison with the corresponding degree of histological regression of the 61

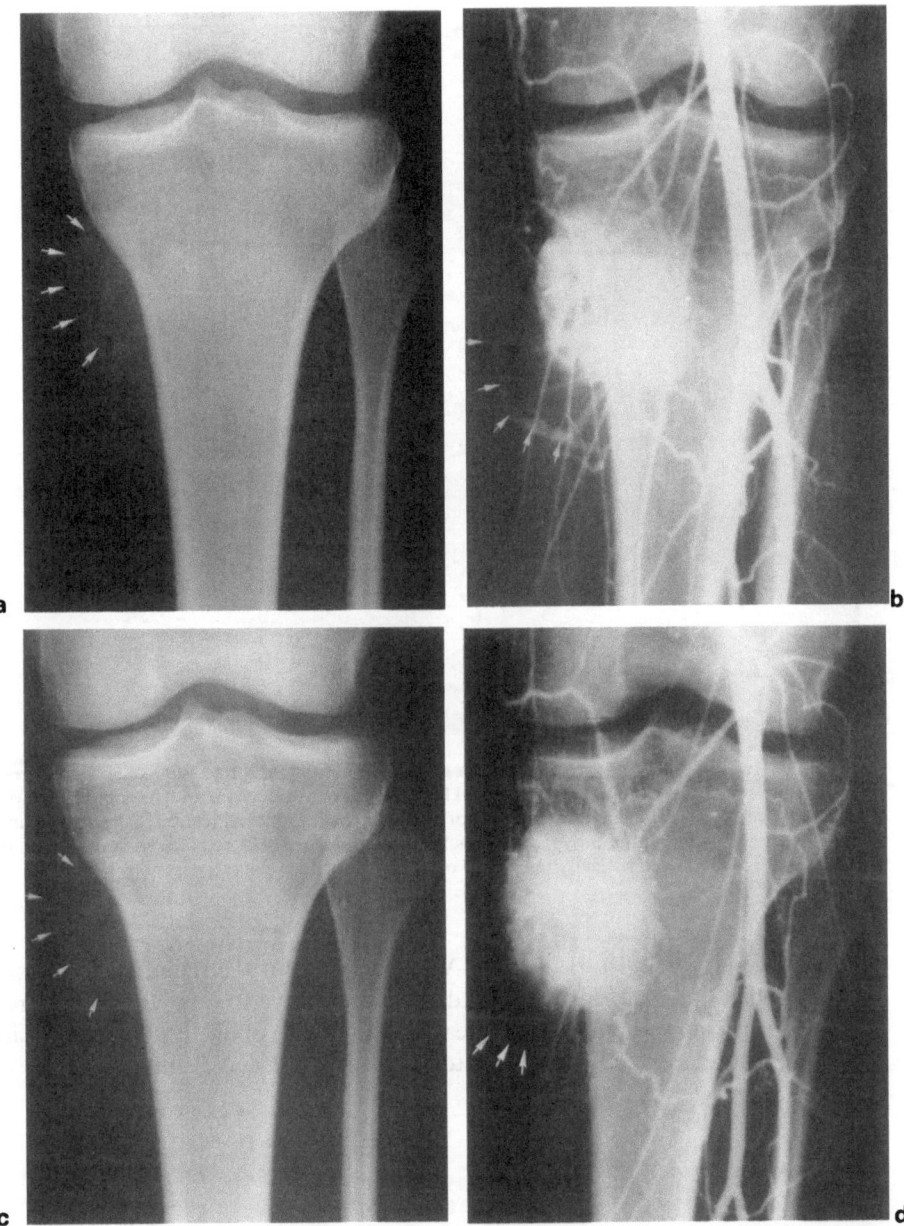

Fig. 2a–d. Atypical osteosarcoma of proximal tibia with poor response (grade V). **a** Initial frontal radiograph. Discrete intraosseous destructions, no typical periostal reactions, smoothly mineralized extraosseous component (*arrows*). **b** Initial angiogram. Extreme pathological hypervascularization with early venous drainage via a-v shunts (*arrows*). **c** After 6 weeks of chemotherapy. Same shape of mineralized extraosseous tumor component without any demarcation and condensation (*arrows*). **d** Angiogram after 6 weeks. Unchanged enormous malignant hypervascularization with persistent early venous filling (*arrows*)

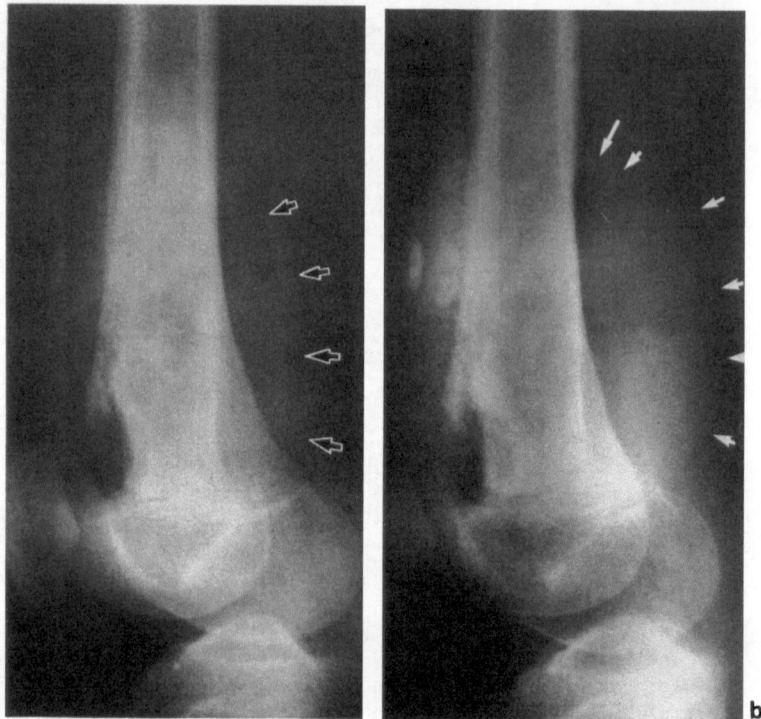

Fig. 3a, b. Huge nonresponding osteosarcoma of distal femur (lateral projection) showing progression despite chemotherapy (grade VI). **a** Initial film. Large extraosseous tumor component (*arrows*). **b** After 6 weeks. Expanding extraosseous tumor component without demarcation (*short arrows*) and condensation, new formation of typical Codman's triangle (*long arrow*), spicules on various sites of bone surface still characteristically remaining or newly formed

osteosarcomas (grades I–III and IV–VI) was found for the radiological assessment of the therapeutic success and clinically relevant subdivision into responders and nonresponders. The greatest congruence of the results occurred in the case of the highly responsive histological grades I and II tumors (93%).

Discussion

In the first few years after the introduction of preoperative chemotherapy for osteosarcomas, the response of the primary tumor was initially demonstrable only by means of conventional radiological techniques and histological studies. The main tasks were, on the one hand, to become familiar with the many and various phenomena of the morphologically different tumors in the course of treatment by means of plain radiograms and angiograms and, on the other, to obtain information about their devitalization even before the operation [3, 4, 13]. This was because only few radiological observations of the course of primarily irradiated osteosarcomas were available from the prechemotherapy era.

Using all plain radiographic procedures (films with various exposures including the soft-tissue technique and in several projections, tomography) and optimal angiographic modalities (high contrast medium doses, long film series, subtraction), detailed basic knowledge was obtained about the morphological change of the various intra- and extraosseous sections of the tumor, which has lost nothing of its importance even today [12]. This knowledge still forms the basis for the interpretation of findings from modern cross-sectional imaging techniques (computed tomography, magnetic resonance imaging). The results of all imaging procedures merely reflect the respective histomorphological status in a qualitatively different form.

The analysis described above of various radiodiagnostic features for assessing regression of osteosarcomas during preoperative chemotherapy has so far been followed by numerous similar studies based on many and varied angiographic, computed tomographic and magnetic resonance examinations [1, 2, 5-7, 9-11, 15, 17, 18]. Even if these new methods allow better, more exact, and in some cases also earlier demonstration of numerous other tumor details than do conventional radiographs (intra- and extraosseous spread, details of soft-tissue compartment, tumor border, etc.), none of them has so far improved to any significant degree the results of the prognostic assessment of the course compared to the results obtained with conventional radiography [5, 7, 11, 15, 18]. In fact, they were even worse in some cases [6, 9]. The basic problem here is that one and the same film finding not only in the radiographic morphology of an osteosarcoma (e.g., lysis–sclerosis) but also in the new cross-sectional imaging techniques can reflect both vital (nonmineralized–mineralized tumor matrix) and devitalized tumor areas (necrosis, connective tissue–reactive bone, devitalized tumor bone or calcified chondroid) [10, 17, 19].

In the analysis of the preoperative regression of an osteosarcoma based on imaging techniques, all valid diagnostic features of an examination technique must always be assessed in combination. In addition, the respective results of various examinations must be compared with each other and their value assessed, while a careful search must be made for the possible causes in the event of incongruences. The subsequent interpretation is done subjectively qualitatively not only in the conventional radiological, but also in the computed and magnetic resonance tomographic and conventional nuclear-medical demonstration of tumors; its validity depends to a not inconsiderable extent on the experience of the examiner. Only a few highly specialized and complicated methods ("parameter-skeletal scintigraphy" [8, 14], "dynamic MRI" [5]) can so far provide objective (semi-)quantitative results. What is more, these results—particularly those of scintigraphy—also display the highest accuracy yet achieved. So far, however, there is a lack of larger comparative studies of the various methods—which must, of course, always be conducted in the same study population. Only then will it be possible to perform a definitive assessment of their validity both individually and combined with each other.

Summary

In terms of all methodological possibilities and combined assessment of relevant diagnostic criteria in osteosarcomas, even radiological (plain radiography, angiography) assessment of the course of chemotherapy allows highly reliable differentiation (87%) between preoperative positive responders (less than 10% vital tumor rest) and inadequate or poor (non-)responders. This great accuracy has not yet been exceeded even with modern cross-sectional imaging modalities. Only the quantitative method of "parameter" skeletal scintigraphy provides better (now up to 100%) and objectively reproducible results. The overall aim in the imaging analysis of local tumor regression is not to view the results of the individual examinations in isolation but to assess all findings in combination and comparison on the basis of an all-embracing histomorphological understanding.

References

1. Bilbao JI, Algarra SM, de Negri JM, Lecumberri F, Longo J, Sierrasesumaga L, Canadell J (1990) Osteosarcoma: correlation between radiological and histological changes after intra-arterial chemotherapy. Eur J Radiol 11: 98–103
2. Carrasco CH, Charnsangeajev C, Raymond AK, Richli WR, Wallace S, Chawla SP, Ayala AG, Murray JA, Benjamin RS (1989) Osteosarcoma: angiographic assessment of response to preoperative chemotherapy. Radiology 170: 839–842
3. Chuang VP, Benjamin R, Jaffe N, Wallace S, Ayala AG, Murray J, Charnsangajev C, Soo C-C (1982) Radiographic and angiographic changes in osteosarcoma after intraarterial chemotherapy. AJR 139: 1065–1069
4. Den Heeten GJ, Thijn CJP, Kamps WA, Schraffordt Koops H, Oosterhuis JW, Oldhoff J (1986) The effect of chemotherapy on osteosarcoma of the extremities as apparent from conventional roentgenograms. Pediatr Radiol 16: 407–411
5. Erlemann R, Sciuk J, Bosse A, Ritter J, Kusnierz-Glaz CR, Peters PE, Wuisman P (1990) Response of osteosarcoma and Ewing sarcoma to preoperative chemotherapy: assessment with dynamic and static imaging and skeletal scintigraphy. Radiology 175: 791–796
6. Holscher HC, Bloem JL, Nooy MA, Taminiau AHM, Eulderink F, Hermans J (1990) The value of MR imaging in monitoring the effect of chemotherapy on bone sarcomas. AJR 154: 763–769
7. Jend HH, Heller M, Boisch ED, Beron G, Winkler K, Delling G (1983) Volumetric and densitometric CT measurements in the evaluation of osteosarcoma. Radiology 149: p 234
8. Knop J, Delling G, Salzer-Kuntschik M, Berberich R, Feine U, Feistel H, Ladenstein R, Müller-Schauenburg W, Schober O, Szabo Z, Wickenhauser J, Winkler K (1989) Nuklearmedizinische Vorhersage des histologischen Tumor-ansprechens beim Osteosarkom. Klin Padiatr 201: 285–292
9. Mail JT, Cohen MD, Mirkin LD, Provisor AJ (1985) Response of osteosarcoma to preoperative intravenous high-dose methotrexate chemotherapy: CT evaluation. AJR 144: 89–93

10. Pan G, Raymond AK, Carrasco CH, Wallace S, Kim EE, Shirkoda A, Jaffe N, Murray JA, Benjamin RS (1990) Osteosarcoma: MR imaging after preoperative chemotherapy. Radiology 174: 517–526

11. Redmond OM, Stack JP, Dervan PA, Hurson BJ, Carney DN, Ennis JT (1989) Osteosarcoma: use of MR imaging and MR spectroscopy in clinical decision making. Radiology 172: 811–815

12. Riebel T (1984) Fortschritte in der Röntgendiagnostik des Osteosarkoms im Rahmen neuer Therapieformen bei Kindern und Jugendlichen. Doctoral dissertation, University of Hamburg

13. Riebel T, Lassrich MA, Kumpan W (1983) Roentgenologic follow-up in primarily conservatively treated osteogenic sarcoma. J Cancer Res Clin Oncol 106 (Suppl): 38–42

14. Riebel T, Knop T, Winkler K, Delling G (1986) Vergleichende röntgenologische und nuklearmedizinische Untersuchungen beim Osteosarkom zur Beurteilung der Effektivität einer präoperativen Chemotherapie. ROFO 145: 365–372

15. Rotte K-H, Kriedemann E, Geyer J, Kunde D, Melcher J, Perlick E, Schmidt-Peter P (1989) Zum Wert der Computertomographie für das Monitoring der präoperativen Chemotherapie des Osteosarkoms. ROFO 150: 8–12

16. Salzer-Kuntschik M, Delling G, Beron G, Sigmund R (1983) Morphological grades of regression in osteosarcoma after polychemotherapy. COSS 80. J Cancer Res Clin Oncol 106 [Suppl]: 21–24

17. Sanchez RB, Quinn SF, Walling A, Estrada J, Greenberg H (1990) Musculoskeletal neoplasms after intraarterial chemotherapy: correlation of MR images with pathologic specimens. Radiology 174: 237–240

18. Shirkoda A, Jaffe N, Wallace S, Ayala A, Lindell MM, Zorzona J (1985) Computed tomography of osteosarcoma after intraarterial chemotherapy. AJR 144: 95–99

19. Sommer H-J, Riebel T, Winkler K, Heise U, Delling G (1985) Vergleich röntgenologischer und histologischer Befunde bei Osteosarkomen nach präoperative Chemotherapie. ROFO 143: 74–83

Significance of Ultrasound for Diagnosis of Recurrences After Radiotherapy of Soft-Tissue Sarcomas of the Limbs and the Thorax Wall

M. Niewald, H.J. Tkocz, and K. Schnabel

Introduction

Regular follow-up examinations are necessary after every radiotherapy of a malignancy to be able to detect late radiation sequelae and for timely diagnosis of recurrences. In the region of the limbs, where, particularly soft-tissues are to be treated, the investigation is very difficult, since extensive scars are generally present after operation and radiotherapy. We therefore compared ultrasound to palpation and computer tomography (CT) in detecting local recurrences in good time and with adequate certainty.

Patients and Methods

Our patients included 49 who presented regularly in our outpatient department for follow-up examinations after operation and radiotherapy of a soft-tissue sarcoma of the limbs and the thorax wall. Between October 1987 and December 1990 these patients underwent a meticulous palpatory and ultrasound investigation of the affected region. In the majority of cases CT was also performed. Ultrasound was carried out with a real-time instrument of the type CS 9000 (Picker). We generally used a 7.5-MHz linear sector scanner in the region of the limbs and in addition a 3.5-MHz convex sector scanner near to the trunk. A water preparatory run was not necessary. The region affected was scanned circularly, parallel and perpendicular to the muscles. Structures appearing spherical to elliptical, hypoechoic compared to surrounding tissue, and readily delimited were regarded as recurrences. The majority of patients afterwards underwent CT. Continuous planigraphic sections of both limbs for comparison between the two sides (collimation 8 mm, forward displacement of the table 8 mm) were prepared on a Somatom DR 2 (Siemens). Contrast medium was administered intravenously only in exceptional cases. Ultrasound and CT were carried out by various physicians, and the results were compared only on the day after the investigations.

Department of Radiotherapy, University Hospital of the Saarland, 6650 Homburg/Saar, FRG

Advanced Radiation Therapy Tumor Response
Monitoring and Treatment Planning
Breit (Editor-in-Chief)
© Springer-Verlag, Berlin Heidelberg 1992

Results

In the ultrasound images 18 recurrences were identified; 14 of these were confirmed histologically as recurrences, and the four others involved scar tissue (Table 1). Of the 18 suspect findings from ultrasound 11 were palpable. Twelve of the 18 were also investigated by CT; of these, nine were demonstrated in the native CT while CT was dispensed with in the others in favor of rapid surgical clearance of the tumor (Fig. 1). Ultrasound thus showed a sensitivity of 100% (CT 75%) and a specificity of 78% (CT 67%).

Discussion

Real-time ultrasound with high frequencies enables a very fine differentiation of tissue structures on the basis of differences in their impedance [1–18]. Local recurrences of soft-tissue sarcomas appear to be mainly hypoechoic, with individual internal echos of varying density. They are spherical to elliptical in form and are readily delimited from the surrounding tissue in most cases [6, 8]. Scars do not spread only in a trabecular or planar manner in connective tissue and the musculature but may also manifest roundish or elliptical forms, and they can thus be distinguished only with difficulty from recurrences. An unclear delimitation of the surrounding tissue is more indicative of a scar than of a recurrence.

In the literature, there is agreement that the diagnostic advantage of ultrasound lies in the easy measurement of a space occupation [2, 4, 9–11, 14, 17]. Moreover, its contents can be appraised and the relationship with bone and tissue represented [2–4, 7–18]. In addition, ultrasound is readily available, can be repeated as often as required, and can be performed within a relatively short time [3, 9, 10].

Table 1. Comparative results of ultrasound and computed tomography

	Histology	
	Positive	Negative
Ultrasound		
Positive	14	4
Negative	0	0
Computer tomography		
Positive	8	1
Negative	3	1
Not performed	3	2

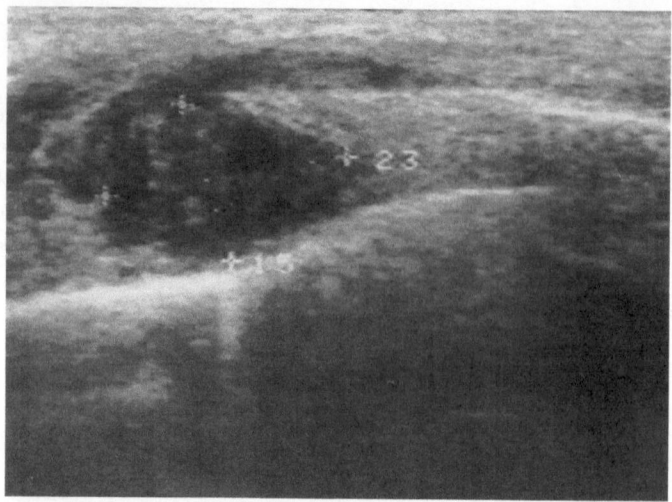

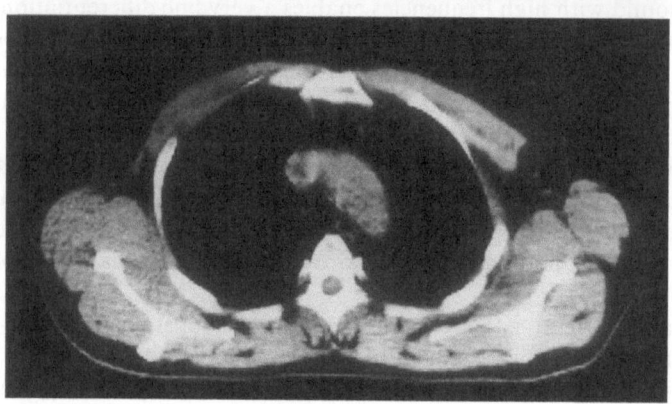

Fig. 1a, b. Recurrence of soft-tissue sarcoma in the right thorax wall. **a** Easily detectable by ultrasound. **b** Almost undetectable on CT

The main diagnostic advantage of CT is that it is largely independent of the investigator and can be better reproduced. It allows easier identification of anatomical structures [7], and neighbouring vessels can be delimited by intravenous administration of contrast medium [2, 3, 8, 9, 16]. Literature references regarding the diagnosis of tumor recurrences are still scanty [2, 10, 15]. Bernardino et al. [2] were able to diagnose two of the five recurrences which they reported exclusively on the basis of ultrasound. Rotte et al. [10] obtained 94% true-positive findings with ultrasound and 82% true-positive findings with CT in 27 patients with soft-tissue sarcomas (including 20 recurrences). Comparison of our own results with these data confirms the superiority of ultrasound. In 12 patients we were able to demonstrate 78% true-positive against 22% false-positive findings by ultrasound; with CT there were 67% true-positive and 33% false-positive findings.

On the basis of these results, patients with suspect findings on ultrasound are generally referred to the surgeon without CT. In the past year nuclear magnetic resonance has also been performed; however, the small number of cases to date does not allow appraisal as to whether this entails advantages in diagnosis.

References

1. Balconi G, Teruzzi P, Ulivi M (1984) Possibilita della ecografia nello studio delle tumefazioni delle parti molli superficiali. Radiol Med (Torino) 70: 878–880
2. Bernardino ME, Jing MS, Thomas JE, Lindell MM, Zornoza J (1981) The extremity soft-tissue lesion: a comparative study of ultrasound, computed tomography and xeroradiography. Radiology 139: 53–59
3. Braunstein EM, Silver TM, Martel W, Jaffe M (1981) Ultrasonic diagnosis of extremity masses. Skeletal Radiol 6: 157–163
4. Graf R, Schuler P (1988) Sonografie bei Weichteiltumoren. Orthopade 17: 128–133
5. Hermann G, Yeh HC, Schwartz I (1984) Computed tomography of soft-tissue lesions of the extremities, pelvic and shoulder girdles: sonographic and pathologic correlations. Clin Radiol 35: 193–202
6. Kuhn E, Stefanits K (1987) Muscular infiltration of the limbs in Hodgkin's disease. Report of three cases. Strahlenther Oncol 163: 6–8
7. Lindell MM, Wallace S, DeSantos LA (1981) Diagnostic technique for the evaluation of the soft-tissue sarcoma. Semin Oncol 8: 160–171
8. Pathria MN, Zlatkin M, Sartoris DJ, Scheible W, Resnick D (1988) Ultrasonography of the popliteal fossa and lower extremities. Radiol Clin North Am 26: 77–85
9. Peters PE, Friedmann G (1983) Radiologische Diagnostik maligner peripherer Weichteiltumoren. Radiologe 23: 502–511
10. Rotte KH, Kleinau H, Kriedemann E, Perlick E, Schmidt-Peter P (1988) Das maligne fibröse Histiozytom der Weichteile. Möglichkeiten und Grenzen der Computertomografie. Fortschr Geb Rontgenstr 148: 520–523
11. Schernberg F, Fernage B, Collin JP, Ameil M, Sandre J (1987) L'echographie en temps reel: une method d'imagerie de la main. Ann Chir Main 6: 239–244
12. Stuhler T, Feige A (eds) (1987) Ultraschalldiagnostik des Bewegungsapparats. Springer, Berlin Heidelberg New York
13. Toolanen G, Lorentzon R, Friberg S, Dahlstrom H, Oberg L (1988) Sonography of popliteal masses. Acta Orthop Scand 59: 294–296
14. Ulivi M, Leonard M, Balconi G, Teruzzi P (1986) Ultrasonography in the diagnosis of soft-tissue tumors. Ital J Orthop Traumatol 12: 109–115
15. Vanel D, Le Treut A (1988) Imagerie des sarcomes des partites molles. Bull Cancer (Paris) 75: 453–458
16. Vincent LM (1988) Ultrasound of soft-tissue abnormalities of the extremities. Radiol Clin North Am 26: 131–144
17. Vulkanovic S, Sidani AH, Ducommun JC, Curati WL (1981) Xerography and ultrasonography in soft-tissue pathology. J Belge Radiol 64: 309–319
18. Yeh HC, Rabinowitz JG (1982) Ultrasonography of the extremities and pelvic girdle and correlation with computed tomography. Radiology 143: 519–515

The Value of Magnetic Resonance Imaging in the Evaluation of Soft-Tissue Sarcomas

R. Schwarz, O. Schneider, M. Heller, R. Maas, V. Nicolas, and E. Bücheler

Introduction

Over the period of 1986–1989, 210 patients with soft-tissue tumors were evaluated with magnetic resonance imaging (MRI). A total of 350 examinations in these patients were performed. These examinations were analyzed retrospectively. Other imaging modalities such as computer-assisted tomography (CAT; 263 examinations in 130 patients), surgical reports, and pathohistological reports were included in the analysis. Sixty patients were treated by radiotherapy. Radiotherapeutic data including treatment plans, dosage, and fractionation were reviewed. The analysis included three fundamental questions: (a) the value of MRI in treatment planning for both surgery and radiotherapy; (b) the value of MRI in detecting recurrences; and (c) changes in normal tissue after surgery and/or radiotherapy.

Subjects and Methods

Of the 210 patients 79 had primary tumors and 75 had recurrence. In 56 cases MRI as follow-up examination for different therapeutic approaches showed no tumor. All tumors were confirmed histopathologically using the system of Enzinger, with malignant, intermediate, or benign tumors. There were 134 patients with malignant tumors, 5 with intermediate, and 72 with benign. In 85 cases MRI demonstrated soft-tissue sarcoma occurring as primary tumor or recurrent tumor. All age groups were represented. The youngest patient was 4 years old, the oldest 90 years old. The mean age of patients was 43 years. All patients were examined using a 1.5-T Gyroscan (Philips). The spine-echo technique was preferred. In all cases images were made in the axial plane and in most cases also in the sagittal or coronal plane. In most cases T1-weighted and T2-weighted images were acquired. In 16% of examinations gadolinium DTPA

Department of Radiology, University Hospital Hamburg, Eppendorf, Martinistr. 52, 2000 Hamburg 20, FRG

Advanced Radiation Therapy Tumor Response
Monitoring and Treatment Planning
Breit (Editor-in-Chief)
© Springer-Verlag, Berlin Heidelberg 1992

(Gd-DTPA) was used for enhancement of soft-tissue tumors in T1 sequences. There were no adverse effects of the Gd-DTPA administration.

Results

Many of the tumors were localized at the lower or upper extremity. Most of the tumors could be defined exactly, with sharp, clearly defined margins. The tumor size was measured and the maximal diameter of the tumor documented. The dimensions of primary and recurrent tumors were comparable; the mean for primaries was 7.1 cm and that for recurrences 6.9 cm. The largest primary tumor was localized at the upper leg and measured 27 cm. The largest recurrent tumor, localized at the upper leg, measured 31 cm. The smallest size of histologically confirmed tumors (primary and recurrent tumors) was 1 cm. A comparison of these predictions with surgical and histopathological reports showed good correlations. Most of the soft-tissue sarcomas with the exception of lipomatous tumors showed the following characteristics. In T1-weighted images tumors of lower intensity could be delineated from fat tissue. In T2-weighted images tumors with higher signal intensity could be delineated from muscle. Tumors may be homogeneous or not. Additional information about tumor extent and tumor vascularization could be achieved by Gd-DTPA enhanced T1 sequences. MRI showed no definite parameters for differentiation of histologies. General criteria such as invasiveness of tumor can be used for this decision.

MRI was less successful for the detection of early recurrences after surgery or radiotherapy of soft-tissue sarcomas than MRI for detection and description of untreated tumors. The analysis shows that the diagnosis for recurrence was true positive in 67 cases, true negative in 47, false positive in 9, and false negative in 8. An analysis of whole population concerning the time between surgical intervention and MRI showed a wide variation, between 1 and 204 months. The time between radiotherapy and MRI showed a variation between 1 and 104 months. An analysis of false predictions showed that the diagnosis was complicated by posttherapeutic changes in the normal tissue, especially radiation fibrosis. Evaluation of cases with false-negative diagnosis demonstrates that all recurrent tumors were smaller than 2 cm at the time of examination. Gd-DTPA enhanced sequences may enable the differentiation between fibrosis and recurrent tumor. Nowadays Gd-DTPA enhanced T1 images are obligatory in the examination of soft-tissue tumors or follow-up examinations of soft-tissue sarcomas. MRI examinations after surgery and radiotherapy demonstrated changes in fat tissue in 89.4% as subcutaneous fibrosis, 53% in muscle, and 6.1% in bone. Subcutaneous fibrosis correlates well with the size of radiation fields. A comparison showed that differences between predictions from MRI and actual size of radiation fields were below 1 cm. Manifestation of changes in normal tissue as shown by MRI occurred within 6 months after radiotherapy.

Discussion and Conclusions

Development of radical surgical techniques combined with radiotherapy and chemotherapy as alternative to amputation in the management of soft-tissue sarcomas has necessitated accurate preoperative staging. Analyses of the value of MRI in evaluation of tumors of the musculosceletal system have been published previously. The goals of MRI include exact definition of the tumor extent and its relationship to surrounding structures [1, 2, 5–7, 9, 10]. Routinely T1- and T2-weighted sequences should be used [1, 2, 5, 6, 9]. Spin-echo sequences should be preferred [1, 3]. Also, Gd-DTPA enhanced T1 sequences should be performed [4]. There are no definite parameters for differentiating benign from malignant lesions [1]. After definite therapy of soft-tissue sarcomas for the further follow-up of these patients a basic documentation with different modalities such as MRI, CAT, and ultrasound should be performed. In the further follow-up these techniques can be used alternatively or sequentially. Most therapeutic changes in normal tissue make the diagnosis of recurrence more difficult [3, 8]. Gd-DTPA enhanced T1 images may assure the decision.

References

1. Aisen AM, Martel E, Braunstein EM et al. (1986) MRI and CT evaluations of primary bone and soft-tissue tumors. AJR 146: 749–756
2. Demas BE, Heelan RT, Lane J et al. (1988) Comparison of MR and CT in determining the extent of disease. AJR 150: 615–620
3. Glazer HS, Lee KT, Levitt G et al. (1985) Radiation fibrosis: differentiation from recurrent tumor by MR imaging. Radiology 156: 721–726
4. Herrlin K, Bi Ling L, Petterson H et al. (1990) Gadolinium-DTPA enhancement of soft tissue tumors in magnetic resonance imaging. Acta Radiol 31: 233–236
5. Kilcoyne RF, Richardson, B, Porter A et al. (1988) Magnetic resonance imaging of soft tissue masses. Clin Ortho 228: 13–19
6. Petasnick JP, Turner DA, Charters JR et al. (1986) Comparison of MR imaging with CT. Radiology 160: 125–133
7. Petterson H, Gillespy T III, Hamlin DJ et al. (1987) Primary musculoskeletal tumors: examination with MR imaging compared with conventional modalities. Radiology 164: 237–241
8. Sundaram M, McGuire MH, Herbold DR (1988) Magnetic resonance imaging of soft tissue masses: an evaluation of fifty-three histologically proven tumors. Magn Reson Imaging 6: 237–248
9. Totty WG, Murphy WA, Lee JKT (1986) Soft-tissue tumors: MR imaging. Radiology 160: 135–141
10. Weekes RG, Berquist TH, McLeod RA et al. (1985) Magnetic resonance imaging of soft-tissue tumors: comparison with computed tomography. Magn Reson Imaging 3: 345–352

Increased Gd-DTPA Enhancement in Malignant Compared with ... in Preclinical Renal Tumors

Methods

For this study we used a 1.5 T superconducting magnet (Siemens Somatom ...) ... a proton-weighted and a T2-weighted SE sequence in a horizontal plane (Spin echo sequence) ... and a T1-weighted SE sequence in a horizontal plane, and a inversion recovery study in a horizontal plane. The dynamic study was carried out with a FLASH two-dimensional gradient echo sequence (TR 40 ms, TE 10 ms, flip angle 90°) ... The technique allows a short acquisition time of 10 s for each image and a high spatial resolution ...

Gd-DTPA was administered manually under standardized conditions after the third sequence (0.1 mmol/kg body weight). The increasing SI of the tumor as well as the increasing SI of the surrounding tissues including cancellous bone ...

Department of Radiology, University ... Publication ...
Department of Radiology ...

Dynamic Gd-DTPA Enhanced Magnetic Resonance Imaging of Musculoskeletal Neoplasms

A.R. Goldmann[1], M. Lehner[1], B. Kladny[1], K. Glückert[1], H. Stöß[2], and F.C. Simm[3]

Introduction

The administration of gadolinium during magnetic resonance imaging (MRI) is a well-established procedure especially in the examination of musculoskeletal tumors. Gd-DTPA produces an increase in signal intensity (SI) in T1-weighted spin-echo images by reducing T1 relaxation time. Zones showing a marked increase in SI after injection of Gd-DTPA are highly vascularized regions, whereas zones with low or no increase in SI are often necrotic areas; however, these areas may also contain viable tumor cells but with little or no vascularization.

Methods

For this study we used a 1.5-T superconducting magnet (Magnetom, Siemens). Before the dynamic study, a routine static study was performed with a T1-, a proton-weighted, and a T2-weighted SE sequence in a longitudinal plane (sagittal or coronal), a T2*-weighted FLASH two-dimensional gradient-echo sequence in an axial plane, and a T1-weighted SE sequence at the end of the dynamic study in a longitudinal plane. The dynamic study was carried out with a FLASH two-dimensional gradient-echo sequence (TR 40 ms, TE 10 ms; flip angle 90°; matrix 256 × 256; one acquisition) which allows a short acquisition time of 10 s for each image and a high spatial resolution. The slice orientation was chosen in the largest intra- and extraosseous extent of the tumor. Twenty images of the same orientation with a delay of 3 s between each image were taken. Gd-DTPA was administered manually under standardized conditions after the third sequence (0.2 ml/kg body weight). The increasing SI of the tumor and, in cases of varying regional uptake, of the different areas within the tumor, as well as the increasing SI of the surrounding tissues including cancellous bone,

[1] Department of Orthopedics, University of Erlangen, Rathsberger Str. 57, W-8520 Erlangen, FRG
[2] Department of Pathology, University of Erlangen, Krankenhaus Str. 8–10, 8520 Erlangen, FRG
[3] Medical Engineering Group, Siemens AG, Hartmann Str. 16, 8520 Erlangen, FRG

Advanced Radiation Therapy Tumor Response
Monitoring and Treatment Planning
Breit (Editor-in-Chief)
© Springer-Verlag, Berlin Heidelberg 1992

muscle, and fatty tissue were determined. For each tissue the values derived from each image were plotted against time. Because of the marked dynamic uptake of Gd the SI increases faster in the vital tumor compared to other tissues. Surrounding tissue that is infiltrated by the tumor also shows a slight increase of SI. On the other hand, the change in SI in normal tissues such as cancellous bone, fatty tissue, central necrosis, or muscle is absent or only insignificant.

To evaluate these different curves of increasing SI, we determined the slopes of the SI increase between different points after the injection of Gd-DTPA and the areas under the curve for different time intervals. When correlating these different values with the different histological findings, the average slope between fourth and seventh points of the curve was the most precise. Therefore in the following this average slope is used. This average slope can be calculated directly on the computer after positioning the region of interest (ROI) on the monitor.

To ensure the correct positioning of the ROI on the MR images during evaluation, we compared the histological findings in specimens after resection with the dynamic images taken immediately before resection. To obtain curves with the fastest and highest increase in SI in the vital tumor, the ROI was positioned in the area of highest SI on the last image of 20-image series. Routinely, additional ROIs were positioned in areas of necrosis in the tumor (or areas of vital tumor with poor perfusion), surrounding tissue infiltrated by the tumor, surrounding edema, normal cancellous bone, muscle, and fatty tissue.

Thirteen patients had benign tumors; these included four enchondromas, two osteoblastomas, two lipomas, two fibrous dyplasias, one giant-cell tumor, one osteoid osteoma, and one nonossifying fibroma. There were 24 patients with malignant tumors; these included eight osteosarcomas, four Ewing's sarcomas, three synoviomas, two chondrosarcomas, two fibrous histiocytomas, two lymphomas, two metastases, and one rhabdomyosarcoma. In eight cases (five osteosarcomas, two Ewing's sarcomas, and one malignant fibrous histiocytoma) the dynamic studies were performed before and after preoperative chemotherapy.

Results

The first question was whether it is possible to grade tumors by this technique. Table 1 shows the average slopes for benign and malignant tumors as graded according to the Enneking classification. The range of values within the groups is relatively wide. However, a value below 3.5 can be taken as a benign and a value over 11 as a malignant lesion. In the broad zone between these values grading by this method is impossible. Malignant synoviomas are not listed here; all three cases showed a very late uptake of Gd-GTPA. Surprisingly, metastases had relatively low values, with an average of 3.2. In two cases we used this

Table 1. Average slopes from curves with dynamic increase in signal intensity after injection of Gd-DTPA obtained in different neoplasms[a]

Grading	n	Mean	Median	Standard deviation	Range
G0	9	3.45	3.11	3.21	0–10.47
G1	4	9.20	9.20	6.38	1.44–16.94
G2	18	6.66	5.99	2.51	3.74–12.24
Metastases	2	3.20	3.20	0.34	2.96–3.44

[a] Excludes three synoviomas.

method to detect local recurrences after preceding chemotherapy and wide exclusions; in all three cases the low average slope (mean 0.76, median 0.80, standard deviation 0.80, lowest value 0, highest value 1.53) made a local recurrence very much unlikely.

The second question was whether it is possible to differentiate between peritumoral edema and infiltration of the tumor in surrounding soft tissue, which is invisible on the standard MRI. The values for these two histological findings differed little (edema: mean 1.29, range 0.80–2.04; tumor infiltration: mean 2.13, range 0.66–3.93). This method provides hints, but the discrimination is not certain.

The third question concerned the assessment of the response of osteosarcomas, Ewing's sarcomas, and malignant fibrous histiocytomas to preoperative chemotherapy (Table 2). Responders and nonresponders were classified according to the degrees of histological regression after chemotherapy (Salzer-Kuntschik: less than 10% viable tumor cells = responders, 10% viable tumors cell or more = nonresponders). Six patients proved to be nonresponders; the values remained almost unchanged, and the quotient of average slope after therapy/average slope before therapy was more than 0.6. Responders, on the other hand, showed a distinct reduction in values, indicating a good response to chemotherapy. The quotient of average slope after therapy/average slope before therapy was less than 0.1 in our two cases.

The response to therapy was compared with sequential bone scanning before and after chemotherapy (Table 2). In this small series, the accuracy of the dynamic Gd-DTPA study was 100%. For the three phases of scintigraphy we determined the quotient T/NT (T = count within the tumor, NT = count measured on the opposite unaffected side). In cases of a reduction in the quotient T/NT from pre- to postchemotherapy (perfusion: reduction $\geq$ 60%; blood-pool phase reduction $\geq$ 50%; osseous phase: reduction $\geq$ 20% of the value before therapy), the tumor was classified as responder. When applying these criteria, the results were incorrect for nonresponders in one case in the blood-pool phase and in two case in the osseous phase. The two responders were classified correctly by sequential scintigraphy.

Recently we have been tesing a new sequence called Turbo-FLASH, supplied by Siemens (TI 100 ms, TR 6.5 ms, TE 3 ms, flip angle 9°, matrix 128 × 128;

Table 2. Assessment of response in eight patients to preoperative chemotherapy (quotient post-therapy/pretherapy)

	Dynamic MRI (slope)	Sequential scintigraphy (T/NT)[a]		
		Perfusion	Blood-pool phase	Osseous phase
Responders (n = 2)				
Mean	0.012	0.387	0.459	0.715
Range	0.000–0.024	0.345–0.428	0.312–0.606	0.530–0.900
Correct	100%	100%	100%	100%
Nonresponders (n = 6)				
Mean	1.057	0.917	0.843	0.932
Range	0.609–1.537	0.381–1.344	0.467–1.132	0.690–1.082
Correct	100%	83%	83%	67%

[a] T, count in the tumor; NT, count in the unaffected opposite side.

number of measurements 40; delay time 0). This sequence allows a reduction in acquisition time from the 10 s of the formerly used FLASH sequence to less than 1 s for one image. Every 3 s three parallel slices are acquired sequentially. Gd-DTPA is administered after the fifth sequence, i.e., after 15 s. The total registration time is reduced from 260 to 120 s.

One advantage of this new procedure is the shorter delay time between the images, and therefore a higher precision or temporal resolution in the interesting time period of about 90 s after the injection of Gd-DTPA, corresponding to the period of dynamic uptake of Gd-GTPA. In addition to this, in the same time three slices are measured in the tumor. On the other hand, the spatial resolution of this Turbo FLASH sequence is comparable to the resolution obtained with the former FLASH sequence.

Conclusions

The indications that we see for this new technique are in a grading of musculo-skeletal neoplasms, however, with the limitations mentioned above. Also, a differentiation of tissue types is possible, especially for vital tumor and necrosis. But the differentiation between surrounding edema and tumor infiltration of surrounding tissue seems to be uncertain. This technique may also be used for the detection of local recurrences. For the assessment of the tumor response to preoperative chemotherapy, this technique appears to be very useful. As in former studies [1, 2], the dynamic Gd-GTPA study was at least as precise as sequential bone scanning. Other techniques such as radiography, computed tomography, and angiography seem to be less accurate for this. Especially non-responders are usually detected with more difficulty using computed tomography or angiography. The combination of three-phase skeletal scintigraphy with the determination of tracer plasma clearance has proven to have a diagnostic accuracy of up to 100%. The value of other methods (MR angiography, opposed-phase MRI for fat/water separation, etc.) for tumor therapy monitoring must be determined in the future.

We see further advantages of this method in the fact that the spatial resolution within the tumor is very good, especially compared with scintigraphy, the method is not invasive, as is angiography, and exposure to radiation can be avoided.

References

1. Erlemann R, Reiser MF, Peters PE et al. (1989) Musculoskeletal neoplasms: static and dynamic Gd-DTPA-enhanced MR imaging. Radiology 171: 767–773
2. Erlemann R, Sciuk J, Bosse A et al. (1990) Response of osteosarcoma and Ewing sarcoma to preoperative chemotherapy: assessment with dynamic and static MR imaging and skeletal scintigraphy. Radiology 175: 791–796

Magnetic Resonance Relaxometry

An Approach to Knowledge-Based Computerized Diagnosis of Tumor Pathology in Quantitative Magnetic Resonance Imaging

S. Meindl, S. Meairs, and G. Bielke

In 1970 Damadian showed in magnetic resonance (MR) experiments with animals that the T_1 values of tumors differ substantially from those of normal tissues, suggesting that it is possible to distinguish the two types of tissues from each other. This has been shown to be true not only for in vitro experiments but also for in vivo examinations especially under imaging conditions, leading to images with high soft-tissue contrast. The hope grew that this would provide better specificity than other imaging modalities. The intrinsic MR tissue parameters represent the biochemical and biophysical characteristics of the tissues and hence could in principle be used to identify them. The extrinsic parameters constitute a tool for combining the multiparametric MRI information in one or more images in the form of signal intensities. Subsequently, many researchers looked for possibilities to use the quantitative differences in relaxation times for diagnostic purposes, and they developed theories about the mechanisms of relaxation effects in biological tissues.

However, while image quality has improved remarkably, the results of studies investigating the value of MR tissue parameters have up to now been more disappointing than encouraging. The use of one- and two-dimensional discrimination methods show a considerable overlap of MR parameters. The questions are: Are the intrinsic parameters not specific enough? or Do we use a wrong model and ask the wrong questions? In some specific fields simple quantitative parameter measurements which can be performed on each commercial magnetic resonance imaging (MRI) unit have already become a routine diagnostic tool.

An example is the assessment of clinical activity in Grave's ophthalmopathy and the detection of its response to therapy with T_2 values. In this case T_2 calculations are performed in the area of each extraocular muscle on a CPMG spin-echo train of eight echoes in the coronal plane. In a study of 28 patients with confirmed moderate to severe ophthalmopathy the T_2 values have been correlated to standard diagnostic parameters and procedures such as tonography values, Hertel exophthalmometry results, and the opthalmopathy index according to Werner's classification. Additionally, the geometric area of the muscles has been calculated in MR images. The evaluations were performed before and after treatment with immunomodulating drugs and after the follow-up period [1]. In all patients there was a significant reduction in intraocular

MR Working Group, Deutsche Klinik für Diagnostik, Aukammallee 33, 6200 Wiesbaden, FRG

Advanced Radiation Therapy Tumor Response
Monitoring and Treatment Planning
Breit (Editor-in-Chief)
© Springer-Verlag, Berlin Heidelberg 1992

pressure during therapy which continued in most of the patients even during follow-up. The overall clinical stage and changes in the mean opthalmopathy indices demonstrated a good to moderate response in all cases. In MRI all patients revealed a strong decrease in T_2 values of the extraocular eye muscles during therapy. After the treatment was stopped, two different types of reaction could be observed; in one group the absence of inflammatory edema was demonstrated by normalized T_2 values while in the other group T_2 values increased again to those measured in the pretreatment period, indicating an unfavorable prognosis (Fig. 1). The data show a high correlation between T_2 values and ophthalmopathy indices, tonography measurements, and mean muscle sizes. The differences at the end of the follow-up period offer a unique opportunity to detect early deterioration.

To quantify not only T_2 alone but also T_1 and proton density we developed a special pulse sequence, called interlaced triple sequence, which consists of a CPMG multiecho train with eight echoes, repeated three times with different recovery times interlaced for each projection. The machine parameters used are optimized for best accuracy for quantification in the area of the most frequent tissue parameter values. This sequence is carried out in single-slice mode at a representative slice location through the tumor to avoid mutual influences of neighboring slices, which can cause significant errors. The technique also has the advantage that the whole acquisition runs without any pause that could lead to patient's movements and destroy the identity of pixel locations in the image

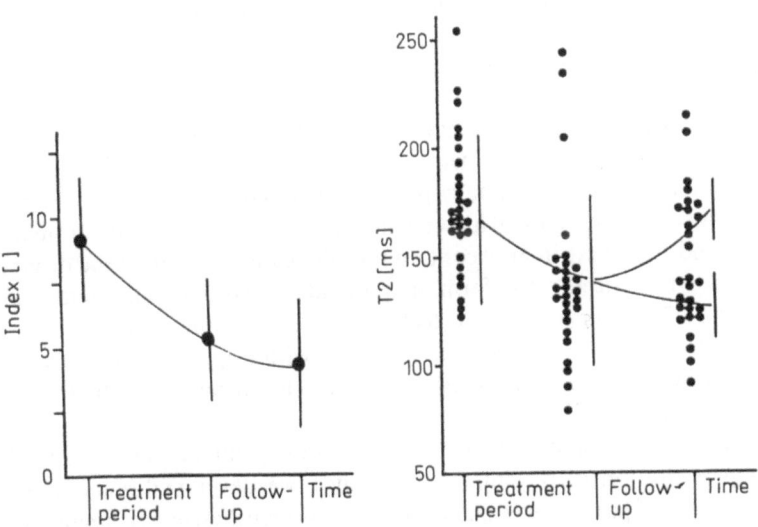

Fig. 1. *Left*, mean ophthalmopathy index, according to Werner's classification. Improvement was observed even after discontinuation of immunomodulating therapy. *Right*, T2 values of affected extraocular eye muscles during therapy. Note increasing values in one group, demonstrating early deterioration of orbitopathy

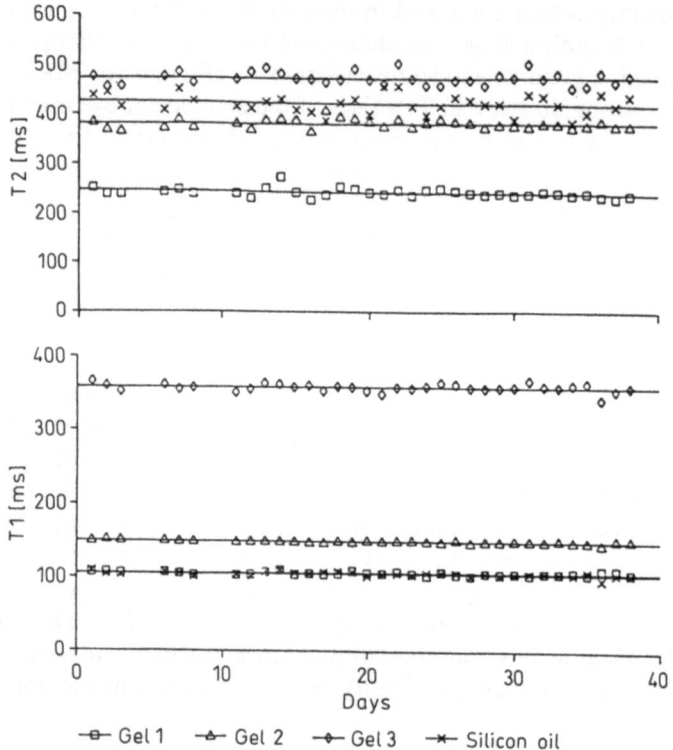

Fig. 2. Stability of the parameter calculation for T1 and T2 relaxation times, measured on a test phantom

series. The resulting 24 pixel-identical images are the basis for all the post-processing and quantification following [2].

After transfer to a powerful image-processing system the parameter estimation is performed on pixel base, which results in a set of three parameter images for Rho, T1, and T2. These images contain the whole information of the original 24-image series in concentrated form. The quality, reproducibility, and long-term stability of the measurement technique and parameter estimation is continuously controlled using a special phantom with doped agarose gels with known parameter values included (Fig. 2). The stability proves to be better than 10% for T_1 and 5% for T_2.

Since these parameter images are a concentrated, but not necessarily the optimal, representation of the interesting tissues, we developed a method to invert the process of parameter calculation and to resynthesize MR images out of the three parameter images with the aid of the simplified solution of the Bloch equation. What we do by this is simulate the imaging process in the computer. The synthesis is done in real time, so that this technique is well suited to analyze the contrast behavior of each tissue and to optimize its contrast to the surrounding. The system is able to calculate synthesized images with good or poor contrast, with extreme parameter values which cannot be measured because of the unacceptably long acquisition time needed and even with parameter combinations that do not exist in reality. We call the latter virtual images. What we can achieve by this is a coherent contrast effect for T_1 and T_2, especially when using short repetition times and negative echo-delay times. These virtual images deliver the total amount of parameter information in a qualitative way and very often the best possible contrast [3].

Another example for the use of, in this case, all three MR tissue parameters for a clinical question has been a study performed some time ago in our group to investigate in vivo the effects of therapeutic brain radiation on the tissue parameters and to confirm the correlation between tumor size and radiation dose. Twelve patients with nonresectable primary and secondary brain tumor were included (eight glioblastoma multiforme, three breast carcinoma metastases, one lung carcinoma metastasis). Diagnosis was histologically confirmed by stereotactic biopsy. All patients underwent photon radiation therapy. Fractionation schedule, estimated total target dose, and systemic steroid therapy were performed according to standardized procedures. An adjuvant chemotherapy was not applied. Each patient was scanned before, at the end of the first (40 Gy), and at the end of the second radiation period (60 Gy) using the described interlaced triple sequence. Mean parameter values were calculated by means of irregular tissue-characteristic regions of interest on the calculated parameter images for solid viable tumor tissue and gray and white brain matter. Due to the limited number of investigated patients an intraindividual evaluation was performed. Tumor volumes were estimated by measuring the three main axes of the tumor and using the formula for ovoid bodies. Compared with the pretreatment estimations, the mean tumor volumes in our study showed a clear reduction . The study also demonstrated a remarkable effect of brain radiotherapy on in vivo MR tissue parameters of tumor tissue even after a dose fraction of 40 Gy. The parameters continued to decrease depending on the X-ray dose administered (Fig. 3). Gray and white matter of the nonaffected contralateral hemisphere showed no significant difference compared with pretreatment measurements, probably because of the high radiation resistance of the brain matter and the carefully administered radiation technique [4].

When we return to our aim of quantitative tissue characterization with MR tissue parameters, we first must solve the problem of segmentation. Segmentation can be understood as the combination of pixels into larger regions called segments which share some common properties, and which are hoped to be tissue characteristic. Several approaches to this problem are possible. One is template matching, which attempts to define beforehand the MR-characteristics of the various tissues and to use this definition to label the pixels within the image. The problems with this method are that reliable tissue signatures are only available for a limited number of normal tissues such as muscle, fat, gray and white matter, and that partial volume effects are a significant problem. The hierarchical methods simulate a property of our visual system simultaneously to

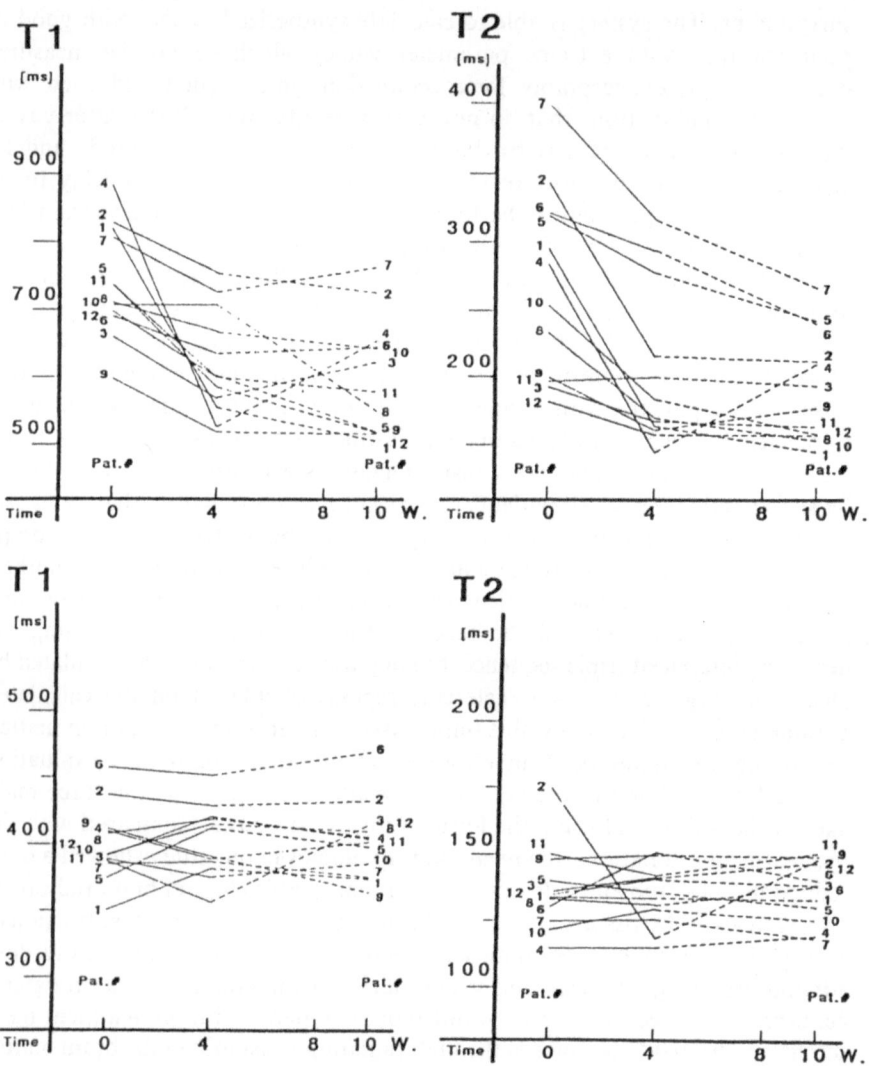

Fig. 3. Calculated relaxation times for viable tumor tissue (*above*) and white brain matter (*below*) during therapy. Note the uniform tendency toward lower values for tumor tissue and the lack of significant effects for brain matter

analyze an image at multiple levels of resolution. While very effective at segmenting over a small local area, problems arise with segments of the same tissue, which are in widely different spatial positions not naturally joined together. Recently, algorithms have been developed based on fuzzy set theory which enable us mathematically to treat uncertainty and imprecision. For each pixel a membership function is calculated which defines its degree of member-ship to a certain cluster, i.e., to a certain tissue. In an iterative process the parameters of the statistical functions are optimized, and each pixel is then assigned to that cluster corresponding to the highest of that pixel's membership function. A method which uses quantitative parameter values and joins widely spaced tissues is based on a clustering procedure in parameter space with a three-dimensional maximum-likelihood classifier. This is the approach to tissue characterization that we use. In the following we present how this method works, and what kind of results can be achieved [5–7].

The relaxation times and the proton density can be seen to span a three-dimensional feature space. Each volume element of the measured slice with its parameter triple is represented by a vector in this feature space. Pixels with a functional neighborhood in the image domain, i.e., pixels belonging to the same tissue, have spatial neighborhood in the feature space, that is, they form clusters. For the classification process a training set must be defined by small regions of interest, representing areas of definite membership to different hitherto possibly unknown tissue types. With this input data the three-dimensional maximum-likelihood classifier sorts all feature vectors into classes, which are displayed in a special color code. Back-transformation into image domain results in a tissue-specific segmented image.

This intraindividual classification can of course deliver only an unspecific tissue discrimination and segmentation. By means of a second run of the classifier, the differential diagnosis of a pathologic area can be achieved by an interindividual classification. In this case the mean vectors and covariance matrices of the statistical distribution of the areas segmented before are compared with a knowledge base containing the interindividually normalized values of a group of histologically confirmed cases. Including a rejection class, to which points are attached, if the probability of the membership to one of the tissue classes in question is low, the class boundaries in feature space have the form of ellipsoids with any given axis ratio and direction of axis in space. In case of displaying the class boundaries of the interindividual tumor clusters in the knowledge base as three-dimensional surface reconstruction, the complicated relation of the angular positions of the ellipsoids and their mutual penetration in feature space become evident. When one considers this complicated inter-relationship one can imagine that it is not possible to characterize tissues well with methods that use projections only of the feature space and disregard the three-dimensional extent of the distribution functions.

If the classifier is able to attach a tissue to any of the classes, the system outputs the area fractions of the successfully classified pixels, which can be interpreted as probability values. As graphic representation a decision board can be constructed showing the results of the classification process. For the purpose of quality control the parameters for the reference probe and the white brain matter are given, and as a main result the position of the mean vectors of the parameter values of the actual region in relation to the ones of the most probable tissue class and to those in second place are shown. Finally, to control the spatial position of the classified pixels, one can tint the intensities of an optimally synthesized image with the code colors of the interesting tissues to achieve a tissue type image. This image represents the total information of the whole study, including high contrasting signal strength and tissue type.

Our experience even with this highly sophisticated classification system has shown that it is not possible to gain reliable results in all imaginable cases. It could be shown that the border conditions and suppositions must be defined very carefully. This means especially that approaches to differentiate individual tumors at the beginning of the decision pathway are not adequate and normally do not correspond to the actual state of diagnostic information which the physician has. The insertion of MR parameters later in the diagnostic decision scheme, for example, for differentiating the best diagnosis from a reduced number of differential diagnoses, seems more effective. Therefore in parallel we have been working on the development of an expert system to include all diagnostic information available, to gain the preselection of differential diagnostic questions influencing the interindividual knowledge base of the classifier, or even to decide on the diagnosis at once if possible.

When we observe a physician using MRI for diagnosis, we realize that he is always using parameter-dependent information by using parameter-weighted images. What we also see is that he interprets these images in a semiquantitative way when he differentiates tissues by a simple rough scale, for example, with the values long, medium, short. So, what he is actually doing is already a kind of qualitative tissue classification. To simulate his decision process we must ask what kind of information he is otherwise using. Besides MR parameter-dependent information he uses localization, anatomical boundaries, texture parameters, behavior of contrast agents, flow, age, sex, time-dependent parameters, and clinical findings. He also uses information about the patient's history and even the family history. Thus, one can imagine that diagnosis is a very complex process, and that all these factors must be taken into account.

In the development phase of the expert system we used a commercial shell for tools to organize and overview the very complex and extensive matter. Most of the points mentioned above have been regarded in our system, especially descriptive facts which can be represented only by uncertain values. The structure of the algorithms now follows modern methods of artificial intelligence in representing the knowledge and decision finding. The system has been transferred to a conventional personal computer in the form of a run time version with an elegant user interface which reduces the restraints to work with it. At the moment it is the task of our diagnostic experts to fill in their knowledge and to specify the diagnostic criteria for the different findings, which can be done easily by selection from a given spectrum. For an actual case similar descriptive values must be inserted, and the system gives its decision with associated probability factors. Additionally, the decision can be supervised by controlling the points that led to the actual diagnosis or ruled out concurrent findings.

In the near future the classification system is to be tested in combination with this expert system on the data of our sample of tumor patients over recent years measured with the described method. We hope that this evaluation will form a further step in defining the diagnostic significance of quantitative MR parameters in vivo.

References

1. Pedrosa P, Neidl K, Higer HP et al. (1990) Assessment of clinical activity in endocrine orbitopathy with T2 values—response to immunomodulating therapy. In: Higer HP, Bielke G (eds) Tissue characterization in MR imaging. Springer, Berlin Heidelberg New York, p 307 ff
2. Meindl S (1987) Entwicklung von Verfahren zur Messung von funktionellen Parametern in biologischen Geweben in vivo unter Ausnutzung von Atomkerneigenschaften. Thesis, University of Mainz
3. Bielke G, Meves M, Meindl S et al. (1984) A systematic approach to optimization of pulse sequences in NMR-imaging by computer simulations. In: Esser PD, Johnston RE (eds) Technology of nuclear magnetic resonance. Society of Nuclear Medicine, New York, p 109ff
4. Pedrosa P, Reis FH, Grigat M et al. (1990) Calculated T1 and T2 in nonresectable brain tumors to monitor the effects of cranial radiation. In: Higer HP, Bielke G (eds) Tissue characterization in MR imaging. Springer, Berlin Heidelberg New York, p 319ff
5. Jungke M, Bielke G, Grigat M et al. (1987) Feature extraction and data preprocessing applied to tissue characterization in NMR-tomography. In: Lemke HU et al. (eds) Computer assisted radiology CAR '87. Springer, Berlin Heidelberg New York, p 48ff
6. Jungke M (1988) Entwicklung eines Systems zur Informationsverarbeitung in der Kernspintomographie. Thesis, University of Mainz
7. Meindl S, Jungke M, Bielke G et al. (1990) Tissue type imaging — an approach to clinical use. In: Higer HP, Bielke G (eds) Tissue characterization in MR imaging. Springer, Berlin Heidelberg New York, p 174ff

Tissue Characterization by Magnetic Resonance Imaging Relaxometry and Texture Analysis in Clinical Oncology

L.R. Schad, I. Zuna, W. Härle, and W.J. Lorenz

Introduction

Prolongation of both the spin-lattice (T1) and spin-spin (T2) proton relaxation times of neoplastic tissue in vitro was first reported by Damadian in 1971 [1]. On the basis of this observation it was hoped that magnetic resonance imaging (MRI) would allow a more precise prediction of tissue characteristics than is possible with computed tomography. However, in vivo evaluation of proton relaxation times of human tumors showed that the range of values of all these parameters was so wide that it is impossible to characterize the tumor-tissue types [2, 3]. Another approach to tissue characterization is based on statistical image texture analysis, which has previously been developed and extensively used for ultrasound tissue characterization [4]. This study was undertaken to evaluate the feasibility of in vivo tissue characterization on the basis of MRI texture analysis using spin-echo and T1 and T2 images of patients with brain tumors.

Materials and Methods

Measurements were performed on a 64-MHz Magnetom (Siemens, Erlangen, FRG) superconducting whole-body imager. A time-saving combined Carr-Purcell/Carr-Purcell-Meijboom-Gill (CP/CPMG) multiple spin-echo sequence with interleaved repetition times $TR_1 = 2000$ ms and $TR_2 = 600$ ms and 30 echoes with $TE = 22$ ms was used for simultaneous determination of T1 and T2. Comparative measurements in the imager and with a spectrometer of relaxation times were performed on phantoms containing fluids of different T1 and T2 values to evaluate accuracy. Twenty tubes with different concentrations of Gd-DTPA were used for measurements in the range of $30 < T1 < 2500$ ms and $25 < T2 < 2200$ ms. A maximum deviation of about 10% was found between the imager and spectrometer relaxation time measurements.

Department of Radiology and Pathophysiology, German Cancer Research Center, Im Neuenheimer Feld 280, 6900 Heidelberg, FRG

Advanced Radiation Therapy Tumor Response
Monitoring and Treatment Planning
Breit (Editor-in-Chief)
© Springer-Verlag, Berlin Heidelberg 1992

Twelve patients (aged 12–71 years) with brain tumors were included in this prospective study. Of these, five had histologically confirmed glioblastomas, five histologically confirmed metastases, and in two patients the histology was not known because no surgery was undertaken. Imaging protocol was as follows. For orientation sagittal FLASH imaging and for diagnosis T1- and T2-weighted spin-echo images in transversal orientation were performed TR/TE 500/35 and TR/TE 1600/35, 70, respectively. The slices with the best visualization of the brain tumor were chosen for the imaging with the combined CP/CPMG multiple spin-echo sequence. For better delineation of the tumor, 0.1 mmol/kg body weight Gd-DTPA was injected intravenously within 15–30 s, and a contiguous slice sequence (TR/TE 500/35) was performed in the same slices imaged with the CP/CPMG sequence. The delay between Gd-DTPA administration and imaging was about 5 min. For each patient, the following image data set was archived: (a) precontrast: 30 echoes at a repetition time of $TR_1 =$ 2000 ms, two echoes at a repetition time of $TR_1 = 600$ ms, one T1 image and one T2 image, yielded from monoexponential evaluation; and (b) postcontrast: one T1-weighted image as reference image for the tumor/edema differentiation.

To describe quantitatively the brightness, micro-, and macrotexture of MR images first- and second-order image texture parameters were used [5]. The first-order texture is sufficiently characterized by the gray-level histogram, which displays the occurrence frequency of all gray levels in the image cluster. The second-order statistics not only gives the occurrence frequency of gray levels but also uses the spatial interdependencies between the image elements (pixels). The most significant parameters are: (a) from first-order gray-level distribution: mean gray level; (b) from the first-order gradient distribution: mean gradient absolute value; (c) from the gray-level cooccurrence matrix: contrast, entropy, and correlation; and (d) the gray-level run length histogram. For a detailed explanation of these parameters see [4].

Results

Classification. A total of 79 regions of interest (ROIs) confirmed by histology were marked to define clinically interesting tissue parts, such as tumor, edema, CSF, white and gray matter. Delineation of the tumor was best in the postcontrast images, i.e., the tumor ROI was defined by regions of Gd-DTPA enhancement in postcontrast images and then transferred to the precontrast relaxation time images. From the T1 and T2 images the previously listed image texture parameters for each ROI were calculated. The classification method used in this study is based on four two-class discriminant tests in a four-layer hierarchical decision tree. In the first layer, a decision is made whether the tissue structure is CSF. In this decision a discriminant function employing only one parameter is used. The parameter is mean gray level, calculated from the T2 image. If the parameter value exceeds a given limit (e.g., 550 ms), the tissue structure is CSF. In the second layer, a decision is made whether to separate the class of white matter from the other classes. Here the discriminant function consisting of two parameters: mean gray levels, calculated from the T1 and T2 images. In the third layer, we separate the class of gray matter from the remaining classes of tumor and edema. The discriminant function used in this decision employs, again, two parameters: mean gray levels, calculated from the T1 and T2 images. In the fourth layer, we separate the class tumor from the edema tissue pattern. The discriminant function used in this last decision employs two parameters: mean gray-level gradient, calculated from the T2 image and correlation of cooccurrence matrix calculated from the T1 image.

Segmentation. The classification results from above were added as discriminant functions together with additional rules, e.g., rules about the correctness and reliability of an image analysis, in the knowledge base of an expert system. The expert system is coded in the IF-Prolog language and running on a central computer (VAX-Workstation/3200, DEC, Maynard, MA, USA). For knowledge representation we chose a frame-based approach. An important fact of the expert system is the interface to the procedural knowledge. Procedural knowledge is the algorithmic knowledge in procedures, which are developed in conventional computer languages. Activated by rules of the expert system, the procedural knowledge delivers facts for the expert system knowledge base. The procedural knowledge exists of: (a) a cluster analysis approach to segmentate the images, (b) procedures to calculate the above first- and second-order texture parameters, and (c) other utility programs, for example, a procedure for cluster fusion. We have used four-feature images for the multivariate cluster analysis: T1 image, T2 image, the fifth spin-echo image (TR/TE 2000/110), and the ninth spin-echo image (TR/TE 2000/198). The inference strategy of the knowledge-based segmentation is as follows. Initially the MR image is divided into two clusters. To check the correctness of the segmented cluster, the image texture parameters and the additional rules about the completeness of an image analysis are used. For example, such a rule might be: an image analysis is at the earliest moment complete when the founded cluster contains background, white and gray matter. If the image analysis is incorrect, the segmentation process is started again by incrementally increasing the cluster number or analyzing a specific cluster. The results of such a knowledge-based segmentation is shown in Fig. 1 in a patient with a glioblastoma multiforme.

Discussion

In conclusion, the main advantage of knowledge-based systems lies in the fact that, after filling the knowledge base with all of the required rules for a given problem, a general problem solving is possible without implementing each

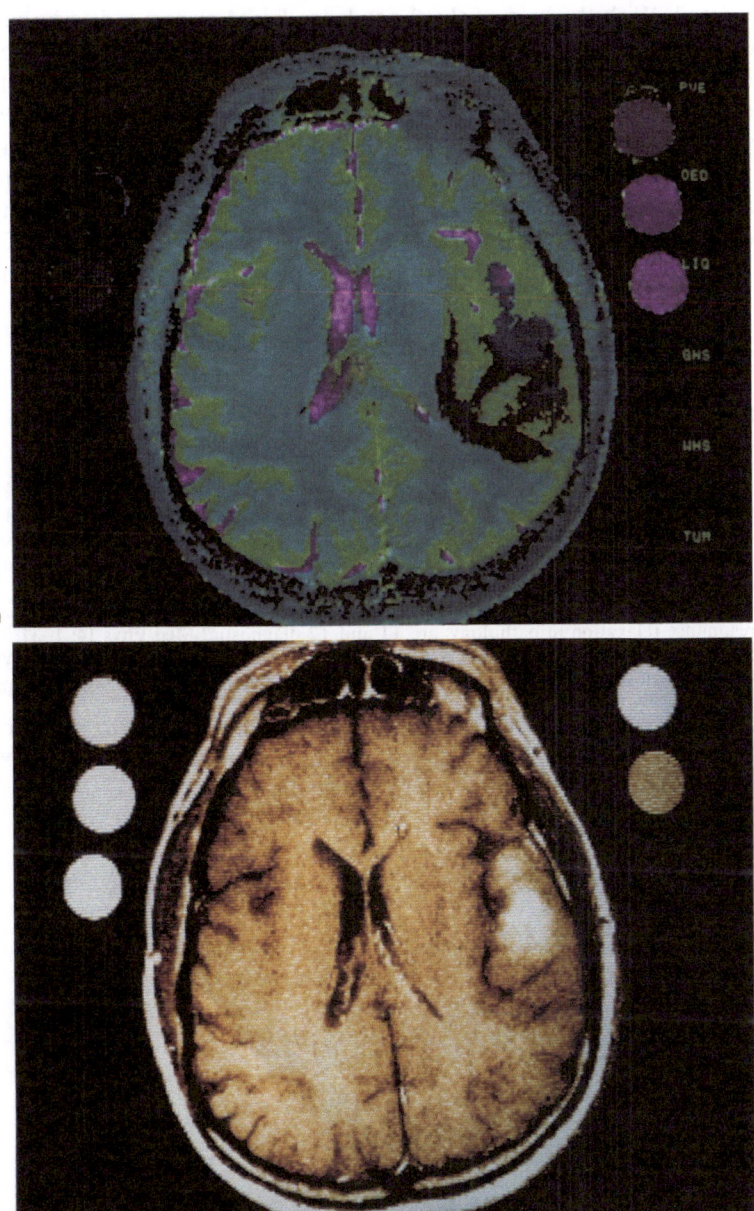

Fig. 1. a Artificial image of a patient with a glioblastoma multiforme after segmentation of
precontrast spin echo, T1 and T2 images. A total of 12 iterative cluster analysis steps were needed.
The correctly found tissues are: white matter (*light blue cluster*), gray matter (*green cluster*),
cerebrospinal fluid (*pink cluster*), edema (*red cluster*), and tumor (*dark blue cluster*). b Postcontrast
spin-echo image (TR/TE 500/35 ms) after intraveneous application of 0.1 mmol/kg Gd-DTPA
(Schering, Berlin, FRG) showing contrast enhancement in tumor tissue

solution in detail. With the help of this knowledge-based system a discrimination between tumor and edema is possible in most patients. Presently, the segmentated images have no greater diagnostic value than postcontrast T1-weighted images. On the other hand, in cases of tumors without Gd-DTPA uptake, segmentated images can support the physicians or therapists by solving nontrivial diagnostical problems, e.g., by supporting the target volume definition in radiation therapy. However, the preliminary results are very promising and suggest that MRI texture analysis can be of help for the in vivo tissue characterization, but a further investigation for the clinical reliability of the method is needed.

References

1. Damadian R (1971) Tumor detection by nuclear magnetic resonance. Science 171: 1151–1153
2. Bottomley PA, Forster TH, Argersinger RE, Pfeifer LM (1984) A review of normal tissue hydrogen NMR relaxation times and relaxation mechanisms for 1–100 MHz. Dependence on tissue type, NMR frequency, temperature, exision and age. Med Phys 11: 425–448
3. Bottomley PA, Hardy CJ, Argersinger RE, Allen-Moore G (1987) A review of 1H nuclear magnetic resonance relaxation in pathology: are T1 and T2 diagnostic? Med Phys 14: 1–37
4. Schlaps D, Räth U, Volk JF, Zuna I, Lorenz A, Lehmann KJ, Lorenz D, van Kaick G, Lorenz WJ (1985) Ultrasonic tissue characterization using a diagnostic expert system. Inf Proc Med Imaging 343–363
5. Haralick RM (1979) Statistical and structural approaches to texture. Proc IEEE 67: 786–804

Part 2

Treatment Planning

Introductory Contribution

Recent Developments in Radiation Therapy Planning

A. Brahme

Introduction

Radiation therapy is a truly multidisciplinary field in which the developments have taken place gradually and almost coherently in many different areas. This is fortunate since a chain is only as strong as its weakest link, and significant developments in one single area are not always sufficient for general improvements in overall performance.

The development of radiation therapy planning during the past decade has been enormous. We have witnessed an unprecedented improvement in three-dimensional diagnostic imaging through the advent of computed tomography (CT), magnetic resonance imaging, single photon emission computed tomography, positron emission tomograpy, and ultrasound techniques. Simultaneously we have seen a considerable improvement in dose planning systems, which now are capable of making use of this new diagnostic information and in some cases of performing true three-dimensional dose planning to improve the accuracy of delivered dose distributions. Since the middle of the 1980s there has also been a considerable improvement in computational algorithms both for electron and photon beams and for treatment optimization in general. The continued development of computer hardware has been an equally important factor in the improved performance.

Quite generally the development can be expressed by the gradual change from two- to three-dimensional therapy planning in a large number of areas of fundamental importance. These include:

- Diagnostic data and patient data
- Target volume definition
- Biological response models
- Treatment objective functions
- Energy deposition kernels
- Dose calculation algorithms
- Dose distribution measurements
- Dose optimization methods

Department of Radiation Physics, The Karolinska Institute and Stockholm University, P.O. Box 60211, 104 01 Stockholm, Sweden

Advanced Radiation Therapy Tumor Response
Monitoring and Treatment Planning
Breit (Editor-in-Chief)
© Springer-Verlag, Berlin Heidelberg 1992

- Treatment simulation
- Diagnostic data and dose display
- Patient fixation aids
- Dose delivery
- Dose verification
- Treatment follow-up

The importance of this change can be seen particularly in diagnostic areas but also in the development of three-dimensional biological response models (Wolbarst 1984; Källman et al. 1991a,b), treatment simulation with CT-augmented simulators (Webb 1990), portal imaging and dose verification with CT capabilities, and computer graphics that make the display of the new images manageable and clear (McShan and Fraass 1987). The understanding of the mechanisms behind fractionated radiotherapy has also increased considerably during the past decade, due partly to an increased knowledge of the time dependence and potential for repair in malignant and normal tissues (Thames and Hendry 1987). Until the past few years the weak link has been radiation therapy equipment capable of true three-dimensional dose delivery. However, most companies are working on various dynamic augmentations of their therapy equipment, developing dynamic asymmetric jaw movements, variable wedge-angle devices, multileaf collimators, scanning beams, and conformation therapy, making in a few cases true three-dimensional dose delivery a reality even today (Brahme 1987; Källman et al. 1988; Ishigaki et al. 1990). At present, the least developed link in the therapy chain, at least regarding commercially available systems, is probably methods capable of performing a true three-dimensional optimization of the dose delivery and the treatment technique.

Unfortunately, all the improvements mentioned here are not generally available at a single clinic and even less so from a single manufacturer, and it is probably in this respect that development will take place during the remaining decade of this century. After a short presentation of some of the most important new algorithms and approaches to treatment planning, the important area of treatment optimization will be briefly discussed.

New Algorithms for Radiation Therapy Planning

From a mathematical point of view, classical radiation therapy planning has been treated as a forward process as it tries to answer the question: how is the absorbed dose in the target volume and surrounding normal tissues distributed for a given target volume, associated patient geometry, and suggested configuration of the incident beams? This is schematically illustrated on the left of Fig. 1. Classical radiation therapy optimization is therefore generally a trial-and-error process, in which gradually improved dose plans can be found by testing an increasing number of beam configurations.

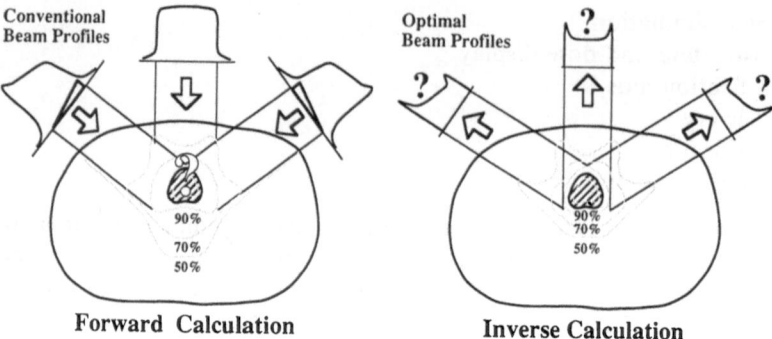

Fig. 1. Illustration of the conceptual difference between conventional forward and inverse radiation therapy planning

However, in mathematical terminology radiation therapy planning is basically an inverse problem. This is because what we really want to find is the optimal combination of incident beams for a given target volume. More exactly, the planning process should answer the question: which configuration and shape of the incident beams are best for controlling the tumor growth with minimal damage to normal tissues? This question is illustrated on the right of Fig. 1. At least on the assumption that the desired dose to the target volume or the geometric and radiobiological properties of the tumor and normal tissues of the patient are known, it should be possible to find the optimal irradiation technique (Brahme and Ågren 1987; Källman et al. 1992a, b). This conceptual difference between the classical forward calculation and the inverse approach may be further clarified by comparing the right and left sides of Fig. 1. The question marks indicate the principal quantity calculated, the isodose distribution in the patient, and the required incident beam profiles by the two methods respectively. Obviously the absorbed dose distribution in the patient is also obtained by the inverse calculation either by an ordinary forward calculation or by the inversion method itself (see Brahme et al. 1990).

Forward Calculation Algorithms

Photons and Neutrons. We look briefly first at the major improvements in forward calculational algorithms. These are summarized in Table 1 and include the transport-oriented methods for electrons (redefinition model, phase space time evolution model, bipartision model) and the direct Monte Carlo calculations (heterogeneous media calculations, treatment head simulations and beam characterization). The most important development is probably the new algorithms that are based on very accurate energy-deposition kernels generally

Table 1. New forward methods for radiation therapy planning

Kernel-based algorithms
  Photon beams
  Neutron beams

Transport oriented methods for electrons
  Redefinition model
  Phase space time evolution model
  Bipartition model

Monte Carlo calculations
  Heterogeneous media calculations
  Treatment head simulations
  Beam characterization therapy

determined by extensive Monte Carlo calculations. Such kernel-based algorithms have been developed mainly for photon and neutron beams, where they are ideally suited due to their property as indirectly ionizing particles. The basic idea involves a very accurate calculation of the energy deposition by photon or neutron interactions at a single point in soft tissue or water and then a superposition of all such energy depositions in the patient to obtain the total dose distribution. Partially integrated point kernels corresponding to physically realizable irradiation geometries such as pencil beams, planar spread sources, or isotropically converging pencil beams are sometimes used to speed up calculations. When these algorithms are fully developed, they result in a quantum leap in calculational accuracy. Today several groups are working on them (Ahnesjö 1984, 1991; Boyer and Mok 1984; Mackie and Scrimger 1984; Chui 1985; Moyers et al. 1988), and at least one is on the way to becoming commercially available. For the first time we will be able to make more accurate calculations than most experimental techniques allow, at least in quasiuniform media.

Electrons. For electron treatment planning the important development of pencil-beam algorithms in the middle 1980s has led to a renewed interest in electron therapy. For recent reviews of this field, see Brahme (1985) and Huizenga (1990). The serious limitation of all pencil-beam methods near extreme heterogeneities such as lung or air cavities and bone is almost the only remaining obstacle. A number of transport-calculation oriented methods are currently under development. Closest to clinical implementation is probably the redefinition model developed by Shui and Hogstrom (1991), in which the beam penetration is followed stepwise into the medium to account accurately for the lateral scatter at inhomogeneities. The phase space time evolution model of Huizenga and Storchi (1989) and the bipartition model developed by Luo Zhengming (1985) and Luo Zhengming and Brahme (1990) can also better handle inhomogeneities. All these models, except possibly the latter, are very time consuming, and their clinical implementation will probably still take several years. However, the very rapid development of workstation-type computers may make these more complex algorithms truly practical in a few years time. Several groups are even studying the possibility of using Monte Carlo calculations for treatment planning (Manfredotti et al. 1990; Mackie et al. 1990; Andreo 1991). However, to achieve a sufficient accuracy the above-mentioned semianalytical approaches will always be one or two orders of magnitude faster. The Monte Carlo method will remain a very important tool for the development, for example, of benchmarks for comparison with more conventional algorithms in complex geometries, to simulate treatment head geometries for accurate beam characterization and to calculate dose distribution kernels in uniform and heterogeneous media.

Inversion Methods and Optimization

General. Many of the problems in the planning and optimization of radiation therapy are linked to inverse problems, as summarized in Table 2. Among these problems are selection of the optimal source density in brachytherapy, generation of the optimal electron or photon depth dose curve by spectral combination, compensation of the beam to obtain high target dose uniformity, and generation of a desired dose distribution in the tumor by scanned beams or dynamic multileaf collimation. In recent investigations (Lind and Brahme 1985, 1987; Brahme 1988; Lind 1991) it has been shown that to shape the delivered isodose distributions in conformity with the shape of the target volume and to minimize the loading of surrounding normal tissues it is necessary to allow each incident beam to be strongly nonuniform. In general, the lateral dose distribution of the incident beam is the single most important property of the radiation field, which is still left largely unused for general optimization of the dose delivery. This is the main reason why the classical dose optimization procedures using, for example, linear or quadratic programming have not been very successful. These have generally relied only on field size, angle of incidence, and wedge angle as free beam parameters. There are several approaches to what may be called inverse radiation therapy planning.

Analytical Approaches. Among the earliest were the purely analytical approaches in which the optimal incident beam was derived using Laplace transformation under the simplifying assumption of rotational symmetry (Lax and Brahme 1982; Brahme et al. 1982). A closer look shows that the assumption of rotational symmetry is not very important (Brahme et al. 1990), but that the major problem with inverse radiation therapy is that there is generally no exact solution. This is simple to understand as the obvious problem of generating a high dose in the tumor of a patient, with zero dose everywhere else, requires

Table 2. Inverse problems in radiation therapy planning

Field	Objective	Kernel	Desired quantity	Mathematical relation
Brachytherapy	Generation of a desired dose distribution; $D(\vec{r})$	Point source dose distribution: $d_p(\vec{r})$	Optimal source density distribution: $\varphi(\vec{r})$	$D(\vec{r}) = \iiint d_p(\vec{r} - \vec{\varrho})\varphi(\vec{\varrho})d^3\varrho$
Arc and conformation therapy	Generation of a desired dose distribution: $D(\vec{r})$	Dose distribution in convergent pencil-beam point irradiation: $d_c(\vec{r})$	Point irradiation density: $F(\vec{r})$, and incident beam profile	$D(\vec{r}) = \iiint d_c(\vec{r},\vec{\varrho})F(\vec{\varrho})d^3\varrho$ Fredholm eq. of first kind
External-beam therapy	Generation of a desired depth dose curve: $D(z)$	Monocromatic depth dose curve: $d(E,z)$	optimal incident particle spectrum: Ψ_E	$D(z) = \int d(E,z)\,\Psi_E dE$ Fredholm eq. of first kind
Photon therapy	Determination of photon beam spectrum from transmission: $\Psi(z)$	Energy dependence of attenuation coefficient: $\mu(E)$	Incident photon spectrum: $\Psi_E(0)$	$\Psi(z) = \int \Psi_E(0)e^{-\mu(E)z}dE$ Fredholm eq. of first kind
Electron therapy	Determination of dose distribution from incident electron fluence: Φ_θ	Scatter distribution in a thin layer: $\varphi_{\Delta t}(\theta)$	Spatial dose and fluence distribution: $\Phi_\theta(\vec{r})$	$\Phi_\theta(\vec{r} + \Delta\vec{r}) = \int \Phi_\theta(\vec{r})\varphi_{\Delta t}(\theta-\theta')d\theta'$
Beam flattening, beam compensation	Generation of a desired lateral dose distribution: $D(x,y)$	Elementary beam dose distribution: $d(x,y)$	Optimal scanning density distribution: $F(x,y)$	$D(x,y) =$ $\iint d(x - \xi, y - \eta)F(\xi,\eta)d\xi d\eta$
Photon dose planning	Determination of dose distribution from incident photon fluence and resultant terma: $T(\vec{r})$	Mean energy imparted point spread function: $h(\vec{r})$	Resultant dose distribution: $D(\vec{r})$	$D(\vec{r}) = \iiint h(\vec{r} - \vec{\varrho})T(\vec{\varrho})d^3\varrho$
Photon dose delivery	Generation of a desired dose profile in a patient: $D(x,y)$	Dose distribution in pencil beam: $d_c(x,y)$	Fluence profile in the incident beam: $(\Phi(\xi,\eta)$	$D(x,y) =$ $\iint d_c(x - \xi, y - \eta)\Phi(\xi,\eta)d\xi d\eta$
External-beam therapy	Generation of a desired lateral dose distribution: $D(\vec{r})$	Collimated slit-beam dose distribution: $H(\vec{r})$	Collimator opening density: $F(\vec{r})$	$D(\vec{r}) = \iiint F(\vec{\varrho})H(\vec{r} - \vec{\varrho})d^3\varrho$
Dosimetry	Determination of true dose distribution from a measurement: $D_m^{(x)}$	Detector response function: $S(x)$	True dose distribution: $D(x)$	$D_m(x) = \int S(x - u)D(u)du$
Tumor imaging in nuclear medicine	Determination true uptake and increase resolution in measured distribution: $I(\vec{r})$	Point source response: $i_p(\vec{r})$	True uptake: $U(\vec{r})$	$I(\vec{r}) = \iiint i(\vec{r} - \vec{\varrho})U(\vec{\varrho})d^3\varrho$

nonphysical negative incident beams when analytical inversion methods are used (Brahme et al. 1982).

Energy Deposition Kernels. A more fruitful approach is therefore to use partially integrated irradiation geometry kernels that can be realized by external beams, as mentioned above. Even if this does not allow an absolutely strict optimization of the dose delivery, it maintains the most important degrees of freedom and allows a very far reaching dose optimization (Lind and Brahme 1985; Brahme 1988; Brahme et al. 1990; Lind 1990, 1991).

Tomography-Related Methods. The required nonuniform incident beams during the realization of the dose delivery make the technique resemble CT (see Fig. 1; Brahme 1987, 1988). This has inspired several researchers to solve the inverse problem of radiation therapy by methods from the field of CT such as filtered-back projection (Brahme et al. 1982; Cormack and Quinto 1989; Mackie et al. 1989; Holmes et al. 1991; Barth 1990; Bortfeld et al. 1990). Unfortunately, due to the very strict requirement of positivity of all delivered dose distributions make this approach less useful. However, it can be used to improve substantially the dose delivery over that achieved by classical techniques, and in combination with more traditional optimization techniques it may still be useful even if it is time consuming (Bortfeld et al. 1990). The same is true for the simulated annealing approach (see Webb 1989).

Radiobiological Approaches

One of the earliest approaches to radiobiologically optimized dose delivery was taken into clinical use by Ulsø (e.g., Ulsø and Brahme 1989). This approach is basically a compensator technique in which each field is compensated so that the probability of achieving uncomplicated tumor control is maximized for all beams together. This is a very practical technique to bring improved radiobiological data into direct clinical use. Similar biological objective functions are being developed by Niemierko et al. (1990) for optimization of dose plans.

One of the most recent contributions to the field of inverse radiation therapy planning is the approach in which the radiobiological properties of tumors and normal tissues are used to maximize the probability of achieving complication-free tumor control (P_+) by external beam radiation. From this point of view, it resembles the compensator technique. This extremely powerful approach is a combination of the irradiation geometry kernel method and a clinically very relevant biological objective function (P_+), as described in more detail elsewhere in this volume (see p. 407). The interesting property of this algorithm is that it opens the door to truly radiobiologically optimized dose delivery. This type of algorithm also has the potential to close the circle of radiotherapy development because, as gradually better dose-response data are collected from clinical trials, this algorithm allows a direct application of the new data to improve future radiation therapy.

References

Ahnesjö A (1984) Application of transform algorithms for calculation of absorbed dose in photon beams. Proc 8th Int Conf on the Use of Computers in Radiation Therapy, Toronto CA, IEE Computer Society, pp 227–230

Ahnesjö A (1991) Dose calculation methods in photon beam therapy using energy deposition kernels. Thesis, University of Stockholm

Andreo P (1991) Monte Carlo techniques in medical radiation physics. Phys Med Biol 36: 861–920

Barth N (1990) An inverse problem in radiation therapy. Int J Radiat Oncol Biol Phys 18: 425–431

Boyer A, Mok EC (1984) Photon beam modeling using Fourier transform techniques. Proc 8th Int Conf on the Use of Computers in Radiation Therapy, Toronto, pp 14–16

Bortfeld T, Bürkelbach J, Boesecke R, Schlegel W (1990) Methods of image reconstruction from projections applied to conformation radiotherapy. Phys Med Biol 35: 1423–1434

Brahme A (1985) Current algorithms for computed electron beam dose planning. Radiother Oncol 3: 347–362

Brahme A (1987) Design principles and clinical possibilities with a new generation of radiation therapy equipment. Acta Oncol 26: 401–412

Brahme A (1988) Optimizations of stationary and moving beam radiation therapy techniques. Radiother Oncol 12: 129–140

Brahme A, Ågren A (1987) Optimal dose distribution for eradication of heterogeneous tumors. Acta Oncol 26: 377

Brahme A, Roos J-E, Lax I (1982) Solution of an integral equation encountered in rotation therapy. Phys Med Biol 10: 1221–1229

Brahme A, Lind B, Källman P (1990) Inverse radiation therapy planning as a tool for 3D dose optimization. Phys Med 6: 53–63

Chui CS (1985) A method for three dimensional gamma ray dose calculations in heterogeneous media and its applications in radiation therapy. PhD Thesis, Columbia University, NY

Cormack AM, Quinto ET (1989) On a problem in radiotherapy: questions on non-negativity. Int J Imaging Systems Technol 1: 120–124

Holmes T, Mackie TR, Simpkin D and Reckwerdt P (1991) A unified approach to the optimization of brachytherapy and external beam dosimetry. Int J Radiat Oncol Biol Phys 20: 859–873

Huizenga H (1990) Electron beam dose calculation algorithms review. Proc X ICCR, Lucknow, India

Huizenga H, Storchi PRM (1989) Numerical calculation of energy deposition by broad high-energy electron beams. Phys Med Biol 10: 1371–1396

Ishigaki T, Itoh Y, Horikawa Y, Kobayashi H, Obata Y, Sakuma S (1990) Computer-assisted conformation radiotherapy. AMPI Med Phys Bull 15: 185–211

Källman P, Lind B, Eklöf A, Brahme A (1988) Shaping of arbitrary dose distributions by dynamic multileaf collimation. Phys Med Biol 33: 1291–1300

Källman P, Ågren A, Brahme A (1992a) Tumor and normal tissue responses to fractionated non-uniform dose delivery. Int J Radiat Biol (in press)

Källman P, Lind BK, Brahme A (1992b) An algorithm for maximizing the probability of complication free tumor control in radiation therapy. Phys Med Biol 37: 871–890

Lax I, Brahme A (1982) Rotation therapy using a novel high-gradient filter. Radiology 145: 473–478

Lind B, Brahme A (1985) Generation of desired dose distributions with scanned elementary beams by deconvolution methods. Proc VII ICMP, Espoo, Finland p 953

Lind B, Brahme A (1987) Optimization of radiation therapy dose distributions with scanned photon beams. Bruinvis IAD, van der Giessen PH, van Kleffens HJ (eds) Proc 9th Int Conf on the Use of Computers in Radiation Therapy. Elsevier, Amsterdam, 235–239

Lind BK (1990) Properties of an algorithm for solving the inverse problem in radiation therapy. Inverse Probl 6: 415–426

Lind BK (1991) Radiation therapy planning and optimization studied as inverse problems. Thesis, University of Stockholm

Luo Zhengming (1985) Improved bipartition model of electron transport. II. Application to inhomogeneous media. Phys Rev 32: 824–836

Luo Zhengming, Brahme A (1990) Generalization of the bipartition model to high energy electrons. Proc X ICCR, Lucknow, India

Mackie TR, Scrimger JW (1984) Computing radiation dose for high energy X-rays using a convolution method. Proc 8th Int Conf on the Use of Computers in Radiation Therapy, Toronto, pp 36–40

Mackie TR, Kubsad SS, Holmes T, Sohn W (1989) New developments in radiotherapy dose planning. Proc 17th ICR, Paris, France, p 30

Mackie TR, Sohn W, Lindstrom M, Kubsad SS, Reckwerdt PJ, Kinsella TJ (1990) The Ottawa-Madison electron gamma algorithm (Omega) project: feasibility of two Monte Carlo techniques. Proc. X ICCR, Lucknow, India

Manfredotti C, Nastasi U, Marchisio R, Ongaro C, Gervino G, Ragona R, Anglesio S, Sannazzari G (1990) Monte Carlo simulation of dose distribution in electron beam radiotherapy treatment planning. Nucl Instr Methods A 258: 1–16

McShan DL, Fraass BA (1987) Integration of multi-modality imaging for use in radiation therapy treatment planning. Lemke HU, Rhodes ML, Jaffe CC, Felix R (eds) Computer assisted radiology. Springer, Berlin Heidelberg New York, pp 300–304

Moyers MF, Horton JL, Boyer AL (1988) A scatter model for fast neutron beams using convolution of diffusion kernels. Rad Prot Dosimetry 23: 475–478

Niemierko A, Urie M and Goitein M (1990) Computer optimization of 3D radiation therapy treatment plans with biological models of tissue response. Int J Radiat Oncol Biol Phys 19 [Suppl 1]: 208

Shiu AS, Hogstrom KR (1991) Pencil-beam redefinition algorithm for electron dose distributions. Med Phys 18: 7

Thames HD, Hendry JH (1987) Fractionation in radiotherapy. Taylor and Francis, London

Ulsø N, Brahme A (1989) Computer-aided irradiation technique optimization. Proc joint US-Scandinavian Symposium on future directions of computer-aided radiotherapy. San Antonio, Texas. National Cancer Institute Bethesda MD, 20892

Webb S (1989) Optimisation of conformal radiotherapy dose distributions by simulated annealing. Phys Med Biol 34: 1349–1369

Webb S (1990) Non-standard CT scanners: their role in radiotherapy. Int J Radiat Oncol Biol Phys 19: 1589–1607

Wolbarst AB (1984) Optimization of radiation therapy. II. the critical-voxel model. Int J Radiat Oncol Biol Phys 10: 741–745

Treatment Planning: New Tools

Present Status of Computed Tomography for Radiation Therapy Planning

Introduction

Availability of Whole-Body CT Scanners for Radiotherapy

Present Status of Computed Tomography for Radiation Therapy Planning

K.-H. Hübener and M. Baumann

Introduction

When one today rereads the papers by Ling and collegues published in 1981 and the book edited by Frommhold and Hübener in 1984, one realizes that almost all the criticisms articulated 10 years ago are applicable to today's status of computed tomography (CT) for treatment planning in radiation oncology. Since 1975 several hundred papers have been published by radiooncologists and radiophysicists, presenting a variety of excellent ideas to improve hard- and software for the special needs of the radiotherapist. However, only limited effort has been made by leading companies to realize these suggestions. Credit must be given to the committed work of small and often poorly equipped groups at universities and in small companies, making possible at least in the software sector some important scientific progress in treatment planning using CT or magnetic resonance imaging (MRI). The most important reason for this disappointing situation is the fact that there is only a small market for radiation therapy hardware but a huge market for diagnostic radiology equipment. Large companies tend to invest only in public relations to boost their products. There is certainly some truth in the criticism that there is no therapeutic counterpart to increasingly sophisticated and expensive diagnostic tools.

Todays most important topics concerning CT and MRI in clinical radiation oncology are: availability of whole-body CT scanners for radiotherapy; intrinsic limitations of diagnostic CT (and MRI) information for oncology; special hardware requirements for radiooncology; software options for data acquisition and processing; and the question of whether treatment planning by CT and MRI can further enhance the results of radiation therapy.

Availability of Whole-Body CT Scanners for Radiotherapy

The use of CT information for treatment planning in radiooncology is obviously possible only if adequate hardware is available to the radiation oncologist.

Department of Radiation Therapy, University Hospital Eppendorf, Martinistr. 52, 2000 Hamburg 20, FRG

Advanced Radiation Therapy Tumor Response
Monitoring and Treatment Planning
Breit (Editor-in-Chief)
© Springer-Verlag, Berlin Heidelberg 1992

However, this is unfortunately not the case in Europe today. Only some privileged departments run their own whole-body scanner. These machines are generally of an older generation, confirming the saying that old CT scanners will be shipped either to Third World countries or, if they would not endure shipping, to the nearest radiation therapy department. Most departments, including most university hospitals, share a CT scanner with the diagnostic radiologists. As a rule of thumb, all necessary maintenance and repairs are performed during the time allotted to the radiation oncologist, and the "emergency" patient must usually also be examined during this time. It is amazing that nearly all cobalt units, which are completely sufficient tools for a variety of treatment situations, have been replaced by linear accelerators while the need of the radiation oncologist for adequate access to a modern-generation whole-body CT scanner is not even generally accepted. In part this may be due to the reservations of some diagnostic radiologists, who are suspicious that their colleagues in the radiation oncology department might misuse modern CT scanners for diagnostic purposes. However, the fact that no one uses even the latest therapy simulator for private diagnostic purposes indicates that this fear is not realistic.

In a recent analysis performed in our department, the average time needed for positioning of patients for CT, aquisition of data, adjustment of skin marks, and storing of data for photographic processing was 45 min per patient. The shortest times — about 10 min — were found in planning of treatment for endocrine orbitopathy and irradiation of the thoracic wall after ablatio mammae; the longest times — more than 90 min — were necessary for three-dimensional treatment planning. The number of scans was 4–40, depending on the complexity of the situation. From this analysis the following suggestions are made:

- Flexible times, not regular hours, should be available for CT planning.
- The CT scanner should be located where it is needed most of the time; if it is used more than half the day for treatment planning, it should be located in the radiation therapy department.
- On the average 45 min is needed per patient; additional times are required if more sophisticated techniques such as three-dimensional treatment planning and stereotactic radiosurgery are performed on a routine basis.
- On the average 1 h of CT scanner availability for treatment planning is necessary for each 200 patients per year.
- A radiotherapy department with more than 1200 new patients per year needs its own CT scanner.

Intrinsic Limitations of Diagnostic CT and MRI Information for Oncology

There is substantial enthusiasm among diagnostic radiologists over increasingly high-resolution capabilities with CT and MRI. This is of course understandable, but the critical evaluation of the relevance of this information for radiation therapy can be performed only by the radiooncologist. Neither today nor in the near future are CT or MR images likely to document the exact extension of tumors. It must be kept in mind that even pixel sizes of less than 0.2×0.2 mm yield less accurate information than a simple magnification lens, and that the fate of a patient may be determined by the geographic miss of a single clonogenic tumor cell with a diameter of about 25 μm. Important information for radiation therapy that at present cannot be obtained by any imaging method include: (a) exclusion of metastasis to lymph nodes that are not enlarged; (b) diagnosis of lymphangiosis carcinomatosa; (c) differentiation among fibrosis, tumor bed, and viable tumor; and (d) differentiation between R0 and R1 situations. There is also no possibility to determine tumor histology, tumor grading, or distant micrometastasis by imaging studies — all questions of great concern in planning radiation therapy. Thus, at present, the merits of imaging studies in treatment planning can be reduced to (a) localization of the macroscopic tumor burden and (b) localization of radiosensitive normal tissues relative to the treatment volume. Extensive and state-of-the-art use of information on those two points of interest, however, allows in many cases the application of higher doses to the tumor without increased toxicity and thereby contributes to improved local control tumor control, quality of life, and survival.

Special Hardware Requirements for Radiooncology

Lichter et al. (1981) described the optimal CT scanner for radiotherapy treatment planning as having the following features:

- Rapid scan time
- Thin slices (5 mm)
- Ability to accumulate 40–60 scans without pause
- "Scout" film — at least AP and lateral — indexed to scans
- Large aperture (> 60 cm)
- Reconstruction in any plane

Their list of the special needs of CT scanners used for therapy planning is presented in Table 1. A further feature which can easily be included is a light beam that directly projects the position of the cursor in the CT scan to the skin of the patient. This simple innovation would greatly improve the reproducibility of later field alignment in the treatment simulator. Especially for the use of three-dimensional treatment planning, stereotactic radiosurgery, and dynamic treatment using multileaf collimators, several other sophisticated features of CT and MRI scanners are urgently needed. However, as outlined above, up to now it has often not even been possible to find companies interested in discussing these special hardware requirements with the radiation oncologist.

Software Options for Data Acquisition and Processing

Also in this sector the market offers no choices that suit the requirements of modern radiotherapy departments. The most important criticism is the lack of compatibility of data obtained using CT scanners of different companies and treatment planning systems. For example, the data obtained using the Somatom Plus (Siemens) must be stored on tape, transformed, and then downloaded before any manipulations can be performed. In the near future the fully digitalized radiodiagnostic department will be a reality; at the present time two-thirds of all large radiotherapy centers in Germany must draw body contours by hand using CT scans projected on a wall — a situation hard to believe. It is of only secondary interest whether data transfer is by floppy disc, tape, or networking, but it is a major priority to obtain a consensus on data formats in imaging technology before further improvements in radiation treatment planning can be used routinely in clinical practice. Since it is expected that other digital diagnostic data will contribute increasingly to radiotherapy, it appears reasonable to integrate treatment planning devices right from the beginning into the picture archiving and communication system.

Can Treatment Planning by CT and MRI Further Enhance the Results of Radiation Therapy?

It is now well established that the use of CT has changed treatment fields for a variety of situations, compared to conventional treatment planning (Tables 1, 2). From this it is expected that local tumor control will improve. Goitein (1979) calculated that a 6%–12% increase in local tumor control should result if CT were used systematically for all treatment planning aimed at cure; their figures are as follows:

- 40% with improved coverage of tumor (40/100)
- 60% of these may achieve local control (24/40)

Table 1. Differences between diagnostic and therapy planning CT scanning

Diagnostic scanning	Therapy scanning
Rounded couch	Flat couch
Positioning not critical	Reproducibility of treatment position critical
Bolus acceptable	No bolus
Accurate reproducibility of patient geometry not necessary	Faithful one-to-one geometric reconstruction a must
No motion for best image	Quiet respiration allowed
External markings not necessary	External markings defines a coordinant system for planning

Table 2. Changes due to CT by tumor site. (From Ling et al. 1983)

Study	Thorax	Abdomen	Pelvis
Brizel et al. (1974)			61% (44/72)
Emami et al. (1978)	53% (17/32)		
Goitein et al. (1979)	44% (7/16)	86% (12/14)	44% (18/41)
Hobday et al. (1979)	30% (9/30)	79% (15/19)	31% (20/65)
Lee et al. (1980)			14% (3/14)
Munzenrider et al. (1977)	67% (14/21)	64% (16/25)	41% (7/17)
Pilepich et al. (1982)			22% (21/97)
Prasad et al. (1981)	26% (13/50)		
Schlager et al. (1979)			29% (6/21)
Seydel et al. (1980)	26% (6/23)		
Total	38% (66/172)	74% (43/58)	36% (119/327)

– 50% of these would have had local control despite poor coverage (chemotherapy, implant, etc.; 12/24)
– 50% of these will succumb to metastases (6/12)

At the same time, reduction of severe complications by overdose to sensitive structures should yield an additional benefit. Considering those tumors which are relatively resistant to radiotherapy, small-volume irradiation using the shrinking field technique offers for the first time a realistic possibility for local tumor control by radiotherapy. It appears worthwhile to organize a multicenter statistical analysis of the extent to which different features introduced to radiotherapy over the past two decades (CT treatment planning, radiobiological knowledge of altered fractionation schedules, more extended surgery) have improved the outcome of radiation treatment. Among the questions that need to be considered in this context are the following:

– Was a similar amount of effort put forth for conventional and CT planning?
– What conventional studies were used — standard radiographs, contrast material, ultrasound?
– If consecutive cases were not studied, what factors influenced case selection?
– If CT planning suggests a change in treatment planning, is it always assumed to be correct?

Rubin in his John Erskine Lecture 1984 showed that improvements in clinical medicine can often be recognized only 15–20 years after their introduction. It was 15 years ago that the first EMI and Delta scanners were used in radiotherapy, and it therefore seems time critically to assess our achievements. If we could demonstrate a significant improvement in local tumor control using CT in radiation treatment planning, this would be an enormous success not only for radiotherapy but also for clinical oncology in general. It would certainly support our demands for the development and installation of more—and more powerful—tools for radiation treatment planning.

Table 3. Changes in treatment plans as a result of CT (all sites) (from Ling et al. 1983)

Study	n	Inadequate or marginal tumor volume		Volume made smaller		Any change[a]	
		n	%	n	%	n	%
Brizel et al. (1974)	72	29	40	4	6	44	61
Emami et al. (1978)	32	10	31	2	7	17	53
Goitein (1979)	77	32	42			40	52
Hobday et al. (1979)	123	29	26	5	4	47	38
Lee et al. (1980)	22	3	14			3	14
Munzenrider et al. (1977)	75	35	47	18	24	41	55
Pilepich et al. (1982)	97	21	22			21	22
Prasad et al. (1981)	50	11	22	2	4	13	26
Schlager et al. (1979)	21	6	29			6	29
Seydel et al. (1980)	23	4	17	2	9	6	26
Van Dyk et al. (1980)	60					36	60
Total	652	180	28	33	5	274	42

[a] Volume larger or smaller, change modality, change intent, etc.

References

Brizel HE, Livingston PA, Grayson EV (1974) Radiotherapeutic applications of pelvic computed tomography. J Comput Assist Tomogr 4: 453–466

Emami B, Melo A, Carter BL, Munzenrider JE, Piro AJ (1978) Value of computed tomography in radiotherapy of lung cancer. Am J Roentgenol 131: 63–67

Frommhold W, Hübener KH (eds) (1986) Computertomographie in der Strahlentherapie. Thieme, Stuttgart

Goitein M (1979) The utility of computed tomography in radiation therapy: an estimate of outcome. Int J Radiat Oncol Biol Phys 5: 1799–1807

Goitein M, Wittenberg J, Mendiondo M, Doucette J, Friedberg C, Ferrucci J, Gunderson L, Linggood R, Shipley WV, Fineberg HV (1979) The value of CT scanning in radiation therapy treatment planning: a prospective study. Int J Radiat Oncol Biol Phys 5: 1787–1793

Hobday P, Hodson NJ, Husband J, Macdonald JS (1979) Computed tomography applied to radiotherapy treatment planning: techniques and results. Radiology 133: 477–482

Lee DJ, Leibel S, Shiels R, Sanders R, Siegelman S, Order S (1980) The value of ultrasonic imaging and CT scanning in planning radiotherapy for prostatic carcinoma. Cancer 45: 724–727

Lichter AS, Fraass BA, Geijn J.v.d., Fredrickson HA, Glatstein E (1983) An overview of clinical requirements and clinical utility of computed tomography based radiotherapy treatment planning. In: Ling CC, Rogers CC, Morton RJ (eds) Computed tomography in radiation therapy. Raven, New York

Ling CC, Rogers CC, Morton RJ (eds) (1983) Computed tomography in radiation therapy. Raven, New York

Munzenrider JE, Pilepich M, Rene-Ferrero JB, Tchakarova I, Carter BL (1977) Use of body scanner in radiotherapy treatment planning. Cancer 40: 170–179

Pilepich MV, Prasad SC, Perez CA (1982) Computed tomography in definitive radiotherapy of prostatic carcinoma. II. Definition of target volume. Int J Radiat Oncol Biol Phys 8:

Prasad SC, Pilepich MV, Perez CA (1981) Contribution of CT to quantitative radiation therapy planning. Am J Roentgenol 136: 123–128

Rubin P (1984) John Erskine Lecture, RSNA, Chicago, USA

Schlager, B, Asbell SO, BAker AS, Sklaroff DM, Seydel HG, Ostrum BJ (1979) The use of computerized tomography scanning in treatment planning for bladder carcinoma. Int J Radiat Oncol Biol Phys 5: 99–103

Seydel HG, Kutcher GJ, Steiner RM, Mohiuddin M, Goldberg B (1980) Computed tomography in planning radiation therapy for bronchogenic carcinoma. Int J Radiat Oncol Biol Phys 6: 601–606

Van Dyk J, Battista JJ, Cunningham JR, Rider WD, Sontag MR (1980) On the impact of CT scanning on radiation planning. Comp Tomogr 4: 55–65

Clinical Experience with Treatment Planning Based on Magnetic Resonance Imaging

P. Lukas

Introduction

Computed tomography (CT) is still the gold standard as imaging modality for treatment planning in radiation oncology. It yields a three-dimensional, exactly scaled matrix of quantitative data and can provide important information on radiation interaction properties correlating directly with X-ray absorption, which is essential for exact dose calculations. Its high spatial resolution often allows localization of the tumor and differentiation of organs that are close to the tumor and should be spared from irradiation. An additional advantage of CT-based treatment planning is ease of use with modern planning systems. Magnetic resonance imaging (MRI) provides spatial resolution comparable to third-generation CT scanners as well as superior soft-tissue contrast. MRI has proved particularly valuable in the depiction of neoplastic disease localized in the central nervous system, head and neck, mediastinum, pelvis, and musculoskeletal system. Although a definite role for MRI in pulmonary and abdominal imaging cannot yet be determined, the range of applications is increasing rapidly.

Preparatory Studies

We began investigating the potential of MRI for radiation therapy management in 1985. Since that time MRI has been integrated into the radiation therapy planning and therapy response control in more than 400 patients. To evaluate it as a tool for monitoring radiation therapy, we examined the changes of signal intensity in a series of 46 breast tumors in mice. Relative signal intensity was measured before and after irradiation with sublethal tumor doses in a given schedule until day 164 after irradiation. We found a high correlation between therapy-induced tumor regression (histologically confirmed denaturation and scarring) and change in MRI signal intensity. The earliest response consisted of

Institut für Strahlentherapie und Radiologische Onkologie, Technische Universität München, Klinikum rechts der Isar, Ismaninger Str. 15, 8000 Munich 80, FRG

Advanced Radiation Therapy Tumor Response
Monitoring and Treatment Planning
Breit (Editor-in-Chief)
© Springer-Verlag, Berlin Heidelberg 1992

necrosis 2–4 days after the onset of radiation therapy. The occurrence of connective tissue or poorly water-containing tissue was visualized 8–12 days postradiation with a maximum of signal decrease on days 24–40. Tumor recurrence could be found on day 164 with a diameter of more than or equal to 3 mm.

Ongoing clinical MRI studies in the course of therapy in rectal, esophageal, and gynecological cancer are confirming these results. According to our experience and that of others, MRI is helpful in detecting early recurrence in rectal carcinoma. Tumors less than 1 cm in diameter may be differentiated from adjacent radiation and surgery-induced scar plates on heavily T2-weighted sequences. No other imaging modalities — including CT and transabdominal/transrectal ultrasound — provide comparable capabilities.

Similar results were observed in our group and by others for gynecological tumors, head and neck neoplasias, and lymphatic disease. In patients with early (< 6 months) therapy-induced changes, such as tumor necrosis and substitution of tumor by granulation tissue, however, a probable increase in tissue fluids can contribute to an increase in signal intensity on T2-weighted images. It thus remains questionable whether MRI can be used to differentiate these entities from tumor recurrence in the early posttreatment stage.

We have proven that MRI is an adequate tool for radiation therapy monitoring. To answer the question whether MRI is capable of replacing CT as a method for radiation therapy planning, we simultaneously calculated dose distributions based on CT and MRI data in a commercial treatment planning system (Mevaplan, Siemens) in more than 60 studies. However, it must be noted that MRI signal intensity is not correlated with tissue absorption coefficients. Absorption coefficients for soft tissue and bone therefore had to be entered interactively for MRI data, while they could be defined automatically for CT data due to the correlation with Hounsfield units. We tested several mean absorption coefficients for MRI and found most adequate coefficients of 1.0 for soft tissue and 1.2 for bone. With these prerequisites, and with patients positioned identically for CT and MRI (on a flat CT table top), the maximum deviation of MRI from CT-based dose calculations was about 2% within the 95% confidence interval. When the original, differently shaped CT and MRI table tops were used, however, the maximum deviation was 5.6% within the 95% confidence interval. This difference includes error due to different patient positioning, to electron density inhomogeneities, and to field distortions. Under optimal conditions the maximal error in the 95% confidence interval could be decreased to 1.6%.

To check and correct for geometric distortions in MR images due to the field inhomogeneity and nonlinearities in the readout gradient, we used special phantoms consisting of tubes filled with copper sulfate. Distortions for small fields of view (up to 200 mm) we found to be less than 2%. For large fields of views (> 400 mm), the range of geometric distortions depended on the plane used. For actual planes the maximum was 3.5%, for coronal 8.3%, and for sagittal 16.2%. Field distortion must be measured in every individual MRI unit for every sequence and every plane and be corrected in coronal or sagittal plane when it is intended for use in radiation therapy planning.

Treatment Planning

There are different approaches to incorporating MRI in treatment planning. Using a projection system with geometrically exact magnification (e.g., ante-scope, Liesegang), MR images of any size can be overlaid on simulation films or isodose plans. If only AP/PA portals are needed for therapy, the contours of the target region and the critical organs can usually be delineated using short TR/short TE coronal MRI series (acquisition time 5–8 min) and can then be transferred to the simulation films. Bony anatomical landmarks, such as ver-tebrae, femoral head, and acetabulum, are crucial for exact fitting. Additional T2-weighted spin-echo or gradient-echo sequences are required when clear tumor discrimination cannot be accomplished. The projection technique in our daily routine requires 10–20 min and may be performed by a technician experienced in MRI and therapy planning. More than half of our MRI-guided therapy plans were based on this approach. Instead of using a projection system, a dual television camera setup (Subtrascope, Siemens) can be used to super-impose MRI and simulation radiographic images, and this may facilitate the procedure.

An advanced approach for MRI-guided treatment planning is the use of a fast image-postpressing system, either in combination with a separate treatment planning unit or with a fully integrated dosimetry software package. Our group is collaborating with Kontron on the latter concept and its future applications. Our goal is to use the full three-dimensional information and high tissue contrast provided by MRI sequences for treatment planning. This allows extensions of tumor, critical organs, and dose distributions to be viewed simultaneously and in arbitrary planes or, if displayed in three dimensions, for arbitrary angles.

In patients with thoracic, abdominal, or pelvic neoplasias MRI changed field extension in up to 70% of the cases when compared to conventional planning. It facilitated the definition of radiation portals with respect to the treatment volume in more than 50% of cases when compared to CT, primarily due to the availability of sagittal and coronal image planes. It improved treatment plan-ning in about 30% of cases compared to CT because of the superior tissue contrast. The usefulness of the method is not restricted to simulation of percutaneous radiation therapy. It also has major implications for the treatment planning of brachytherapy. Specially designed plastic afterloading applicators that do not induce image artifacts are positioned in situ before the imaging procedure and can be easily visualized on MR images in any desirable orienta-tion. The imaging information of the applicator position relative to tumor and critical organs serves as basis for exact dose calculation and procedure determination.

Useful Applications

According to our experience in more than 400 cases, MRI-guided treatment planning is superior to CT planning in tumors of the following regions.

Brain and Spinal Chord. Treatment planning can be done easily on the basis of CT for a number of brain tumors. When dealing with neoplasms of the posterior fossa or the craniocervical junction, however, MRI enables the therapist to delineate the abnormality exactly and to use this information for precise treatment planning. Moreover, imaging the tumor perpendicular to the assumed treatment portals provides a straightforward approach to accomplish easy treatment simulation. If required, T2-weighted sequences or administration of Gd-DTPA may deliver sufficient contrast to discriminate tumor from brain edema and may possibly prevent the radiation oncologist from using more extended fields.

Head and Neck. We consider MRI the superior approach for treatment planning in head and neck tumors on account of its power to depict not only space-occupying processes but also small neoplastic extensions and infiltration of normal tissue. If certain imaging parameters are used, such as inversion recovery multislice sequences, MRI provides a unique and sensitive screening technique for abnormal lymph nodes. The exact depiction of tumor and lymph node metastases is essential for the planning of electron or photon boost irradiation.

Musculoskeletal and Soft Tissue. Due to high sensitivity for tumor invasion into adjacent structures and for peripheral edema of soft-tissue tumors, MRI is the only approach to adequately simulate radiation therapy. Perifocal edema in soft-tissue tumors must be considered ill defined, and therefore field enlargements result more often when MRI rather than CT is used for treatment planning. We perform MRI routinely as a basis for treatment management in neoplasias of the axial skeleton and of large bones of the extremities. In a 2-year study of 100 patients in our institution, we compared MRI to conventional radiographs, bone scans, and CT (if available) with respect to the maximum tumor involvement and extent. In over 40% of cases MRI changed the therapeutic management due to tumor extensions not seen in other imaging modalities. We discovered that short TR/short TE spin-echo sequences in combination with T2*-weighted gradient-echo sequences (total acquisition time about 10 min) provide sufficient information for treatment management.

Pelvis. Based on the large quantity of available data on MRI of the pelvis, it is apparent that this is the imaging modality of choice for depiction and staging of many tumors in the male and female pelvis. In our experience, MRI is useful particularly for radiation treatment planning in tumors of uterine origin because tumor extensions and lymph node involvement can be readily assessed with high contrast and in multiplanar display. It has not yet been proven whether MRI is superior to CT in the diagnosis of prostatic carcinoma except for the depiction of tumoral invasion of the prostatic capsule and the seminal vesicles. In the management of tumors of the bladder, MRI fully replaces invasive techniques such as catheterization to determine residual urine and retrograde opacification of the bladder lumen. The extraluminal tumor mass can easily be appreciated and included in the therapy plan. Another important pelvic application of MRI concerns recurrent rectal carcinoma. The role of MRI for its depiction is discussed below. However, the exact differentiation of the recurrence from postoperative scarring, not provided by CT, is the clue to adequate radiation therapy.

Large Fields. MRI is a valuable tool when extended fields must be used for treatment, for example, in lymphomas or seminomas. It provides information about the size and location of lymph nodes as well as anatomical information about the location and contours of important organs such as spleen, kidneys, bladder, and the large blood vessels. If an abdominal bandage and intravenous glucagon or butyl-scopolamine derivatives are used, movement artifacts due to respiration and peristalsis can be reduced considerably, resulting in high image quality. All important information is usually obtained with a single, large field-of-view sequence (10-min acquisition time) and can easily be used for field design and beam blocking in regions of critical organs.

Future Developments

The ultimate clinical value of MRI in radiation therapy management should be determined by further comparative and prospective studies. As with any new technique, advantages must be weighed against limitations and costs. However, the preliminary experience gained so far indicates that MRI offers a promising and exceptionally versatile tool in treatment planning and evaluation of tumor response or recurrence.

In treatment planning, special attention must be focused on quality control of the imaging equipment. For instance, geometric distortions in MR images of an individual scanner must be analyzed and documented. Suitable algorithms can then be employed for compensation.

Current and future developments include the implementation of automatic or semiautomatic contour-finding algorithms to facilitate the input of absorption coefficients and a real three-dimensional treatment planning system by use of simultaneous multiplanar reconstructions or three-dimensional display based on 1 mm^3 isotropic voxels of three-dimensional Fourier transform data sets.

In a number of centers worldwide, efforts are being directed toward new hardware and software developments to make treatment planning with MRI an easy and most adequate technique in radiation oncology — which may eventually be integrated into the network of modern image archiving and communication systems. In addition, if three-dimensional rendering of MRI data is used, volumetric quantification of neoplastic tissue will possibly provide new diagnostic and therapeutic information to the oncologist that may supplement the biochemical information provided by MR spectroscopy.

Treatment Planning:
Biological Models

Application of Radiation-Biological Data for Dose Optimization in Radiation Therapy

A. Brahme, B.K. Lind, and P. Källman

Introduction

From a mathematical point of view, radiation therapy planning is in principle an inverse problem. This is because with a given target volume one wants to find the optimal combination of incident beams. More exactly, the planning process should answer the question: for a given target volume and location of surrounding organs at risk, which configuration and shape of the incident beams are best for controlling tumor growth and minimizing damage to normal tissues? At least on assumption that the geometric and radiobiological properties of the tumor and of the patient are known, it should be possible to find the optimal irradiation technique [1]. Classical radiation therapy planning, however, is essentially a forward process: for a given configuration of the incident beams and associated patient geometry, what does the dose distribution in the target volume and surrounding normal tissues look like? Conventional therapy planning is therefore by necessity a trial-and-error process in which gradually improved dose plans may be found by iteratively testing an increasing number of beam configurations. However, inverse therapy planning results directly in an optimized dose plan for a given irradiation technique. Optimal incident beams in this context generally mean those beams that deposit the smallest possible dose in normal tissues outside the tumor. Recent general solutions to this inverse problem have the potential of greatly improving the dose delivery, especially in the treatment of large, complex, or deep-seated target volumes. However, they rely on the assumption that the best possible dose distribution in the target volume can be specified by the prescribing physician.

The new algorithm presented here is based rather on knowledge of the dose-response relationships for the tumor and surrounding normal tissues and on the accurate delineation of target volume and possible organs at risk. From these basic volume and dose-response relationships the algorithm optimizes the incident beam profiles and directions such that the probability of achieving complication-free tumor control is maximized. Today we are gradually obtaining better information about the dose-response relationships for many tumors

Department of Radiation Physics, The Karolinska Institute and Stockholm University, P.O. Box 60211, 104 01 Stockholm, Sweden

Advanced Radiation Therapy Tumor Response
Monitoring and Treatment Planning
Breit (Editor-in-Chief)
© Springer-Verlag, Berlin Heidelberg 1992

and most normal tissues. Therefore this new algorithm will allow a more accurate and biologically based optimization of the delivered dose distributions. In general there is a need to consider in detail both the volume irradiated and the sensitivity and heterogeneity of the normal tissues as well as the tumor. The volume dependence of the radiation response of the tumor is fairly simple to handle as it depends basically on the eradication of all clonogenic tumor cells. From a structural point of view, the tumor is therefore a perfect parallel tissue because all clonogenes must be eliminated to control the tumor. The problem with the response of the tumor is rather to know the radiation sensitivity of the most resistant clonogenic cells. Today it is well known that they dominate the result of therapy. Furthermore, it has recently been shown that even if they make up only as little as 10^{-4} of the clonogenes, their distribution will completely determine the shape of the optimal dose distribution and the required dose level for tumor eradication [2]. Normal tissues cannot be well described simply by a parallel infrastructure, and injury is normally induced well before all stem cells are eradicated. Models for normal tissue reactions must therefore consider the higher complexity of normal tissue organization.

In the most general case the algorithm can even take the varying cell density of the tumor and surrounding normal tissue into account. Today the cell density of the tumor and normal tissues can be quantified using positron or single photon emission computed tomography. In some cases it may also be possible to use ordinary computed tomography or magnetic resonance imaging to quantify the cell densities. With such data available a very strict dose optimization should be possible with minimal clinical uncertainty. It is also clear that as various predictive assays for radiation sensitivity of the tumor and normal tissues are being developed, such data can be used directly in the dose optimization process. As better predictive assays and dose-response models for tumors and normal tissues are being developed, the present algorithm allows a very strict biological optimization of the delivered dose distribution during radiation therapy.

Classical Dose-Response Relationships

Traditionally a large number of different mathematical functions have been used to describe the dose-response relationship for tumors and normal tissues. To allow a straightforward comparison of them we write them here in a standard format using only the 50% control or complication dose (D_{50}) and the maximum value of the normalized dose response gradient (γ) as descriptors. The probit, logit, and Poisson models, respectively, they take the forms:

$$P(D) = \tfrac{1}{2}\left\{ 1 - \operatorname{erf}\left[\sqrt{\pi}\gamma\left(1 - \frac{D}{D_{50}}\right)\right]\right\} \tag{1}$$

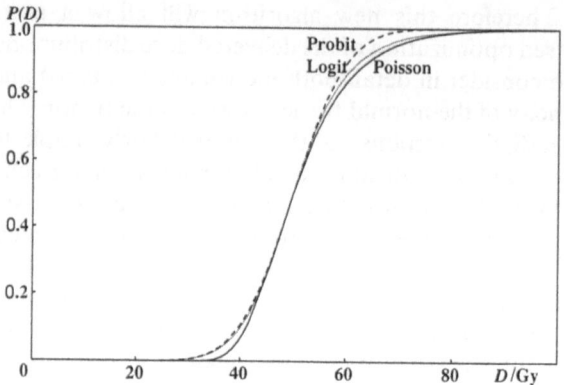

Fig. 1. The three different dose-response curves based on Eqs. 1–3. *Dashed curve*, probit; *dotted curve*, logit; *solid curve*, Poisson expression. In this case $D_{50} = 50$ Gy, and $\gamma = 2.5$

$$P(D) = \left[1 + \left(\frac{D_{50}}{D} \right)^{4\gamma} \right]^{-1} \tag{2}$$

$$P(D) = 2 - e^{[e^{\gamma}(1 - D/D_{50})]} \tag{3}$$

It is only the last of these models which has a strict radiobiological background since it is based on the Poisson statistical model of cell kill. The probit and, in particular, the logit model have a shape of the response curve which rather well approximates that of the radiobiologically more relevant Poisson model. The merit of the probit model is that it is most simple to use when calculating the influence of dosimetric and biological uncertainties [2–4]. The probit and logit models also are mathematically easier to use when analyzing a large clinical material, but less desirable as these models are not biologically coherent [5]. An example is the point at which the normalized dose response gradient $\gamma = D \cdot dP/dD$ has its maximum value just above D_{50} for the probit model and precisely at D_{50} for the logit model but just above the 37% probability level for the Poisson model (see Fig. 1).

Volume Dependence of Dose-Response models

The effect of irradiating an entire tumor or organ at risk with a homogeneous dose is described by the dose-response relationships given above (Eqs. 1–3). Normally only a fraction of each organ is irradiated at a high dose, a situation which cannot be directly covered by these equations. To calculate the injury caused by partial irradiation, the organ could be divided into a structure of sensitive subunits. The classical model treats a tumor as a completely uniform and parallel tissue, so the probability to control a fraction of the whole tumor volume ($v = V/V_{ref}$) of known response $P(1)$ for the reference volume $V_{ref}(v = 1)$ is given by:

$$P(v) = [P(1)]^v \tag{4}$$

For the Poisson model (Eq. 3) the dose- and volume-dependent expression becomes especially simple:

$$P(D, v) = 2 - e^{[e\gamma(1 - D/D_{50}) + \ln v]} \tag{5}$$

This expression may be rewritten to express the volume dependence of the γ and D_{50} values:

$$P(D, v) = 2 - e^{[e\gamma_v (1 - D/D_{50,v})]} \tag{6}$$

where

$$\gamma_v = \gamma\left(1 + \frac{\ln v}{e\gamma}\right) \tag{7}$$

and

$$D_{50,v} = D_{50}\left(1 + \frac{\ln v}{e\gamma}\right) \tag{8}$$

This illustrates the fact that the normalized dose-response gradient increases with the logarithm of the volume or the number of tumor cells [3] and so does the dose, yielding 50% control probability [2]. These relationships derived for tumors which have an accurately parallel tissue organization may be generalized to approximate the volume dependence also for normal tissues (which may have partly serial structure) by inserting a constant (k) in front of the logarithmic terms in Eqs. 5, 7, and 8. For normal tissue Eq. 5 may thus be generalized to:

$$P(D, v) = 2 - e^{[e\gamma(1 - D/D_{50}) + k \ln v]} \tag{9}$$

The constant k is equal to unity for tumors but generally has a more or less negative value for normal tissues depending on the internal organization and seriality of the tissue. This effect is obtained because when a smaller volume of normal tissue is irradiated, the risk of injury decreases, which is artificially handled in Eq. 9 by increasing the colonogen number $N_0 (\ln N_0 \approx e\gamma)$ [3]. Data on γ, k, and D_{50} for some representative tissues are given in Table 1 by fitting to some recent clinical data [6].

To obtain a more realistic description of the radiation sensitivity of a structured organ it may be divided into subcompartments. Methods for describing an organ as composed by a number of subcompartments has been discussed by several workers. Morphologically, the elementary compartment can be structurally well defined or undefined. The term "functional subunit" [7] is well suited for structurally well-defined tissue compartments such as the nephron, but for structurally quasihomogeneous tissues such as the skin the "tissue-rescuing unit" [8] or the "regenerative unit" [9] is a more valid descriptor. For further details on the mathematical model employed the reader is referred to the recent work of Källman et al. [10].

Table 1. Radiobiological data for the cervix tumor and associated normal tissues

Tissue	D_{50}/Gy	γ	k
Cervix tumor	52	4	1
Lymph nodes	39	3	1
Rectum	55	3	
Bladder	80	3	-2.9
Small bowel	80	1.5	

Complication-Free Tumor Control

To judge the clinical merits of a given dose distribution it is important to be able to compare its advantages in terms of tumor control with its disadvantages in the form of normal tissue complications. In the general case this is very hard to do as the tissue effects generally are incomparable entities. However, for fatal normal tissue injuries that cannot be salvaged by surgery a strict comparison is possible, as this end point is as undesirable as an irresectable tumor recurrence. For this special case it was shown by Ågren et al. [1] that the probability of tumor control without fatal complications, P_+, may be expressed by:

$$P_+ = P_B - P_I + \delta P_I (1 - P_B) \tag{10}$$

where the probability of benefit (P_B) is the tumor control probability and that of injury (P_I) is the probability of normal tissue complications. The parameter $\delta(\approx 0.2)$ specifies the fraction of patients in whom benefit and injury are statistically independent endpoints. Here P_B and P_I could be taken from Eq. 9.

The Inversion Algorithm

Optimization of the delivered dose distribution in radiation therapy can be performed to very different degrees of sophistication. Brahme et al. [11] developed an optimization procedure that minimizes the discrepancy between desired and resultant dose distributions and always avoids underdosage. The present algorithm, rather, maximizes a biological objective function, namely the probability of achieving complication-free tumor control, as defined above by Eq. 10. An objective function of this kind can be maximized by various procedures, for example, least-squares search or randomized procedures such as stimulated annealing. With the present algorithm P_+ from Eq. 10 is maximized directly by an effective gradient method. The resultant dose distribution from an elementary kernel $h(r, r')$ and a kernel density $f(r')$ can be described by a

Fredholm equation of the first kind:

$$D(r) = \int h(r, r')f(r')\, dr' \tag{11}$$

If the kernel h is assumed to be spatially invariant, i.e., $h(r, r') = h(r - r')$, Eq. 11 becomes a convolution integral,

$$d = Hf \tag{12}$$

where a matrix notation is used so that lowercase boldface letters denote column vectors and uppercase letters denote operators or their matrix representation. Thus H is a convolution operator represented by a positive definite matrix constructed from the kernel h. For a given desired dose distribution $D(r)$ the optimal kernel density, f_∞ is calculated with an iterative procedure, using the following algorithm:

$$f_{k+1} = C[f_k + a(d - Hf_k)] \tag{13}$$

or, which may be rewritten as:

$$f_{k+1} = C[f_k - a\nabla_f F(f_k)] \tag{14}$$

where

$$F(f_k) \equiv \tfrac{1}{2} f_k^T H f_k - f_k^T d \tag{15}$$

According to the Kuhn-Tucker theorem, it can be shown that F is minimized by the limit value f_∞ of the iterative schemes in Eqs. 13 and 14 [12, 13]. If, instead of trying to generate a desired dose distribution $D(r)$, we want to generate the dose distribution which maximizes P_+ or minimize $1 - P_+$ we only need to replace F above by $-P_+(d) = -P^+(Hf)$ according to:

$$f^{k+1} = C(f^k + a\nabla_f P_+(d_k)) \tag{16}$$

where C is the positivity constraint operator assuring that the kernel density remains nonnegative. Here the gradient of P_+ can be expanded using the chain rule and Eq. 12, since:

$$\nabla_f P_+(d) = \frac{\partial d}{\partial f}\frac{\partial P_+(d)}{\partial d} = \frac{\partial Hf}{\partial f}\nabla_d P_+(d)H\nabla_d P_+(d) \tag{17}$$

It is now possible to write Eq. (16) as:

$$f^{k+1} = C(f^k + aH\nabla_d P_+) \tag{18}$$

which contains the gradient of P_+ with respect to the dose and a convolution that can easily be calculated with fast Fourier transform routines. For further details the reader is referred to Källman et al. [14] and Lind [13].

Clinical Application

We now apply this algorithm on an advanced cervix cancer. Figure 2 illustrates the primary cervix tumor (Fig. 2a) and the target volume due to lymphatic

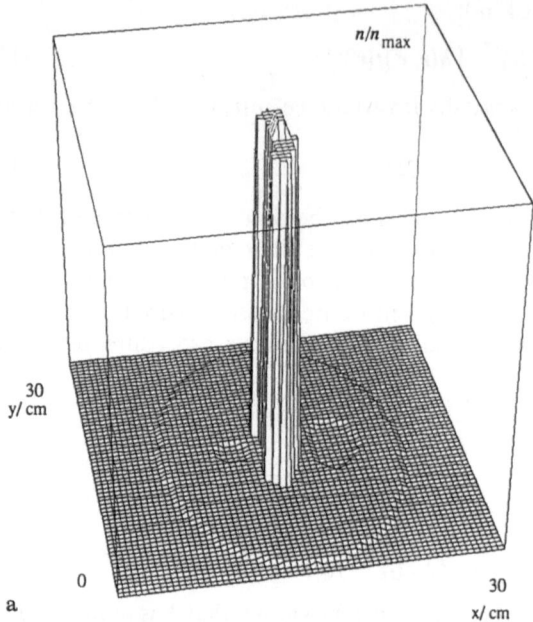

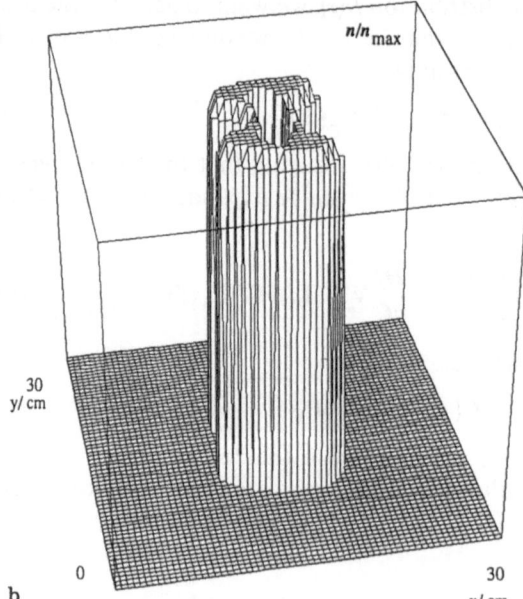

Fig. 2. **a** The primary target volume for a cervix tumor. Also seen by relief effect are the organs at risk: rectum and bladder. **b** The secondary target volume including the locally involved lymph nodes. Everything outside the mentioned organs are considered to be small bowel

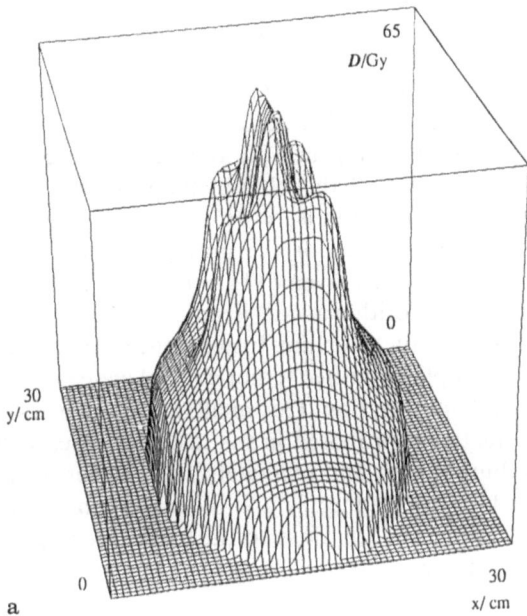

a

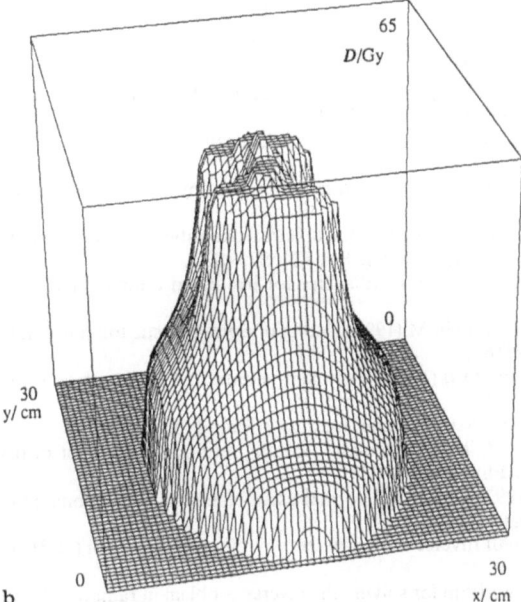

b

Fig. 3. a The resultant optimal dose distribution with the biological algorithm ($P_+ = 0.91$). By comparison with Fig. 2 it is seen that the dose on the rectal side is lowered to reduce complications in the most sensitive organ. **b** This figure is analogous to **a** but pertains to a desired dose distribution given by targets $1 + 2$ in Fig. 2 ($P_+ = 0.87$; see [11]). It is interesting to note that the dose distribution in **a** has a smoother shape than that in **b** because of the restrictions imposed by the steps in the desired dose from Fig. 2

spread (Fig. 2b). Also included in Fig. 2a are the organs at risk, rectum, bladder, and the small bowel. These tissues are described in our calculations by the approximate clinical data in Table 1 (see Eq. 9). With these parameters as input to P_+ (the probability of achieving complication-free tumor control) the algorithm above has been used to optimize P_+. The presently used dose distribution kernel h is that produced by a 10-MeV pencil photon beam rotated 360° around isocenter in the rotational plane of the photon target of the rotary gantry. The resultant optimal dose distribution $d_\infty = Hf_\infty$ is shown in Fig. 3a. For comparison, the analogous distributions for the previously treated case when the desired dose distribution $D(r)$ was given [11], are shown in Fig. 3b. From these figures it is clear that the algorithm avoids irradiating the rectal side of the lymph nodes to a high dose to protect rectum. Instead, the bladder side is given a slightly higher dose. The complication-free tumor control increases from about 87% to 91% with biological optimization. This small improvement is due partly to the rather advanced treatment proposed in the reference case, with a desired nonuniform dose distribution with approximately 10% higher dose to the primary tumor than to the surrounding lymph nodes. With a more conventional reference case assuming uniform dose to the target the improvements would in general be much larger.

References

1. Ågren A, Brahme A, Turesson I (1990) Optimization of uncomplicated control for head and neck tumors. Int J Radiat Oncol Biol Phys 19: 1077–1085
2. Brahme A, Ågren A (1987) Optimal dose distribution for eradication of heterogeneous tumors. Acta Oncol 26: 377
3. Brahme A (1984) Dosimetric precision requirements in radiation therapy. Acta Radiol Oncol 23: 379–391
4. Lindborg L, Brahme A (1990) Influence of microdosimetric quantities on observed dose-response relationships in radiation therapy. Radiat Res 124: S23–S28
5. Porter EH (1980) The statistics of dose/cure relationships for irradiated tumours, part I. Br J Radiol 53: 210–227
6. Burman C, Kutcher GJ, Emami B, Goitein M (1991) Fitting of normal tissue tolerance data to an analytic function. NCI-CM-47316
7. Withers HR, Taylor JMG, Maciejewski B (1988) Treatment volume and tissue tolerance. Int J Radiat Oncol Biol Phys 14: 751–759
8. Hendry JH, Thames HD (1986) The tissue-rescuing unit. Br J Radiol 59: 628–630
9. Archambeau JO, Shymko RM (1988) Tissue population configuration as a modifier of organ response. Int J Radiat Oncol Biol Phys 15: 727–734
10. Källman P, Ågren A, Brahme A (1992) Tumor and normal tissue responses to fractionated nonuniform dose delivery. Int J Radiat Biol (In press)
11. Brahme A, Lind B, Källman P (1990) Inverse radiation therapy planning as a tool for 3D dose optimization. Phys Med 6: 53–63
12. Lind BK (1990) Properties of an algorithm for solving the inverse problem in radiation therapy. Inverse Prob 6: 415–426
13. Lind BK (1991) Radiation therapy planning and optimization studied as inverse problems. Thesis, University of Stockholm
14. Källman P, Lind BK, Brahme A (1992) An algorithm for maximizing the probability of complication free tumor control in radiation therapy. Phys Med Biol 37: 871–890

Elimination of Artefactual Distribution in Bone Marrow

Introduction

Radioimmunotherapy is a potentially useful therapeutic tool in achieving a uniform dose. The dose distribution within the target volume around the radioactive point sources. This is due to the rapid dose fall-off around these sources. In this paper we confine ourselves to the problem of finding the optimal dose from the variation of given source position and orientation.

Material and Methods

A serious problem in radioimmunotherapy is to eradicate all cancerous tumor cells. To minimize the radiation therapy there is a certain fraction of this may be lost by the surviving fraction of tumor cell, within the total volume around the position of the point sources, a decrease in the crystallization cell can always be removed by simply increasing the dose. However, at the same time the method employed is limited by the total dose. Therefore it seems necessary to introduce some kind of normalization of one wants to compare different activity of the same distribution in different regions. By taking the number of activity is given by the well is expressible in other words by the product $(A \times t)$ of activity (A) and irradiation time (t). If we have two different sources with different dwell times these can be normalized to one:

$$A = \frac{n \cdot A_s}{V \cdot t}$$

where n is the number of sources, A_s is the activity of a source, and t is the dwell time. If a source is such a measured quantity for a given activity distribution, within the surrounding tissue per tumor cell, within the target volume V. The size of the

Optimization of Activity Distribution in Brachytherapy*

P. Kneschaurek, C. Hugo, and R. Wehrmann

Introduction

Optimization in brachytherapy is a very complex process. The usual goal of achieving a homogeneous dose distribution within the target volume cannot be reached using point or line sources. This is due to the rapid dose fall-off around these sources. In this paper we confine ourselves to the problem of finding optimal dwell times for the source(s) of given source positions and target volumes.

Material and Methods

A Measure of Quality for a Given Activity Distribution. The ultimate goal in radiation therapy is to eradicate all clonogenic tumor cells (Thames et al. 1983). Because cell killing is a stochastic process, this means that the surviving fraction of tumor cells within the target volume should be as low as possible. In principle, a decrease in the survival fraction (SF) can always be achieved by simply increasing the dose. However, in clinical practice this method is limited by normal tissue tolerance. Therefore it seems necessary to introduce some kind of normalization if one wants to compare different activity or dose distributions. In classical radium therapy this normalization is given by the well-known *mghr*, in other words by the product (AT) of activity (A) and irradiation time (T). If we have multiple sources with different dwell times, this can be generalized to give:

$$AT := \sum_{i=1}^{n} A_i T_i$$

where n is the number of sources, A_i is the activity of source i, and T_i is the dwell time of source i. As a measure of quality for a given activity distribution, we use the survival rate for tumor cells within the target volume. For the sake of

Institut für Strahlentherapie und Radiologische Onkologie, Technische Universität München, Klinikum rechts der Isar, Ismaninger Strasse 15, 8000 Munich 80, FRG
* This research was supported in part by Deutsche Forschungsgemeiuschaft grant Br-678/6-1.

Advanced Radiation Therapy Tumor Response
Monitoring and Treatment Planning
Breit (Editor-in-Chief)
© Springer-Verlag, Berlin Heidelberg 1992

simplicity we take a simple exponential dose-response curve:

$$sf = \exp[-\alpha \times D(r)]$$

However, in principle a more realistic and more complicated survival curve $sf[D(r)]$ could be used alternatively. To calculate the mean SF one must know the tumor cell distribution $n(r)$ within the target volume. Usually this distribution is not known, and a constant tumor cell density n_0 is assumed. Therefore the general formula for the surviving fraction SF:

$$SF = \frac{1}{N} \times \int_V sf[D(r)] \times n(r)\, dV$$

where N is the number of tumor cells and V is the target volume, can be simplified and yields:

$$SF = \frac{1}{V} \times \int_V \exp\{-\alpha \times [D(r)]\, dV\}$$

The dose distribution can be calculated straightforwardly if the positions, activities, and dwell times of the sources are known. Using an afterloading technique with a single stepwise moving source of activity and assuming the inverse quadratic law to be valid for this source, the dose distribution is given by:

$$D(r) = \sum_{i=1}^{n} \Gamma \times A \times t_i / (r - r_i)^2$$

where r_i is the position of stopping point i, t_i is the dwell time at stopping point i, and Γ is the activity to dose conversion factor for the used isotope. In this case, keeping AT (the equivalent to the classical $mghr$) constant means that the total irradiation time is constant.

Correlations Between Dose Values and Surviving Fractions. Assuming that SF is a reasonable measure of quality, we tried to determine whether different dose values (which might be easier to calculate than SF) can give a good approximation for the quality of a given dose distribution. We calculated the mean volume dose D_V, the mean surface dose D_S, and the minimal target dose D_{min} for randomly distributed sources within a spherical target volume with a radius of 2 cm. The radiosensitivity parameter was assumed to be $1/\alpha = 2$ Gy. We investigated two different types of source arrangements: one consisting of 10 sources, each with an activity of 37 GBq, and the other consisting of 100 sources with an activity of 3.7 GBq. The irradiation time was 1000 s in both cases; therefore the normalization factor AT was the same. The calculation was performed for an ^{192}Ir source. Figure 1 shows the results of the calculation. Obviously neither D_V nor D_S correlate with SF, but there is a strong correlation between SF and D_{min}. This shows clearly that the "cold spots" of a dose distribution have a great influence on the value of SF. Because of the inverse quadratic law, the local minima of the dose distribution are quite flat. Therefore, the "cold spots" have a considerable spatial extension.

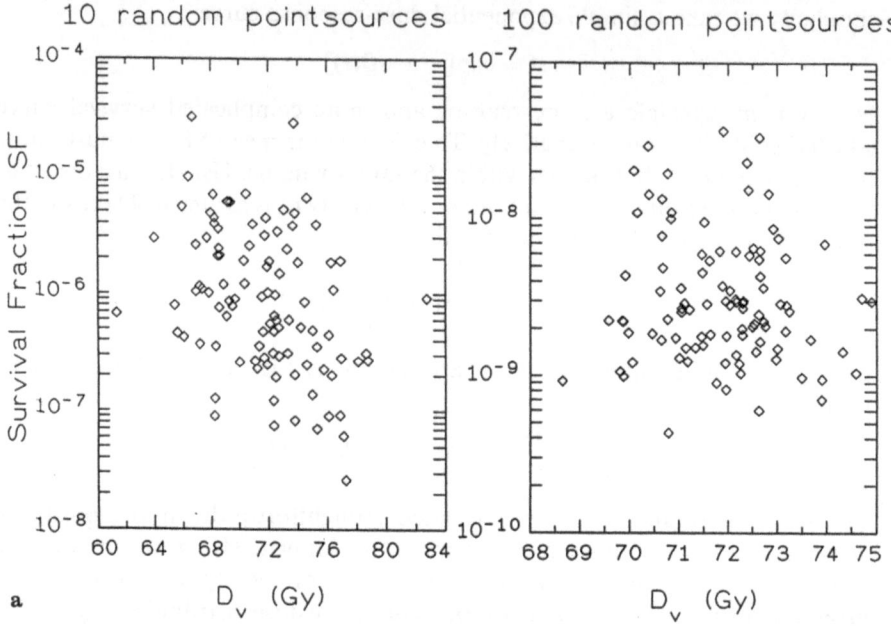

a

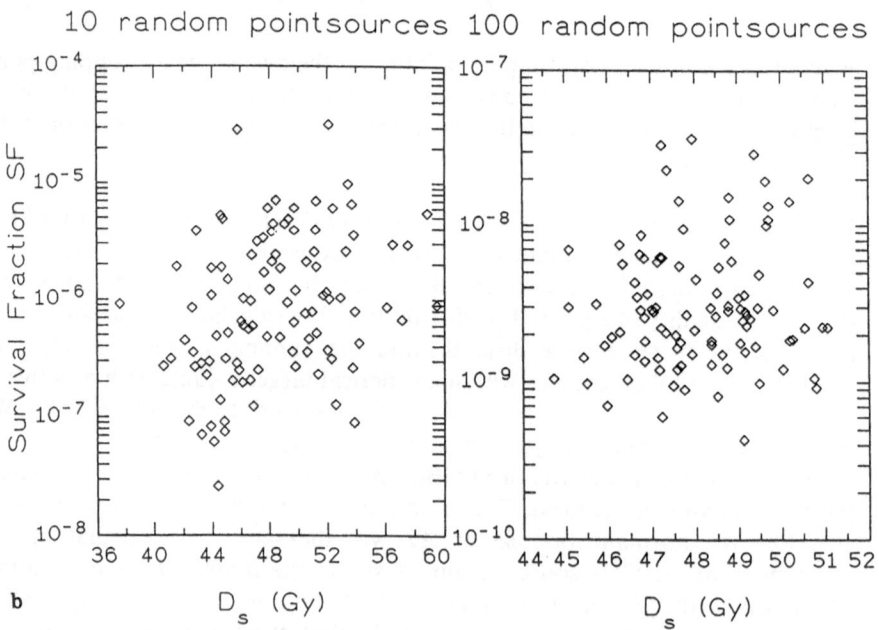

b

Fig. 1. (a) and (b).

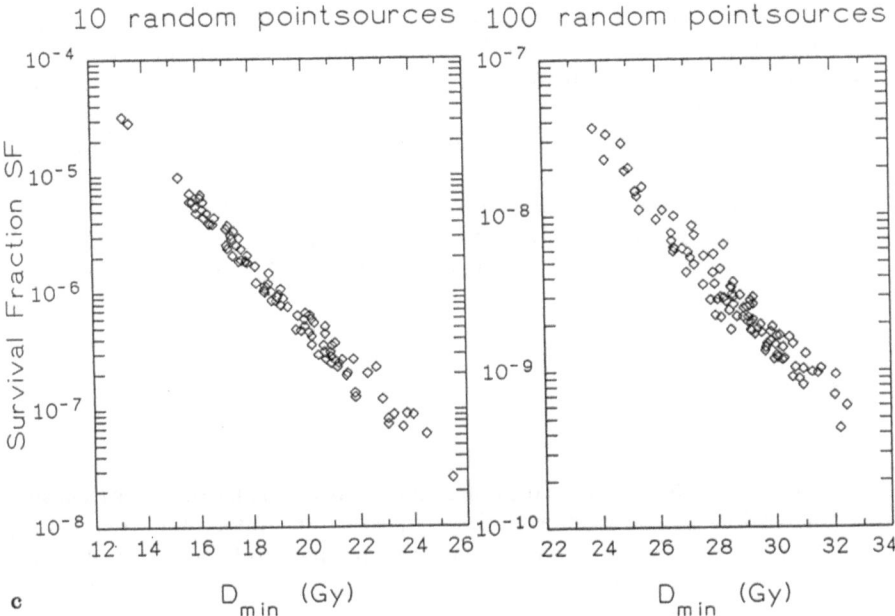

Fig. 1. Surviving fraction (SF) as a function of the mean volume dose (D_V; **a**), mean surface dose (D_S; **b**), and minimum dose (D_{min}; **c**) for a sphere with a radius of 2 cm. The constant $1/\alpha$ in the exponential surviving curve is assumed to be $1/\alpha = 2$ Gy. *Left*, the results for 100 different arrangements of sources. Each arrangement consists of 10 sources with an activity of 37 GBq. The sources have a random distribution inside the sphere. *Right*, the corresponding results for 100 sources with an activity of 3.7 GBq. The total irradiation time is 1000 s.

Optimization of Dwell Times. Numerous methods (Anderson 1985; Busch 1984; Wehrmann and Kneschaurek 1987) have been described for optimizing the dwell time in afterloading brachytherapy. In this paper we compare the results of the different algorithms.

In the case of constant dwell times, the dwell times at the different source positions are equal. The dwell time is calculated simply by dividing the total irradiation time by the number of stopping points.

There are various methods described in the literature for fitting the dose to prescribed values at reference points (Busch 1984; Tölli and Ragnhult 1987). We used a method which minimizes the sum of the logarithmic ratios of the resultant and prescribed dose values (Wehrmann and Kneschaurek 1987). When using these methods, the resulting normalization factor (AT) in general depends on the position and number of reference points.

As we have shown, D_{min} is strongly correlated with SF. We developed an algorithm which maximizes D_{min} for given source positions, target volume, and normalization factor (Wehrmann and Kneschaurek 1988). This algorithm works as follows. The total time of irradiation (T) is divided into m equal time portions: $t = T/m$ ($m = 1000$ is a reasonable choice). The first time portion refers to the source position closest to the center of the target volume. The resulting dose distribution is calculated, the minimum within the target volume is determined, and the next time portion refers to the source position closest to the dose minimum. This procedure is repeated $m - 1$ times until all time portions refer to source positions.

An algorithm has been developed which minimizes the surviving fraction. This algorithm is described elsewhere (Wehrmann et al. 1991). In principle, the method is similar to the method of simulated annealing (Webb, this volume).

Results

To demonstrate the quality of the different optimization algorithms, we chose an example which is close to a clinical situation, the interstitial treatment of prostatic carcinoma. The target volume was assumed to be a sphere of 4 cm in diameter. Six almost parallel needles were placed into the target. In each needle five stopping points at a distance of 1 cm were allowed. An ^{192}Ir source with an activity of 370 GBq was used. The total irradiation time was 1000 s. The radiation sensitivity α of the tumor cells was assumed to be $1/\alpha = 2$ Gy.

Constant Dwell Times. In total there were $6 \times 5 = 30$ stopping points. Therefore the individual dwell time was 33.3 s. As in all the following cases, all calculations were done on a cubic grid with $80 \times 80 \times 80$ points. The distance between two neighboring points was 4 cm/80 = 0.5 mm. Because of the very nonlinear behavior of SF, the approximate result for SF depends to a large degree on the grid constant. Therefore we developed a numerical procedure which allows a calculation of lower and upper limits for the exact value of SF. The mathematical details of our method are discussed elsewhere (Wehrmann 1991). For the given source geometry the minimal dose was $D_{min} = 22.06$ Gy; for SF we found $1.25 \times 10^{-7} < SF < 1.34 \times 10^{-7}$.

Fitting the Dose to Prescribed Values at Reference Points. We investigated two different sets of reference points. The first set consisted of six points on the surface of the target volume which formed a regular octahedron. The second set consisted of the same points plus eight additional points on the surface of the target. The reference dose on these positions was chosen as 30.75 Gy. This value corresponds to a single central source with 370 GBq and 1000 s dwell time. For the first set (six reference points) the optimization method for the dwell times yielded the prescribed dose values exactly. For the second set (14 reference points) this was not the case. Another remarkable difference is the fact that the sum of the dwell times in the first case was 1050 s compared to 893 s in the second case. The survival rates were $7.84 \times 10^{-9} < SF < 8.46 \times 10^{-9}$ and

$1.85 \times 10^{-7} <$ SF $< 1.98 \times 10^{-7}$, respectively. The minimal doses were 27.68 Gy and 22.28 Gy, accordingly. With the individual dwell times of the two cases increased or decreased proportionally in such a way that the total irradiation time was 1000 s, the survival rates were $1.69 \times 10^{-8} <$ SF $< 1.83 \times 10^{-8}$ and $3.94 \times 10^{-8} <$ SF $< 4.21 \times 10^{-8}$, which are much now closer. The minimum doses were 26.36 Gy and 24.92 Gy, respectively. In general, choosing different sets of reference points to define a prescribed reference isodose surface results in different dwell times, minimal doses, and SF.

Maximizing D_{min}. Applying our method for maximizing D_{min} we obtained $D_{min} = 29.11$ Gy and $8.84 \times 10^{-9} <$ SF $< 9.53 \times 10^{-9}$.

Minimizing the Surviving Fraction. With the minimal dose calculated as 28.58 Gy, SF was given by $6.14 \times 10^{-9} <$ SF $< 6.62 \times 10^{-9}$.

Discussion

We compared different methods for optimizing the activity distribution in brachytherapy. All of these methods are especially suited for stepwise moving sources as used in high dose rate brachytherapy equipment. As a measure of quality for dose distributions, the resulting SF were used. We showed that these correlate very well with the minimal doses in the target volume if the same normalization factor is used. Compared with the simplest method, in which all possible dwell times are equal, all of the more elaborate optimization methods give improved results.

Care must be taken if methods are used in which one tries to fit the doses at given reference positions to given values. This is due to the fact that usually these points are chosen arbitrarily, and the number and position of points determine to a great extent the distribution of dwell times. The inherent problems of all these methods are threefold. First, the usually very limited number of reference points is not sufficient to determine accurately the whole target. Second, nearly all of these methods try to minimize the variances between the actual and the prescribed doses. This leads to an overweighting of dwell times at stopping points which are far from the reference points. In a very extreme and artificial case in which a possible source point is very far from the reference points, all the activity is given to this point, and if this point is far outside the patient, we have the situation of percutaneous therapy. The third problem is due to the fact that it is very cumbersome to prescribe doses in regions with a very high dose gradient because the position of the reference points determines the absolute dose to a high degree. This very trivial effect is sometimes overlooked. In the simple case of a single source, increasing the distance between source and reference point from 1.0 to 1.1 cm results in an increase in the activity-time product of 21%.

Table 1. Optimization of dwell times

	D_{min} (Gy)	SF (lower limit)	SF (upper limit)
Equal dwell times	22.06	1.25×10^{-7}	1.34×10^{-7}
Reference points = 6	26.36	1.69×10^{-8}	1.83×10^{-8}
Reference points = 14	24.92	3.94×10^{-8}	4.21×10^{-8}
D_{min} optimized	29.11	8.84×10^{-9}	9.53×10^{-9}
SF optimized	28.58	6.14×10^{-9}	6.67×10^{-9}

$T_{total} = 1000$ s, $A = 370$ GBq; $1/\alpha = 2$ Gy; radius = 2 cm.

Therefore it is much better to prescribe the activity-time product (e.g., *mghr*) for the known target volume, as it is usually performed in classical brachytherapy treatment schemes (e.g., Manchester, Paris, Quimby systems).

The methods which either maximize the minimum dose or minimize the SF are truly three-dimensional. This corresponds to the fact that the target is a three-dimensional volume and not only a finite set of 0-dimensional reference points. As shown in Table 1, these methods lead to an improvement in the minimal dose and to a reduction in SF. The main difficulty with these methods is that they depend on detailed information about the size and shape of the target volume. However, using the new imaging modalities such as computed tomography, magnetic resonance imaging, and ultrasound, it seems possible to improve the definition of the target volume. The same methods may also be used to determine accurately the position of the applicators within the target volume. More powerful computers allow the reduction in calculation times for these optimization routines.

References

Anderson LL (1985) Physical optimization of afterloading techniques. Strahlentherapie 161: 264–268

Busch M (1984) Analytic optimization method for afterloading techniques. In: Cunningham JR, Ragan D, van Dyk J (eds) Proceedings of the 8th international conference on the use of computers in radiation therapy, Toronto, Canada. IEEE Computer Society, Los Angeles, pp 398–402

Thames HD, Peters LJ, Withers HR, Fletcher GH (1983) Accelerated fractionation vs hyperfractionation: rationales for several treatments per day. Int J Radiat Oncol Biol Phys 9: 127–138

Tölli H, Ragnhult I (1987) An analytical method to solve an optimization problem in brachytherapy. In: Bruinvis et al. (eds) The use of computers in radiation therapy. Elsevier, New York, pp 123–126

Wehrmann R, Kneschaurek P (1987) Use of a portable personal computer for treatment planning in intraoperative high-dose-rate brachytherapy. In: Bruinvis IAD et al. (eds) The use of computers in radiation therapy. Elsevier, New York, pp 91–94

Wehrmann R, Kneschaurek P (1988) Ein neues Verfahren zur Optimierung der Dosisverteilung in der Brachytherapie. Zentralb Radiol 136: 635

Wehrmann R, Hugo C, Kneschaurek P (1991) (to be published)

Maximizing Local Control by Customized Dose Prescription for Pelvic Tumours*

A.E. Nahum[1] and D.M. Tait[2]

Introduction

Currently a great deal of effort is being expended on ways of increasing the dose to the target volume in external beam radiotherapy as it is generally accepted that this will lead to increased local control and, in certain cases, to higher cure rates for certain tumours (Suit and Westgate 1986). Conformal therapy (CFRT) is seen as the way to achieve this (Tait and Nahum 1990), through the optimization of photon and electron beam arrangements (Brahme 1988; Webb 1989), the development of accelerator technology (Brahme 1987; Boesecke et al. 1988) or through exploiting the superior depth-dose characteristics of proton beams (Slater et al. 1988).

Parallel with the above, three-dimensional treatment planning systems of increasing sophistication have been developed (McShan et al. 1990); such systems are in use in many more clinics than can presently benefit from advanced techniques of CFRT still under development. Thus it is possible to calculate and visualize the dose distribution throughout the target volume and the critical normal tissues. A recent analysis of normal tissue sparing achievable by simple blocking techniques for pelvic tumours (Tait et al. 1988) showed clearly the considerable variation in dose distribution in the rectum, for example, between one patient and another. Dose-volume histograms (DVHs) demonstrate this very clearly. Put another way, some patients "conform" already. Nevertheless, it is almost universal practice to prescribe a standard target dose, for example, 32 fractions of 2 Gy. To our knowledge there is only one published study on prescribing the target does according to the information in normal tissue DVHs (Lawrence et al. 1990). We report here on a study of the potential for increased tumour control probability (TCP) by customized dose prescription in pelvic malignancies; we have applied the Kutcher-Burman normal tissue complication probability (NTCP) model (Kutcher and Burman 1989) to DVH data for 51 patients entered into an on-going clinical trial.

[1] Joint Department of Physics, Royal Marsden Hospital and Institute of Cancer Research, Sutton SM2 5PT, UK
[2] Department of Radiotherapy, Royal Marsden Hospital, Sutton SM2 5PT, UK
* This research was supported by the Cancer Research Campaign, UK

Patient Material

A clinical trial is presently underway at the both sites of the Royal Marsden Hospital to determine differences in both acute and late complication rates when pelvic malignancies (prostate, bladder, cervix, rectum) are treated radically using 6 MV photons, with "conventional" (i.e. minimally blocked) fields in one arm and beam's eye view customized blocked fields in the other. The target volume and the critical normal tissues rectum, small and large bowel and bladder are outlined on computed tomography slices, with 0.5 or 1 cm spacing, and the DVHs computed for both the blocked and unblocked plans (using the IGE Target system).

The DVH data for the custom blocked plans for 51 patients accrued to date have been used in this study. The trial will continue until 200 patients have been treated.

Normal Tissue Complication Probability Model

Lyman (1987) proposed a model for NTCP for the particular case of the partial (fractional) volume (V) of an organ uniformly irradiated to a dose (D):

$$\text{NTCP} = 1/\sqrt{2\pi} \int_{-\infty}^{t} \exp(-t^2/2)dt \tag{1}$$

where

$$t = [D - \text{TD}_{50}(V)]/[m * \text{TD}_{50}(V)] \tag{2}$$

and

$$\text{TD}_{50}(V) = \text{TD}_{50}(1) * V^{-n} \tag{3}$$

The NTCP expression has the expected sigmoid form; it is the integration of a gaussian with standard deviation $\sigma = m \times \text{TD}_{50}(V)$, m being the slope parameter and $\text{TD}_{50}(V)$ the dose resulting in a 50% complication rate (for some specific endpoint). The parameter n expresses the crucial relation between partial and whole volume irradiation.

We have used the clinically based data of Burman et al. (1991) fitted to the above model: for the rectum with the endpoints of severe proctitis, necrosis, stenosis and fistula, the whole-volume tolerance dose $\text{TD}_{50}(1) = 80$ Gy, $m = 0.15$, and $n = 0.12$; for the small intestine (bowel) with the endpoints of obstruction and perforation, $\text{TD}_{50}(1) = 55$ Gy, $m = 0.16$, and $n = 0.15$.

Further, we have followed the method developed by Kutcher and Burman (1989) for reducing the non-uniform irradiation of normal tissues to the uniform partial irradiation required in the model: one operates on each volume ΔV_i in bin i receiving dose D_i to calculate an effective partial volume V_{eff} irradiated to dose D_{max} according to:

$$V_{\text{eff}} = \Delta V_{\text{max}} + \Delta V_1(D_1/D_{\text{max}})^{1/n} + \Delta V_2(D_2/D_{\text{max}})^{1/n} + \ldots \tag{4}$$

Tumour Control Probability Model

The study involves estimating the change in TCP when the target dose is changed. The TCP for a mean dose D to the target volume is based on the following expressions:

$$N_s = N_o \exp[-\alpha D] \tag{5}$$

where N_o is the initial number and N_s the surviving number of clonogenic cells (we are assuming that the influence of β is negligible for 2-Gy fractions), and:

$$TCP = \exp[-N_s] \tag{6}$$

We have made one important modification to the above standard model. It is well known (e.g. Brahme 1984) that unrealistically steep dose-response curves result from Eqs. 5 and 6 (Fig. 1). We have therefore assumed that the radiosensitivity parameter α is distributed normally among the patient population with standard deviation σ_α. Note that we have based the calculation of TCP on the *mean* dose to the target volume rather than on the DVH data as the latter allows for a margin where the clonogenic cell density is (ideally) close to zero.

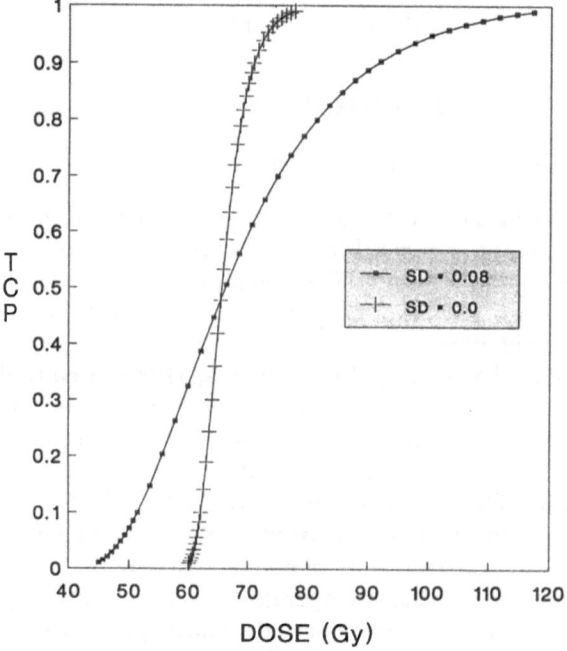

Fig. 1. Tumor control probability (*TCP*) as a function of target dose, derived from Eqs. 5 and 6, with $\alpha = 0.35$ $\rho_c = 10^7$ for a volume of 320 cm^3, for $\sigma_\alpha = 0.0$ (+) and for the clinically realistic $\sigma_\alpha = 0.08$ ($\square$)

For all the pelvic tumours in the study we have used $\alpha = 0.35\ \mathrm{Gy}^{-1}$ that Deacon et al. (1984) give for bladder tumours. Additionally we have taken the clonogenic cell density ρ_c to be 10^7 (G.G. Steel private communication) which enables us to estimate N_0 from $\rho_c \times V_{\mathrm{tgt}}$, the target volume. It has been found that the value $\sigma_\alpha = 0.08\ \mathrm{Gy}^{-1}$ results in a dose-response curve (Fig. 1) very similar to the one derived from clinical data for photon irradiation of T4B bladder tumours (Batterman et al. 1981); so this volume has been adopted.

Calculational Scheme

1. NTCPs were calculated from the (custom-blocked) DVH data using the model and parameters described above, for the rectum ($\mathrm{NTCP_R}$) and for the small bowel ($\mathrm{NTCP_{SB}}$) only, as these are the most important dose-limiting structures. The total target dose, D_{tgt} was set at 64 Gy for all patients.

2. A combined NTCP was computed according to:

$$1 - \mathrm{NTCP_{tot}} = [1 - \mathrm{NTCP_R}] * [1 - \mathrm{NTCP_{SB}}] \tag{7}$$

It was considered that the complication endpoints were equally serious for both structures, which is consistent with the equal weighting implied in Eq. 7.

3. The target dose D_{tgt} was adjusted so as to make $\mathrm{NTCP_{tot}}$ equal to 0.05, resulting in an optimized dose ($D_{0.05}$).

4. An optimized TCP ($\mathrm{TCP_{0.05}}$) was calculated corresponding to target dose ($D_{0.05}$).

Results

For the 51 patients in the DVH database, the rectum was involved in 44 of them, the small bowel in only 11. There was a very large distribution in both target and

Table 1. Mean values of the key quantities

64 Gy:	
$\quad \mathrm{TCP_{64}} = 0.45$	$\approx$ Consistent with clinical results
$\quad \mathrm{NTCP_{64}} = 0.11$	Very large spread
Optimized at NTCP = 0.05:	
$\quad D_{0.05} = 66\ \mathrm{Gy}$	All patients
$\qquad\quad = 70\ \mathrm{Gy}$	Only rectal DVHs
$\qquad\quad = 51\ \mathrm{Gy}$	Small bowel present
$\quad \mathrm{TCP_{0.05}} = 0.58$	All patients
$\qquad\quad = 0.68$	Only rectal DVHs
$\qquad\quad = 0.12$	Small bowel present

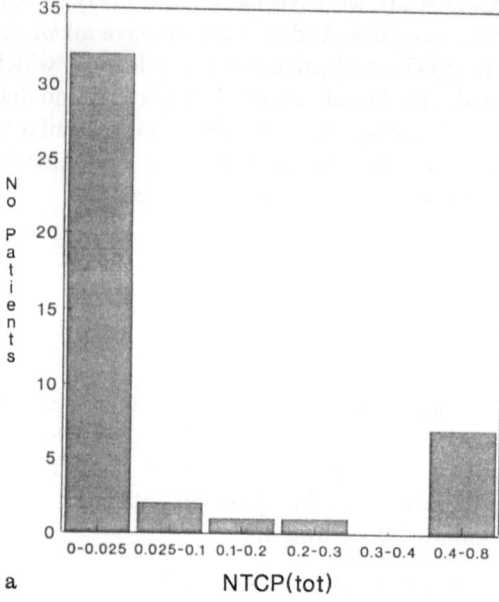

a   NTCP(tot)

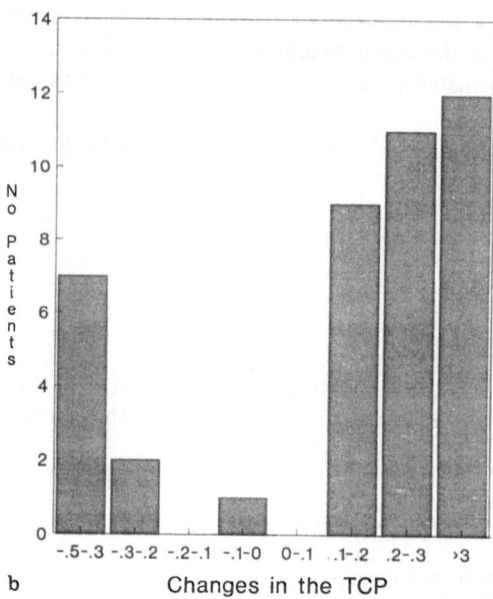

b   Changes in the TCP

Fig. 2 a,b. Frequency distributions of NTCP$_{tot}$ (**a**) at 64 Gy and the change in TCP (**b**), TCP$_{64}$ − TCP$_{0.05}$ resulting from changing the dose from 64 Gy to $D_{0.05}$

rectal volumes, with means of 320 and 77 cm³ resp. The major findings are set out in Table 1. Frequency distributions of NTCP$_{tot}$ at 64 Gy and the change in TCP resulting from customizing the dose to $D_{0.05}$, ΔTCP, are shown in Fig. 2a and Fig. 2b, respectively.

Discussion and Conclusions

A very large variation in $NTCP_{tot}$ at 64 Gy was found, with no less than 12 patients (all of whom had DVH data for rectum, small bowel or both) having a value less than 0.005. The surprisingly high mean value of 0.11 (Table 1) was due to a few patients having appreciable small bowel involvement (Fig. 2a); the $TD_{50}(1)$ value for the small bowel was only 55 Gy. Customizing the dose so that $NTCP_{tot} = 0.05$ resulted in a 29% increase in the mean TCP from 0.45 to 0.58 (Table 1) though at the same time the mean NTCP actually *decreased* from 0.11 to 0.05. Figure 2b shows the very wide range in ΔTCP; the patients without small bowel involvement *gained* by as much as 0.3.

The clinical data on which the model is based are far from complete; for example, the marked split between patients with and those without small bowel involvement is almost certainly unrealistic. In order to gauge how critically the results depend on the volume effect parameter n we performed recalculations varying the value for the rectum (0.12 so far) between 0.01 and 0.50. We found that $TCP_{0.05}$ increased steadily from 0.4 for $n = 0.01$ (negligible volume effect) to 0.9 for $n = 0.5$ for those patients with only rectal involvement. This should caution us not to take the results of this study too literally.

In conclusion, we have shown that there is considerable potential for increasing the TCP by customizing the target dose based on critical normal tissue DVH data.

Acknowledgements The help of the physics staff in carrying out the DVH calculations and of the radiographers in entering this data into the database is gratefully acknowledged.

References

Batterman JJ, Hart GAM, Breur K (1981) Dose-effect relations for tumour control and complication rate after fast neutron therapy for pelvic tumours. Br J Radiol 54: 899–904

Boesecke R, Doll J, Bauer B, Schlegel W, Pastyr O, Lorenz WJ (1988) Treatment planning for conformation therapy using a multi-leaf collimator. Strahlenther Onkol 164: 151–154

Brahme A (1984) Dosimetric precision requirements in radiation therapy. Acta Radiol Oncol 23: 379–391

Brahme A (1987) Design principles and clinical possibilities with a new generation of radiation therapy equipment. Acta Oncol 26: 403–412

Brahme A (1988) Optimization of stationary and moving beam radiation therapy techniques. Radiother Oncol 12: 129–140

Burman C, Kutcher GJ, Emami B, Goitein M (1991) Fitting of normal tissue tolerance data to an analytic function. Int J Radiat Oncol Biol Phys 21: 123–136

Deacon J, Peckham MJ, Steel GG (1984) The radioresponsiveness of human tumours and the initial slope of the cell survival curve. Radiother Oncol 2: 317–323

Kutcher GJ, Burman C (1989) Calculation of complication probability factors for non-uniform normal tissue irradiation: the effective volume method. Int J Radiat Oncol Biol Phys 16: 1623–1630

Lawrence TS, Tesser RJ, Ten Haken RK (1990) An application of dose volume histograms to the treatment of intraheptic malignancies with radiation therapy. Int J Radiat Oncol Biol Phys 19: 1041–1047

Lyman JT (1987) Complication probability as assessed from dose-volume histograms. Radiat Res 104: S13–S19

McShan DL, Fraass BA, Lichter AS (1990) Full integration of the beam's eye view concept into clinical treatment planning. Int J Radiat Oncol Biol Phys 18: 1485–1494

Slater JM, Diller DW, Archambeau JO (1988) Development of a hospital-based proton beam treatment center. Int J Radiat Oncol Biol Phys 14: 761–775

Suit HD, Westgate SJ (1986) Impact of improved local control on survival. Int J Radiat Oncol Biol Phys 12: 453–458

Tait D, Nahum A (1990) Conformal therapy. Eur J Cancer 26: 750–753

Tait D, Nahum A, Southall C, Chow M, Yarnold JR (1988) Benefits expected from simple conformal radiotherapy in the treatment of pelvic tumours. Radiother Oncol 13: 23–30

Webb S (1989) Optimisation of conformal radiotherapy dose distributions by simulated annealing. Phys Med Biol 34: 1349–1370

Retrospective Analysis of Complication Probabilities Induced by Radiation Treatment of the Esophagus

G. Becker[1,2], R. Lohrum[1], F. Hensley[3], W. Schlegel[1], J.T. Lyman[4], U. Weischedel[3], and W.J. Lorenz[1]

Introduction

Technical improvements in hardware, computer graphic devices, and dose calculation algorithms have made possible a new generation of three-dimensional treatment planning systems [17]. However, the amount of information provided by a three-dimensional dose distribution can substantially complicate the process of selecting the best plan [2]. While a number of tools have been developed for presenting the physical dose distribution, the question of what biological effect the doses have on the tumor and the surrounding healthy tissues remains unanswered.

Our goal was to quantify the optimization of three-dimensional treatment planning in comparison with the two-dimensional procedure and to identify the irradiation technique for esophageal cancer with the lowest complication probability. For this purpose a number of methods have been developed which for a given dose distribution calculate tumor control probabilities (TCP) and normal tissue complication probabilities (NTCP), thus leading to a quantitative measure helping to select the optimal plan [13]. At the German Cancer Research Center (DKFZ) an algorithm developed by Lyman which calculates TCPs and NTCPs on the base of dose-volume histograms has been implemented in the treatment planning system VOXEL-PLAN.

In a retrospective trial involving 13 patients with esophageal cancer the original two-dimensional treatment planning (combination of fixed opposed and moving fields) was reconstructed and calculated in three dimensions. The same irradiation technique was three-dimensionally optimized by means of beam's eye view, and the dose distribution was compared with that of the original plan. In addition, the possibility of further improvement of the dose fitting by three-dimensionally planned isocentric fixed fields was examined. To

[1] *Current address*: German Cancer Research Center, Im Neuenheimer Feld 280, 6900 Heidelberg, FRG

[2] Department of Radiotherapy, University Clinic for Radiology, University of Tübingen, Hoppe-Seyler-Str. 3, 7400 Tübingen, FRG

[3] Department of Radiotherapy, University Clinic for Radiology, University of Heidelberg, Im Neuenheimer Feld 400, 6900 Heidelberg, FRG

[4] Lawrence Berkeley Laboratory, University of California Berkeley, CA 94720, USA

Advanced Radiation Therapy Tumor Response
Monitoring and Treatment Planning
Breit (Editor-in-Chief)
© Springer-Verlag, Berlin Heidelberg 1992

what extent this approach is suitable for the biological treatment planning of esophageal cancer is examined here.

Materials and Methods

Hardware

At the Institute for Radiology and Pathophysiology of the DKFZ medical workstations (DEC VAX stations 3200 and 3520) are available. They are used in a local area VAX cluster with a DEC 3600 as node. Imaging data from computed tomography, magnetic resonance image, and positron emission tomography are transferred directly to this network (Ethernet with DECNET protocol). As operating system VMS is used; the software language is FORTRAN.

Software

Three-Dimensional Treatment Planning. In the last few years the computer-based three-dimensional radiotherapy planning system VOXEL-PLAN-Heidelberg was developed at the DKFZ. Computer tomographic data on tumor, target volume, lungs, cor, and spinal cord are interactively defined and marked. Graphic systems such as beam's eye view and others allow virtual radiotherapy simulation [3]. For the calculation of the primary component and two-dimensional convolution for the consideration of the scattering dose, a fast voxel based three-dimensional dose calculation algorithm including three-dimensional ray tracing is used [6,16]. A special feature of this software is the ability to calculate noncoplanar and irregular field irradiation techniques [4,5]. All these technical and software components have been described in more detail elsewhere [1, 8, 16].

*Complication Probability .*The dose distributions on volumes of interest for various organs (heat, spinal cord, lung, etc.) were used to calculate dose-volume histograms. An algorithm based on a simple biological model calculates complication probabilities as a function of dose and irradiated volume [11]. The algorithm calculates complication probabilities for each step in the dose-volume histogram. By interpolation the N step histogram is reduced to an N-1step histogram. This interpolation is repeated recursively until arriving at a single-step histogram, the complication probability of which is taken as an estimate for the NTCP of the complete irradiated volume [11,12]. Table 1 lists the tolerance doses for 50% complication probability (TD_{50}) used in these calculations for the different organs listed in the table, referring to the indicated clinical endpoints.

Table 1. Normal tissue complication probabilities: $TD_{50/5}$

Organ	RBE	$TD_{50/5}$	Endpoint
Heart	1	48.0 GY	Pericarditis
Spinal cord	1	66.5 GY	Myelitis/necrosis
Lung	1	24.5 GY	Pneumonitis
Contour minus target	1	60.0 GY	

The calculation was performed for 2 Gy single-dose administration five times a week for 40 days, up to dose maximum of 60 Gy.

Patients

All patients who underwent irradiation for esophageal cancer between 1984 and 1986 in Heidelberg were analyzed retrospectively. On the basis of computed tomography data the original treatment planning was reconstructed. However, in only 13 cases did all technical and medical features allow a correct evaluation. One patient had a cervical and 12 a thoracic esophageal carcinoma.

Irradiation Technique

Because of numerous radiotherapeutic difficulties the esophagus is very well suited for such a study. For example, it is difficult to fit the dose exactly to the target volume because of the curvature of the esophagus and the kyphosis of the thoracic spine. Thus the topographic neighborhood of esophagus and spinal cord leads to a high radiation burden to the upper parts of the spinal cord. Moreover, the target volume is surrounded by other sensitive structures such as the mediastinum, lungs, and heart [18]. A safety distance of at least 5 cm craniad and caudad to the tumor leads to rather long fields. However, up to 80% of patients die of locally recurrent disease and aspiration pneumonia caused by the persisting cancer [7, 15]. Concerning solutions to this problem there is no agreement on the technical treatment aspects in the international literature [7].

Three-Dimensional Reconstructed Original Plan (2D). In Heidelberg a solution to these problems has been attempted by combining two different irradiation techniques. At first the patients were irradiated with two large opposing fixed fields, mainly to cover the carcinoma lymphomatosa. However, this causes a high radiation burden of the mediastinum and spinal cord; therefore only 28–34 Gy were applied. The remaining dose was administered by means of moving technique and reduced field length and width. In most cases a monoaxial moving technique from $\pm 120°$ to $-120°$ was selected. This combined irradiation was developed by Kuttig [9, 10, 14].

Three-Dimensional Optimized Original Plan (3D). The same irradiation technique for the patients has been optimized with the help of the three-dimensional treatment planning program. Rotation angles and gantry positions were not changed, i.e., field length and width were fitted by means of beam's eye view.

Three-Dimensional Optimized Three Isocentric Fixed Fields (3 Iso). In addition, the possibility of further improvement of the dose fitting by three-dimensionally planned isocentric fixed fields ($O°$, $+120°$, $-120°$) was examined. For this the beam's eye view is an essential help, allowing exact individual fitting of the field to the target volume while maximally sparing the spinal cord by optimal collimator setting.

Results and Discussion

First the different dose distributions were compared by means of dose-volume histograms, beginning with the target volume (Fig. 1a). It turned out that in two-dimensional treatment planning the 80% isodose covered only about 80% of the target volume, i.e., 20% of the target volume is underdosed. With three-dimensional treatment planning this can be avoided regardless of the irradiation technique. The dose-volume histogram of the spinal cord (Fig. 1b), however, clearly demonstrates the difference. Because of fitting the field length and width by the combination of ventrodorsally opposing fields and moving technique the spinal cord becomes clearly more burdened, so that the total spinal cord receives more than 60% of the dose. As can be seen clearly, the spinal cord is protected by the three-dimensionally planned fixed fields, receiving only the half of the dose burden. The irradiation burden of the lungs appears to be different (Fig. 1c). With the combination of fixed fields and moving technique there are no essential differences in two- and three-dimensional treatment planning, but because of the segmental burdening of the two lateral fixed fields the total dose burden of the lungs is higher with the three-dimensionally planned isocentric fixed fields.

What does this mean from the medical point of view? Which of these treatment plans can be recommended for the treatment of patients; which one has — assuming a sufficient dose for the target — the smallest NTCP? Table 2 shows the calculated NTCPs of the different organs of one patient. For better interpretation they are also represented as relative NTCPs.

Based on calculations based on the approach of Lyman, three-dimensional optimization of the combined fixed fields and moving technique causes a 1.6-fold increase in the NTCP of the spinal cord, whereas that of the NTCP is only

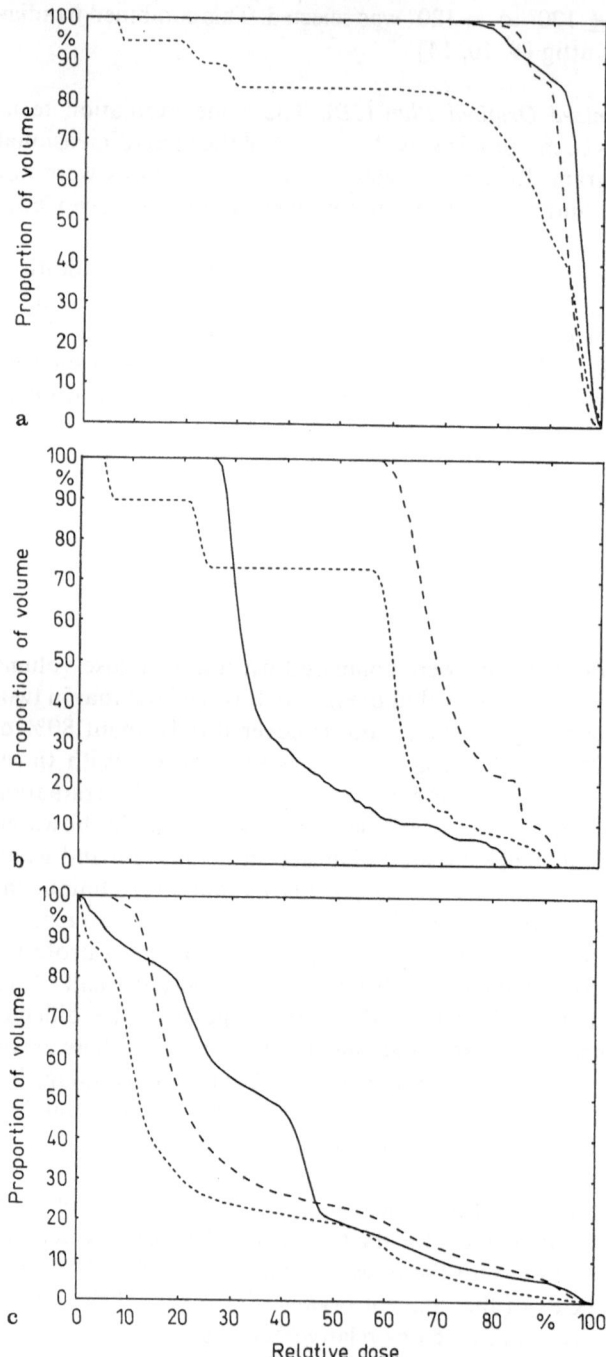

Fig. 1a–c. Dose-volume histograms. **a** Target volume. **b** Spinal cord. **c** Lung. *Dotted curve*, three-dimensionally reconstructed original plan; *dashed curve*, three-dimensionally optimized original plan; *solid curve*, three-dimensionally planned three isocentric fixed fields

Table 2. Normal Tissue Complication Probabilities in one patient

	2D	3D	3 Iso
Observed values			
Spinal cord	0.03642	0.05744	0.01708
Heart	0.0037	0.21603	0.00063
Right lung	0.0066	0.12161	0.28445
Left lung	0.00215	0.02925	0.08509
Volume-target	0.00007	0.00062	0.00007
Ratios			
Spinal cord	1	1.6	0.5
Heart	1	58.4	0.17
Right lung	1	18.4	43.0
Left lung	1	13.3	9.6
Volume-target	1	8.9	1.0

2D, Three-dimensionally reconstructed original plan; 3D, three-dimensionally optimized original plan; 3 Iso, three-dimensionally optimized isocentric fixed fields.

0.5 for the three isocentric fixed fields. Referring to the sufficient dose coverage of the target volume this means that the risk of myelitis or necrosis is only one-third that with irradiation by three-dimensionally planned isocentric fixed fields, assuming a TD_{50} of 66.5 Gy. This difference even more dramatic in the case of the heart. With the combined irradiation technique the risk would increase 58-fold, while with the fixed fields it would amount to only a fraction (0.17). The disadvantage of the fixed field technique is the two lateral fields which lead to a high segmental burdening of the lung. Thus, calculation for the left lung results in an almost threefold complication probability compared to the combined irradiation technique (13.6:39.6). With the technique of Kuttig the surrounding healthy tissue as a whole is more burdened; for the difference between total body volume and target volume the complication probability is ninefold compared to the fixed field irradiation.

Table 3 presents the mean NTCPs all 13 patients as ratios of the two-dimension treatment planning. With combined fixed fields and moving technique the risk to the spinal cord increases to 3.3-fold. Compared to this the risk with the three-dimensionally planned isocentric fixed fields is minimal. Referring to the heart, the differences are even greater. For the lungs the reduction algorithm based on the Lyman dose-volume histogram leads surprisingly to somewhat smaller complication probabilities compared with two-dimensional treatment planning, although the dose-volume histograms clearly demonstrate the segmental burdening of the lung. Thus the dose-volume histograms of the fixed field irradiation are inferior. Whether this specific finding is the result of a mistake or is clinically correct cannot be determined with certainty. Whether

Table 3. Normal tissue complication probabilities: mean ratios ($n = 13$)

	2D	3D	3 Iso
Spinal cord	1	3.3	0.075
Heart	1	15.5	0.004
Lung	1	24.6	0.93
Volume-target	1	9.8	0.06
Target	25%	100%	100%

2D, Three-dimensionally reconstructed original plan; 3D, three-dimensionally optimized original plan; 3 Iso, three-dimensionally optimized isocentric fixed fields.

such numbers actually have a clinical correlate must be examined in numerically larger prospective studies.

Conclusion

In summary, this retrospective evaluation shows that two-dimensional treatment planning is not sufficient for the irradiation of the esophagus. In 75% of cases the target volumes were underdosed. In contrast to this, three-dimensional treatment planning is always indicated for complex target volumes such as the esophagus. The combination of ventrodorsally opposing fixed fields and moving technique leads to a high tissue complication probability of healthy tissue. Concerning both spinal cord and heart the average NTCPs of the 13 patients are significantly lower with three-dimensionally planned isocentric fixed fields. In contrast to this the NTCPs of the lung must be considered particularly carefully, because no clinical data can as yet confirm these calculations, and because at these volumes of interest there was a difference between the dose-volume histograms and the NTCPs. Because in the retrospective comparison of two- and three-dimensional treatment planning the physical dose distribution and the dose-volume histograms were so clearly different, these data were used to introduce the Lyman algorithm into the Heidelberg software and as a first plausibility test with a dataset on esophagus irradiation. The results presented here permit the conclusion that this could be a possibility for "biological treatment planning." However, the corresponding clinical data for examining the calculated NTCPs are still lacking. An essential premise of Lyman is the TD_{50} value taken from the literature. Large and exact prospective studies are necessary to determine especially the crucial ratio between dose and volume relating to the exact localization. Thus, as long as exact data and exact biological-mathematical models are lacking, this remains a first approach which will have its first, careful clinical application at the DKFZ.

References

1. Bauer-Kirpes B, Schlegel W, Boesecke R, Lorenz WJ (1987) Display of organs and isodoses as shaded 3d objects for 3d therapy planning. Int J Radiat Oncol Biol Phys 13: 135–140
2. Becker G, Lohrum R, Werner T, Bürkelbach J, Nemeth G, Boesecke R, Schlegel W, Lorenz WJ (1989) Presentation and evaluation of 3D dose distribution in radiotherapy planning, In: Lemke HU, Rhodes ML, Jaffe CC, Felix R (eds) Computer assisted radiology. Springer, Berlin Heidelberg New York, pp 254–261
3. Becker G, Gademann G, Schlegel W, Lohrum R, Boesecke R, Lorenz WJ (1990) Medical aspects of 3D treatment planning of brain tumors with Voxel-Plan-Heidelberg. In: Hukku S, Iyer PS (eds) The use of computers in radiation therapy. Proceedings of the Xth ICCR, Alpana Arts, Lucknow, India, pp 147–151
4. Boesecke R, Hartmann GH, Scharfenberg H, Schlegel W (1986) Dose calculations for irregular fields using three-dimensional first-scatter integration. Phys Med Biol 3: 291–298
5. Boesecke R, Becker G, Alandt K, Pastyr O, Doll J, Schlegel W, Lorenz WJ (1991) Modification of a three-dimensional treatment planning system for the use of multi-leaf-collimators conformation radiotherapy. Radiother Oncol 21: 261–268
6. Bortfeld T, Boesecke R, Schlegel W, Bohsung J (1990) 3-D dose calculation using 2-D convolutions and ray tracing methods. In: Hukku S, Iyer PS (eds) The use of computers in radiation therapy. Proceedings of the Xth ICCR, Alpana Arts, Lucknow, India, pp 238–241
7. Flores AD (1989) Cancer of the esophagus and cardia: overview of radiotherapy. Can J Surg 32 (6): 404–409
8. Gademann G, Schlegel W, Becker G, Romahn J, Höver KH, Pastyr O, van Kaick G, Wannenmacher M (1990) High precision radiotherapy of head and neck tumors by means of an integrated stereotactic and 3D planning system. Int J Radiat Oncol Biol Phys 19 [Suppl 1]: 135
9. Kuttig H, Schnabel K, Bark R (1977) Die Pendelbestrahlung des mittleren Ösophagus mit schnellen Elektronen und ultraharten Röntgenstrahlen. Strahlentherapie 153: 533–537
10. Kuttig H (1980) Die klinischen Applikationsverfahren zur Erzielung einer geeigneten räumlichen Dosisverteilung. In: Scherer E (ed) Strahlentherapie. Radiologische Onkologie, 2nd edn. Springer, Berlin Heidelberg New York, pp 97–126
11. Lyman TJ (1985) Complication probability as assessed from dose-volume histograms. Radiat Res 104: 13–19
12. Lyman TJ, Wolbarst AB (1987) Optimization of radiation therapy. III. a method of assessing complication probabilities from dose-volume histograms. Int J Radiat Oncol Biol Phys 13: 103–109
13. Lyman TJ, Wolbarst AB (1989) Optimization of radiation therapy. IV. a dose-volume histogram reduction algorithm. Int J Radiat Oncol Biol Phys 17: 433–436
14. Ne'meth G, Kuttig H (1981) Isodose atlas for use in radiotherapy. Nijhoff, Den Haag
15. Rosenberg JG, Roth JA, Lichter AS, Kelson DP (1985) Cancer of the esophagus, 621–657. In: De Vita VT, Hellmann S, Rosenberg SA (eds) Cancer principles and practice of oncology, Vol 1, 2nd edn. Lippincott, Philadelphia
16. Schlegel W, Scharfenberg H, Doll J, Hartmann G, Sturm V, Lorenz WJ (1984) Threedimensional dose planning using tomographic data. In: Cunningham JR (ed) Proceedings of the 8th international conference on the use of computers in radiation therapy. IEEE Computer Society Press, Silver Spring, pp 191–195
17. Schlegel W, Pastyr O, Boesecke R, Bortfeld T, Becker G, Schad L, Gademann G, Lorenz WJ (1990) Computer systems and mechanical tools for stereotactically guided conformation therapy with linear accelerators. Int J Radiat Oncol Biol Phys 19 [Suppl 1]: 133
18. Zum Winkel K, Adolph J, Kuttig H, Weischedel U (1986) Spezielle Therapieplanung bei Tumoren des Mediastinums und des Oesophagus. In: Frommhold W, Hübener KH (eds) Computertomographie in der Strahlentherapie. Thieme, Stuttgart, pp 187–193

Biological Treatment Planning: Calculation of Normal Tissue Complication Probabilities Based on Dose-Volume Analysis of Three-Dimensional Treatment Plans*

F.W. Hensley[1], G. Becker[2], R. Lohrum[2], J.T. Lyman[3], G. Gademann[1], D. Fehrentz[1], W. Schlegel[2], M. Flentje[1], and W.J. Lorenz[2]

Introduction

Future applications of biological treatment planning in routine clinical work may include, on the one hand, the design and comparison of fractionation schemes with planned and unplanned treatment pauses and, on the other, alternate schemes with hyperfractionated or accelerated treatment for improving therapeutic results. This kind of planning may utilize radiobiological models such as linear quadratic formalism [1, 2], which can be extended to account for individual effects of cell repair and kinetics such as incomplete repair and repopulation [3, 4]. The second issue in biological treatment planning is the consideration of volume effects on normal tissues and tumors. For this purpose several methods have been developed which calculate normal tissue complication probabilities (NTCP) and tumor control probabilities for inhomogeneously irradiated volumes of tissue.

Materials and Methods

At the German Cancer Research Center an algorithm has been incorporated into the treatment planning system Voxel-Plan [5] which uses a simple model to calculate complication probabilities as a function of dose and volume [6]. The volume dependence of tolerance doses (for example, the tolerance dose, TD_{50}, which results in 50% complication probability within 5 years) is described by the power-law relationship:

$$TD(V) = TD(1)/V^n$$

[1] University Clinic for Radiology, University of Heidelberg, Im Neuenheimer Feld 400, 6900 Heidelberg, FRG
[2] German Cancer Research Center, Im Neuenheimer Feld 280, 6900 Heidelberg, FRG
[3] Lawrence Berkeley Laboratory, University of California, 1 Cyclotron Road, Berkeley, California, 94720, USA
* This research was supported by Deutsche Forschungsgemeinschaft grant Fe-269/1-1.

Advanced Radiation Therapy Tumor Response
Monitoring and Treatment Planning
Breit (Editor-in-Chief)
© Springer-Verlag, Berlin Heidelberg 1992

where TD(V) is the tolerance dose for a given partial volume, TD(1) is the tolerance dose for the full volume, and n is a fitted parameter. The sigmoid curve describing complication probability as a function of dose is approximated by the integral of a normal distribution:

$$P(D) = \frac{1}{\sqrt{2\pi}} \int_{-\infty}^{t} e^{-t^2/2}\, dt$$

where $t = (D - TD_{50}(V))/\sigma(V)$. The mean of the distribution is given at $TD_{50}(V)$, and its standard deviation $\sigma(V)$ is approximated by a constant fraction $m \times TD_{50}$. Complication probability as function of dose and volume is then completely defined by the three parameters, $TD_{50}(1)$, n, and m.

Calculations of NTCP are performed on the basis of dose-volume histograms which are provided by Voxel-Plan for any volume of interest (VOI) defined in the treatment plan. The algorithm calculates complication probabilities for each step of the histogram. By interpolation, the histogram, which initially has N steps on the dose axis, is reduced to an $N - 1$ step histogram providing (nearly) the same complication probability when applied to the VOI. This interpolation is repeated recursively until one arrives at a single-step histogram, the complication probability of which is taken as an estimate of the NTCP of the irradiated volume [7, 8]. The program can in principle, account for non-standard fractionation by correcting the TD_{50} according to the linear quadratic model. For simplicity, however, all calculations here were performed for a standard scheme of 2 Gy per fraction.

As a first trial the algorithm was applied to existing three-dimensional dose distributions calculated to simulate different treatment techniques for irradiation of the paraaortic lymph nodes [9, 10]. Two different techniques, a biaxial rotation and a four-field box technique were compared with respect to complications of the kidney. Figure 1 shows dose-volume histograms of the two

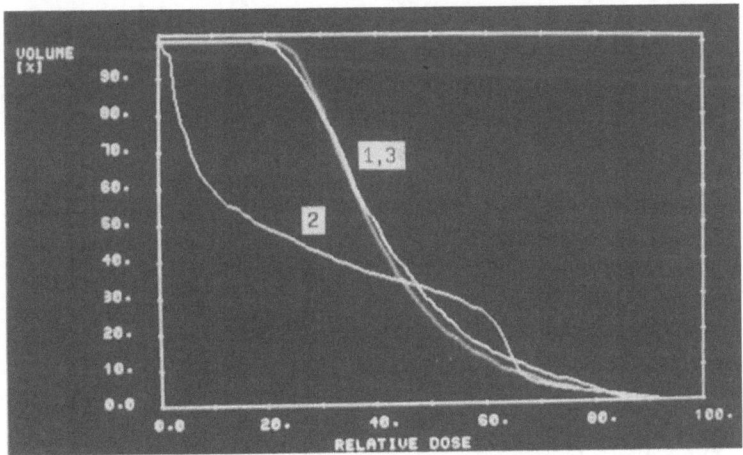

Fig. 1. Dose-volume histograms for the treatment of paraaortic lymph nodes. *No. 1*, Biaxial rotation; *no. 2*, four-field box; *no. 3*, conformal rotation using a multileaf collimator

methods (together with a third histogram for a conformal rotation simulating a multileaf collimator continuously matched to the target shape for every gantry angle). The histograms reflect the information of the complete three-dimensional dose distribution on both of the kidneys. The rotation technique provides a dose distribution which covers the complete kidney with 30%–35% of the target dose. In contrast, the box technique delivers 65% of the target dose to approximately 30% of the kidney but almost completely spares the remaining 70% of the organ. These dose-volume histograms together with histograms for homogeneous dose distributions calculated for parallel opposed beams including the entire kidney were analyzed with Lyman's algorithm. NTCPs were calculated for a range of kidney doses between 15 and 25 Gy for the rotation technique, 40 and 60 Gy for the box, and 20 and 40 Gy for the opposed beams.

Results and Discussion

Complication probabilities were calculated for an endpoint of clinical nephritis occurring within 5 years. The results are presented in Table 1. Calculated NTCPs for the opposed beams are 0.2% for 20 GY and 2.2% for 25 Gy. Above

Table 1. Complication probabilities for the kidney in radiotherapy

Technique	Maximum dose in distribution (Gy)	Total dose to kidney (Gy)	NTCP (%)	Method
Opposed beams (15 MeV photons)	20	20	0.2	Calculation
	25	25	2.2	
	28	28	14.6	
	30	30	34	
	35	35	88	
	40	40	100	
Biaxial rotation[a] (15 MeV photons)	45	15–23	0.6	Calculation
	60	20–30	17–20	
	75	25–33	90	
Four-field box[b] (15 MeV photons)	60	40	1.4	Calculation
	92.5	60	15–33	
Opposed beams[c] (Co-60, 4 MeV)		21–30	22	Patient data[d]
		30–40	57	
		41–48	100	
Opposed beams (X-rays)		20	37	Patient data[e]

Model parameters: $TD_{50} = 28$ Gy; $n = 0.7$, $m = 0.1$
[a] 30% of maximum dose to 90% of kidney;
  50% of maximum dose to 30% of kidney.
[b] 65% of maximum dose to 30% of kidney.
[c] 50%–100% of left kidney in beam portal.
[d] See [12].
[e] See [13].

this, NTCP is predicted to rapidly increase to 14.6% for 28 Gy, 34% for 30 Gy and 88% for 35 Gy. At doses above 40 Gy to the kidney 100% NTCP is calculated. These results are rather low compared with the TD_5 of 23 Gy and TD_{50} of 28 Gy used to determine the model parameters. This discrepancy may be caused by an overestimation of the volume effect. Consistant NTCPs of 5% at 23 Gy and 50% at 28 Gy would trivially be calculated for an ideally homogeneous dose distribution (leading to a single-step dose-volume histogram). The realistic histograms used in the calculations, however, also include regions of lower dose which will reduce the NTCP. Possibly these disagreements can be corrected by adjustment of the volume parameter n; however, they may also indicate an error in the calculations, or even in the model, and require further examination. Recent calculations by Niemierko and Goitein [11] show that for large complication probabilities, and for doses comparable to or larger than TD_{50} Lyman's algorithm does deviate from other models (critical element model) and may lead to an overestimation of NTCP.

For the rotation technique in which 30%–40% of the maximum dose is directed to over 90% of the kidney volume, organ doses of 25 Gy are calculated to give 90% NTCP. This, in contrast to the results for the opposed beams, appears extremely high. However, the rotational dose distribution for 25 Gy kidney dose included doses as high as 40 Gy in 40%, and 50 Gy in 15% of the organ which raise the NTCP. Again, these results may indicate an overestimation of the volume effect. Below 25 Gy, NTCP is predicted to sink rapidly, and for 15 Gy to 90% of the kidney an NTCP of 0.6% remains. For the box technique which covers 30%–35% of the kidney with dose the calculations predicted far lower complication probabilities of 15%–33% for kidney doses as high as 60 Gy. For doses of 40 Gy NTCP was calculated to sink to 1.4%. These findings suggest that the box method may entail a lower risk to the kidney even though the partial volume lying within the fields is covered by substantially higher doses than would occur in a comparable rotational technique.

The results of two publications are listed in Table 1. From the follow-up of 18 patients who received doses between 21 Gy and 48 Gy to 50%–100% of the left kidney during irradiations of gastrointestinal and retroperitoneal non-Hodgkin's lymphoma, Kim observed nephropathy in 22% (2/9) of a group receiving 21–30 Gy. The complication occurred in 57% (4/7) of a group receiving 30 Gy–40 Gy, and in all patients with doses larger than 40 Gy (3/3) [12]. These frequencies are comparable to the NTCPs calculated for the opposed beams, especially keeping in mind that the patient data reflect dose groups spread over ranges of 9–10 Gy.

Thompson reports complications in 37% (22) of a group of 84 patients treated for peptic ulcer with doses between 15 Gy and 20 Gy [13]. These irradiations were performed between 1948 and 1956 with opposed beams of X-rays. The dose distributions of this method were probably similar to the distribution delivered to the kidney by the rotation. For the rotation, the calculated NTCPs lie in the same region of up to 20%.

Conclusions

A number of requirements concerning the documentation of treatments must be fulfilled to verify theoretical models for calculating radiation treatment outcome by comparison with clinical data. To understand the dose distributions to organs at risk one needs an exact documentation of the treatment technique. This is essential if a reconstruction of the distribution is necessary, for instance, for the calculation of dose-volume histograms. In treatments causing a high risk to certain tissues it would be helpful to document additionally the dose to the respective organs. Guidelines for dose specification in organs at risk are included in the recommendations of ICRU [14]. The calculation and documentation of dose-volume histograms would also provide a valuable help in choosing among alternate treatment plans for new patients and in the follow-up of the patients, allowing an immediate correlation between dose load and radiation effect.

Finally, substantial help in testing radiobiological models would be provided by standardization in the follow-up and documentation of patients regarding definitions of complications that include a correlation with radiobiological endpoints and regarding regular examination for their occurrence. In any case radiobiological models, including that examined here, must also be carefully verified concerning both relative and absolute predictions before they can be clinically applied. Only then can they provide a rationale for decisions in the optimization of radiotherapy.

References

1. Douglas BG, Fowler JF (1976) The effect of multiple small doses of X-rays on skin reactions in the mouse and a basic interpretation. Radiat Res 66: 401–426
2. Barendsen GW (1982) Dose fractionation, dose rate and isoeffect relationships for normal tissue responses. Int J Radiat Oncol Biol Phys 8: 1981–1999
3. Thames HD (1985) An 'incomplete repair' model for survival after fractionated and continuous irradiations. Int J Radiat Oncol Biol Phys 47: 319–339
4. Fowler JF (1988) What do we need to know to predict the effectiveness of fractionated radiotherapy schedules? Caldwell Memorial Lecture 1988. In: Paliwal BR, Fowler JF, Herbert DE, Kinsella TJ, Orton CG (eds) Prediction of response in radiation therapy. AAPM Symp Proc 7 (1): 1–24
5. Schlegel W, Scharfenberg H, Doll J, Hartmann G, Sturm V, Lorenz WJ (1984) Three dimensional dose planning using tomographic data. In: Cunningham JR (ed) Proceedings of the 8th international conference on the use of computers in radiotherapy. IEEE Computer Society Press, Silver Spring, pp 191–195
6. Lyman JT (1985) Complication probabilities as assessed from dose-volume histograms. Radiat Res 104: S13–S19
7. Lyman T, Wolbarst AB (1987) Optimization of radiation therapy. III. a method of assessing complication probabilities from dose-volume histograms. Int J Radiat Oncol Biol Phys 13: 103–109

8. Lyman JT, Wolbarst AB (1989) Optimization of radiation therapy. IV. a dose-volume histogram reduction algorithm. Int J Radiat Oncol. Biol. Phys. 17: 433–436; 1989
9. Mechler J (1988) Quasi-dreidimensionale Bestrahlungsplanung für die paraaortale Lymphknotenbestrahlung. Dissertation, University of Heidelberg
10. Becker G (1990) Klinische Aspekte der dreidimensionalen Bestrahlungsplanung und der Konformationstherapie. Dissertation, University of Heidelberg
11. Niemierko A, Goitein M (1991) Calculation of normal tissue complication probability and dose-volume histogram reduction schemes for tissues with a critical element architecture. Radiother Oncol 20: 166–176
12. Kim TH, Somerville PJ, Freeman CR (1984) Unilateral radiation nephropathy — the long-term significance. Int J Radiat Oncol Biol Phys 10: 2053–2059
13. Thompson PL, Mackay IR, Robson GSM, Wall AJ (1971) Late radiation nephritis after gastric X-irradiation for peptic ulcer. Q J Med XL (157): 145–157
14. International commission on radiation units and measurements (1978) Dose specification for reporting external beam therapy with photons and electrons. ICRU Rep 29; Bethesda, Maryland

Fractionation Treatment Planning for Sequential Half-Body Irradiation of Small-Cell Lung Cancer

K. Merkle and W. Schmidt

Introduction

Early recurrence after sequential half-body irradiation (SHBI) of patients with small-cell lung cancer (SCLC) is still of crucial importance. The need to spare normal lung tissue prohibits a further increase in total dose for improving therapeutic results. However, changing the current fractionation schedules can improve the efficacy of radiation treatment by making use of the different repair capacities of normal lung tissue and SCLC cells. Choosing among different variations of the time-dose relationship is an empirical process in the treatment of SCLC by SHBI, and the consideration of peculiarities in proliferation kinetics of this tumor type is unsatisfactory. To improve fractionation schedules in the palliative radiotherapy of SCLC we therefore developed a model on the basis of the present experimental and clinical data for facilitating the systematic evaluation of current and future clinical investigations.

Methods

Due to complications of the dose-limiting organ (lung) upper half-body irradiation is considered primary. A lower half-body irradiation carried out some 6 weeks later can be considered in almost the same way.

We sought to answer the following question: Given the best available estimates of the radiosensitivity of SCLC cells and a proven isoeffect model for the normal lung, what schedules are most appropriate for the treatment of SCLC by SHBI? This kind of radiation therapy is used as a palliative. During the treatment sessions SCLC cells can disseminate from the upper body to the lower and vice versa. Independently of this, the focus should be on the greatest possible cell kill and the avoidance of radiation pneumonitis.

The radiobiological assumptions involved in our approach are as follows.

1. The fractionation schedule in lung is taken to be of crucial importance and the lung to be the dose-limiting organ. The SCLC cell population is assumed to obtain a uniform dose equal to that of the lung.

Department of Clinical Radiobiology, Max-Delbrück-Center for Molecular Medicine, Robert-Rössle-Str. 10, 1115 Berlin-Buch, FRG

Advanced Radiation Therapy Tumor Response
Monitoring and Treatment Planning
Breit (Editor-in-Chief)
© Springer-Verlag, Berlin Heidelberg 1992

2. Enough time is left after every radiation session to complete the repair of radiation damage of the lung. To achieve this at least 6 h between fractions must be allowed.

3. The linear-quadratic (LQ) model adequately describes the radiation damage to the normal lung tissue. The α/β ratio was defined as 2.857 Gy by a special evaluation method from the first clinical experience in our clinic (Eichhorn et al. 1983) concerning radiation pneumonitis after SHBI with high single doses and was similar to the ratios used elsewhere (e.g. Fowler 1989).

4. The killing of SCLC cells by radiation is also described by the LQ model. The values for α and β were taken from in vitro experiments (Malaise et al. 1986) and have mean values of $\alpha = 0.65 \text{ Gy}^{-1} \pm 37\%$ and $\beta = 0.081 \text{ Gy}^{-2} \pm 183\%$.

5. The effective doubling time (T_{eff}) of a human SCLC cell population needed for our analysis was calculated from the data of Muggia et al. (1974) and amounted to about 40 days (960 h). This value is in agreement with results of other researchers (Salazar et al. 1976; Strauss 1974).

6. It is assumed that SCLC cells proliferate exponentially between radiation fractions.

7. Only high dose-rate irradiation is considered, and variations in dose rate are neglected.

For the calculation of fractionation schedules we used the concepts of extrapolated response dose (ERD; Barendsen 1982) and relative effectiveness (RE; Dale 1985), with:

$$\text{ERD} = D \cdot \text{RE}(F_n)$$

and

$$\text{RE}(F_n) = 1 + \frac{1}{n} \cdot \frac{\alpha}{\beta} \cdot D$$

where D is the total dose and F_n is the fractionation schedule with n equal fractions.

The program first finds the total dose (D) for a given number of fractions (n) using $\text{ERD} = D \cdot \text{RE}(F_n)$. SCLC cell survival $S(D)$ is then defined by the LQ model using the formula $S(D) = \exp(-\alpha \cdot D/n - \beta \cdot D^2/n^2)$. Since tumor cells grow exponentially between treatment sessions, the relative tumor kill can be calculated. In the program all fractionation schedules from 1 to 60 treatment sessions with equal fractions are taken into account. Furthermore, the number of treatment weeks, single and total doses, and the presumed time interval needed to regrow to the original tumor volume are calculated by the program.

Results

Using the computer program the following fractionation schedules were analyzed: one, two, three, and four fractions per day with and without the weekend (up to 60 fractions each). The results indicate that the treatment with or without the weekend did not have any essential influence on the result in terms of SCLC cell kill. Furthermore, the radiotherapy with two, three, or four sessions per day had almost no influence on the effect on SCLC. Hence for further analysis of treatment schedules one and two fractions per day and treatment without using the weekend were compared.

Figure 1 presents the results of calculations for one treatment session daily. Using several effective tumor doubling times results in very different fractionation curves. The variation in T_{eff} from 72 to 5016 h corresponds to the range reported by several researchers (Strauss 1974; Lenhard et al. 1981; Fowler 1990). In very rapidly proliferating tumors (T_{eff} = 72 h) the optimal treatment effect is achieved after the fifth session. More fractionation leads to less effective results. After 21 fractions the results are even worse than after a single irradiation. With increasing T_{eff} the maximum of the curves shifts in the direction of increasing numbers of fractions, and this is not reached before 60 fractions considering very high T_{eff}. The latter shows very little improvement with increasing numbers of fractions beyond a certain value. Using the one-fraction per day schedule it is not recommended to administer more than ten fractions within 2 weeks if T_{eff} is not precisely known.

The effect improves when two fractions per day are used. Figure 2 shows that the two-fraction per day schedule has essentially the same shape for every T_{eff} considered; however, the cell kill for tumors with little T_{eff} is higher. After ten fractions (5 days) a cell kill is reached which almost covers a reduction in tumor volume for low as well as for high T_{eff} near the maximum. With the shorter treatment time into account with two fractions per day and the more favorable characteristic of fractionation curves for that schedule, ten fractions in 5 days are recommended (2 sessions per day) with single doses of 1.8 Gy.

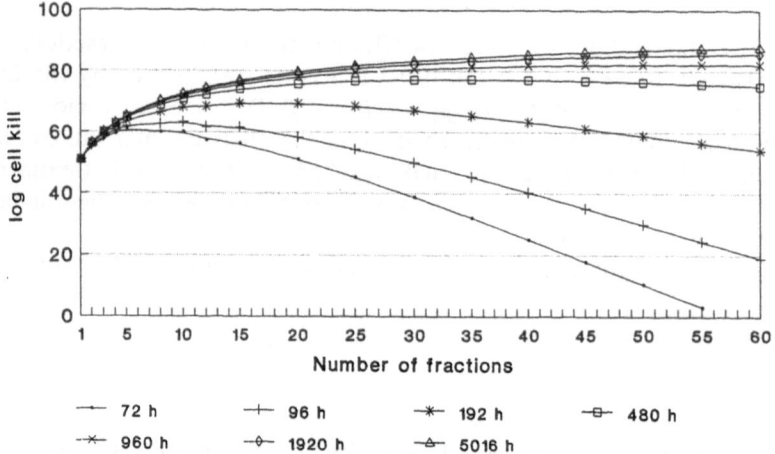

Fig. 1. Treatment efficiency depending on number of fractions for a one-session per day regime. SCLC has an effective doubling time of 960 h. For comparison, possible variations in this parameter from 72 to 5016 h are given. ERD = 30 Gy. *Ordinate,* log cell kill · (− 5 · ln 10)

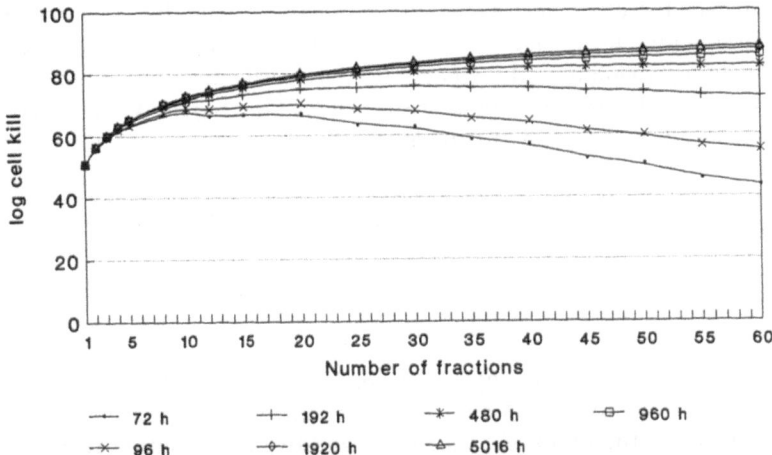

Fig. 2. Treatment efficiency depending on number of fractions for a two-session per day regime. SCLC has an effective doubling time of 960 h. For comparison, possible variations in this parameter from 72 to 5016 h are given. Especially for fast proliferating tumors this treatment regime shows better results compared to the one fraction per day schedule. ERD = 30 Gy. *Ordinate*, log cell kill $\cdot(-5\cdot\ln 10)$

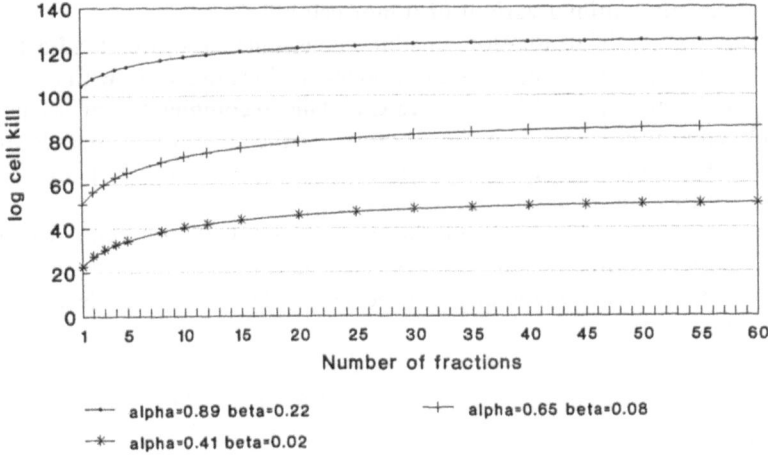

Fig. 3. *Middle curve*, treatment efficiency of a two fraction per day regime for an effective doubling time T_{eff} = 960 h. *Upper and lower curves*, the same parameters but α and β are used with the variation limits found experimentally (Malaise et al. 1986). Considering the possible variations in these parameters the treatment effect can be changed drastically, but the character of the curves remain the same. *Ordinate*, log cell kill $\cdot(-5\cdot\ln 10)$

Figure 3 shows three curves with T_{eff} = 40 days (960 h) and the two-fraction per day schedule considering the relatively high coefficients of variation in determination of α and β for SCLC cells (Malaise et al. 1986). Figure 3 indicates that possible variation in α and β in the given limits leads to very different values of cell kill, but the character of the curves remains essentially the same. The middle curve represents the mean values of α and β. The upper and lower curves give a rough approximation of the possible confidence interval. Even under the conditions of extreme variation in the parameters of the LQ model ten fractions in 5 days may lead to good treatment results considering the short overall treatment time.

Conclusions

1. The currently used and empirically confirmed fractionation schedules for SHBI of SCLC lead to a great reduction in radiation pneumonitis rates. The early recidivism of the tumor calls for more effective fractionation regimes.

2. By a better exploitation of differing repair capacities of normal lung tissue and tumor cells an improvement of palliation can be expected.

3. The concept of extrapolated response dose can be used as a basis for a computer program to calculate optimized fractionation schedules.

4. The calculation indicates that a treatment consisting of only one or two fractions (which are currently used) can be worse by some orders of magnitude compared with the optimal variant of tumor cell kill.

5. An analysis of the irradiation schedules determined as optimal indicates a two fraction per day regime up to ten treatment sessions in 5 days with a single dose of 1.8 Gy and a total dose of 18 Gy. This recommendation seems a reasonable compromise between the duration of the treatment schedule and total cell kill considering the great variation in T_{eff} and the lack of exact knowledge of this parameters in individual patients.

6. An acceleration of radiotherapy using more than two fractions per day and the inclusion of the weekend did not result in an essential increase in the effect on the tumor. A possible gain can be seen only in a further decrease in treatment time.

References

Barendsen GW (1982) Dose fractionation, dose rate and isoeffect relationships for normal tissue responses. Int J Radiat Oncol Biol Phys 8: 1981–1999

Dale RG (1985) The application of the linear-quadratic dose-effect equation to fractionated and protected radiotherapy. Br J Radiol 58: 515–528

Eichhorn H-J, Hüttner J, Dallüge K-H, Welker K (1983) Preliminary report on "one time" and high dose irradiation of the upper and lower half-body in patients with small cell lung cancer. Int J Radiat Oncol Biol Phys 9: 1459–1465

Fitzpatrick PJ, Rider WD (1976) Half-body radiotherapy. Int J Radiat Oncol Biol Phys 1: 197–207

Fowler JF (1989) The linear-quadratic formula and progress in fractionated radiotherapy. Br J Radiol 62: 679–694

Fowler JF (1990) How worthwhile are short schedules in radiotherapy? A series of exploratory calculations. Radiother Oncol 18: 165–181

Lenhard RE, Woo KB, Freund JS, Abeloff MD (1981) Growth kinetics of small cell carcinoma of the lung. Eur J Cancer Clin Oncol 17: 899–904

Malaise EP, Fertil B, Chavandra N, Guichard M (1986) Distribution of radiation sensitivities for human tumor cells of specific histological types: comparison of in vitro to in vivo data. Int J Radiat Oncol Biol Phys 12: 617–624

Muggia FM, Krezoski SK, Hansen HH (1974) Cell kinetic studies in patients with small cell carcinoma of the lung. Cancer 34: 1683–1690

Salazar OM, Rubin P, Brown JC, Feldstein MI, Keller BE (1976) Predictors of radiation response in lung cancer. Cancer 37: 2636–2650

Steel GG, Peacock JH (1989) Why are some human tumors more radiosensitive than others? Radiother Oncol 15: 63–72

Strauss MJ (1974) The growth characteristics of lung cancer and its applications of treatment design. Semin Oncol 1: 167–174

Efficacy of Biological Isoeffect Distributions in Clinical Practice

R. Schwarz[1], D. Rades[1], R. Schmidt[1], H.-P. Beck-Bornholdt[2], and K.-H. Hübener[1]

Calculation of Biological Isoeffect Distributions

The calculations described below permit a comparison of the biological effects of different fractionation schemes, with different doses per fraction (d), overall treatment times (t), total doses (D), and numbers of fractions (N). Since the tolerance doses (TD) for the various tissues are generally given in the literature [5, 6] in terms of treatments with fractions of 2 Gy administered with five fractions per week, it is convenient to relate all the different treatment schemes to this standard fractionation schedule. The calculations are based on the linear-quadratic model. However, analogous calculations can be performed with any other model that describes dose and time effects in fractionated radiotherapy.

The linear-quadratic model [3] describes many biological effects of ionizing radiation. In this model the effect is given as a linear-quadratic function of dose:

$$\text{Effect}(D) = \alpha D + \beta D^2 \tag{1}$$

where α and β are the corresponding coefficients for the linear and quadratic terms, respectively. For a fractionated irradiation with N fractions, the total dose D is given by $D = Nd$, where d represents the dose per fraction. If we assume that all fractions are isoeffective, i.e., that the same fractions of cells are inactivated with any fraction, the effects of subsequent treatments are additive, and the biological effect is given by [2, 4]:

$$\text{Effect} = N(\alpha d + \beta d^2) \tag{2}$$

if we assume that the time interval between the various fractions is sufficient to allow for complete repair of sublethal and potentially lethal damage. The linear-quadratic model does not include repopulation. Thus, this effect must be considered separately. It can be added to the linear-quadratic equation as follows:

$$\text{Effect} = N(\alpha d + \beta d^2) - \gamma t \tag{3}$$

[1] Department of Radiotherapy, University Hospital Eppendorf, Martinistr. 52, 2000 Hamburg 20, FRG

[2] Institute of Biophysics and Radiobiology, University Hospital Eppendorf, Martinistr. 52, 2000 Hamburg 20, FRG

Advanced Radiation Therapy Tumor Response Monitoring and Treatment Planning
Breit (Editor-in-Chief)
© Springer-Verlag, Berlin Heidelberg 1992

where γ represents the proliferation rate. In some tissues proliferation does not start until some time (*tlag*) after start of irradiation. This can be considered by replacing t in Eq. (3) by $(t - tlag)$.

If a given treatment schedule is to be compared to a reference schedule with a different number of fractions, dose per fraction, and overall treatment time, isoeffectivity is achieved when:

$$\alpha Nd + \beta Nd^2 - \gamma t = \alpha N_{ref} d_{ref} + \beta N_{ref} d_{ref}^2 - \gamma t_{ref} \tag{4}$$

In general, it is relatively easy to determine the α/β ratios for the various tissues, whereas the absolute values of α and β are almost unknown. Thus, it is useful to transform this equation as follows:

$$\frac{\alpha}{\beta}D + dD - \frac{\gamma}{\beta}t = \frac{\alpha}{\beta}D_{ref} + d_{ref}D_{ref} - \frac{\gamma}{\beta}t_{ref} \tag{5}$$

$$D = \frac{(\alpha/\beta + d_{ref})D_{ref} - \gamma/\beta(t_{ref} - t)}{\alpha/\beta + d} \tag{6}$$

where d_{ref} represents the total dose applied in the reference schedule. Reference schedules in tolerance calculations have also been used by others [2, 4, 7].

As already mentioned, tolerance doses are generally given for treatments with 2 Gy per fraction. Equation (6) can be transformed to calculate tolerance doses for treatments with different doses per fraction:

$$TD = \frac{(\alpha/\beta + d_{ref})TD_{ref} - \gamma/\beta(t_{ref} - t)}{\alpha/\beta + d} \tag{7}$$

where TD_{ref} represents the tolerance dose of the reference treatment with a dose per fraction of 2 Gy.

The biological isodose (BI) expressed as percentage of the tolerance dose is given by:

$$BI = \frac{100D}{TD} = \frac{100D(\alpha/\beta + d)}{(\alpha/\beta + d_{ref})TD_{ref} - \gamma/\beta(t_{ref} - t)}. \tag{8}$$

From Equation (8) the biological isodose for different fractionation schedules can be calculated by normalization to a standard treatment and the corresponding tolerance doses of the various tissues involved.

Methods and Material

To evaluate the efficiency of biological isoeffect distributions we analyzed the data on 28 patients suffering from bronchial carcinoma and two patients suffering from non-Hodgkin lymphoma who were irradiated over the period from 1987 through 1990. Eight patients had small-cell lung cancer, 20 had non-small-cell lung cancer, and two had non-Hodgkin lymphoma. Tumor stage for patients with bronchial carcinoma was: stage I, 12 patients; stage II, two; stage IIIa, six; stage IIIb, three; and stage IV, five. Before radiotherapy ten patients had surgical interventions. Lobectomy was used in eight cases and pneumectomy in two. Ten patients received chemotherapy before. In all cases radiotherapy was planned on the basis of computed tomography (Philips Tomoscan 350). The treatment planning in terms of absorbed dose was performed by the system SIDOS-U1 (Siemens) on a PDP 11/45 computer and the system Mevaplan (Siemens). The body contours and the anatomical topography of the patients' cross-sections were obtained from computed tomography and entered into the computer by digitizer and stored as polygons. In the course of treatment planning the technique of irradiation and the radiation qualities were chosen and modified to optimize physical dose distributions. The dose calculation was performed within a 50×60 matrix, which was stored for further use. As the code for the treatment planning is written mainly in FORTRAN, modifications could easily be made to enable the calculations of the biological isoeffect distributions based on the algorithm described above. For these calculations, the stored topographical and dose distribution data were reprocessed. In a dialogue procedure the polygons corresponding to the different organs were displayed, and a code number corresponding to the type of biological tissue was assigned to the contour polygons. Subsequently a code matrix was generated, based on the same grid as the dose matrix, allowing definition of the type of tissue for every element of the matrix. After defining the total dose corresponding to the 100% level, the number of fractions, and the overall treatment time, the dose matrix and the code matrix were used to calculate the biological isoeffects and were normalized to the corresponding tolerance dose of the respective organ for each matrix element separately. For every normal tissue considered these calculations require the following biological parameters: tolerance dose (5% incidence of intolerable normal tissue damage), α/β ratio, overall treatment time, time exponent for slow repair in lung as 0.05. The following tolerance doses and, respectively, α/β ratios were used for the tissues: Lung, 36 Gy, 3.7 Gy (γ/β ratio, 2.2 Gy^2/day); spinal cord, 50 Gy, 1.8 Gy; and bone, 60 Gy, 3.5 Gy.

Different treatment schedules were used for the analyzed patients. Total doses ranged from 30 to 60 Gy, single doses from 1.7 to 2.5 Gy, and treatment time from 24 to 57 days. Based on these parameters and the stored physical treatment plans, biological isoeffect distributions were calculated for all patients. For all patients clinical data, X-ray films of the chest, and computerized assisted tomography (CAT) scan of the chest before and after therapy were analyzed to measure lung fibrosis and look for radiation myelitis.

Lung fibrosis was graded on PA X-rays of the chest using a scoring system described by Arriagada [1]. In correspondence to CAT scan of the chest areas of lung fibrosis were related to the calculated biological isoeffect distributions.

Results

The survival rate in patients with bronchial carcinoma was 63% 1 year after radiotherapy and 30% 2 years after radiotherapy. The local recurrence rate was 23.3%. Twenty patients died. The analysis included 186 X-ray examinations of the chest and 16 CAT examinations in 30 patients. The longest follow-up time was 42 months after radiotherapy. No patient died of radiotherapy-related problems. No one developed neurological deficits as side effect after radiotherapy. The effects on the spinal cord were well below tolerance dose in all patients. In all cases the lung was subjected partially to a dose above the 100 units tolerance level. Eight patients developed pneumonitis; 28 developed lung fibrosis within irradiated parts of the lung. The onset of lung fibrosis ranged from 1 to 9.8 months, with a mean of 4.1 months. Scoring of lung fibrosis showed the following distribution: score 1, three patients; score 2, two; score 3, four; score 4, five; score 5, three; score 6, three; score 7, one; and score 9, one. A comparison with biological isoeffect distributions shows that lung fibrosis occurred in areas with a minimal biologically effective dose of 20 units; the range was between 20 and 190 units. Summarizing all patients, lung fibrosis in areas with biologically effective doses of 20 units occurred in one patient, 100 units in 11, 125 units in four, 150 in five, and 190 units in one. The risk of lung fibrosis seems to increase with higher biologically effective doses.

Discussion

Treatment planning is widely understood today as the process of optimizing dose distributions in time and space. For considering the dose-time relationship different analytical approaches can be used. Some efforts have been made to calculate the biological influence of different fractionations in order to make irradiation treatment comparable. These calculations are routinely performed for some discrete reference points. Some authors have modified the model to include volume effects and heterogeneities, although it is extremely difficult to derive the corresponding parameters from analysis of clinical results. It can be stated that the available biological data are not sufficient to enable a complete correlation between physical and biological dose distributions. Our own results obtained in patients with bronchial carcinomas are preliminary and experimental. Further investigations in a great number of patients is necessary to reach conclusions on the efficacy of biological isoeffect distributions. All clinical and radiobiological parameters which could influence the effects on normal tissues should be evaluated. Calculation of biological isoeffect distributions is a simple technique to facilitate the transfer of new radiobiological and clinical findings into routine clinical treatment planning. The use of biological isoeffective distributions may help to visualize risks for normal tissues according to different treatment schedules. At this time data are not sufficient to quantify these effects or to make predictions on defined biological isoeffect distributions.

References

1. Arriagada R, de Guevra JCL, Mouriesse H, Hanzen C, Couanet D, Ruffie P, Baldeyrou P, Deway J, Lusinchi A, Martin M, le Chevalier R (1989) Limited small cell lung cancer treated by combined radiotherapy and chemotherapy: evaluation of a grading system of lung fibrosis. Radiother Oncol 1: 1–8
2. Barendsen GW (1982) Dose fractionation, dose rate and iso-effect relationships for normal tissue responses. Int J Radiat Oncol Biol Phys 8: 1981–1997
3. Chadwick KH, Leenhouts HP (1973) A molecular theory of cell survival. Phys Med Biol 18: 78–87
4. Fowler JF (1984) What next in fractionated radiotherapy? Br J Cancer 49 [Suppl VI]: 285–300
5. Rubin P, Casarett GW (1968) Clinical radiation pathology. Saunders, Philadelphia
6. Sack H, Leetz HK (1987) Bestrahlungsplanung. In: Scherer E (ed) Strahlentherapie. Radiologische Onkologie, 3rd edn. Springer, Berlin Heidelberg New York
7. Van Dyck J, Keane TJ (1989) Determination of parameters for the linear-quadratic model for radiation-induced lung-damage. Int J Radiat Oncol Biol Phys 17: 695–698

A Biological Therapy Planning System for Use in Remote High Dose Rate Afterloading

K. Baier

Introduction

In radiotherapy treatment planning only spatial dose distributions are generally calculated very accurately. Often planning is done without taking into account the influence of dose rate, number of fractions, or other more time-dependent factors. This leads to the distinction between two types of treatment planning: the physical and the biological. Although the time factor is accepted as being very important, no treatment planning system has provided a solution with a general approach to biological treatment planning. The reason for this lies in the complexity of the problem and the special architecture of the planning systems for physical dose planning. However, there are some investigations made by different authors to overcome these problems. There are at least two different points of view: in analogy to physical treatment planning, one considers lines of biological isoeffect (Licht and Leetz 1986; Schmidt et al. 1988); the other takes into account at least the effects in the organs at risk (Baltas 1988; Baier 1987). The first of these approaches implies an enormous amount of calculation time whereas the second encourages rather the comparison of the effectiveness of different treatment plans.

Biological Treatment Planning in Clinical Routine

One of the main differences between physical and biological treatment planning is that the former normally finishes with the first treatment plan; the doses are linearly additive and do not depend on the time of administration. For the latter, this is not true. The biological effect of radiation varies with numerous parameters, such as dose rate, time of administration, number of fractions, and the dose per fraction; none of these parameters are calculated in physical dose planning. As a result, biological treatment planning must be carried out over the whole treatment period, which entails a tremendous amount of work in a normal radiation department. In practice, therefore, biological treatment planning can be compared to physical planning only in retrospective studies. The

Strahlenabteilung, Universitäts-Frauenklinik, Josef-Schneider-Str. 4, 8700 Würzburg, FRG

Advanced Radiation Therapy Tumor Response
Monitoring and Treatment Planning
Breit (Editor-in-Chief)
© Springer-Verlag, Berlin Heidelberg 1992

only way to carry out biological planning during clinical routine is to use a computer.

The success of incorporating a biological treatment planning system into clinical routine depends on the way in which the system is implemented. There are three different methods to integrate such a system into a radiotherapy department. One is through the use of a conventional physical treatment planning system. Although most of these planning systems are powerful machines, this task is inconvenient for the staff. In most cases, the physical treatment planning system is not in close proximity to the therapy units. Also, only one case at a time can be handled, and in general these cases are different for the different therapy units and planning systems. The second is integration into a verification system. Most treatment machines use verification systems. These systems report and control the complete status of the machine. However, if there are different treatment machines in the same department. one must deal with the problem of linkage. The third method involves an independent system. Using a freely programmable computer with interfaces to the treatment planning systems and treatment units, it is possible to create a highly sophisticated and reliable planning system.

The Planning System Biodoc

The biological treatment planning system used in the radiation department of the Universitäts-Frauenklinik in Würzburg is based on the third method discussed above and is described elsewhere (Baier 1987, 1989). Since starting in 1985 this system has been used in clinical routine with a high degree of acceptance by the staff. The basic concepts of the system are (a) every treatment unit uses its own workstation, which means that all relevant data concerning the time schedule and physical treatment plan of a patient are collected; (b) all relevant data of an individual treatment are stored in a central database, which means that all data of a patient even for different treatment machines and treatment regimes are available simultaneously. Therefore it is very easy to calculate changes in the biological effect caused by machine breakdown or other events (fever or holidays). Also, there is no restriction to the use of any known radiobiological model. Up to 20 parameters are handled for up to 50 different models. At least two independent biological effects calculated by these models are displayed at the workstation. All inputs are made online into the planning system with any changes in the treatment plan depicted in a calendar form. The system presents up to 2 months of the radiotherapy timetable and all relevant data. The system consists of five modules which include all of the necessary features for a planning system: biological treatment planning, organizational tool, documentation, archiving, and customizing. Each of these modules is subdivided into many different functions and modules.

Biological Treatment Planning in Gynecological Brachytherapy

The main difference between external-beamtherapy and gynecological remote high dose rate afterloading is that the latter is not a multiple administration of the same dose distribution. While it is usual in external-beam therapy to administer 20–25 times the once-calculated dose distribution, in brachytherapy every fraction needs its own treatment planning because of the changed geometry. Thus not all of the relevant parameters for calculating the biological effect are constant. One of the most important factors is dose rate. Due to the dominant influence of the inverse square law in brachytherapy the dose rate is modulated by this effect. Therefore each particular region in the patient is treated with a different dose rate. To take this into account the treatment planning system must be able to calculate biological effects in the administered dose rate regions. Volume effects are also very important because of the inhomogeneous dose distribution. At a closer look, it is not the dose delivered to the whole volume of the hollow organ at risk—such as bladder and rectum— but the dose administered to the wall of these organs which must be taken into account. Moreover, as an effect of the combination of the different treatment modalities such as external beam and brachytherapy, the problem of summarizing dose effects in the same anatomical region arises, for the anatomical geometry may be disturbed by applicators and tamponades.

The Modified Biodoc System

To overcome these problems, the main modification in the Biodoc system used in external beam therapy is the introduction of up to ten regions of interest (ROIs) representing organs at risk. These ROIs are attached to specific anatomic structures or organs. It is thereby possible to superimpose different treatment regimes in an accurate way. According to the ICRU (1985), for example, the doses in bladder and rectum are to measure directly (in vivo) by semiconductor probes in the case of brachytherapy. The biological effect in each ROI is calculated by its individual radiobiological model and parameters. The results are displayed as percentages of deviation from the corresponding reference. Thus it is very easy to estimate the changes of effects forced by each individual afterloading administration directly to the target and to the organs at risk.

Discussion

It has been shown that it is possible to handle biological treatment planning also in brachytherapy, even when combining it with external radiation. This treatment planning system is a powerful utility for clinicians especially when treating a large number of patients. Future investigations will involve adapting the system to a PC-based local area network. Operating in such a network, it will be easy to interchange data between physical treatment planning systems. This makes it possible to perform volume or surface analysis based on three-dimensional patient models. It will also be able to transfer data to patient databases for follow-up and reasearch.

References

Baier K (1987) Ein biologisches Planungssystem für die routinemäßige klinische Strahlentherapie. Rontgenberichte 16: 180–191

Baier K (1989) A biological treatment planning system. In: Martinez AA, Orton CG, Mould RF (eds) Brachytherapy HDR and LDR. Proceedings of remote afterloading: state of the art, Dearborn, pp 217–228

Baltas D (1988) Ein Rechenprogramm zur Berücksichtigung von Dosis und Zeit nach dem NSD- und dem linearquadratischen Modell in der Strahlentherapie. Thesis, University of Heidelberg

ICRU (1985) Dose and volume specification for reporting intracavitary therapy in gynaecology. Report no 38 (International Commission on Radiation Units and Measurements, Bethesda, Maryland, USA)

Licht N, Leetz HK (1986) Biologische Bewertung von Energiedosiverteilungen durch prob- lemorientierte Bildverarbeitung. Medizinische Physik, pp 19–26

Schmidt R, Beck-Bornholdt HP, Schwarz R (1988) Biologische Isoeffekt-Verteilungen. Medizinische Physik, pp 481–487

Biological Treatment Planning Based on the Multi-Powerlaw Model

L. Voigtmann

Assessing the biological effect of radiotherapy must consider both the intended tumor control and the undesired normal tissue damage and likewise not only the spatial but also very importantly the temporal conditions of dose delivery. The goal of biological treatment planning in expanding the customary physical treatment planning consists in optimizing not only the spatial but also the temporal dose distribution to achieve a maximum of tumor control with a minimum of normal tissue damage. In addition to this, a suitable reference quantity is necessary, which encompasses both the spatial and the temporal conditions of dose delivery and quantifies tumor control as well as normal tissue damage. At the present time such a reference quantity which fulfills all four of these requirements is unknown.

Absorbed dose, the reference quantity of physical treatment planning, considers only the spatial dose distribution and does not quantify biological effects. The cell survival rate as a possible reference quantity for biological treatment planning can encompass both spatial and temporal conditions of dose delivery and quantify tumor control, but the inadequacy of individual values for model parameters means that these possibilities have not made their way into clinical use.

Presently the linear-quadratic (LQ) model is generally preferred for quantifying the biological effect of fractionated irradiations to normal tissues because of its claim of having a scientific basis. However, the concept of extrapolated response dose in this model is of only limited suitability for biological treatment planning because it does not include the temporal dose distribution.

The multi-power law (MP) model is formulated as follows:

$$\text{BEN} = \left(\sum_{i=1}^{N} d_i^a \, \Delta t_i^b \right)^c$$

where BEN means the biological effect on normal tissue, d_i is the dose for the i fraction (given in Gy $\times$ 100), Δt_i is the time interval between the i and $i+1$ fractions (given in days), and N is the number of fractions. The values of the exponents in early-reacting tissues are: $a = 1.538$, $b = -0.169$, $c' = 0.65$; and in late-reacting tissues: $a = 1.587$, $b = -0.080$, $c = 0.63$. This model results from a generalization of Ellis's nominal standard dose (NSD) equation with the

Department of Radiotherapy, Clinic and Policlinic of Radiology, Medical Academy Carl Gustav Carus, Fetscherstr. 74, O-8019 Dresden, FRG

Advanced Radiation Therapy Tumor Response
Monitoring and Treatment Planning
Breit (Editor-in-Chief)
© Springer-Verlag, Berlin Heidelberg 1992

change of the global quantities of total dose (D) and total treatment time (T) to the mathematically independent and biologically more relevant quantities of dose per fraction and especially time interval to the administration of the next fraction (Voigtmann 1984). The quantity of BEN encompasses both the spatial and the temporal dose distribution and quantifies the biological effect on normal tissues. The exponent values a, b, c for early-reacting tissues result from Ellis's original exponents 0.24 for N and 0.11 for T. For late-reacting tissues, on the other hand, they result from investigations of radiation-induced pneumopathy (Herrmann et al. 1986, 1987), with findings for exponent values of 0.32 for N and 0.05 for T (Voigtmann et al. 1988).

In the context of the time-dose-fractionation problem the definition of total treatment time is a most important question. In the literature the following three definitions are used (Fig. 1): elapsed time: $T1 = t_N - t_1$; nominal time: $T2 = t_N + 1 - t_1$; overall treatment time: $T3 = t_{N+1} - t_1$. The MP model is based on the third of these definitions, elaborated by Orton and Ellis (1974). Only this definition considers the last fraction in the biological evaluation in the same way as all preceding fractions, concretely with the middle time interval between all other fractions. In accordance with the recommendation of Goitein (1976), the uniform and exclusive use of only this definition for total treatment time must be claimed.

The BEN for two series is calculated using Kirk's "equivalence condition at the junction between consecutive fractionation schemes" (Kirk et al. 1971). In terms of this, the biological effect of the preceding series is expressed in an equivalent number ($\bar{n}_2$) of fractions of the succeeding series, which can then be added to the number (n_2) of true fractions of this series:

$$n_1 d_1^{1.538} \Delta t_1^{-0.169} = \bar{n}_2 d_2^{1.538} \cdot \Delta t_2^{-0.169}$$

$$\mathrm{BEN}_{1+2} = [(\bar{n}_2 + n_2) d_2^{1.538} \Delta t_2^{-0.169}]^{0.65}$$

$$\mathrm{BEN}_{1+2} = (n_1 d_1^{1.538} \Delta t_1^{-0.169} + n_2 d_2^{1.538} \Delta t_2^{-0.169})^{0.65}$$

To include a consideration of rest periods, Ellis's method of gap correction for one series with a succeeding gap of P days (Ellis 1968) is adapted:

$$\mathrm{BEN}_{1+P} = (n_1 d_1^{1.538} \Delta t_1^{-0.169} Z_1)^{0.65}$$

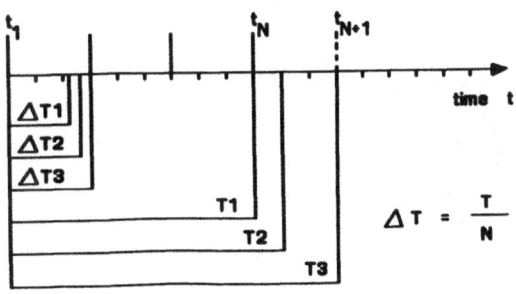

$$\Delta T = \frac{T}{N}$$

Fig. 1. Schematic representation to the different definitions of total treatment time

with

$$Z_1 = \left(\frac{n_1 \Delta t_1}{n_1 \Delta t_1 + P}\right)^{0.169} \qquad \text{("decay factor")}$$

A generalization of this principle for two or more series before the gap is possible in the following way (Voigtmann 1984):

$$Z_{1+2} = \left(\frac{(\bar{n}_2 + n_2)\Delta t_2}{(\bar{n}_2 + n_2)\Delta t_2 + P}\right)^{0.169}$$

The decay factor for the period in which the biological effect before the gap occurs must consider the effective time in terms of Kirk's equivalence condition. Additionally, Ellis's maximum gap length of 100 days is replaced by a minimum value for the decay factor of 0.5. The iterative use of this method allows the BEN to be calculated for any complex radiotherapy course with gaps and different fractionation schemes (Voigtmann 1989).

A formal description of a therapy course was developed for the practical calculation of BEN distributions in cross-sections for biological treatment planning. With this the calculation algorithm can evaluate biologically the actual spatial and temporal conditions of dose delivery at each calculation point in the body region. This formal description contains a numbered list of all fractional dose distributions and a line vector, the number of components in which is equal to the number of days in the therapy course (including the last fraction). The vector components contain the number of the fractional dose distribution, administered on a given day and zeros for days without dose delivery. Gaps are recognized by differences in the beginning and final dates of series. This algorithm was added to the software package of the treatment planning system SIDOS-U2, version 8.2. (Siemens). The following example illustrates the calculation of BEN distributions.

A patient with a gynecological tumor was treated by biaxial moving beam therapy (Fig. 2) and the following fractionation scheme: 30 fractions of 2 Gy at maximum, one fraction per day, five fractions per week. After 7 years a second

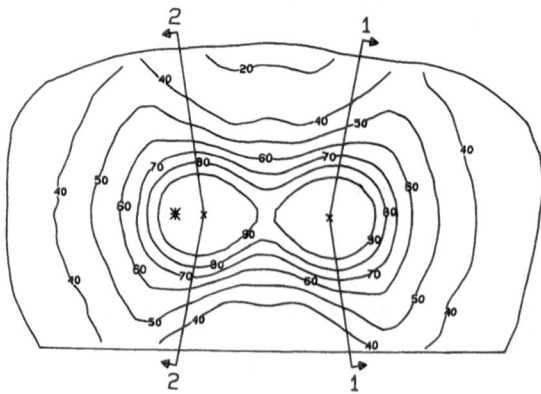

Fig. 2. Dose distribution for a biaxial moving beam therapy (first series, 60 Gy at maximum)

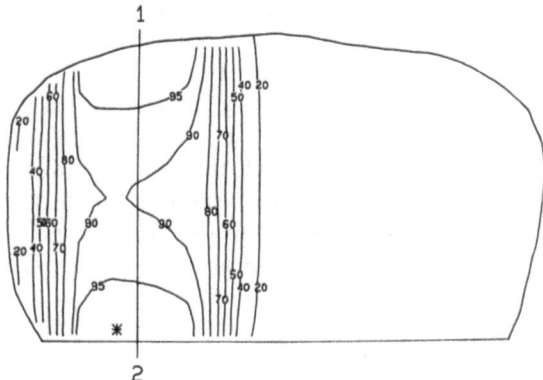

Fig. 3. Dose distribution for a treatment with opposing fields (second series, 25 Gy at midline)

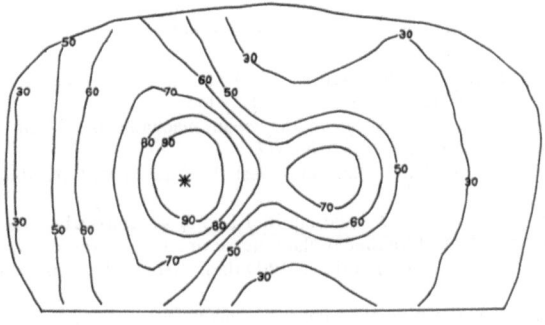

Fig. 4. Distribution of total dose for both series (87 Gy at maximum)

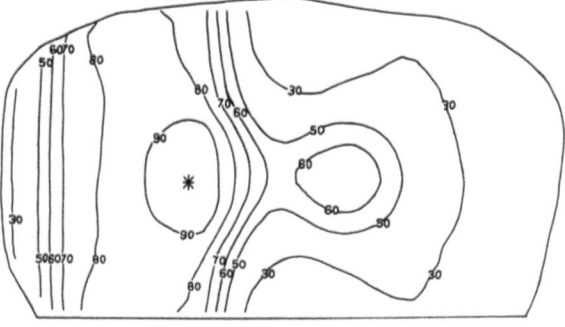

Fig. 5. The ret dose distribution for the whole treatment with two series

series was necessary because of a large metastasis in the right pelvic bones. This was performed with opposing fields (Fig. 3) and the following fractionation scheme: five fractions of 5 Gy at midline, one fraction per day, five fractions per week. Figure 4 presents the resulting distribution of total dose for both series, normalized to the maximum value of 87 Gy. The corresponding BEN distribution for early reactions (Fig. 5) is normalized to the maximum value of 1875 beu (biological effect unit), which lies only 4% over the tolerance level of 1800 beu. Comparison of the two distributions shows large differences between biological effect and total dose.

It should be pointed out finally, that — although these possibilities for biological treatment planning are based on a model, which is certainly yet insufficient — they should be used already now and methodically improved upon, until a better model for the description of biological effects of radiotherapy can be substituted in this algorithm.

References

Ellis F (1968) Time, fractionation and dose rate in radiotherapy. Front Radiat Ther Oncol 3: 131–140

Goitein M (1976) Review of parameters characterizing response of normal connective tissue to radiation. Clin Radiol 27: 389–404

Herrmann T, Voigtmann L, Knorr A, Lorenz J, Johannsen U (1986) The time-dose relationship for radiation-induced lung damage in pigs. Radiother Oncol 5: 127–135

Herrmann T, Voigtmann L, Knorr A, Lorenz J (1987) On the repair mechanisms of lung — experimental and clinical results. Strahlentherapie 163: 370–377

Kirk J, Gray WM, Watson ER (1971) Cumulative radiation effect. I. Fractionated treatment regimes. Clin Radiol 22: 145–155

Orton CG, Ellis F (1974) Definition of T in the NSD-equation. Br J Radiol 47: 200–201

Voigtmann L (1984) Computer-assisted biological treatment planning for oncological radiotherapy based on a measure of the biological effect on normal tissue. PhD thesis, Humboldt University, Berlin

Voigtmann L (1989) To the evaluation of the biological effect of unconventional fractionation schemes. Radiobiol Radiother 30: 299–301

Voigtmann L, Herrmann T, Knorr A, Lorenz J (1988) Dose-time-studies on radiogenic pneumopathy, 5-th information: character and quantitative registration of the radiogenic lung reaction. Radiobiol Radiother 29: 77–99

Treatment Planning:
Mathematical Models

Potential Applications of Invariant Kernel Conformal Therapy*

A.L. Boyer, G.E. Desobry, and N.H. Wells

Introduction

A conformal therapy technique with a complementary inverse treatment planning methodology is described here based on concepts introduced by Brahme et al. (1990). The methodology is based on the use of the three-dimensional fast Fourier transform to convolve an energy deposition kernel with a weighting distribution. Brahme originally considered the energy deposition kernel due to the cylindrically symmetric rotational dose distribution developed by a rotating X-ray pencil beam. Here we compare this type of treatment with a conformal therapy technique based on multiple fixed-gantry-angle noncoplanar fields. Either approach can be planned using a spatially invariant kernel. The kernels are to be convolved with a weighting distribution calculated by a constrained iterative deconvolution procedure.

It should be noted that the approach here assumes that the desired dose distribution is known. This technique does not attempt to modify the physical dose distribution based on a chosen radiobiological model. It simply provides a means to deliver a dose distribution that comes as close as possible to the desired physical distribution of dose, $D'(\mathbf{r})$, defined in a three-dimensional calculation volume at points $\mathbf{r}$.

Implementation of the technology under discussion is a major undertaking. Motivation for such an effort must be provided from a clear perception of the benefits of such dose distributions. The purpose of the work described here was to investigate the potentials and limitations that one anticipates from such a conformal therapy.

Methods and Materials

If the rotational kernel is invariant, then one should be able to calculate the dose distribution using a convolution, such as:

$$D(\mathbf{r}) = \int_V \Psi(\mathbf{r}_0)\, \Lambda(\mathbf{r} - \mathbf{r}_0)\, dV_0, \tag{1}$$

Department of Radiation Physics, University of Texas M.D. Anderson Cancer Center, Houston, TX 77030, USA

* This research was supported in part by PHS grant R01 CA-43840 awarded by the National Cancer Institute, United States Department of Health and Human Services

where we have introduced a weighting factor distribution $\Psi(\mathbf{r}_0)$ for the kernel at point $\mathbf{r}_0$, and the invariant kernel is defined as:

$$A(\mathbf{r}) = \int_{E=0}^{E_{max}} \int_{\theta=0}^{2\pi} \int_{V'} \frac{d\phi}{dE} \cdot R(\mathbf{r}'; \theta) \cdot k_\theta(\mathbf{r} - \mathbf{r}') dV' d\theta dE \qquad (2)$$

A spectral collimator fluence $d\phi/dE$ is specified for a pencil beam in the direction kernel center, and a ray-trace factor $R(\mathbf{r}'; \theta)$ accounts for attenuation from the surface of the medium to the kernel center. The sum of energy-specific kernel distributions weighted by the X-ray spectrum yields a pencil-beam dose distribution. Rotating the distribution through continuous or discrete values of θ and superposing evaluates Eq. 2. This is the rotational kernel.

The line from the X-ray target to a particular point within the calculation array is the pencil beam angle vector $\mathbf{\Omega}$. This vector is a function of the gantry angle θ. A desired value of the collimator fluence is achieved by the proper selection of a differential monitor unit weight $MU(\mathbf{\Omega})$. The collimator fluence is proportional to monitor units and an output factor OF, for each value of the angle vector $\mathbf{\Omega}$:

$$\phi(\mathbf{\Omega}) = MU(\mathbf{\Omega}) \cdot OF(\mathbf{\Omega}, E) \cdot \phi_0, \qquad (3)$$

where ϕ_0 is a scaling factor.

The total collimator fluence distribution for a fixed gantry angle is calculated as

$$\phi(\mathbf{\Omega}) = \int_0^1 \frac{\Psi(\mathbf{r}_0)}{2\pi} \cdot \exp\left[\int_{\mathbf{r}_t(\theta)}^{\mathbf{r}_0} \mu(\mathbf{r}) d\mathbf{r} \right] d\alpha, \qquad (4)$$

where $\mathbf{r} = \mathbf{r}_t(\theta) + \alpha[\mathbf{r}_0 - \mathbf{r}_t(\theta)]$. This is a ray trace through the calculation volume and is the inverse of a computed tomographic back-projection algorithm. The function ϕ is the superposition of sinograms in $\mathbf{\Omega}$ space due to each of the non-zero points in the weighting distribution. There will be regions in $\mathbf{\Omega}$ space where ϕ is equal or close to zero. These regions define the limits at which the multileaf collimators should be set. Contouring the ϕ functions provides an automated method for calculating the collimator settings as a function of gantry angle. The values of ϕ within these limits define the in-field compensation necessary to create the optimized dose distributions.

A practical approach to finding $\Psi(\mathbf{r})$ proposed by Lind and Brahme (1987) employs an iterative calculation described by van Cittert (1931). The weighting distribution is calculated iteratively by the recursion relation:

$$\Psi_{n+1}(\mathbf{r}) = \Psi_n(\mathbf{r}) + \Delta\Psi_n(\mathbf{r}), \qquad (5)$$

based on the dose difference:

$$\Delta\Psi_n(\mathbf{r}) = a \cdot \Delta D_n(\mathbf{r}) = a \cdot [D'(\mathbf{r}) - D_n(\mathbf{r})], \qquad (6)$$

where dose is obtained by the convolution:

$$D_n(\mathbf{r}) = \Psi_n(\mathbf{r}) \otimes A(\mathbf{r}). \qquad (7)$$

This sequence will converge on some weighting distribution that produces the best "fit" to the desired dose distribution allowed by the rotational kernels. An adaptive recursion constant a_n can be used to normalize the results to the desired dose value:

$$a_n = \frac{\sum_r \Delta D_n(\mathbf{r}) \cdot [\Delta D_n(\mathbf{r}) \otimes \Lambda]}{\sum_r [\Delta D_n(\mathbf{r}) \otimes \Lambda]^2}. \tag{8}$$

In order to evaluate Eq. 8 one must convolve the dose error with the rotational kernel. Thus to carry out this algorithm, two convolutions are required for each iteration. The sums in Eq. 8 are calculated to find a new convergence factor a_n for each iteration. Even so, the procedure will occasionally drive the rotation center fluence Ψ to take negative values. This is avoided by placing an algorithmic constraint on these weighting values to force them to remain nonnegative. Note that this procedure is self-normalizing in the sense that whatever values of D' are selected, the algorithm will determine values of the weighting distribution that will produce a dose distribution that approaches the desired dose distribution values absolutely.

Carrying out these calculations over arrays of the order of $64 \times 64 \times 64$ would require unreasonable amounts of time were it not possible to use an array processor and the fast Fourier transform. However, we have implemented this scheme using an array processor with 16 megabytes of memory (Model NMX-332, Numerix, Newton, MA, USA). We have found that after 40–50 iterations there is little subjective improvement in the calculated dose distributions. Our implementation of the technique takes advantage of the symmetry in the kernel, the real nature of the input data, and other algorithmic optimizations (Wells et al. 1990). The time required to carry out the 40 iterations is 30 min.

Results

Use of this algorithm allowed the study of conformal therapy treatment techniques which were embodied in the convolution kernels used in the calculation. Kernels were created from point energy spread-array kernels and beam spectra calculated using Monte Carlo techniques. The conformal therapy kernels included continuous coplanar rotation kernels, noncoplanar skip arc rotation kernels, and multiple fixed field coplanar and noncoplanar kernels. An example of an isodose distribution calculated in the central transverse plane for 18-MV X-rays using a conventional four-field box to treat a 10-cm diameter right cylindrical target volume (indicated by shading) is given in Fig. 1a. In this and the following cases, isodoses were calculated for the delivery of unit dose to the target volume to within 10%. For comparison here we show the isodose distributions for two conformal therapy techniques for the same cylindrical target volume. Figure 1b shows a coplanar continuous arc conformal therapy

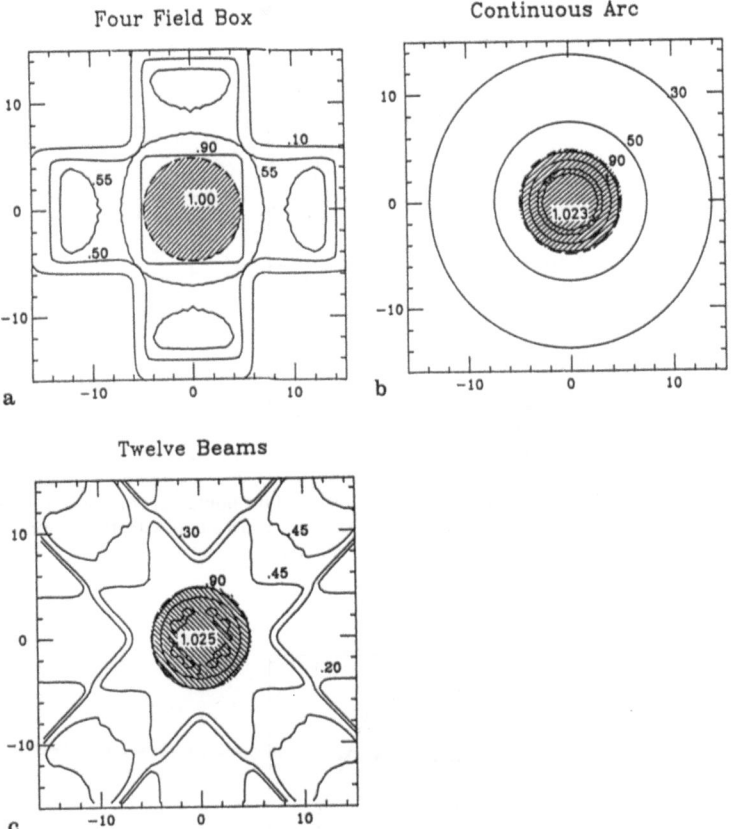

Fig. 1. Dose distributions in the central transverse plane for treating a cylindrical target volume 10 cm in diameter and 10 cm in height (*shaded area*) using: a conventional four-field "box" technique (**a**), a continuous rotation conformal therapy technique (**b**), and a static field conformal therapy technique using 12 noncoplanar fields (**c**)

technique, and Fig. 1c shows a noncoplanar conformal therapy technique using 12 fixed beams.

The dose volume histograms in Figs. 2 and 3 compare the conformal therapy plans with the conventional plan for the 10-cm diameter target. All of the dose in the calculation array outside the target volume was included in the nontarget volume for the purpose of dose volume histogramming. Figure 2 compares the conventional plan (dot-dash lines) to the coplanar continuous arc conformal therapy plan (solid lines), and Figure 3 compares the coplanar continuous arc conformal therapy plan (solid lines) to the noncoplanar fixed field conformal therapy plan (dot-dash lines). In these cases the target volume was treated about equally by all techniques. The major differences between the techniques are in the nontarget dose-volume histograms. In Fig. 2 the rotational conformal therapy plan is demonstrated to treat a larger nontarget volume to doses less

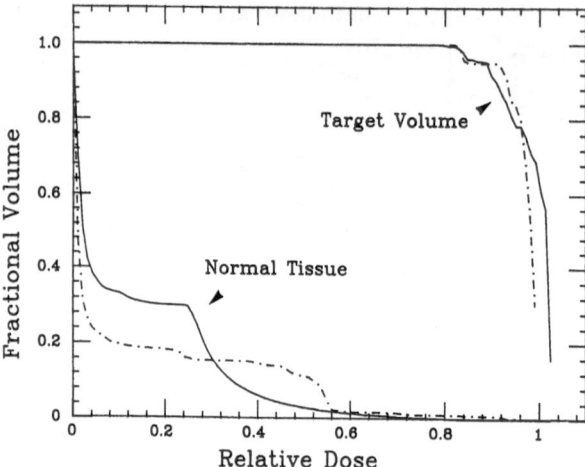

Fig. 2. Integral dose-volume histograms for the target volume and the nontarget volume comparing the conventional four-field "box" dose distribution of Fig. 1a (*dashed lines*) with the continuous rotation conformal therapy dose distribution of Fig. 1b (*solid lines*)

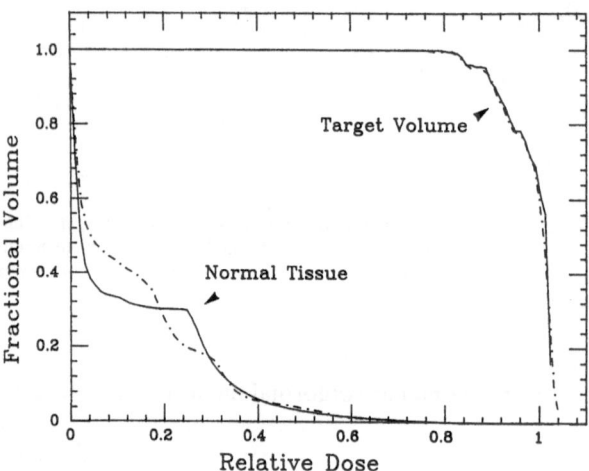

Fig. 3. Integral dose-volume histograms for the target volume and the nontarget volume comparing the continuous rotation conformal therapy dose distributions of Fig. 1b (*solid lines*) with the static noncoplanar conformal therapy technique of Fig. 1c (*dashed lines*)

than 30% of the target dose than the conventional plan, whereas the conventional plan treats a larger nontarget volume to doses above 30% of the target dose.

In order to be successful, a conformal therapy technique must deliver an escalated dose to the tumor target volume to enhance the probability of local tumor control without raising the normal tissue complication rate to an unacceptable level. A theoretical estimation of the potential for target dose escalation can be made by using the normal tissue complication probability function (Goitein and Schultheiss 1985):

$$\text{NTCP} = cVD^k, \tag{9}$$

where V is a volume of normal tissue that receives a dose D, and $k = 7$. We have used this relation to estimate the dose escalation that the nontarget volume would allow with the conformal therapy dose distributions which we have calculated. The conventional treatment delivers a dose D_t to the target volume and a dose D_n to the nontarget tissue in a volume V_n. On the other hand, the conformal treatment delivers a dose D'_t to the target volume and a dose D'_n to all the normal tissue in the volume V'_n.

From our three-dimensional dose distributions we have obtained the non-target tissue protection factor, the ratio between the target dose and the average nontarget dose, $R_1 = D_t/D_n$ for a conventional technique and $R_2 = D'_t/D'_n$ for the conformal technique. The ratio of the normal tissue volumes $R_3 = V'_n/V_n$ was also determined. These ratios applied to Eq. 9 lead to a relation (Schultheiss 1987, private communication) for the dose escalation factor for the same nontarget complication probability:

$$\frac{D'_t}{D_t} = \frac{R_2}{R_1} e^{1/k \ln (1/R_3)}. \tag{10}$$

We found that the conventional plans yielded a nontarget tissue protection factor of $R_1 \approx 2$ while the conformal plans provided nontarget protection with a factor of $R_2 \approx 3.5$–4.0. However, the conformal plans treated about twice the nontarget volume as the conventional plans. When these factors were applied to Eq. 10 the dose escalation potential was estimated to be 50%–80% for the same normal tissue complication rate, even though more normal tissue had been irradiated to a lower dose. It is dubious that the normal tissue stroma within a tumor volume could sustain an increase of this magnitude over current conventional therapy treatment doses.

Conclusions

If the estimate that we have made of the potential dose escalation is correct, the clinical significance of a practical and reliable conformal therapy technique would be that the tolerance to treatment would be set by the normal tissue stroma in the target volume rather than by the normal tissue structures outside the treatment volume. Assuming that some dose escalation can be achieved by implementing a conformal therapy technique (Fig. 3) the dose-volume histo-grams of the multiple field noncoplanar conformal therapy plan and of the coplanar continuous arc conformal therapy plan are seen to be quite similar. We conclude that if the radiobiology is favorable for conformal therapy, then the more easily implementable multiple fixed field technique should be pursued.

References

Brahme A, Lind B, Källman P (1990) Inverse radiation therapy planning as a tool for 3D dose optimization. Phys Med 6: 53–68

Goitein M, Schultheiss TE (1985) Strategies for treating possible tumor extension: some theoretical considerations. Int J Radiat Oncol Biol Phys 11: 1519–1528

Lind B, Brahme A (1987) Optimization of radiation therapy dose distributions using scanned electron and photon beams and multileaf collimators. In: Bruinvis IAD, van der Gressen PH, van Kleffens HF, Wittkamper FW (eds) Proceedings of the 9th international conference on use of computers in radiation therapy. North Holland, Amsterdam, pp 235–239

Mackie TR, Bielajew AF, Rogers DWO, Battista JJ (1988) Generation of photon energy deposition kernels using the EGS Monte Carlo code. Phys Med Biol 33: 1–20

Van Cittert PH (1931) Einfluss der Spaltbreite auf die Intensitätsverteilung in Spektrallinien. II. Z Physik 69: 298–308

Wells NH, Burrus CS, Desobry GE, Boyer AL (1990) Three-dimensional Fourier convolution with an array processor. Comp Phys 4: 507–513

Characterisation of Photon Beams
for Kernel-Based Dose Calculation Via ...

A. Ahnesjö and M. Aspradakis

Introduction

Characterization of Photon Beams
for Kernel-Based Dose Calculation Methods

A. Ahnesjö[1,2] and M. Saxner[2]

Introduction

In three-dimensional radiotherapy, the need for photon models general enough
to handle complex situations with patient heterogeneities, irregular field shapes,
etc. is best met by models that calculate the dose through integration of energy
deposition kernels [1–5]. The basic idea of such models is to calculate as much
as possible of the particle transport with analytical methods and approximate
the remaining part by means of Monte Carlo calculated [6–8] kernels. Several
types of kernels dependent on the irradiation geometry have been defined
(Fig. 1). A fast algorithm using point spread functions is the collapsed cone
convolution [5] that constrains the flow of secondary particles onto a lattice of
lines on which the points of dose calculation are located. Models based on the
use of pencil beam kernels are, due to less overhead, better suited for interactive
dose calculations, but corrections for patient outline and tissue heterogeneities
must be handled separately [9]. Planar spread functions are useful for derivation of heterogeneity correction factors. Rotated pencil beam kernels find
applications in beam optimization using inverse methods [10, 11].

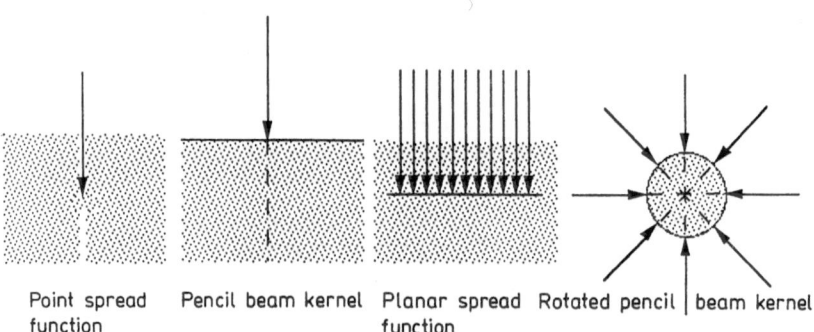

Point spread   Pencil beam kernel Planar spread   Rotated pencil | beam kernel
function   function

Fig. 1. Irradiation geometries for different types of energy deposition kernels

[1] Department of Radiation Physics, Karolinska Institute and Stockholm University, Box 60211,
104 01 Stockholm, Sweden
[2] Helax, Box 1704, 751 47 Uppsala, Sweden

Advanced Radiation Therapy Tumor Response
Monitoring and Treatment Planning
Breit (Editor-in-Chief)
© Springer-Verlag, Berlin Heidelberg 1992

Through integration, all types of kernels could be derived from the basic point spread functions, provided knowledge of the beam quality [12]. In this paper, we summarize the procedures for derivation of all the necessary beam data for the clinical use of kernel-based dose calculations. The procedure is divided into four main parts: (a) calculation of energy deposition kernels and attenuation coefficients by using an effective spectrum from depth dose data, see Fig. 2; (b) describing lateral dose characteristics by acquiring the lateral energy fluence distribution for the largest possible open beam; (c) modeling dose from contaminant particles; and (d) calibration of output factors.

The Effective Spectrum and Charged Particle Contamination

Calculation of energy deposition kernels, attenuation coefficients, and stopping power ratio etc. is straightforward, provided one knows the beam spectrum. Unfortunately, there is no practical method available for direct measurement of therapeutic beam spectra in a clinic. Several investigators have unfolded transmission data for narrow beams [13] by means of least-square methods. In practice, all methods proposed so far involve unfolding techniques with substantial uncertainties. Realizing this, methods should be used that minimize the errors of the entities for which the spectrum is intended. This entity for radiation treatment planning is, of course, dose. Methods for determination of depth dose effective spectra have been proposed by Ahnesjö and Andreo [14] and Sauer and Neumann [15]. Through iteration, both methods minimize the difference between convolution-calculated and measured depth doses by varying the spectrum. As the problem is ill conditioned, both methods include constraints on the spectrum. Simultaneously, the difference between the convolution-calculated and the measured dose at shallow depths is determined and used to represent the dose from contaminant charged particles.

The Lateral Energy Fluence Distribution

The effective spectrum discussed in the previous section is a mean entity for the whole beam cross-section, i.e., it is not differentiated in location. In theory, provided knowledge of the energy fluence distribution differential in energy $\psi_E(x, y)$, the dose is calculated by the convolution:

$$D(x, y, z) = \iiint \Psi_E(x', y') \frac{p}{\rho}(E, x - x', y - y', z) \, dE \, dx' \, dy' \tag{1}$$

where $\frac{p}{\rho}(E, x - x', y - y', z)$ is the pencil beam kernel for photons of energy E.

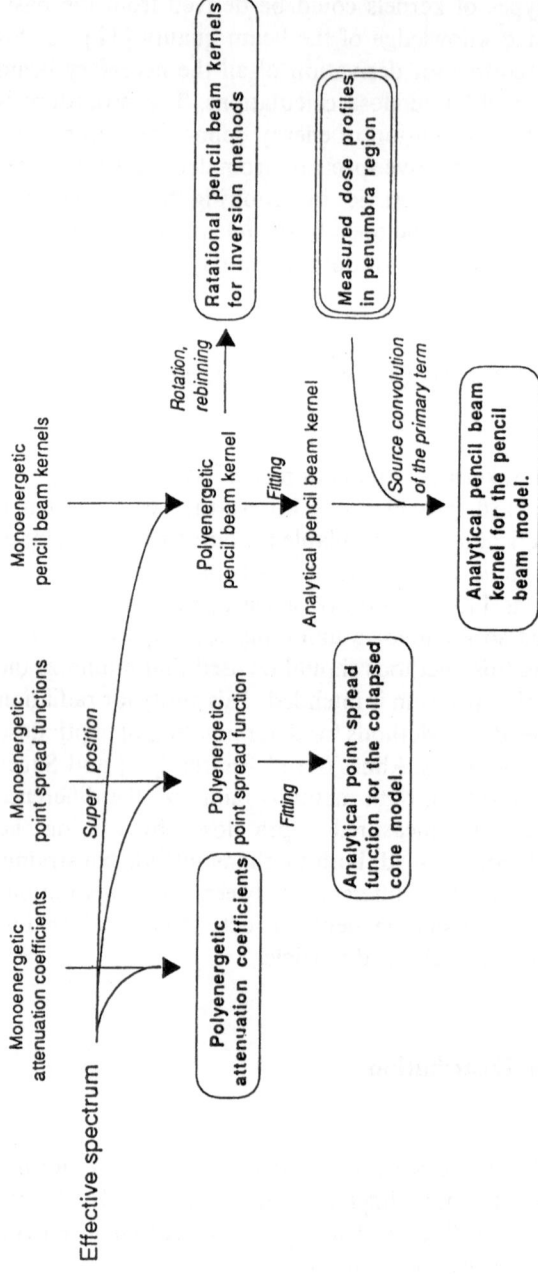

Fig. 2. The use of the effective spectrum for calculation of attenuation coefficients and energy deposition kernels

As there are no means available to derive $\Psi_E(x, y)$, and if it could be derived it would be impractical to use due to extensive integrations over energy, the convolution and integration over energy in Eq. 1 is replaced by a convolution of effective entities:

$$D(x, y, z) \approx \iint \hat{\Psi}(x', y') \frac{\hat{p}}{\rho}(x - x', y - y', z)\, dx'\, dy' \tag{2}$$

The effective pencil beam kernel is given by:

$$\frac{\hat{p}}{\rho}(x, y, z) = \frac{\int \hat{\Psi}_E \frac{p}{\rho}(E, x, y, z)\, dE}{\int \hat{\Psi}_E\, dE} \tag{3}$$

in which $\hat{\Psi}_E$ is the effective spectrum discussed in the previous section. The concepts of effective entities in Eq. 2 is greatly facilitated by the weak energy dependence of the kernel when it is normalized to the energy of the impinging photon. Ahnesjö and Trepp [16] have developed a method that, based on the inverse of Eq. 2, determines $\hat{\Psi}(x, y)$ through deconvolution of a lateral dose distribution measured at the reference depth.

Before deconvolving, both the measured dose distribution and the pencil beam kernel must be given in the same discrete cartesian system. Considering that the measured dose should be obtained for the largest field, 40×40 cm^2 on most machines, and at a desired resolution of 2–5 mm, the number of required measure points ranges from 6400 to 40 000. This is far too large for most single detector systems to acquire in clinical routine. Therefore a method has been developed [16] that interpolates the dose from relatively sparse measurements acquired by scanning with a single detector along radial lines arranged in a star-shaped pattern. As each scan line passes the origin, the variance of the dose at the origin can be used to check the reproducibility of the accelerator and the measurement set-up. In practice, feasible step lengths are about 0.2 cm in the gradient region and 0.2–1 cm in the flatter parts. With an angular increment of 10°–20° between adjacent scan lines, the number of measure points is reduced to approximately 1500. The dose values at the cartesian grid points are extracted using specifically developed interpolation algorithms, different for different dose regions to minimize artifacts.

The pencil beam kernel as derived from the Monte Carlo method is given in cylindrical bins. These are rebinned into a high-resolution cartesian pixel grid using an area-overlap technique [12] before filtering and downsampling to the same cartesian grid as the dose distribution. This, rather complicated, scheme for representation of the kernel in a cartesian grid is due to the high gradients around the symmetry axis.

In real beams, the mean energy of the spectrum decreases with increasing off-axis distance, a phenomenon known as off-axis softening. Dose calculation using the acquired energy fluence matrix reconstructs the measured dose at the depth of measurement. Due to off-axis softening, the dose calculated at the rim of large fields is underestimated at depths less than the characterization depth and vice versa at greater depths. Using a characterization depth of 10 cm, the error was less than 1.5% for the rim of a 20×20 cm^2 field at 8 MV [16]. This is less than expected from attenuation data computed by Mohan et al. [17]. There are several effects that counteract the influence on dose from off-axis softening. The most important is probably the decreasing primary-to-scatter ratio with increasing depth. However, off-axis softening might be worse for higher beam energies as the overall primary-to-scatter ratio increases. Hence, care should be taken when designing flattening filters to chose media combinations that equalize the spectrum as much as possible.

The Dose from Contaminant Particles

The dose from contaminant particles in photon beams is not intrinsically modeled through convolution of energy deposition kernels for the primary photon beam. However, both dose from contaminant charged particles and dose from contaminant photons can be described by means of separate analytical kernels [9]. Several approximations are necessary, but the contaminant dose is only a fraction of the primary dose and may therefore be modeled with less absolute accuracy.

Charged Particle Contamination. Contaminant charged particles are released from filters, block trays, and the air column. They are subject to multiple scattering before they enter the patient. At the surface of the patient, the impinging fluence of contaminant charged particles around a primary photon pencil beam can be approximated by a gaussian distribution. Further scattering in the tissue is unlikely to increase the radius significantly, and the dose is given by a gaussian pencil beam kernel with depth-independent radius as proposed by Nilson [18]. The broad beam depth dose behavior of contaminant charged particles has been shown to be almost exponential [1]. Combining these effects, the pencil beam kernel is given by:

$$p_{c \pm}(r, z) = \alpha e^{-\beta z} e^{-\gamma r^2} \tag{4}$$

where α, β, and γ are machine-dependent parameters. Integrating, the charged particle contaminant dose at depth z on the beam axis of a square field of size f becomes

$$\alpha e^{-\beta z} \int_{-f/2}^{f/2} \int_{-f/2}^{f/2} e^{-\gamma(x^2 + y^2)} \, dx \, dy = \alpha e^{-\beta z} \frac{\pi}{\gamma} \operatorname{erf}^2 \left(\sqrt{\gamma} \frac{f}{2} \right) \tag{5}$$

By least-squares fitting of Eq. 5 to the charged particle depth dose obtained when determining the effective spectrum the values of α, β, and γ are determined. It follows that the kernel is normalized per unit of incident primary photon energy.

Photon Contamination. Contaminant photons are treated as part of the primary photon beam when the effective spectrum is determined. The dose outside of the geometrical beam is caused mainly by photons scattered from the irradiated part of the patient, but significant contributions also come from photons scattered in the treatment head and from photons transmitted through the collimators. The scatter dose is modeled by use of Monte Carlo kernels in the convolution models, whereas the sum of treatment head scattered photons and those transmitted through the collimators is generally referred to as contaminant photon dose and requires explicit modeling. The main source of scattered photons in the treatment head is the flattening filter [19]. The contaminant photon dose is estimated by taking the difference between measured dose profiles and convolution calculated profiles outside of the primary beam. These data are used to derive the parameters ξ and ζ of a gaussian pencil beam kernel:

$$\frac{p}{\rho_{chv}}(r, z) = d_z \xi \, e^{-\zeta r^2} \tag{6}$$

where d_z is the sum of the equilibrium primary dose at depth and the scatter dose at the point of calculation. A small constant dose level must be added to account for collimator transmittance.

Output Factors

The output factor for a clinical beam is defined, at a reference position, as the dose per monitor reading relative to the ratio of the dose per monitor reading at the same position in a reference field. Convolution models compute, in absolute units, the dose per incident energy fluence and enable therefore direct calculation of output factors. In a recent work [20] measured and convolution-calculated output factors were compared and differences as great as 5% were found. Significant perturbations are caused by backscatter from the collimators to the monitor and forward scatter from the filter and collimators in the treatment head. The forward scatter adds an "unmonitored" contribution to the total energy fluence of the beam. Characterizing these perturbations from measurements of the "output in air," and using a model based on view factors, the field size dependence of these perturbations can be modeled and output factors predicted with high accuracy [20].

Results and Discussion

Speed and accuracy are central concepts in dose calculation models for treatment planning, however seldom possible to achieve simultaneously. Close at hand is to include two algorithms into a treatment planning system, one where some accuracy is traded for computional speed and one focusing on accuracy rather than speed. For consistency (and convenience) it is important that both models are based on the same set of data. The pencil beam model [9] has been implemented in the TMS-Radix system and tested clinically for a wide range of machines with accelerating potentials ranging from 4 to 50 MV. Comparisons in homogeneous water phantoms show very small deviations in the exponential region, i.e., the region within the field boundaries but at depths greater than d_{max}. In the buildup region the displacement error is generally less than 1 mm. The uncertainties in the buildup region extend somewhat into the region around d_{max}. In a clinical environment, with changing of block trays, etc. there are always uncertainties connected to the contaminant dose and consequently also to the dose at d_{max}. To reduce dosage errors, normalization should, whenever possible, be made at depths greater than the maximum penetration depth of contaminant particles. A preferable choice is the depth of 5 or 10 cm, as used in most dosimetry protocols for absolute dose calibration.

Lateral comparisons, also for rather inhomogeneous fields, show excellent agreements due to the use of an energy fluence matrix [16]. When testing output factors (at 10 cm depth versus 10×10 cm^2 field) for 147 fields ranging from 4×4 to 40×40 cm^2 on two different accelerators at three beam energies (5.6 and 18 MV), including also very elongated fields, the standard deviation of the difference between calculated and measured output factors was 0.86% [20].

Conclusions

Provided a depth dose effective spectrum, an effective energy fluence matrix, and separate models for dose from contaminant particles, photon dose calculation for treatment planning can be performed by convolution models with excellent results. These models are based on first principles and hence general enough to model complex three-dimensional treatments with great accuracy. From the same sets of data measured along scan lines in water phantoms the beam characterization process can deliver data for different types on models, including three-dimensional optimization based on inverse methods, which facilitates beam data acquisition and quality assurance.

References

1. Mackie TR (1984) A study of charged particles and scattered photons in megavoltage X-ray beams. Thesis, University of Alberta, Edmonton
2. Boyer A, Mok EC (1985) A photon dose distribution model employing convolution calculations. Med Phys 12: 169–177

3. Chui CS (1985) A method for three dimensional gamma ray dose calculations in heterogeneous media and its application in radiation therapy. Thesis, Colombia University, New York
4. Ahnesjö A (1984) Application of transform algorithms for calculation of absorbed dose in photon beams. Proc 8 Int Conf Comp Rad Ther, VIII ICCR, pp 17–20
5. Ahnesjö A (1989) Collapsed cone convolution of radiant energy for photon dose calculation in heterogeneous media. Med Phys 16: 577–592
6. Ahnesjö A, Andreo P, Brahme A (1987) Calculation and application of point spread functions for treatment planning with high energy photon beams. Acta Oncol 26: 49–56
7. Mackie TR, Bielajew AF, Rogers DWO, Battista JJ (1988) Generation of photon energy deposition kernels using the EGS Monte Carlo code. Phys Med Biol 33: 1–20
8. Mohan R, Chui C, Lidofsky L (1986) Differential pencil beam dose computation model for photons. Med Phys 13: 64–73
9. Ahnesjö A, Saxner M, Trepp A (1992) A pencil beam model for photon dose calculations. Med Phys 19: 263–273
10. Lind BK (1991) Radiation therapy planning and optimization studied as inverse problems. Thesis, Stockholm University, Stockholm, Sweden
11. Brahme A (1988) Optimization of stationary and moving beam radiation therapy techniques. Radiother Oncol 12: 129–140
12. Eklöf A, Ahnesjö A, Brahme A (1990) Photon beam energy deposition kernels for inverse radiotherapy planning. Acta Oncol 29: 447–454
13. Huang P, Kase KR, Bjärngard BE (1983) Reconstruction of 4-MV bremsstrahlung spectra from measured transmission data. Med Phys 10: 778–85
14. Ahnesjö A, Andreo P (1989) Determination of effective bremsstrahlung spectra and electron contamination for photon dose calculations. Phys Med Biol 34: 1451–1464
15. Sauer O, Neumann M (1990) Reconstruction of high-energy bremsstrahlung spectra by numerical analysis of depth-dose data. Radiother Oncol 18: 39–47
16. Ahnesjö A, Trepp A (1991) Acquisition of the effective lateral energy fluence distribution for photon beam dose calculations by convolution models. Phys Med Biol 36: 973–985
17. Mohan R, Chui C, Lidofsky L (1985) Energy and angular distributions of photons from medical linear accelerators. Med Phys 12: 592–597
18. Nilsson B (1985) Electron contamination from different materials in high energy photon beams. Phys Med Biol 30: 139–151
19. Nilsson B, Brahme A (1981) Contamination of high-energy photon beams by scattered photons. Strahlentherapie 157: 181–187
20. Ahnesjö A, Knöös T, Montelius A (1992) Application of the convolution method for calculation of output factors for therapy photon beams. Med Phys 19: 295–301

Implementation of a Pencil Beam Model in the TMS-Radix Treatment Planning System

M. Saxner and A. Ahnesjö

Introduction

We present here an implementation of a photon dose pencil beam algorithm (Ahnesjö et al. 1991a) in the TMS-Radix (Helax) treatment planning system. It is intended for interactive dose calculation with a minimum of overhead to specified points including two-dimensional grids in an interactive environment in which field shapes, gantry angles, wedges, and treatment units may be changed in the search for an optimal treatment plan. Although the dose can also be calculated in three-dimensional grids, the algorithm is not primarily intended for such bulk dose calculation, as better performing algorithms exist for that purpose (Ahnesjö 1989). The algorithm is based on first physical principles as far as possible. In this way the number of characterizing measurements is kept to a minimum, and yet the algorithm is flexible enough to handle nonstandard cases such as arbitrary field shapes, inhomogeneities, and laterally varying energy fluence from the radiation head. The characterizing measurements required are summarized elsewhere (Ahnesjö and Saxner, this volume).

Pencil Beam Kernels

In the pencil beam formulation the dose at a given point is obtained by integration of a pencil beam kernel over a plane through the dose point and perpendicular to the beam axis. The depth variation is implicitly contained in the precalculated pencil beams.

For the present algorithm a database of monoenergetic pencil beams has been derived from Monte Carlo calculated point spread functions. Together with a spectrum for the treatment unit the pencil beams are used to construct spectrally integrated pencil beam kernels appropriate for the given treatment unit. These spectrally integrated pencil beams can be accurately represented by

Helax, Box 1704, 751 47 Uppsala, Sweden

Advanced Radiation Therapy Tumor Response
Monitoring and Treatment Planning
Breit (Editor-in-Chief)
© Springer-Verlag, Berlin Heidelberg 1992

the analytical formula:

$$\frac{p}{\rho}(r) = \frac{A e^{-ar}}{r} + \frac{B e^{-br}}{r} \tag{1}$$

where the parameters A, a, B, and b are functions of the depth z. In the present version of the Monte Carlo database only the total dose is scored. The separation into two terms in Eq. 1 is thus purely numerical, but physical arguments indicate that the first term ($a > b$) can be ascribed to the primary dose and the second term to the scatter dose. This interpretation of the terms has been verified by Monte Carlo calculations in which the two dose contributions have been separated.

The primary dose in the penumbra region is influenced by the geometrical penumbra and the diffusion of primary charged particles in the medium. The former component is a consequence of the finite size of the radiating source. Both these effects are modeled by convolving the first term in Eq. 1 by a gaussian function whose width is determined by the "size" of the radiating source. The result of this convolution is that the primary dose is expressed as a linear combination of an exponential over r and a gaussian function, i.e.:

$$P_{prim}(r) = w A' \frac{e^{-a'r}}{r} + (1 - w)A'' \, e^{-a''r^2} \tag{2}$$

where the new parameters a', a'', A', A'', and w are functions of A, a, and the source size. As mentioned above the scatter dose is described by the second term in Eq. 1:

$$P_{scat}(r) = B \frac{e^{-br}}{r} \tag{3}$$

The Monte Carlo calculations are done for an ideal beam and do not consider secondary effects due to contaminating particles. In the present algorithm these additional dose contributions are also modeled through the use of pencil beam kernels. One such contribution is the dose outside of the geometrical beam which results partly from photons leaking through the collimators and photons scattered in the treatment head. The pencil beam kernel for this photon contamination contribution is assumed to be described by a broad gaussian function:

$$P_{phcontam}(r) = C \xi e^{-\zeta r^2} \tag{4}$$

where the parameters ξ and ζ are determined by fitting measured dose profiles outside the geometrical beam. The parameter C describes the depth variation of the contamination dose. It is set equal to the sum of the equilibrium primary dose at the actual depth and the amplitude of the local scatter dose. The photon contamination is, of course, also present inside the beam. In this region, however, it is not considered explicitly but is included in the primary dose due to the construction of the spectrum. Another additional dose contribution in the surface layers comes from charged particles emanating from photon interactions in the collimator, filters, and air before reaching the patient. Since these particles have been multiply scattered before reaching the patient, the charged particle contamination is also modeled as a broad gaussian equation:

$$P_{chcontam}(r) = \alpha e^{-\beta z} e^{-\gamma r^2} \tag{5}$$

where α, β, and γ are parameters that are characteristic of the treatment unit and the energy used.

Ray Trace

The calculation of the dose in a specified point starts with a ray trace to the point. The physical properties of the patient are defined by a density matrix which is based on one or more parallel computed tomographic slices and constitutes a three-dimensional matrix containing Hounsfield numbers (scaled to a one byte representation to save memory). All parts of the patient involved in the ray trace must be contained within the density matrix. Voxels exterior to the patient are marked as air voxels.

The ray trace is divided into two parts. First the entrance point into the density matrix is found, and the density matrix is traced until a patient voxel is reached. From this point a new ray trace is performed using a Bresenham algorithm to sample patient interior voxels along the ray. During the ray trace the total attenuation to the dose point is calculated as the sum of the linear attenuation coefficients for each voxel passed, and the geometrical and radiological depths are determined.

The linear attenuation coefficient is obtained in real time by looking up in a precalculated table for the spectrally averaged attenuation coefficient corresponding to the Hounsfield value of the voxel. The attenuation table has been constructed in the following way. For a number of organic tissues and other materials of given physical density the electron density and linear attenuation coefficients were calculated. Using the calibration of Knöös et al. (1986) of electron density as a function of Hounsfield number, the corresponding Hounsfield numbers were determined. Linear attenuation coefficients for intermediate Hounsfield numbers were obtained by interpolation.

Sievert Integration

To obtain the dose the pencil beam kernels must be integrated over the field. By definition we have said that the dose in a point with position (x, y) in the field is obtained from:

$$D(x, y) = \iint\limits_{Field} \Psi(x', y') \frac{p}{\rho}(x - x', y - y') \, dx' dy' \tag{6}$$

where the integral is taken over the geometrical field. $\tilde{\Psi}$ is the energy fluence at the depth of the dose point and p/ρ is the pencil beam kernel. The field is represented by a polygon and may be decomposed into a number of triangles with one vertex at the dose point position (x, y) and the opposite side equal to one of the polygon segments. Assuming the energy fluence to be constant over each such triangle the dose may be expressed as:

$$D(x, y) = \sum \Psi \iint_{\text{Triang}} \frac{p}{\rho}(x - x', y - y') \, dx' dy' \tag{7}$$

For pencil beam kernels of the form described above the integral in Eq. 7 may be expressed in terms of Sievert integrals of the first and second kind.:

$$S_1(t, \theta) = \int_0^\theta e^{-(t/\cos x)} \, dx \tag{8a}$$

$$S_2(t, \theta) = \int_0^\theta e^{-(t/\cos x)^2} \, dx \tag{8b}$$

These standard integrals have been evaluated numerically for the relevant parameter range and tabulated. Thus the integrals of the pencil beam kernel are looked up in the Sievert tables, and the results of all triangles of the field are summed. The sign of the different terms in this sum depends on the orientation of the field polygon. Structures representing open field shape constraints, such as collimators and mantles, are represented by positively oriented polygons whereas blocking structures have negatively oriented polygons.

For the primary dose the energy fluence used in Eq. 7 is taken to be the local value in the direction of the dose point. This is justified by the short range of the primary electrons causing the primary dose to be deposited close to the primary photon pencil beam. The scatter dose, on the other hand, contains contributions from all parts of the field. For the scatter we therefore calculate a weighted mean of the energy fluence in a selected number of points within each triangle. For the contamination dose contributions we take a mean value over the entire field to represent the energy fluence.

Inhomogeneity Corrections

The pencil beam kernels defined above have been derived from calculations and measurements in homogeneous water. We now discuss how the methods described above are extended to situations in which the medium is not homogeneous. The corrections for inhomogeneities are preferably one-dimensional for this type of interactive algorithm. Hence the primary dose is obtained by evaluating the pencil beam at the radiological depth. For the scatter dose we employ a method which is similar to the Batho method but does not require any measured depth dose curve for the particular field. The amount of forward-scattered photons at the dose point is estimated through a one-dimensional convolution along the ray and compared to the corresponding quantity at the same geometrical depth in water. The ratio between these two quantities is used as a correction factor by which the scatter pencil beam data evaluated at the geometrical depth is multiplied. The contaminant dose contributions are both evaluated at the radiological depth.

Absolute Dose

All pencil beam kernels used in the algorithm are normalized to unit incident energy fluence at the isocenter distance. The algorithm is therefore well suited for the calculation of absolute dose. The delivery of a specified absolute dose to the patient is tracked by the reading of a monitor chamber inserted in the beam. From the calculational point of view the absolute dose in a point is proportional to the energy fluence since the algorithm gives the dose per unit energy fluence. Unfortunately the energy fluence itself cannot be measured. The absolute dose per monitor unit for a reference field is measured in a reference geometry and the dose is calculated for the same reference conditions. The algorithm delivers the dose per unit energy fluence, and the ratio between the measured and calculated quantities gives the desired scale factor between energy fluence and the readings of the monitor chamber.

In practice there are different kinds of perturbations that cause deviations from the simple scaling described above. First, we have the contaminant photons, which are created below the monitor chamber and therefore constitute an unmonitored contribution to the fluence at the patient. Secondly, some photons are scattered backwards from the collimator into the monitor chamber, thereby increasing the monitored fluence without any corresponding fluence at the patient. A method, based on viewing factors, to handle these perturbations has been proposed by Ahnesjö et al. (1990b). The method has been incorporated into the algorithm, which is therefore able to produce the number of monitor units required to give a specified absolute dose.

Results

The properties of the photon dose algorithm described above are summarized in Table 1. Comparison of depth dose curves for a number of treatment units and energies indicate that the algorithm agrees with measurements to within less than 1% in the exponential region. In the dose maximum region the maximum error is about 1%. In the build-up region the deviation is larger, but the corresponding displacement is less than 1 mm in almost all cases.

Table 1. Summary of photon pencil beam algorithm properties

Fraction	Region	Radial variation	Depth variation	Energy fluence	Inhomogeneity correction
Primary	Inside geometric field	None (charged particle equilibrium)	$PB(z_{rad})$	Local	1D (z_{rad})
	Penumbra	$A'w\,e^{-a'r}/r + A''(1-w)e^{-a''r^2}$			
Scatter	Whole volume	e^{-br}/r	$PB(z_{geom})$	Weighted mean	1D (z_{geom}, SCF)
Photon contamination	Inside geometric field	–	–	Output factor calibration	–
	Outside geometric field	$e^{-\zeta r^2}$	Primary equilibrium + local scatter	Mean	–
Electron contamination	Surface layers (build-up region)	$e^{-\gamma r^2}$	$e^{-\beta z}$	Mean	–

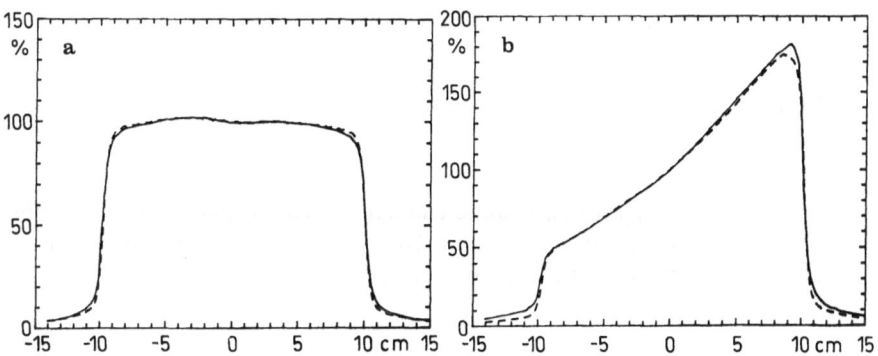

Fig. 1a, b. Profiles for a 20×20 field at 10 cm depth in water for a photon energy of 16 MV. *Solid lines*, measured profiles; *dashed lines*, calculated profiles

In Fig. 1 we compare measured and calculated profiles for an open beam and a wedged beam. The agreement between the two sets of profiles is very good, and the difference is within a few percent. The largest deviation occurs at the field edges of the wedged field. It is probably caused by an insufficiently realistic treatment of the photon contamination dose. The deviation for wedges is due partly to the spectral variation over the wedge which has not been considered.

An example of the performance in inhomogeneous cases is given in Fig. 2, where the dose has been calculated for a slab geometry with densities and compositions chosen to mimic a lung. The resulting depth dose distribution is compared to the results of Monte Carlo simulations and to calculations using the Batho method. The diagram shows that the present algorithm performs as well as the Batho method. The calculation time for one point is around 5 ms on

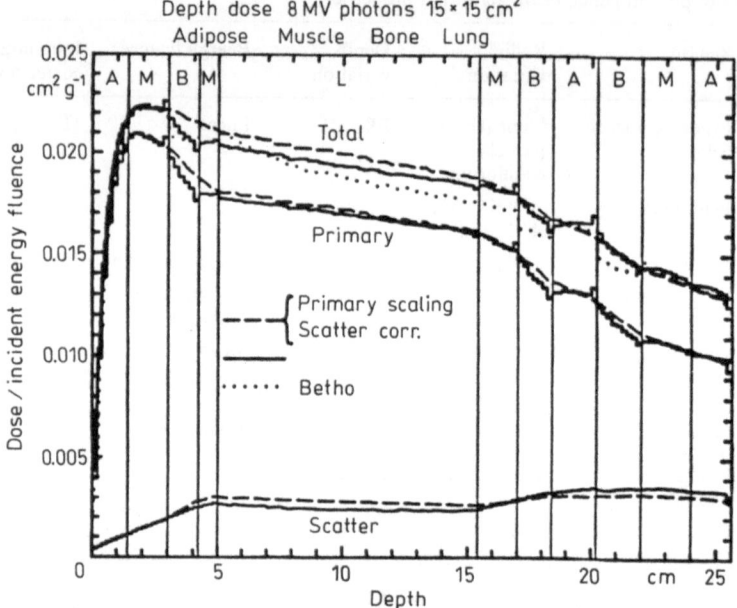

Fig. 2. Comparison for inhomogeneous slab calculation

a MicroVAX 3100, which is quite enough to make it interactive; an ordinary two-dimensional matrix containing 1000 points is calculated in 5 s. The algorithm is used clinically at a number of installations in Sweden.

References

Ahnesjö A (1989) Collapsed cone convolution of radiant energy for photon dose calculation in heterogeneous media. Med Phys 16: 577–592

Ahnesjö A (1991) Dose calculation methods in photon beam therapy using energy deposition kernels. Thesis, Stockholm University, Stockholm, Sweden

Ahnesjö A, Saxner M, Trepp A (1991a) A pencil beam model for photon dose calculation Med Phys (to be published)

Ahnesjö A, Knöös T, Montelius A (1991b) Application of the convolution method for calculation of output factors for therapy photon beams (to be published)

Knöös T, Nilsson M, Ahlgren L (1986) A method for conversion of hounsfield number to electron density and prediction of macroscopic pair production cross sections. Radiother Oncol 5: 337–345

Optimised Three-Dimensional Treatment Planning for Volumes with Concave Outlines, Using a Multileaf Collimator

S. Webb

Introduction

The aim of curative radiotherapy is to deliver a high dose, as uniformly as possible, to a target volume (TV) which encompasses the tumour, any marginal spread of disease and perhaps a border of safety, whilst minimising the dose to radiosensitive structures lying nearby. The widespread availability of tomographic medical images including X-ray computed tomography and magnetic resonance tomography enables sensitive volumes (SV) and TV to be accurately determined in three-dimensions (e.g. Fraass et al. 1991). The goal of conformal radiotherapy is to tailor the treatment fields so that the differential between the high-dose TV and the low-dose SV is as wide as possible. Under these circumstances dose escalation may be appropriate, thus increasing the probability of local control. A recent review of conformal therapy sets out the issues (Tait and Nahum 1990).

Three-dimensional conformal radiotherapy may be achieved by using a combination of geometrically shaped radiation fields from different orientations around the patient. A convenient way of shaping the fields to the beam's eye view (BEV) of the treatment volume is to use a multileaf collimator (MLC). The problem is then to find the optimum distribution of beam weights to apply to each field to minimise the dose to sensitive structure whilst aiming towards a uniform dose distribution in the treatment volume. This paper provides a method of optimising the choice of beamweights. The method is based on the well-known optimisation technique of simulated annealing. Either an optimal set of single beamweights per field is generated, or the intensity is spatially modulated across the field at each orientation (two weights per field) depending on whether there is only TV or both TV and SV in the line of sight. It is shown that the dose matrix resulting from the latter optimisation is closer to the dose prescription than that obtained by using either an optimal set of single weights per field or uniform beamweights.

Joint Department of Physics, Institute of Cancer Research and Royal Marsden Hospital, Downs Road, Sutton, Surrey SM2 5PT, UK

Advanced Radiation Therapy Tumor Response
Monitoring and Treatment Planning
Breit (Editor-in-Chief)
© Springer-Verlag, Berlin Heidelberg 1992

Three-Dimensional Treatment Plan Optimisation

If the TV has convex borders, and the SV is somewhat remote from the TV, then it is largely a simple matter to determine a set of entry angles whereby the primary beam never intersects SV. However, if the TV has concave borders, and sensitive structure lies within these concavities, this cannot achieve the goal. Unlike what is possible in the two-dimensional planning problem (single slices irradiated by lines of radiation with different profiles) we cannot easily overcome this problem by spatially varying the intensity of the irradiation across the geometrically tailored two-dimensional field with variations on a small spatial scale. The two-dimensional analogue of one-dimensional highly modulated beam profiles (see e.g. Bortfeld et al. 1990; Brahme 1988; Webb 1989) would be too difficult to deliver at present.

In this paper each beam port is considered "open" [in the sense of unwedged and of uniform (or dual — see below) intensity], but of course the beam may be switched on for different times per field or part-field. This will be referred to as the beamweight for that field or part-field. The question then arises, to which a solution is presented in this paper: what is the optimum distribution of beam weights for MLC fields (or part-fields) to achieve as high a differential as possible between the dose in a TV with concave borders and the dose in a SV at least partly encased by the TV? In the method presented here the distinction is made between the beamweight attached to that part of a MLC field "seeing" only TV and that "seeing" both TV and SV.

Method (Description of the New Treatment-Planning Technique)

The optimisation proceeds by the following steps.

Dose Specification. The three-dimensional dose prescription was represented digitally by $D_{pres,ijk}$ — specified on a 32^3 matrix, where i, j, k label the elements in the x, y, z directions of a right cartesian coordinate system with the y axis being the long axis of the patient (Fig. 1). This allows volumes of interest (VOI) to be placed on the distributions (specified by the appropriate i, j, k values) for determining features such as the mean dose and the uniformity of dose in, for example, the TV and SV.

Specification of the Multileaf Collimator. The direction in space of the MLC was specified by the angle θ to the positive y axis and the angle ϕ between the projection on the x-z plane and the positive z axis of a line from the origin of dose space to the centre of the face of the MLC (Fig. 1). The MLC was also represented as a two-dimensional digital matrix of elements $M_{i',j'}$ which are

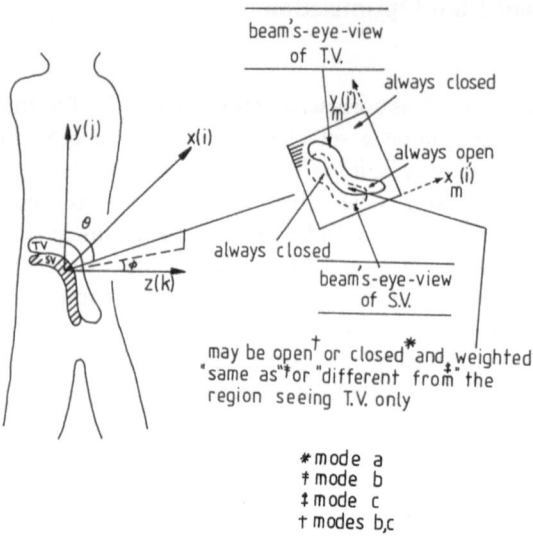

Fig. 1. The x, y, z coordinate system used to specify the dosimetry $D_{pres, i, j, k}$, together with the relationship between this system and the position of the multileaf collimator. The MLC coordinates are x_M, y_M, the leaves being parallel to the x_M direction. The position of the MLC is such that a line from the origin of dose space to the centre of the face of the MLC makes an angle ϕ with the positive y axis and its projection on the x-z plane makes an angle ϕ with the positive z axis. The target volume (TV) is shown *unshaded* and the sensitive volume (SV) is shown *shaded* in the patient. The figure also shows how the areas in the MLC space may be labelled separately depending on whether they "connect" to only TV, only SV, TV plus SV, other tissue. *Dotted line*, beam's eye view of the SV (shown *shaded* in the patient); *solid line*, beams eye view of the TV (shown *unshaded* in the patient)

either open or shut depending on whether radiation is to pass through or be blocked. In practice of course the pattern $M_{i', j'}$ is constrained such that it can be realised practically by an arrangement of leaves with different openings per pair of leaves in the well-understood way. There were P ϕ values equispaced in $0-2\pi$ (which are labelled ϕ_p, $p = 1 \ldots P$), and at each ϕ position there were T θ values (labelled θ_t, $t = 1 \ldots T$) equispaced in $\pi/3-2\pi/3$. Typically odd P and T were selected so that no two views face each other (e.g. $P = 7$ and $T = 3$, i.e. there was a ring of seven coplanar equatorial positions and two other rings of non-coplanar positions). The $\theta = \pi/2$ plane is the conventional transaxial plane.

Relation Between Dose Space and MLC Space. For each location of the MLC specified by θ, ϕ, each position (voxel) in dose space may be mapped to an element on the collimator. BEV-mapping equations, specifying the order of rotations, are given in full in Webb (1991). The optimisation has been implemented in three modes (see Figure 1). (a) Only the MLC elements connecting to the TV are open. They receive different weights per MLC position. In this mode the SV can never receive primary radiation, but the opportunities for irradiating the TV are limited (and, it will be shown, too restricted). (b) The MLC elements connecting to both TV and SV are open, receive the *same* weight at any one position, but different weights per MLC position. (c) The MLC elements connecting to both TV and SV are open, receive *different* weights at any one position and different weights per MLC position. It may be appreciated that mode b is akin to "conventional" multiport treatment but with geometrically shaped (BEV) fields. Mode c begins to have some of the merits of fields with spatially modulated beam intensities as proved so successful in two dimensions.

Optimisation by Simulated Annealing. Starting from some initial distribution of beamweights, the optimisation by simulated annealing (Press et al. 1988) proceeds by randomly polling MLC positions. (If the mode a or mode b choice is in operation, each MLC position has a single beamweight assigned to all the i', j' pixels in the open field. If, on the other hand, the mode c choice is invoked, the i', j' groups of pixels in the two separate parts of each MLC field are also randomly polled and assigned independent beamweights.) After determining a particular open area at a particular MLC orientation (θ_t, ϕ_p), a grain of beamweight was added to all the open i', j' pixels in that area. The cycles of iteration were labelled by N so that the set of beam weights at this cycle is $B_{i',j'}^N(\theta_t, \phi_p)$. With this in place the new (pseudo-) dose distribution corresponding to including this addition was determined via

$$D_{\text{ps},i,j,k}^N = \sum_{i',j' \to i,j,k} B_{i',j'}^N(\theta_t, \phi_p) \exp - (\mu l_{i,j,k,i',j'}), \tag{1}$$

where $i', j' \to i, j, k$ means the sum is taken over all those i', j' MLC elements connecting to ($\to$) dose elements i, j, k. $l_{i,j,k,i',j'}$ is the set of distances from each i, j, k dose point to the external patient boundary in the direction of each i', j' on the collimator. A quadratic cost function was defined by:

$$V_N = \left[\frac{1}{32^3} \sum_{i=1}^{32} \sum_{j=1}^{32} \sum_{k=1}^{32} w_{i,j,k}(D_{\text{pres},i,j,k} - D_{\text{ps},i,j,k}^N)^2 \right]^{0.5} \tag{2}$$

being the weighted rms difference at iteration N between the digital dose prescription $D_{\text{pres},i,j,k}$ and the pseudo-dose distribution $D_{\text{ps},i,j,k}^N$. The aim is to reduce this to as low a value as possible. The parameter $w_{i,j,k}$ is a weight which can be used to emphasise differentially the importance of matching prescription and calculation. The progress of the iteration is determined by the behaviour of the cost function. The change in cost function at each iteration is:

$$\delta V = V_N - V_{N-1} \tag{3}$$

If the addition of a grain of beamweight reduces the cost function, then that grain is accepted. If, on the other hand, it increases the cost function, a random number is generated to decide whether to accept the grain with a reduced probability:

$$\exp - (\delta V)/k\Theta \tag{4}$$

where k is the Boltzmann constant and Θ is a temperature. Both positive and negative grains of beam weight were randomly selected. Typically grains of size

0.05 were used. Initially the temperature was high so that there is a wide search of the options available for the MLC beamweights. As the iteration proceeded, and typically some 100 000 iterations were performed, the temperature was gradually reduced more slowly than the logarithm of the cycle number. This guarantees a convergence to the global minimum cost function (sometimes also called a potential function). The best distribution of beamweights gradually "crystallizes out", giving the dose distribution $D_{\text{opt},i,j,k}$ which is closest to the prescription $D_{\text{pres},i,j,k}$.

Quantifying the Resultant Dose distribution. As well as computing the optimum dose distribution $D_{\text{opt},i,j,k}$ in this way, all the coding exists to obtain quickly the distribution $D_{\text{unif},i,j,k}$ which would be obtained if all the open parts of each field were set to a constant value. This is the distribution corresponding to switching on the X-ray beam for the *same time* for each MLC field. The improvements depend on the mode chosen for the optimisation. To express this numerically define:

$$\psi_1 = \left[\frac{1}{32^3} \sum_{i=1}^{32} \sum_{j=1}^{32} \sum_{k=1}^{32} w_{i,j,k}(D_{\text{pres},i,j,k} - D_{\text{opt},i,j,k})^2 \right]^{0.5}, \tag{5}$$

and

$$\psi_2 = \left[\frac{1}{32^3} \sum_{i=1}^{32} \sum_{j=1}^{32} \sum_{k=1}^{32} w_{i,j,k}(D_{\text{pres},i,j,k} - D_{\text{unif},i,j,k})^2 \right]^{0.5}. \tag{6}$$

For all the optimisations performed $\psi_2 > \psi_1$, the ratio ψ_1/ψ_2 characterising the improvement of $D_{\text{opt},i,j,k}$ over $D_{\text{unif},i,j,k}$. All computations were made on a DEC VAX 3900 computer.

Illustrative Results

Figure 2 shows a schematic of the dose prescription in the model problem. The TV is crescent shaped in any one transaxial x, z plane and is "wrapped around" a SV which is circular in transaxial cross-section. Twenty-one MLC positions were considered, seven ϕ positions equispaced in $0-2\pi$ and three θ positions at $\pi/3$, $\pi/2$ and $2\pi/3$ for each ϕ position.

The results of optimisations in all these modes are shown in Table 1 for one of many model problems studied. For mode a, i.e. the beam switched on only for that part of each MLC field 'seeing" only TV, the SV received no primary dose. The uniformity (ratio: standard deviation to mean) in the TV was, however, is poor ($\simeq 40\%$). The optimised distribution showed little improvement on the distribution from uniform weights $[(\psi_1/\psi_2) \simeq 0.981]$.

For mode b, i.e. the beam switched on for all of each MLC field "seeing" both TV only and TV together with SV, the SV received considerable primary dose.

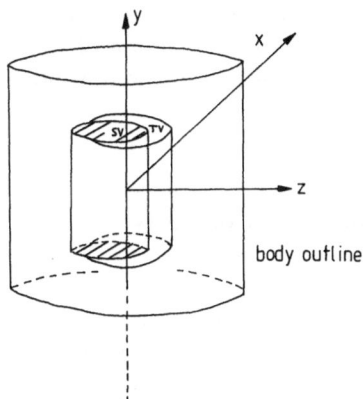

body outline

Fig. 2. The geometry of the model planning problem showing the target volume and the sensitive tissue. The target volume has a concave border and "wraps around" the sensitive structure

Table 1. The statistics for a model problem in VOI placed within target volume (TV) and sensitive volume (SV) following computation of dose distributions from either uniform or optimum beam weights[a]

Method	ψ_1/ψ_2	(SD/mean) TV	(Mean SV/mean TV)	(Max SV/max TV)
Mode a				
Uniform weights		38.5%	0	0
Optimum weights	0.981	37.8%	0	0
Mode b				
Uniform weights		0.9%	85.7%	98.1%
Optimum weights	0.912	3.0%	77.4%	93.6%
Mode c				
Uniform weights		0.9%	85.7%	98.1%
Optimum weights	0.866	10.8%	60.0%	55.0%
Mode d				
Uniform weights		0.9%	85.7%	98.1%
Optimum weights	0.822	11.9%	44.0%	77.0%

[a] Modes a, b, c and d are defined under "Relation Between Dose Space and MLC Space", and ψ_1 and ψ_2 are defined in Eqs. 5, 6.

The uniformity in the TV was, however, much better ($\simeq 3\%$). The optimised distribution was an improvement on the distribution from uniform weights [$(\psi_1/\psi_2) \simeq 0.912$]. This was also reflected by the ratio of the mean dose in the full SV to the mean dose in the full TV falling from 85.7% with uniform weights to 77.4% with optimised weights. The improvement was small but significant.

In mode c, i.e. the beam switched on for all of each MLC field "seeing" TV and SV but the separate parts of each MLC field differentially weighted, the SV received considerably less primary dose than for mode b. The uniformity in the TV now becomes acceptable ($\simeq 11\%$). The optimised distribution is a greater improvement on the distribution from uniform weights [$(\psi_1/\psi_2) \simeq 0.866$]. This was also reflected by the ratio of the mean dose in the full SV to the mean dose in the full TV falling from 85.7% with uniform weights to 60.0% with optimised weights.

The mode c result is a "half-way house" between modes a and b, i.e. it provides a means to gain simultaneously *both* acceptable dose uniformity in the TV *and* a reduction in the dose to SV. Dose-volume histograms were routinely produced to check for absence of hot and cold spots.

Results from Full Modulation of Two-Dimensional Intensity

Very recently the option ("mode d") has been added to the code to allow full spatial modulation of intensity across the MLC ports as a computational exercise. One must emphasise that this is impractical at present. The results (Table 1) give 12% dose uniformity to the TV with the ratio of the mean SV dose to the mean TV dose now falling to 44%.

Conclusions

The method presented in this paper is an attempt to allow a small amount of spatial modulation per beam (only two values) and gain the advantages of fully three-dimensional field shaping with the MLC. The beam orientations need not be coplanar. The work is a logical development of the method presented by Webb (1989). The method has been tested for model three-dimensional distributions of three-dimensional TV with concave boundaries entwined with sensitive structures which cannot be simply disconnected from the TV by judicious selection of beam orientations.

It was found that by "switching off" that part of the MLC field connecting to both TV and SV, allowing only the part connecting to TV only, the dose to the SV could be reduced to exactly zero (of course, in a primary-dose only model), but that the dose uniformity in the TV was unacceptably much greater than the generally allowable 10%. Conversely, "switching on" all the MLC port "seeing" both TV and SV with only one weight per field gave an acceptable dose uniformity in the TV but an unacceptable dose to the SV. In between, by using the differential weighting to the two parts of each MLC field, and optimising such weights, an acceptable dose uniformity ($\simeq 10\%$) and a lower dose to SV was achievable.

References

Bortfeld T, Burkelbach J, Boesecke R, Schlegel W (1990) Methods of image reconstruction from projections applied to conformation therapy. Phys Med Biol 35: 1423–1434

Brahme A (1988) Optimisation of stationary and moving beam radiation therapy techniques. Radiother Oncol 12: 129–140

Fraass BA, McShan DL, Ten Haken RK, Lichter AS (1991) A practical 3D treatment planning system: overview and clinical use for external beam planning. Int J Radiat Oncol Biol Phys (in press)

Press WH, Flannery BP, Teukolsky SA, Vetterling WT (1988) Numerical recipes: the art of scientific computing. Cambridge University Press, Cambridge, pp 326–334

Tait DM, Nahum AE (1990) Conformal therapy. Eur J Cancer 26: 750–753

Webb S (1989) Optimisation of conformal radiotherapy dose distributions by simulated annealing. Phys Med Biol 34: 1349–1369

Webb S (1991) Optimisation by simulated annealing of three-dimensional, conformal treatment planning for radiation fields defined by a multileaf collimator. Phys Med Biol 36: 1201–1226

Three-Dimensional Solution of the Inverse Problem in Conformation Radiotherapy

T. Bortfeld, J. Bürkelbach, and W. Schlegel

Introduction

Several recently published papers deal with the so-called inverse problem of radiation therapy (Brahme 1988; Webb 1989; Barth 1990; Goitein 1990; Lind and Källman 1990; Bortfeld et al. 1990a). Most of the authors define this as the problem of directly determining treatment parameters on the basis of the desired dose distribution, which is the inverse process to that in conventional radiotherapy planning. Usually, the term inverse problem is used in conjunction with a new treatment technique using modulated irradiation fields, where the treatment parameters are the modulation profiles for each beam direction. Also, in this context, the term inverse problem is justified because the problem of calculating the modulation profiles is in principle a matrix inversion problem.

For the solution of the inverse problem, several approaches have been proposed. The resulting dose distributions are very promising. However, there are still some unsolved difficulties and open questions. Among these is the fact that, for physical reasons, the ideal dose distribution (a uniform dose distribution within the target and no dose outside) is generally not achievable. Thus, also in the case of modulated irradiation fields, the dose distribution must be a compromise between applying a high and uniformly distributed dose to the target and sparing the surrounding normal tissue. Earlier investigations have shown that a very satisfying compromise can be found for some complexly shaped targets. However, the general question remains of how to define the compromise, and how to find an *optimal* compromise.

Another difficulty with currently known approaches to the solution of the inverse problem lies in the fact that these are two-dimensional solutions. Although it should in principle be possible to achieve a three-dimensional solution by solving the two-dimensional problem slice by slice, this approach presumably runs into the following problems: (a) the beam divergence cannot be taken into consideration, (b) noncoplanar techniques cannot be applied, and (c) the calculation time is very long.

In this paper we present a truely three-dimensional algorithm for the solution of the inverse problem. The algorithm is based on the very effective and

Department of Radiology and Pathophysiology, German Cancer Research Center, Im Neuenheimer Feld 280, 6900 Heidelberg, FRG

Advanced Radiation Therapy Tumor Response
Monitoring and Treatment Planning
Breit (Editor-in-Chief)
© Springer-Verlag, Berlin Heidelberg 1992

well-established image reconstruction methods known from computed tomography (Bortfeld et al. 1990a). Due to this, the calculation time could be kept within very reasonable limits. The inverse problem is regarded as an optimization problem. Clinical data such as the tolerance dose for organs at risk are taken into consideration as constraints on the optimization.

Methods

Mathematical Formulation. To obtain a mathematical formulation of the problem, the two-dimensional intensity modulation profiles are seen as composed of small pencil beams with different intensities. All of the pencil beam intensities for one two-dimensional irradiation field k are written as components of a vector $\mathbf{x}^k$. (The values are stored in the same way as a two-dimensional image is stored in a one-dimensional computer array.) Then a bigger vector $\mathbf{x}$ is created, comprising all pencil beam intensity vectors $\mathbf{x}^k$ for all N irradiation fields:

$$\mathbf{x} = (\mathbf{x}^1, \mathbf{x}^2, \ldots, \mathbf{x}^N)'$$

Now the tissue is split into a great number of small voxels (volume elements), and the dose values for each of these voxels are written as another vector $\mathbf{d}$. Because of the validity of the superposition principle, there is a linear relationship between $\mathbf{x}$ and $\mathbf{d}$:

$$\mathbf{d} = \mathbf{D}\mathbf{x} \tag{1}$$

$\mathbf{D}$ could be termed a "dose calculation matrix" whose component D_{ij} is the dose contribution of pencil beam j to tissue point i. Now, if the inverse of $\mathbf{D}$ were known, a solution of the inverse problem would be easy: one writes the desired dose values (for instance, 100% within the target and 0% elsewhere) as $\mathbf{d}$ and calculates $\mathbf{x} = \mathbf{D}^{-1}\mathbf{d}$. However, besides the problem that $\mathbf{D}$ generally cannot be inverted, there is the problem that this solution would result in a vector $\mathbf{x}$ which contains negative elements. This is, of course, an unphysical result, because negative intensities cannot be realized. The following methods have been published to overcome this problem: the negative values can either simply be cut off, i.e., set to zero (Barth 1990), or the dose outside the target can be set to a value greater than zero (Webb 1989). However, both of these approaches are somewhat critical, as other considerations have shown (Goitein 1990).

Since it is impossible to solve the inverse problem exactly, we treat it as an optimization problem. The following optimization criteria are taken into consideration: (a) minimization of the deviation between prescribed and calculated dose in the target; (b) a large value of the dose gradient at the target boundary; and (c) reduction of the dose in organs at risk to a tolerable value. The first criterion is translated into mathematical form by defining an objective function

F_1 which is to be minimized:

$$F_1 = \sum_{i \in T} (d_i - p)^2 \overset{!}{=} \min \tag{2}$$

where d_i is the calculated dose in tissue element i, and p is the prescribed dose. The summation is taken over all target points. Introducing a "target operator" T which extracts only the target points from all tissue points and using the expression from Eq. 1, this can be written as a squared vector norm:

$$F_1(\mathbf{x}) = \|T(\mathbf{Dx} - \mathbf{p})\|^2 \tag{3}$$

The second criterion concerning the dose gradient at the target boundary is considered by stating that the dose at a given distance to the target (and at greater distances) should be less than 60% of the maximum dose. The mathematical formulation of this criterion is similar to the third criterion and is not elaborated further. The third criterion can be written as an optimization constraint in the simple form $d_i \le u_i$ for points in organs at risk where u_i is the upper dose limit. It is considered by the definition of a "penalty function" which is added to F_1 to obtain a new objective function F:

$$F(\mathbf{x}) = \|T(\mathbf{Dx} - \mathbf{p})\|^2 + r\|\mathbf{R}^+(\mathbf{Dx} - \mathbf{u})\|^2 \overset{!}{=} \min$$

In this equation $\mathbf{u}$ is a vector which contains the upper dose limits for all points within all organs at risk, $\mathbf{R}^+$ extracts those points in the organs at risk where the dose is too high $(d_i > u_i)$, and r is a parameter which controls the strength of the constraint.

For the solution of the optimization problem, i.e., for the minimization of F, we use the "scaled gradient projection algorithm," which is defined by the iteration equation

$$\mathbf{x}(t + 1) = \mathbf{x}(t) - \frac{1}{N}\mathbf{S}^{-1}[\mathbf{D}'T(\mathbf{Dx}(t) - \mathbf{p}) + r\mathbf{D}'\mathbf{R}^+(\mathbf{Dx}(t) - \mathbf{u})]. \tag{5}$$

$\mathbf{S}$ is the scaling matrix and $\mathbf{D}'$ denotes the transposed matrix of $\mathbf{D}$. More details concerning the penalty function technique and the scaled gradient algorithm are given by Bortfeld et al. (1990a). In the present paper, however, we want to emphasize the computer implementation of the algorithm.

A Three-Dimensional Inversion Program. When the two-dimensional modulation profiles for a three-dimensional target volume are to be optimized, the size of the matrix $\mathbf{D}$ becomes huge. For a typical application we have a relevant tissue area of 10 000 voxels, and the modulation profiles (typically nine) consist of 1000 pencil beams each, resulting in a total number of 9000 pencil beams. Then $\mathbf{D}$ consist of $10\,000 \times 9000$ elements, which is too many for any of today's computers. In order to overcome this problem, we do not store the whole matrix $\mathbf{D}$ but instead calculate the elements of $\mathbf{D}$ during each iteration step with a simplified dose calculation algorithm. Also, the pencil beam intensities and dose values are stored in another way than that described above.

The computer program uses the three-dimensional arrays $d(i,j,k)$ and $d\_pre(i,j,k)$ to store the dose data. At program start, $d\_pre(i,j,k)$ is loaded with the prescribed dose in the target for all target voxels and with the upper dose limits for organs at risk; $d(i,j,k)$ is initialized to zero. In addition, there are the three-dimensional arrays $x(m,n,f)$ and $x\_upd(m,n,f)$ which contain the pencil beam intensities (i.e., the elements of $\mathbf{x}$). The index f refers to the field number: $f = 1 \ldots N$. The first program step is the calculation of an initial estimate of $x(m, n, f)$ with the method of filtered projection (Bortfeld et al. 1990a). Then the resulting dose distribution is calculated. This is done by ray-tracing the depth dose distribution calculated by an analytic expression (Schoknecht 1968) through the three-dimensional dose array $d(i, j, k)$. The rays are followed in a fanline geometry. Each ray is weighted with the corresponding pencil beam intensity. Doing this, the interference between the pencil beams is not taken into consideration, i.e., the pencil beams are assumed to be δ-like in the lateral extension, and scatter is not adequately accounted for. A more sophisticated approach has been developed (Bortfeld et al. 1990b) but not yet implemented. In the next step, the difference between $d(i,j,k)$ and $d\_pre(i,j,k)$ is calculated for target voxels and stored in $d(i, j, k)$. Within organ-at-risk voxels this difference is multiplied by r and the result is also stored in $d(i, j, k)$ if the dose is greater than the upper limit. Otherwise, $d(i, j, k)$ is set to zero. Outside the target and organs at risk $d(i, j, k)$ is also set to zero. Referring to Eq. 5 we have now calculated $\mathbf{T(Dx - p)}$ and $r\mathbf{R}^+(\mathbf{Dx - u})$. Now the transposed matrix $\mathbf{D'}$ is applied to these expressions. Referring to our program again, this means that $d(i, j, k)$ must be ray-traced backwards onto the update profiles $x\_upd(m, n, f)$. This step is performed in the same way as the forward ray-tracing. In a last step these profiles are scaled (which cannot be explained in detail here), divided by the number of fields N, and subtracted from the starting profiles $x(m, n, f)$.

The process described above is repeated iteratively. Several investigations have shown that seven iteration steps are sufficient for almost all cases. The program is currently implemented on a VAX station 3200 (Digital Equipment). On this computer the calculation time for one iteration step is about 3 min. Thus, the whole optimization process requires only a little more than 20 min.

Results

The clinical case of a patient with a carcinoma of the nasopharynx was examined. Since this was a very fast-growing tumor, it was necessary to define an unusually large target volume, at least in the slice shown in Fig. 1. Due to the close vicinity of the very radiation-sensitive eye lenses to the target contour, the treatment planning for this case was especially complicated. Figure 1 compares

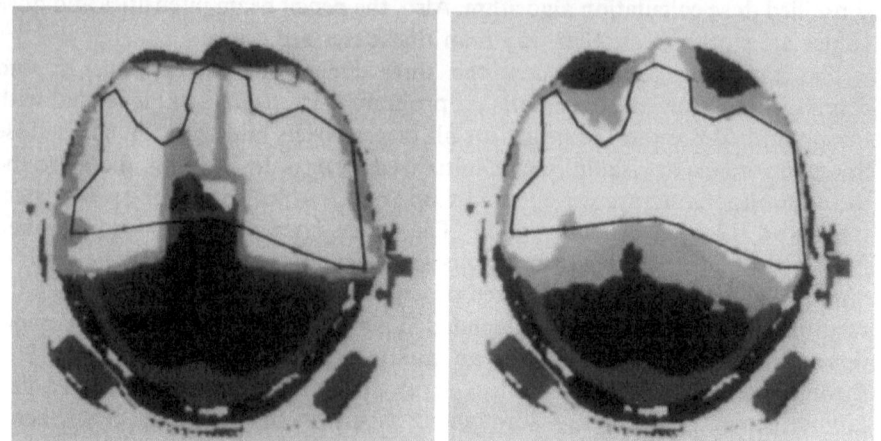

Fig. 1. a Dose distribution resulting from "conventional" planning. **b** Optimized dose distribution

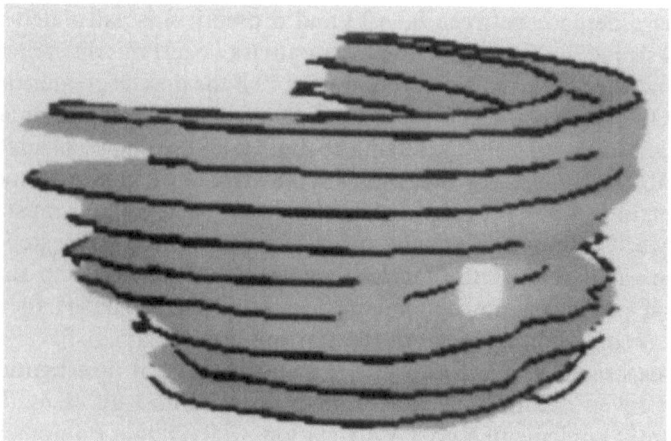

Fig. 2. Three-dimensional shaded surface display of the optimized dose distribution. *Light gray,* target; *white,* eye lenses; *black ribbons,* 80% isodose lines

the dose distribution resulting from a "conventional" plan with a plan which was optimized with the methods described above. The contour of the target volume is shown by black lines. The white area marks the therapeutic dose range (between 80% and 100% of the maximum dose) and the light grey area shows the 60%–80% dose range. The eye lenses are marked as organs at risk.

Figure 1a shows the result of a "conventional" plan. The term conventional is placed in quotation marks because the plan is conventional only in comparison to the described methods of inverse planning. However, today's most sophisticated treatment techniques have been applied, i.e., noncoplanar beam directions, irregular field shaping with a multileaf collimator and three-dimensional treatment planning. The figure shows that with all of these techniques it is not possible to adequately fit the dose distribution to the target. The dose to the eye lenses is much too high, and other parts of the tumor are underdosed.

The result which can be achieved by an optimized treatment with nine modulated fields is shown in Fig. 1b. The much better fit of the dose to the target is evident. The eye lenses are spared at maximum, and there is no underdosage. A three-dimensional display of this optimized dose distribution is shown in Fig. 2. It demonstrates how exactly the therapeutic dose range (black ribbons) can be fitted to the target, which is shaded in light grey, while at the same time the eye lenses (displayed in white) are clearly outside the therapeutic dose range.

The clinical case described above should not be mistaken as a precedent for the application of modulated fields and optimized inverse planning. However, it shows that there are some very complicated cases where even today's most advanced treatment techniques fail, but where inverse planning gives satisfying results.

References

Barth NH (1990) An inverse problem in radiation therapy. Int J Radiat Oncol Biol Phys 18: 425–431

Bortfeld T, Bürkelbach J, Boesecke R, Schlegel W (1990a) Methods of image reconstruction from projections applied to conformation radiotherapy. Phys Med Biol 35: 1423–1434

Bortfeld T, Boesecke R, Schlegel W, Bohsung J (1990b) 3-D dose calculation using 2-D convolutions and ray-tracing methods. In: Hukku S, Iyer PS (eds) Proceedings of the 10th international conference on the use of computers in radiation therapy (ICCR). Alpana Arts, Lucknow (India)

Brahme A (1988) Optimization of stationary and moving beam radiation therapy techniques. Radiother Oncol 12: 129–140

Goitein M (1990) The inverse problem. Int J Radiat Oncol Biol Phys 18: 489–491

Lind BK, Källman P (1990) Experimental verification of an algorithm for inverse radiation therapy planning. Radiother Oncol 17: 359–368

Schoknecht G (1968) Die Beschreibung von Strahlenfeldern durch Separierung von Primär- und Streustrahlung. Strahlentherapie 136: 24–32

Webb S (1989) Optimisation of conformal radiotherapy dose distributions by simulated annealing. Phys Med Biol 34: 1349–1369

A New Source Model for Linear Accelerators

E. Ihnen[1] and J.M. Jensen[2]

Introduction

The dose at a given point in a phantom is the result of three components: the primary dose, the scattered dose influenced by the surrounding material, and the scattered dose produced in the radiation head of a linear accelerator. While the primary dose depends only on the constant photon flux emerging from the target, the number of scattered photons varies with the field size. However, the dose of central ray in the maximum dose in a phantom is the result of only two components: the primary dose and the head scatter dose, provided the backscatter factor is neglected. After normalization of all measured dose values to those of a 10×10 cm^2 field, it is possible to obtain the machine-specific, output factor by varying the field size. The output factor, so defined, depends on several sources of scattered radiation, such as collimator scatter, backscatter into the monitor chamber, and scatter from the beam flattening filter. Kubo and Lo [1] reported that there is very little influence of the backscattering effect, (about 1%). In contrast, we found up to 13% variation (even more with CGR Saturne) by increasing the field size from 4×4 cm^2 to 40×40 cm^2. Here we studied the influence of the collimator and flattening filter. The most important influence on scattered radiation is that due to the flattening filter, as suggested by Kase [2].

In a computer simulation using an area source localized at the bottom edge of the flattening filter and an additional line and area source at the position of the collimator edge and bottom, we constructed a model for the scatter-producing radiation head elements. We report here on the principal shape of the output factor function and the output factors of rectangular fields and on the interdependence of the different sources and their relative strength.

Theory

The central idea in creating a source model to explain the mode of action of the output factor is to add a scatter-producing area source at a defined distance to

---

[1] Department of Radiotherapy and Nuclear Medicine, Medical University of Lübeck, Ratzeburger Allee 160, 2400 Lübeck, FRG
[2] Department of Radiotherapy and Radiooncology, University of Kiel, Arnold-Heller-Str. 9, 2300 Kiel, FRG

Advanced Radiation Therapy Tumor Response
Monitoring and Treatment Planning
Breit (Editor-in-Chief)
© Springer-Verlag, Berlin Heidelberg 1992

the focus. Since at the center of the bottom of the flattening filter there is a high, unavoidable photon attenuation (factor of 2–5) — necessarily combined with a high proportion of photon scattering — the best place to locate the scatter-producing area source appears to be there. The assumption of a volume source offers only little advantage in terms of accuracy compared to the disadvantage of increasing calculation time.

The projected field (PF) at the bottom of the flattening filter is defined by the isocenter and the collimator setting. Figure 1 shows how this model works. It can be seen that from a square light field there results a rectangular field. The reason must be seen in the different focus distances to the lower and upper jaws. It is suggested that the defined area produces mainly the scatter radiation which is visible at the isocenter by the output factor function. The output factor therefore depends on the length (A') and the width (B') of PF, not on its rotation, and on an area source function (ASF), which has yet be defined. Assuming a symmetrical ASF, we chose a sum of three gaussian probability functions, symmetrical to the central axis of the beam flattening filter with a center maximum and minimum at the edge:

$$ASF = \Sigma\, A_i * exp[-(x^2 + y^2)/2*S_i] \quad i = 1, 2, 3 \tag{1}$$

This function contains only a small number of parameters. Dimensions for the amplitudes have been chosen arbitrarily because the output factor itself is relative. Other scattering sources must also be included. The jaws themselves are area sources. Measurements show that the influence on the output factor is not more than 1% (transparency and scatter). The measurement was performed by closing the lower jaw and varying the upper jaw, and vice versa, to separate the edge radiation of the collimator. Another source is the scatter radiation

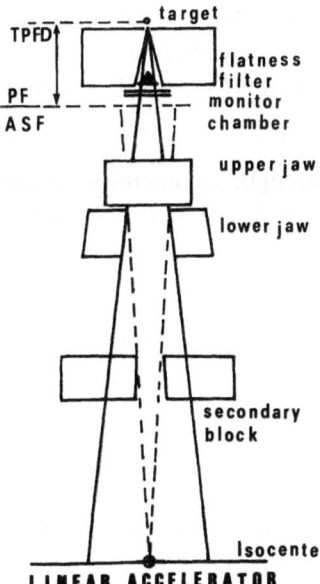

Fig. 1. Area scattering source of the radiation head and measurement geometry. *TPFD*, Target-projected field distance; *PF*, projected field; *ASF*, area source function

produced by the collimator edges. In accordance with Rosen et al. [3], we assumed a line source at the upper edge of each collimator jaw. This type of radiation is produced by an already flattened field. Therefore it should be nearly proportional to the length of the field edges. This would result in a linear increase function at larger field sizes. However, the output factors remain nearly constant, except for CGR Saturne 20.

To study whether the main part of scatter radiation originates from a small area near the focus, we installed secondary collimators with three different small square fields. The PF of the secondary fields were slightly smaller than the area source to show their influence on the output factor. Only the smallest secondary field, which with the PF just covers parts of the flattening filter, decreases the output factor at greater field sizes. If the secondary collimator is of relevance as an additional area source, the output factor should increase according to a square function. However, it was not possible to demonstrate such an effect.

Material and Methods

The theoretical model mentioned in Eq. 1 was used. The procedure was a reconstruction of the output factor defined in the following formulas for square light fields at the isocenter by means of a computer-aided integration process. The parameters have been fixed by trial and error. The choice is not critical because the integration is a smoothing process. Another function instead of Eq. 1 is also possible. We defined the output factor (OF) by:

$$OF = (F_x + p)/(F_{10} + p) \qquad (2)$$

where F_x is the computer-integrated ASF, x is the edge of square light field in the isocenter, and p is the constant intensity of the focus. The output factor becomes 1 for $x = 10$. Reducing Eq. 2 by F_{10} and substituting p/F_{10} with P we obtain:

$$OF = (F_x/F_{10} + P)/(1 + P) \qquad (3)$$

where P is now the ratio of focus to area source strength. An interesting feature is the possibility of an extrapolation to field size 0, $F_x = 0$. If P is known, we obtain the output factor for zero fields:

$$OF = P/(1 + P) \qquad (4)$$

Also P has been determined by trial and error.

Results

We studied the Mevatron 74-10X, Clinac 20-15X, SL 25-6X, and SL 25-15X linear accelerators. The set of parameters for ASF and the ratio P is given in Table 1. For the Mevatron 74 we show the output factor for square and

Table 1. Area source function parameter values and ratio of point source to area source

	A_1	A_2	A_3	S_1 (cm)	S_2 (cm)	S_3 (cm)	P	TPED
Mevatron 74	2.5	17.0	15.0	1.9	0.9	0.3	10	10
Clinac 20	2.0	15.0	15.0	4.5	1.0	0.4	10	12.6
SL 25-6X	3.5	0.0	300	2.5	--	0.4	5	16
SL 25-15X	4.5	10.0	30.0	2.5	1.0	0.5	11	16

P, Ratio of point source to area source; TPED, target-projected field distance.

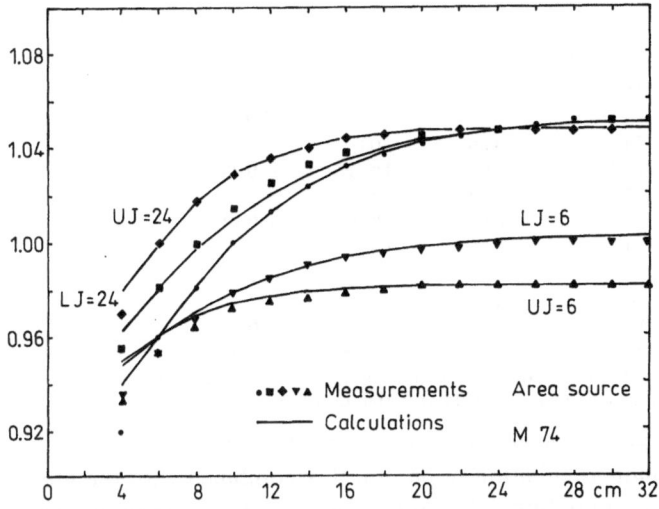

Fig. 2. Output factor for square and rectangular fields, Mevatron 74: measurements and calculations

rectangular fields with fixed jaws (6 or 24 cm) plotted in Fig. 2. It is typical for linear accelerators, except CGR Saturne. In Table 2 we demonstrate the differences of the dose measurements for PF with A' and B' for different collimator settings to verify our theory.

Discussion

The data presented show that in our model the output factor for square and rectangular fields at the isocenter was reproduced within 1.01% using identical parameter sets. The effect of collimator scattering can be neglected. This also holds for collimator block scattering. It is obvious that the most scattered radiation is produced in the flattening filter itself. This is plausible because there

Table 2. Differences in measurements for the same projected field but different collimator settings (with block tray)

A (cm)	B (cm)	Equivalent square	A' (cm)	B' (cm)	Dose difference (%)
4	4	4	0.932	1.416	
6.1	2.6	3.67	1.416	0.932	− 0.72
6	6	6	1.398	2.124	
9.1	3.9	5.46	2.124	1.398	− 0.54
8	8	8	1.864	2.832	
12.2	5.3	7.35	2.832	1.864	− 0.22
10	10	10	2.33	3.54	
15.2	6.6	9.11	3.54	2.33	− 0.08
12	12	12	2.796	4.248	
18.2	7.9	11.02	4.248	2.796	− 0.24
15	15	15	3.495	5.31	
22.8	9.9	13.77	5.31	3.495	− 0.47
20	20	20	4.66	7.08	
30.4	13.2	18.37	7.08	4.66	− 0.25
25	25	25	5.825	8.85	
38.0	16.5	23.0	8.85	5.825	− 0.17
6	20	9.23	1.398	7.08	
30.4	3.9	6.9	7.08	1.398	+ 1.01
20	6	9.23	4.66	2.124	
9.1	13.2	10.77	2.124	4.66	− 0.54

A, Upper jaw at isocenter; B, lower jaw at isocenter; A', upper jaw, projected field at flattening filter; B', lower jaw, projected field at flattening filter.

is the greatest absolute attenuation of photon flux combined with the greatest dose rate of scattered radiation. The output factor of CGR Saturne 20 mentioned by Kase [2] with its unique collimator design shows the effect that PF covers parts of the upper irradiated trimmers. Those with PF-covered trimmer area increase linearly with fields size, and so does the output factor.

For future investigations this new source model may be helpful in calculating output factors in irregular field techniques, in the use of asymmetrical jaws, and with the multileaf collimator.

References

1. Kubo H, Lo KK (1989) Measurements of backscattered radiation from Therac-20 collimator and trimmer jaws into beam monitor chamber. Med Phys 16: 292
2. Kase KR (1986) Head scatter data for several linear accelerators (4-18MV). Med Phys 13: 530
3. Rosen II, Loyd MD, Lane RG (1990) Collimator scatter in modeling radiation beam profiles. Med Phys 7: 422
4. Ihnen E, Jensen M, Brandenburg B, Tänzer B (1990) Untersuchungen zum Verhalten des 'Outputfactor' am Mevatron-74 Linearbeschleuniger, Medizinische Physik (Gemeinsame Jahrestagung Göttingen 1990), 248

Computer-Aided Photogrammetry for Precise Localization of Applicators in Brachytherapy*

R. Wehrmann and P. Kneschaurek

Introduction

In our hospital we use interstitial high dose rate brachytherapy for the treatment of recurrent tumors in the ears, nose, and throat region. To do this, the physician places hollow steel needles (length 20 cm; diameter 3 mm) percutaneously into the tumor. These needles are connected via plastic tubes to a remote-control afterloading machine (Gammamed IIi). A small ^{192}Ir source with an activity of about 370 GBq is mounted at the tip of a flexible steel wire. Using remote control, this source is first pushed through the tubes to the tip of each needle and then drawn back in a user-defined manner. It is possible to define up to 20 equidistant stopping points for each needle, and an individual dwell time for each stopping point can be chosen.

For optimized treatment planning the coordinates of the stopping points must be known in a patient-fixed system. It is sufficient to determine the position of the needles, which can be achieved by measurement of two significant points per each needle. Two video cameras, a frame grabber, and a personal computer are employed to fulfill this task using an optical method. The algorithm allows the reconstruction of the needle positions with X-ray pictures as well.

Materials and Methods

Hardware. A cube made of transparent plastic (length of edges 10 cm) is used to define the patient-fixed system of coordinates. This cube is placed at the patient close to the needles. From this arrangement, we need two images from different directions. The choice of these directions is in principle almost arbitrary. However, for reasons of numerical stability it is advantageous to use almost orthogonal directions of view. To acquire the pictures we use two video cameras connected to a personal computer based video frame grabber. The video

Institut für Strahlentherapie und Radiologische Onkologie, Technische Universität München, Klinikum rechts der Isar, Ismaninger Strasse 15, 8000 Munich 80, FRG
* This research was supported in part by Deutsche Forschungsgemeinschaft grant Br-678/6-1.

Advanced Radiation Therapy Tumor Response
Monitoring and Treatment Planning
Breit (Editor-in-Chief)
© Springer-Verlag, Berlin Heidelberg 1992

cameras (Hamamatsu C3077-01) are equipped with a high-resolution CCD-chip
with $756*581 = 439\,236$ square pixels and an almost distortion-free object lens
(Schneider Xenoplan 1.9/35 mm). The video digitizer board (Imaging Technologies VS 100) has connectors for four cameras and is able to digitize images with
$768*512$ pixels and 256 gray levels at a rate of 25 pictures per second. The frame
memory has a size of $1024*1024$ pixels and is therefore able to hold two images
at a moment. This frame grabber is hosted by a Compaq 386/20e equipped with
5 MB of RAM and a 40-MB fixed disk drive. To avoid errors induced by
movements of the patient, the pictures from both cameras are digitized to within
0.1 s.

Algorithm. We start our evaluation by marking in each picture the eight corners
of cube A–H. A mouse-driven cursor is used to do this. The same technique is
used to define every point of interest. We choose two points of interest for each
needle, the end of the needle, and the point at which the needle transverses the
skin. If we know the coordinates of these points, it is easy to calculate the
location of the needle tip and the position of the stopping points for the source.
To calculate the coordinates of a given point P, we proceed as follows (Fig. 1). In
the first image we choose four corners of the cube which form a square, for
example, A, B, C, and D. These points define a plane which we initially regard as
the object plane. Now we introduce point P′ into the object plane by requiring
that the image of P′ coincide with the picture of P. Our next step is to calculate
the coordinates of P′. The relationship between the object plane and the image
plane can be described as a projective transformation. If we use coordinates X
and Y for the object plane and x and y for the image plane, we have the following
equations [1]:

$$X = \frac{u_1{}^*x + u_2{}^*y + u_3}{w_1{}^*x + w_2{}^*y + 1}$$

$$Y = \frac{v_1{}^*x + v_2{}^*y + v_3}{w_1{}^*x + w_2{}^*y + 1} \qquad (1)$$

In these equations, the eight unknown parameters u_1, u_2, u_3, v_1, v_2, v_3, w_1,
and w_2 describe the interior and exterior orientation of the picture. The object
coordinates and the image coordinates are known for the four points A, B, C,
and D. Thus from Eq. 1 one obtains a system of eight equations with eight

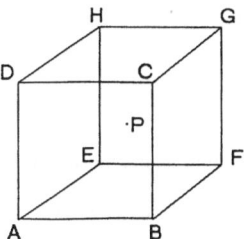

Fig. 1. Sketch of the cube and the point of interest

unknown quantities. It is possible to solve this system numerically. Then, by inserting the picture coordinates of P' (which are by definition the same as those of point P) into Eq. 1, we can calculate the object coordinates of P'. However, we have developed a special method based on ideas of Finsterwalder [2] and Rinner [3]. In the "Appendix" we demonstrate the calculation of the object coordinates of P' without any explicit calculation of the unknown parameters.

Now, in the same picture, we again choose four corners of the cube which form a square, for example, E, F, G, and H. These points define a second object plane which must not coincide with the first one. Point P" in this second object plane is defined by requiring again that this picture coincide with the picture of P. Using the algorithm described above, we calculate the object coordinates of P". According to the laws of central projection, P must be situated at some point on the straight line defined by P' and P". Now we go on to the second picture. In the same way as described above, we calculate another two points, P''' and P'''', which define another straight line. From a theoretical point of view, the object coordinates for P can now be found simply by calculating the point of intersection of the two straight lines. However, in practical calculations the two lines almost never intersect because of the limited accuracy of the input data. In this case, on each line one point is chosen in such a way that the distance between them becomes minimal. The length of the straight line between these two points gives us some information about the accuracy of the measurement, whereas the center of the line gives an approximation for P.

Conclusion

The method discussed in this paper allows a quick and accurate determination of the position of the needles relative to a patient-fixed coordinate system. With the help of skin marks the contour of the body can be determined. We are now working on the problem of how to translate the tumor volume, which is determined either by computed tomography or magnetic resonance imaging, into the patient-fixed coordinate system.

References

1. Kraus K (1986) Photogrammetrie, Vol 1. Dümmler, Bonn
2. Finsterwalder S (1899) Über die Konstruktion von Höhenkarten aus Ballonaufnahmen. Jahresb Dtsch Math Verein 6: 149
3. Rinner K (1972) Photogrammetrie. In: Jordan W, Eggert O, Kneißl M (eds) Handbuch der Vermessungskunde, Vol III a/1 Metzler'sche Verlagsbuchhandlung, Stuttgart

Appendix

Here we use uppercase letters for the object plane and lowercase letters for the image plane. For vectors we use boldface type. For the object plane, we use the X-Y coordinate system as shown in Fig. 2a. Therefore we have:

$$\mathbf{A} = (1, 0), \quad \mathbf{B} = (0, 1), \quad \mathbf{C} = (-1, 0), \quad \mathbf{D} = (0, -1). \quad (2)$$

For the image plane, we use the x-y coordinate system in such a way that the origin of the system coincides with the intersection of the diagonals of the quadrangle formed by the four image points $\mathbf{a}$, $\mathbf{b}$, $\mathbf{c}$, and $\mathbf{d}$ (Fig. 2b). Because each straight line in the object plane is transformed into a straight line in the image plane, it follows for this that the origin of the object plane is transformed into the origin of the image plane. Therefore Eq. 1 leads to $u_3 = v_3 = 0$. From Fig. 2b we obtain the relations:

$$\mathbf{a} = a^*(\cos\alpha, \sin\alpha), \quad \mathbf{b} = b^*(\cos\beta, \sin\beta),$$

$$\mathbf{c} = -c^*(\cos\alpha, \sin\alpha), \quad \mathbf{d} = -d^*(\cos\beta, \sin\beta) \quad (3)$$

Now we insert Eqs. 2 and 3 into Eq. 1. If we introduce the substitutions:

$$k_1 := u_1^*\cos\alpha + u_2^*\sin\alpha, \quad k_2 := u_1^*\cos\beta + u_2^*\sin\beta,$$

$$k_3 := v_1^*\cos\alpha + v_2^*\sin\alpha, \quad k_4 := v_1^*\cos\beta + v_2^*\sin\beta,$$

$$k_5 := w_1^*\cos\alpha + w_2^*\sin\alpha, \quad k_6 := w_1^*\cos\beta + w_2^*\sin\beta \quad (4)$$

we obtain the following equations:

$$\frac{a^*k_1}{a^*k_5+1} = \frac{b^*k_4}{b^*k_6+1} = \frac{c^*k_1}{1-c^*k_5} = \frac{d^*k_4}{1-d^*k_6} = 1$$

$$\frac{a^*k_3}{a^*k_5+1} = \frac{b^*k_2}{b^*k_6+1} = \frac{c^*k_3}{1-c^*k_5} = \frac{d^*k_2}{1-d^*k_6} = 0 \quad (5)$$

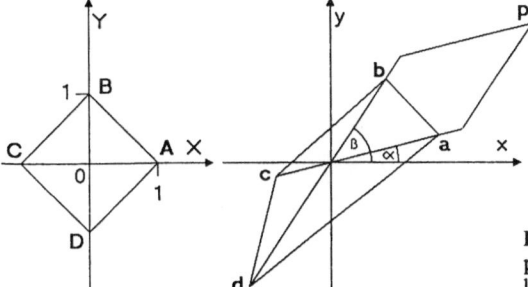

Fig. 2. Transformation of the different points from the object plane (uppercase letters) to the image plane

This system has the following solution:

$$k_1 = \frac{a+c}{2\,ac}, \qquad k_2 = 0, \qquad k_3 = 0, \qquad k_4 = \frac{b+d}{2\,bd},$$

$$k_5 = \frac{a-c}{2\,ac}, \qquad k_6 = \frac{b-d}{2\,bd} \tag{6}$$

Now we write **p** as a linear combination of **a** and **b**:

$$\mathbf{p} = m*\mathbf{a} + n*\mathbf{b} \tag{7}$$

If we insert this into Eq. 1, we can easily obtain the coordinates for point
$\mathbf{P'} = (X_{p'}, Y_{p'})$:

$$X_{p'} = \frac{u_1(m*a*\cos\alpha + n*b*\cos\beta) + u_2(m*a*\sin\alpha + n*b*\sin\beta)}{w_1(m*a*\cos\alpha + n*b*\cos\beta) + w_2(m*a*\sin\alpha + n*b*\sin\beta) + 1}$$

$$= \frac{a*m*k_1 + b*n*k_2}{a*m*k_5 + b*n*k_6 + 1}$$

$$= \frac{m*d*(a+c)}{2*c*d + m*d*(a-c) + n*c*(b-d)} \tag{8}$$

An analogous calculation for $Y_{p'}$, yields:

$$Y_{p'} = \frac{n*c*(b+d)}{2*c*d + m*d*(a-c) + n*c*(b-d)} \tag{9}$$

Treatment Planning:
Quality Assurance

Quality Assurance Tests of the ... Treatment Planning System

Introduction

The calculation of dose planning system by Hogstrom has been used in clinical routine at the University Hospital in Lund for more than a year. As originally
was one electron beam per plan. An interactive test program was created to
before the system was used in the clinic. Five different therapy machines are in
use at the University Hospitals. The beam sizes possible to have and the
consist of ... The x-ray quality available were 4, 6, 10, and 21 MV, and the
electrons available range from 4 to 21 MeV. Also, a satellite unit consisting of
therapy machines between about 20 MeV are now operational. In 6 MV and have
been subjected to tests. This paper deals with tests of the dose calculation model
for photon and electron beams.

Dose Calculation Models for Photons and Electrons in TMS Beam

The photon dose model is a pencil beam model developed for the treatment
planning system used in Chicago 1979. Ahnesjö and Saxner. The calculation
is based on know electron energy pencil-related therapy dose distributions
and on dose distributions measured in a water phantom. A pencil beam
algorithm is also used for electrons. Ahnesjö and Saxner 1991, personal
communications. The three-dimensional dose integration in this model is based
on an intentional symmetry of the pencil beam kernels. The dose to a point is
calculated by superposition, the kernel most where in turn is distributed into
several separate around the boundary from the source to the calculation point.

The Test System

The tests were computationally between dose distribution data obtained with a
small algorithm to interpret the three-dimensional matrix in the ... The other

Quality Assurance Tests of the TMS-Radix Treatment Planning System

A. Montelius, B. Jung, G. Rikner, A. Murman, and K. Russell

Introduction

The TMS-Radix treatment planning system by Helax has been used in clinical practice at the University Hospital in Uppsala for more than a year. As Uppsala was one of the two test sites for TMS, an extensive test program was undertaken before the system was used in the clinic. Five different therapy machines are in use at the University Hospital: one ^{60}Co unit, three linear accelerators, and one microtron. The X-ray qualities available are 5, 6, 8, 16, and 21 MV, and the electron energies range from 5 to 22 MeV. All X-ray qualities and a number of electron energies between 8 and 20 MeV are now implemented in TMS and have been subjected to tests. This paper deals with tests of the dose calculation models for photon and electron beams.

Dose Computation Models for Photons and Electrons in TMS-Radix

For photon dose calculations, a pencil beam model designed for three-dimensional dose planning is used (Ahnesjö 1991; Ahnesjö and Saxner, this volume). This model is based on Monte Carlo precalculated energy deposition kernels and on dose distributions measured in a water phantom. A pencil beam algorithm is also used for electrons (Ahnesjö and Saxner 1991, personal communication). The three-dimensional dose integration in this model is based on rotational symmetry of the pencil beam kernels. The dose to a point is calculated by integration over the beam area, which in turn is divided into circular segments around the ray from the source to the calculation point.

The Test System

The tests were comparisons between dose distribution data obtained with a small semiconductor detector in a three-dimensional scanner (RFA-7, Therados)

Department of Hospital Physics, University Hospital, Akademiska sjukhuset, 751 85 Uppsala, Sweden

Advanced Radiation Therapy Tumor Response
Monitoring and Treatment Planning
Breit (Editor-in-Chief)
© Springer-Verlag, Berlin Heidelberg 1992

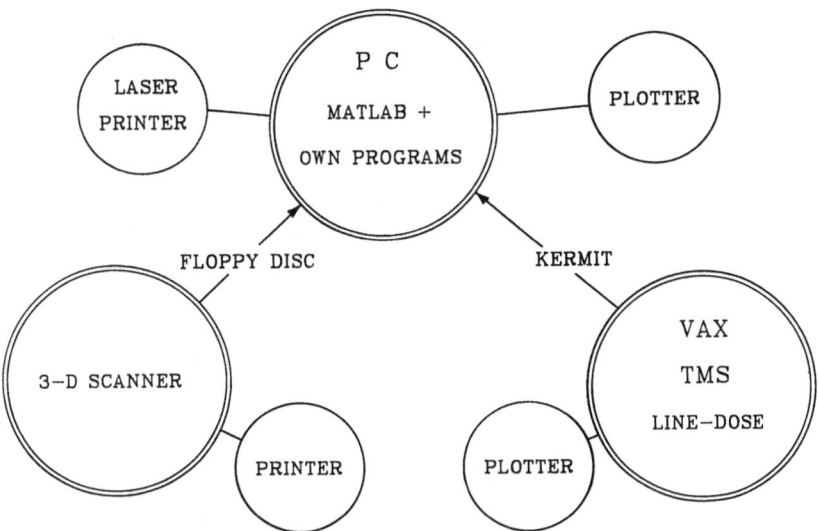

Fig. 1. Configuration of the system

and TMS-calculated dose distribution data. The line-dose routine of TMS gives the dose along a line between two arbitrarily selected points in the irradiated object. External users of the dose planning computer (in our case a Microvax II) can obtain the line-dose data as ASCII files exported from the TMS system. The three-dimensional scanner exports measured dose curves in ASCII format via floppy disc to an IBM-compatible personal computer. Also, the line-dose files are transferred from the dose-planning computer to the personal computer, here with the general transport code Kermit. In the personal computer, our own computer codes together with the program Matlab (Borland) are used to display dose curves and for quantitation of data, such as penumbra widths and maximum deviations between curves. The configuration of the test system is illustrated in Fig. 1.

Results and Discussion

Tests were made for all implemented beam qualities and energies in water phantoms and measured depth dose distributions, and dose profiles were compared to the corresponding line-doses from TMS. Tests were also made for oblique incidence, irregular phantom surfaces, and inhomogeneous phantoms containing air cavities and bone equivalent materials.

A detailed account for all tests of the different TMS versions cannot be given here; however, examples of dose distribution tests are discussed in the following.

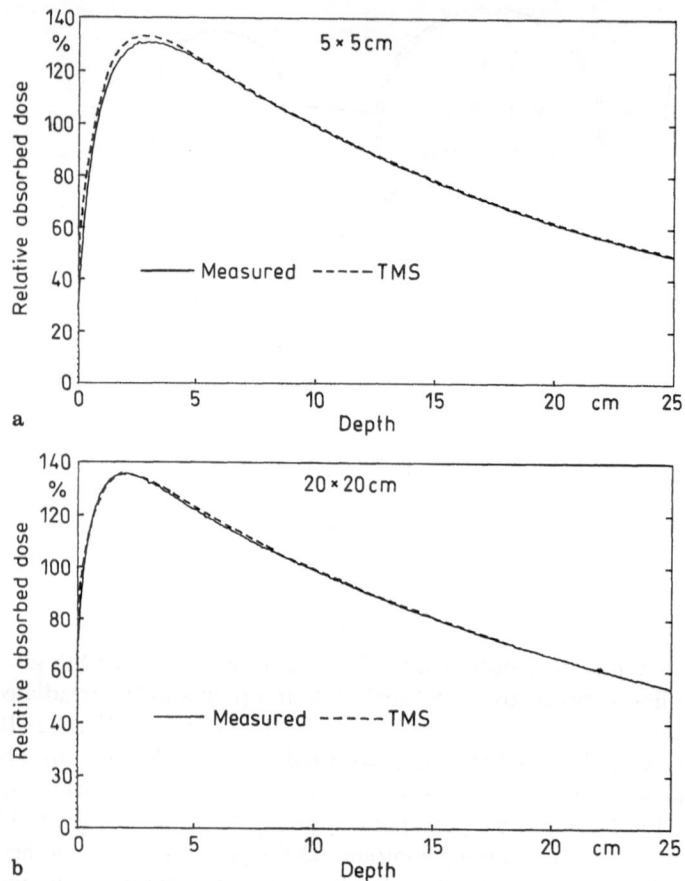

Fig. 2. Measured and TMS-calculated depth dose distributions for 21-MV X-rays for 5×5 cm² (**a**) and 20×20 cm² (**b**) fields. The source-to-phantom distance was 90 cm. All curves are normalized to 10 cm depth

Figure 2 shows measured and calculated depth dose curves from 21-MV X-rays for the field sizes 5×5 and 20×20 cm². This beam has a relatively strong contamination of electrons, especially for large field sizes. As a result of the electron contamination, the dose maximum moves toward the surface as the field size increases. Figure 2 shows that the gross effects of the electron contamination can be described with the model. For 20×20 cm² the deviations from measurements are small, but for smaller field sizes the deviations become larger. In the worst cases the deviations at dose maximum can reach 3%. For other therapy machines and X-ray qualities, with less electron contamination, the dose deviations at dose maximum are around 1% (Ahnesjö 1991). It is assumed in the model that the contaminating electrons emanate from one source, located at the position of the flattening filter. In reality, many sources contribute to the electron fluence, for example, the air volume between the

photon source and the phantom surface, the collimators, and the flattening filter
(Nilsson 1985a, b; 1985b; Nilsson and Brahme 1979). A more accurate and
detailed modeling of the contaminating electron sources might improve the
calculated dose distributions in the build-up and dose maximum regions.

A second example of a dose distribution comparison is shown in Fig. 3. Here,
a broad 20-MeV electron beam impinges on an inhomogeneous phantom. A
cross-section of the phantom is also shown in Fig. 3. It consists of a lucite block
containing a long air cavity with a rectangular cross-section. The lucite block
was placed in contact with the water surface of a tank, in which dose profiles and
depth dose curves were measured. Figure 3 shows dose profiles, both measured
and calculated, in water 5 mm below the air cavity. The strong effects on the
dose distribution caused by the difference in attenuation and scattering between
air and lucite, are well described by the pencil beam model. This encourages us
to use high-energy electrons also in inhomogeneous tissues such as in the head
and neck region.

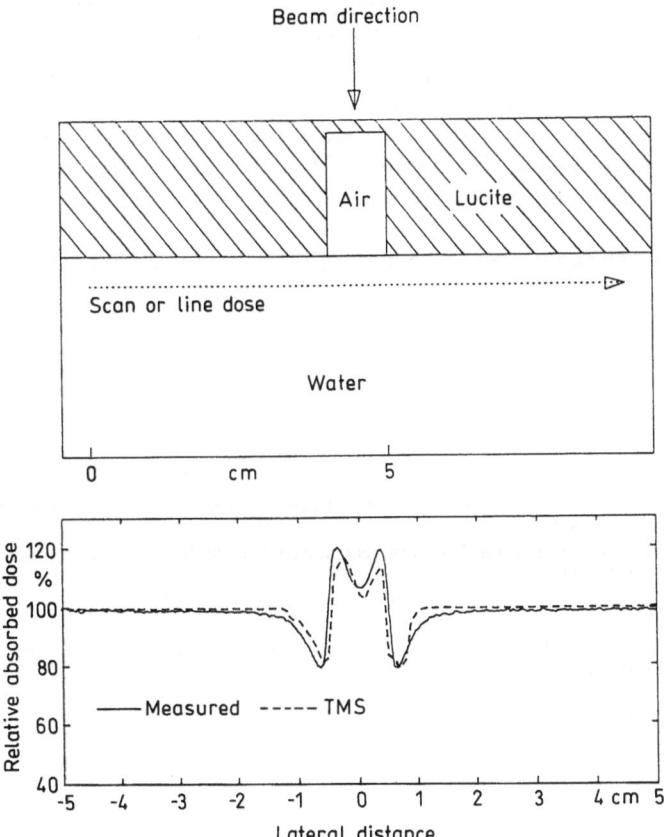

Fig. 3. Irradiation geometry along with measured and TMS-calculated dose profiles in an inhomogeneous lucite-water-air phantom

Conclusions

A treatment planning system such as TMS-Radix is constantly being developed with the implementation of new, improved dose calculation models and the introduction of new therapy machines into the system. It is important to have the necessary tools for rapid evaluation and verification of large quantities of dose distribution data. The line-dose function in the treatment planning system in combination with a three-dimensional scanner are important tools in this respect as well as computer programs for display and quantitation of dose distribution data.

It is also concluded from the results shown in Fig. 2, that it is difficult accurately to simulate the dose distribution in the build-up and dose maximum regions for X-ray beams which are contaminated by electrons. If the dose distributions calculated with the treatment planning system are normalized to the dose maximum along the central axis and if this point is used as a reference point for calibrating the monitor units for therapy machines, this may lead to an error in the tumor dose of a few percent for deep-seated tumors. This can be avoided if the reference point is chosen at a greater depth, for example, at 10 cm.

The overall experience from our tests of the dose distributions from the TMS-Radix system is that the dose calculation models satisfactorily simulate the photon and electron dose distributions. Also, the dose distributions for rather complicated inhomogeneities are well predicted by the models.

Acknowledgements. The advice on computer problems from Håkan Sjöstrand is gratefully acknowledged.

References

Ahnesjö A (1991) Dose calculation methods in photon beam therapy using energy deposition kernels. Thesis, University of Stockholm

Nilsson B (1985a) Electron contamination from different materials in high energy photon beams. Phys. Med. Biol. 30: 139–151

Nilsson B (1985b) Analysis of quality characteristics of radiotherapeutic photon beams. Thesis, University of Stockholm

Nilsson B, Brahme A (1979) Absorbed dose from secondary electrons in high energy photon beams. Phys Med Biol 24: 901–912

Verification of Radiation Therapy Plans Using Computed Tomography*

M. Gbordzoe, O. Sauer, K. Baier, and M. Herbolsheimer

Introduction

Electron beam therapy of the chest wall has acquired a permanent role as adjuvant radiotherapy in the treatment of breast cancer. As such, it has been in use in clinical routine in the Universitäts-Frauenklinik Würzburg for a number of years now [1]. An effective treatment planning takes into account, among other factors, the geometry of the chest wall, any additional regions of missing tissue which may have resulted from the preceding mastectomy, and the presence of healthy lung and heart tissue under the chest wall. Thus, the need often arises for the use of bolus material to assist in optimizing the delivery of the prescribed dose. In this regard, it is essential to design an appropriate radiation treatment verification method.

In the special situation of electron beam arc therapy of the chest wall, the treatment verification methods currently in use in clinical routine — involving simulators, portal radiography with therapy films, and portal verification methods employing solid-state detectors or ionization chambers in conjunction with digital imaging systems [2, 3] — cannot be easily applied. In this special situation computed tomography (CT) can be used as a verification method in addition to any direct dose measurements which may be performed on the patient.

Materials and Methods

The radiation treatment planning is based on the use of CT slices. The CT slices of the patient's chest wall are made with a Philips Tomoscan 300, in scanning distances of about 35 mm with a slice thickness of 12 mm. Usually five slices over the region of interest are made for the postmastectomy radiotherapy plan. The radiation treatment plan (RTP) is calculated using Philips Oncology Support System, which allows the generation of three-dimensional patient models.

Strahlenabteilung, Universitäts-Frauenklinik, Josef-Schneider-Str. 4, 8700 Würzburg, FRG
* This research was supported by Deutsche Forschungsgemeinschaft grant RO-795/1-1.

Advanced Radiation Therapy Tumor Response
Monitoring and Treatment Planning
Breit (Editor-in-Chief)
© Springer-Verlag, Berlin Heidelberg 1992

The therapy unit is a Philips linear accelerator model SL75/14 with six electron energies, ranging from 4 to 14 MeV in steps of 2 MeV, available. The technique applied for almost all chest wall treatment plans is arc therapy. A focus to isocenter distance of 100 cm and an applicator with an exit field dimension of 15 cm × 5 cm are used in all cases. Collimation is 75 cm.

In cases in which dents — resulting usually from mastectomy — are present in the chest wall, the effect of missing tissue or tissue inhomogeneity in that area on dose distribution can be significant. A considerable amount of radiation can penetrate into the underlying healthy lung tissue. Selecting an electron beam with a lower energy for the arc segment in question does not necessarily lead to a better overall dose distribution. In such cases, boluses (moulage) made from beeswax have been employed to compensate for missing tissue. In a few cases of patients with very thin chest walls, it has been found necessary, in addition to using electron beams with the lowest energies available to cover the whole chest wall with a bolus. In such a case, the bolus material Superflap with the appropriate thickness is employed.

Patient positioning on the couch of the linear accelerator is in accordance with the CT-based treatment plan. This involves, among other things, fixing the source-to-skin distance, drawing a reference line parallel to the sternum, and marking the horizontal and vertical isocenter positions as well as the start and stop gantry angles of the individual electron beam segments in the central plane — and any other planes of interest — on the patient. The horizontal isocenter corresponds to the depth of the axis inside the patient while the vertical isocenter defines the horizontal displacement of the isocenter from the reference line.

CT slices are made for a treatment verification plan (TVP) with the markings on the patient as at the first delivery of radiation therapy. Thin copper wires of 1 mm diameter are used to indicate the markings. Normally two slices, one of which must be identical with the RTP central slice, are required for calculating a TVP. When boluses are used, slices covering the bolus domain and the adjacent slices below and above are needed.

Comparison between an RTP and its TVP is carried out with respect to reproducibility of isodoses, dose homogeneity, monitor units, horizontal and vertical isocenter positions (respectively, the surface-to-axis distance and the horizontal displacement of the axis from the reference line), and the angular positions of the individual beams. Where bolus material has been used, comparison is made to ascertain the effectiveness, or otherwise, of the bolus, its influence on the dose distribution, and the correctness of its positioning.

Results

Figure 1 shows a CT slice made for calculating a TVP. It represents the case of a patient who had a mammary carcinoma of the right breast in stage pT4pN2M0 after mastectomy. The markings can be seen as extended points on the patient

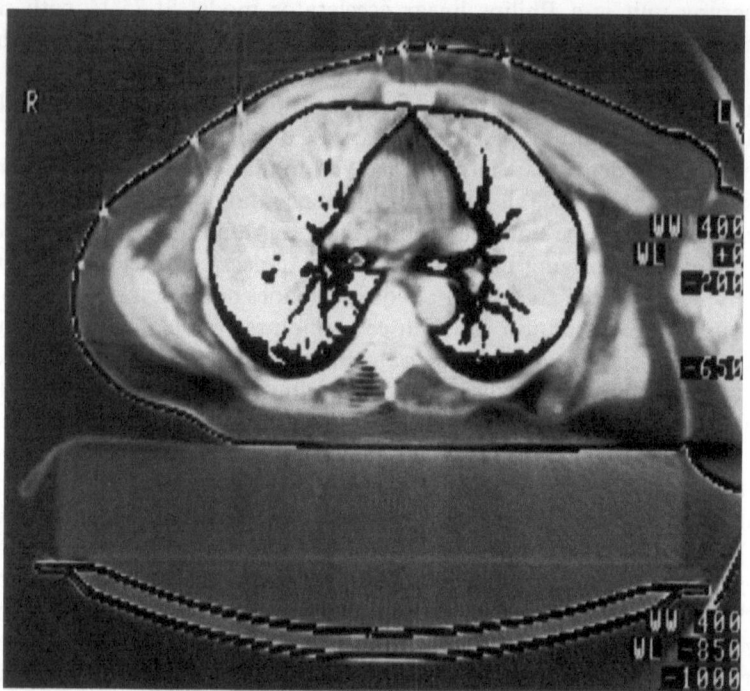

Fig. 1. A computer tomography slice for a verification plan

outline (external contour). The first point on the right of the patient at 90° to the focus-axis direction indicates the horizontal isocenter position. The seven points which can be seen at angles of 280°, 290°, 310°, 320°, 350°, 355°, and 15° mark the start and stop gantry angles of the six electron beams used for the arc therapy. The point at 0° denotes the vertical isocenter and the reference line positions; the two coincide in this example.

Figure 2 shows the central slice of an RTP. In Fig. 2a, the changing thickness of the chest wall with a very thin section can be seen. Figure 2b shows the dose distribution indicating the penetration of unwarranted radiation into the healthy lung tissue where no bolus was administered.

Figure 3 represents the slices of a verification plan corresponding to the RTP of Fig. 2 with a bolus made from beeswax used to compensate for missing tissue. The extension of the bolus is indicated by crosses in Fig. 3. This figure also shows a very good coincidence of the beams of the verification plan with the expected positions given by the markings of the original RTP (the angle between IH and IV is 90.6° compared with the expected 90°, which is well within acceptable limits). In Fig. 3B, it is evident that the use of the bolus has successfully prevented the penetration of radiation into the lung.

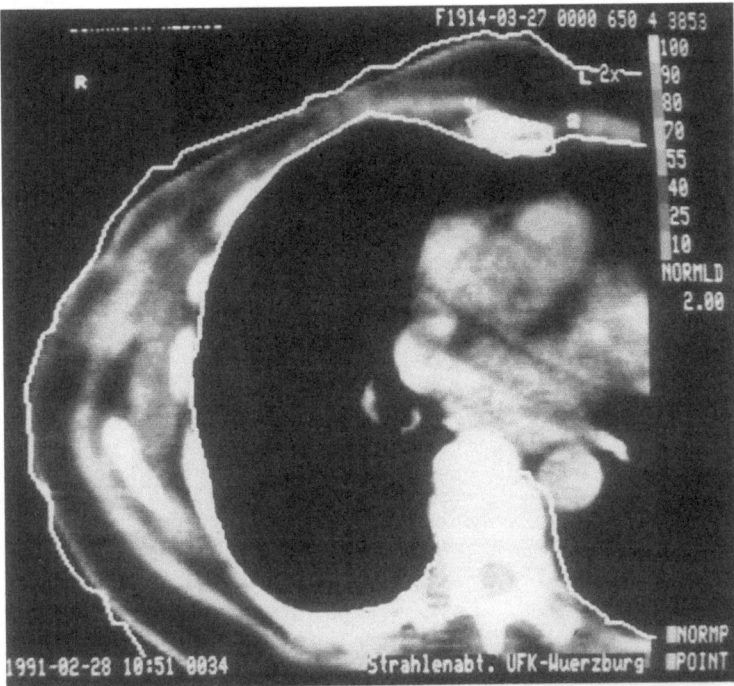

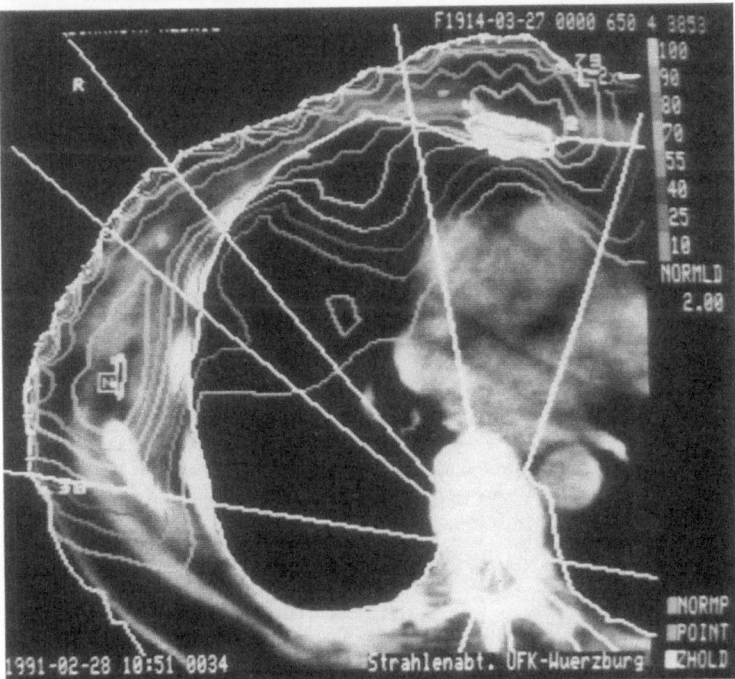

Fig. 2a, b. Central slice for a radiation therapy plan. **a** Changes in the thickness of the chest wall.
b Penetration of radiation into healthy lung tissue

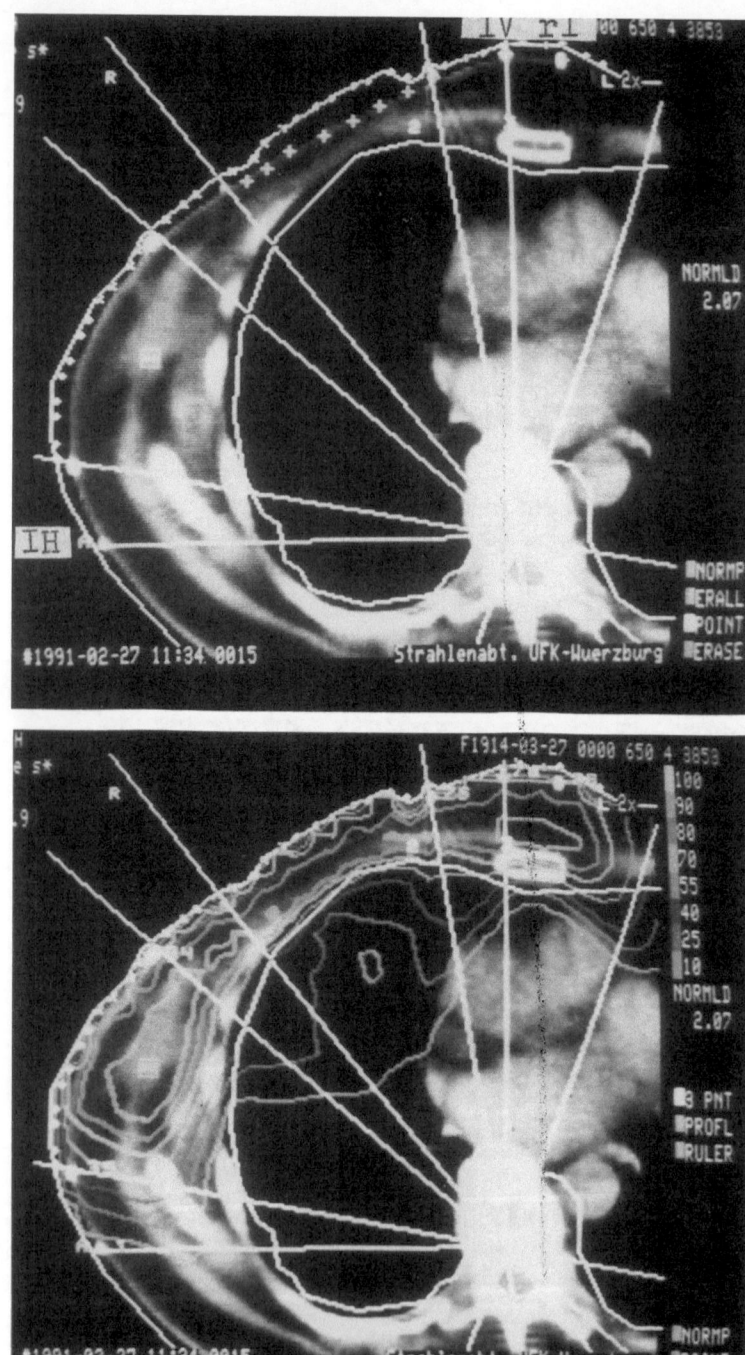

Fig. 3a, b. Central slice of a verification plan for the therapy plan of Fig. 2. **a** Demonstration of the use of bolus material. **b** Removal of undesirable radiation from the lung. *IV rl*, Vertical isocenter reference line

Discussion

A total of forty patient cases was selected for analysis. In nine of these, bolus material was used to compensate for missing tissue. The implementation of a treatment plan was accepted when the TVP satisfied the following conditions: (a) the monitor units for the same electron beam did not differ by more than $\pm 5\%$; (b) the difference between prescribed and actual angles was less than $2°$; and (c) variation in the surface-to-axis distance and in the vertical isocenter position on the patient did not exceed 0.5 cm. In 73% of the cases analyzed, these conditions were fulfilled. In 15% of all cases a bolus had to be modified. In 12% of cases, there was the need to check patient positioning for possible corrections, and, if necessary, for further verification plans to be calculated. In several exceptional cases characterized by unusual difficult patient positioning due, for example, to patient obesity, differences of up to $4°$ in angular positions occurred. The usefulness of the method is limited by the accuracy with which the patient can be positioned on the couch for CT and at the linear accelerator.

Conclusion

In addition to direct dose measurements on the patient, CT offers an adequate facility for verifying the degree of accuracy with which CT-based radiation treatment plans are implemented in the postmastectomy irradiation of the chest wall.

References

1. Löffler E (1984) Multisegmentale postoperative Bewegungsbestrahlung der Thoraxwand mit schnellen Elektronen. In: Schmidt T (ed) Medizinische Physik. Deutsche Gesellschaft für Medizinische Physik, pp 435–444
2. Van Herk M, Meertens H (1987) A digital imaging system for portal verification. In: Bruinvis IAD, van der Giessen PH, van Kleffens HJ, Wittkämper FW (eds) The use of computers in radiation therapy. North-Holland, Amsterdam, pp 371–373
3. Morton EJ, Swindell W (1987) A digital system for the production of radiotherapy verification images. In: Bruinvis IAD, van der Giessen PH, van Kleffens HJ, Wittkämper FW (eds) The use of computers in radiation therapy. North-Holland, Amsterdam, pp 375–377

Comparative Measurements of Homogeneity and Dose Distribution Cobalt-60 and 9-MeV X-Ray Beams in the Mamma and the Chest Wall

E. Standke and U. Jahn

Introduction

In radiotherapeutic practice the homogeneity of the dose distribution has an important influence on the tumor killing rate. After mastectomy or conservative operation in patients with breast cancer, irradiation of the mamma and thoracic wall requires substantial attention to treatment planning due to varying topographic features in the thoracic area. Problems concerning dose distribution and homogeneity often result from an uneven course of the body surface or a different volume of the mamma after lumpectomy or quadrantectomy. This leads to a number of questions, for example: What radiation quality should be used in irradiation of the chest wall? Is there a change in the build-up effect upon altering the angle of incidence? While there are no physical problems in depth dose distribution when administering a vertical beam to the body surface, clinical experience shows that the build-up effect does not seem to be that expected from tangential rotation or opposed field techniques for mammary or chest wall tumors. In general, this margin effect is not a consideration in radiation treatment planning systems. We therefore attempted to find a qualitative scale for isodoses of cobalt-60 and 9-MeV X-rays in patients with tumors near the body surface and to draft practical guidelines for clinical routine, especially for linear accelerators, in this energy range.

Material and Method

Measurements were initially performed in a rectangular water phantom with a wall thickness under 1 mm and using an automatical semiconductor probe. We registered the course of the depth dose curve and the change in dose maximum upon altering the incidence angle between 0° and 85°, measured in steps of 10° and at increasing distance to the phantom wall at a field size of 4×15 cm and source-to-skin distance (SSD) of 97 cm.

Department of Radiotherapy, Central Institute for Cancer Research, Lindenberger Weg 80, 1115 Berlin-Buch, FRG

Advanced Radiation Therapy Tumor Response
Monitoring and Treatment Planning
Breit (Editor-in-Chief)
© Springer-Verlag, Berlin Heidelberg 1992

The goal of our investigations was to describe the dependence of the build-up effect on beam incidence. The field width of only 4 cm was selected to avoid interference in the measurements from the phantom corners. If the thoracic wall and mammary organ had a vaulted surface, we continued the measurements with a cylindrically shaped water phantom of plastic glass with a wall thickness of 0.5 mm and a diameter of 20 cm and the same semiconductor probe. The investigations were conducted using cobalt-60 energy of 1.2 MeV (field size 10 * 15 cm, SSD 76 cm) and photon energy of 9 MeV delivered by the linear accelerator Neptun 10p with the same field size. We determined the depth dose curves for these energy levels in vertical and tangential beam directions and at different distances to the phantom surface.

Results

At a photon energy of 9 MeV the measured depth dose curve had the expected course at vertical incidence in the rectangular phantom. However, a relative surface dose of about 45% was registered immediately behind the phantom wall, and this value increased with depth, reaching a maximum at 20 mm. Altering the incidence angle each 10° caused a further increase in the relative surface dose with higher angles and a shifting of the dose maximum near the surface. We observed a relative surface dose of about 65% at an incidence angle of 60° and a

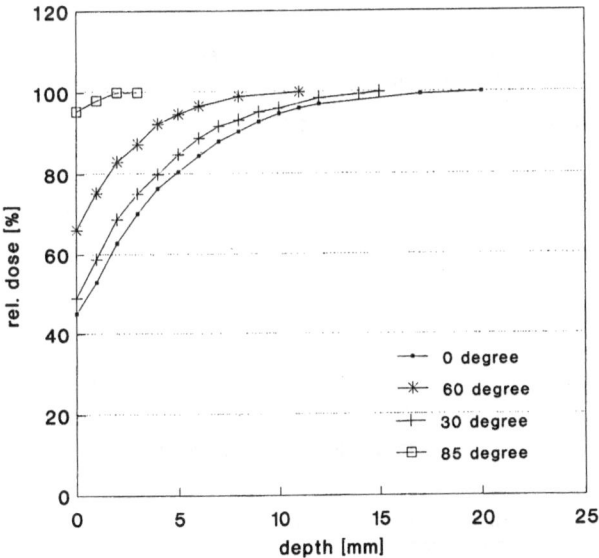

Fig. 1. Build-up effect according to beam incidence

dose maximum at a depth of 12 mm. With quasihorizontal incidence at an angle of 85° only small differences were observed in the dose distribution. The relative surface dose was 95%, and the dose maximum was at a depth of about 2 mm. The relationship between the shift in the build-up effect near the surface and the direction of incidence is presented in Fig. 1; the increase in relative surface dose varied from about 45% at vertical to 95% at tangential beam direction. A typical depth dose curve was found for cobalt-60 radiation in the cylindrically shaped phantom with a dose maximum of 0.5 cm and followed by a slow decrease in dose. With tangential beam incidence the build-up effect was not confirmed, and the decrease in dose was less steep than in the vertical direction (Fig. 2).

At a photon energy of 9 MeV the observed depth dose curve (Fig. 3) was similar to the curve in the rectangular phantom. The relative surface dose was only about 38%, and the dose maximum varied in a range of 15–20 mm. At horizontal beam incidence the relative surface dose had a value of 80% and a dose maximum at a depth between 5 and 8 mm.

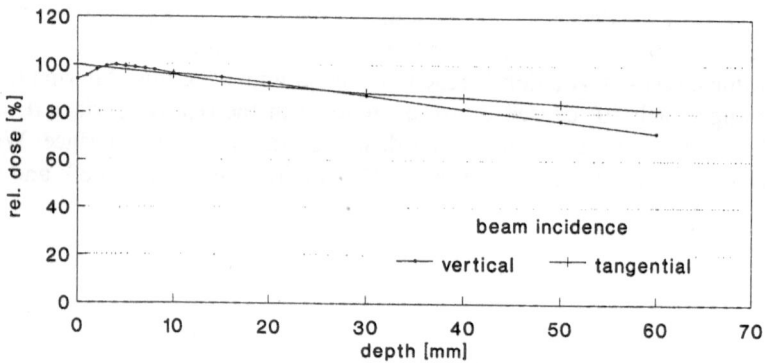

Fig. 2. Depth dose in a cylindrical phantom. Cobalt-60, 1.2 MeV

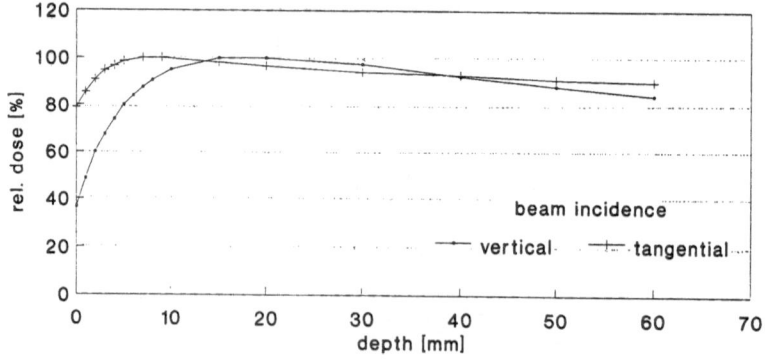

Fig. 3. Depth dose in a cylindrical phantom. Photon energy, 9 MeV

Discussion

The postoperative irradiation of the thoracic wall after mastectomy or of the mamma after lumpectomy or quadrantectomy with axillary lymph node dissection in patients with breast cancer requires a total dose of 50 Gy in single doses of 1.8–2.0 Gy five times per week. A problem in this is the homogeneous dose distribution because of the irregularly shaped thoracic wall and the varying thickness of the mammary organ. Therefore we used a tangential pendulum technique with cobalt-60 energy and changing incidence angle to the chest wall. In most cases a satisfactory dose distribution was reached. In our phantom measurements we established only a small difference between the depth dose curves with vertical versus tangential radiation incidence (Fig. 2). However, our question was: Can a photon energy of 9 MeV delivered by a linear accelerator for a tangential or an opposed-field technique be used in view of its unfavorable build-up effect? The investigations with a rectangular phantom showed an increase in the relative surface dose from 45% (at 0°) to 95% (at 85°) depending on the beam incidence angle. Simultaneously the dose maximum shifted from the depth to surface at increasing tangential beam incidence and was situated at a depth of only 2 mm with the quasi-tangential beam direction. Similar effects were observed in a cylindrically shaped phantom. Therefore we conclude that the actual dose distribution in the mamma and thoracic wall is better than the dose distribution calculated by radiation planning systems. In addition, we also considered the breathing course of the patients, which contributes to dose homogeneity.

Summary

Initial measurements of the dose distribution in mamma and thoracic wall were performed with a rectangular water phantom and later continued using a cylindrically shaped phantom; irradiation was with cobalt-60 and 9 MeV delivered from a linear accelerator. With cobalt-60 energy we detected only small differences in the depth dose curves of vertical and tangential radiation incidence, but the 9-MeV photon energy showed a shifting of the dose maximum from the depth to the surface with increasing tangential beam incidence.

Measurement of Electron Beam Dose Distributions Using Ferrous Sulfate Gels and Magnetic Resonance Imaging*

J.D. Hazle, L. Hefner, W. Baker, V.A. Otte, and A.L. Boyer

Introduction

The clinical implementation of complex radiotherapy dose delivery techniques necessitates the development of proportionally powerful dose computation models. Traditional techniques (i.e., ion chambers, thermoluminescence dosimetry, radiographic film) used to measure single-field electron beam dose distributions are not capable of obtaining integral, multiple-field dose distributions over large volumes with high spatial resolution in a reasonable time frame. It is therefore necessary to explore new dosimetry techniques to measure these multiple-field three-dimensional doses. Imaging methods are believed to be capable of addressing this problem, once a suitable dosimeter system is developed.

Aqueous ferrous sulfate systems (Fricke and Hart 1966) were first used to evaluate the radiolytic conversion of Fe^{2+} to Fe^{3+} using nuclear magnetic resonance (NMR) by Gore et al. (1984). It has since been shown that the iron atoms can be "trapped" in organic gel matrices, permitting the determination of spatial dose distributions (Appleby et al. 1987). A number of semisolid systems have been characterized and appear to be potentially useful for measuring these distributions (Olsson et al. 1989, 1990; Schulz et al. 1990; Hazle et al. 1991). The steps necessary to implement a ferrous sulfate magnetic resonance imaging (FeMRI) system for measuring absorbed dose distributions include choosing a semisolid material for immobilizing the iron centers (gelatin or agarose), determining the dose-response characteristics, optimizing the NMR data acquisition parameters, verifying the results for single fields, and building more complex phantoms for determining three-dimensional dose distributions. The dose-response characteristics of the system used to measure electron beam depth dose have been described elsewhere (Hazle et al. 1991). Electron beam depth dose curves were determined using region-of-interest (ROI) type measurements, and single-field electron beam "dose images" were calculated on a pixel-by-pixel basis.

Departments of Radiation Physics and Diagnostic Radiology, The University of Texas M.D. Anderson Cancer Center, 1515 Holcombe Blvd., Box 235, Houston, TX 77030, USA
* This research was supported in part by PHS grant CA 43840 awarded by the National Cancer Institute, United States Department of Health and Human Services.

Materials and Methods

Gels were generally prepared following Olsson et al. (1989) using 5% gelatin and inorganic components including 0.1–2.0 mM FeSO$_4$, 1 mM sodium chloride, and 0.05 M sulfuric acid. After the gelatin had been allowed to melt completely at 55°C, heating was discontinued, and the solution containing the inorganic components was added. The gel was then allowed to cool with continual mixing for about 60 min, poured into appropriate containers for either dose response or electron beam profile measurements, and then cooled overnight at room temperature.

NMR experiments were carried out on a 1.5-T whole-body scanner (Signa, General Electric Medical Systems, Waukesha, WI). R_1 relaxation rates were calculated from as many as seven images of the same location acquired with different repetition times (TR). Typical repetition times were 150, 300, 600, 1000, 1500, 3000, and 5000 ms. T1 was calculated using a three-parameter fit of the saturation recovery data. Input pixel intensity values for the R_1 calculation were obtained using either the standard Signa ROI software or by an iterative technique carried out on a Sun workstation for generating dose images.

For dose response measurements, tubes containing FeMRI gel were exposed in a ^{137}Cs irradiator (3975 cGy/min). Electron beam irradiations were carried out on a Clinac 2100C (Varian Associates, Palo Alto, CA). Approximately 21 volumes of the gel were irradiated at 100 cm source-to-skin distance to a maximum dose of approximately 45 Gy and immediately imaged to reduce diffusion effects.

Results

The dose-response characteristics of the gel system used for these electron dose profiles have been shown to be approximately linear in the range of 0–50 Gy (Hazle et al. 1991). The slope of the dose response curve for the gelatin system was found to be approximately constant (0.0425 s^{-1} Gy^{-1}) at concentrations greater than 0.2 mM. Because the slope of the dose response curve is constant at concentrations above 0.2 mM, and only the initial or zero-dose relaxation time is affected by increasing ferrous sulfate concentrations, gel preparation is not critical, nor likely to introduce appreciable uncertainties into the dose calculations.

Depth dose distributions for 6–20 MeV electron beams were measured using the FeMRI system. All FeMRI depth dose curves were in good agreement with ion chamber data at depths greater than d_{max}. Depth dose data from ROI calculations (approximately 5 × 5 × 7 mm) from FeMRI data and ion chamber measurements of a 12-MeV electron beam are shown in Fig. 1. There remains a

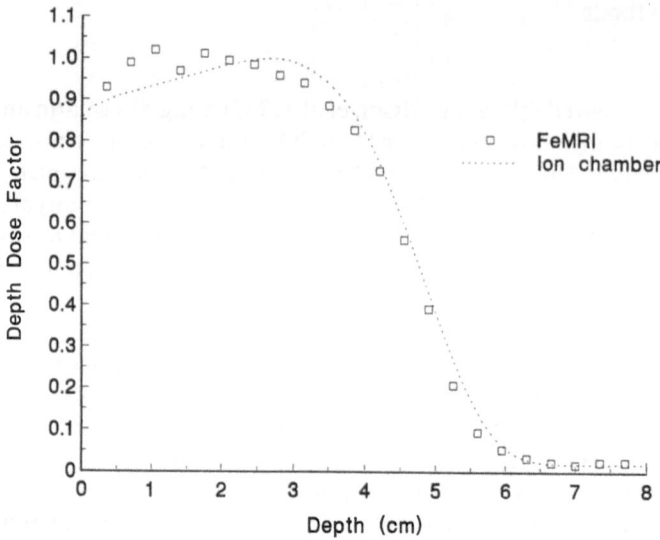

Fig. 1. FeMRI and ionization chamber depth dose measurements for a 12-MeV electron beam. The FeMRI data points are from ROI relaxation rate determinations and result from a volume approximately $1.5 \times 1.5 \times 7$ mm

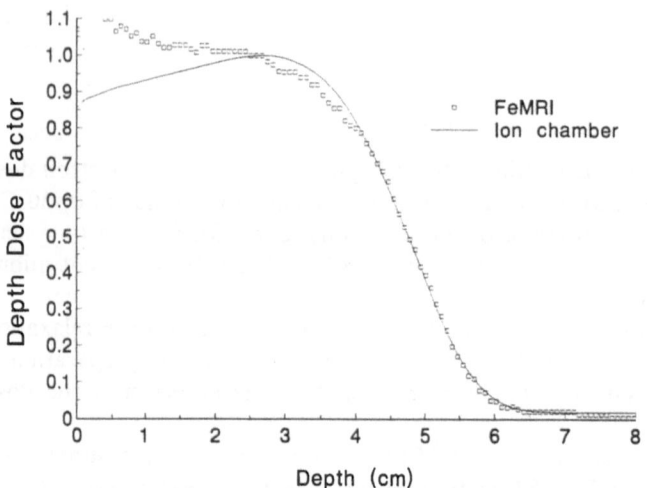

Fig. 2. FeMRI-derived depth dose plot for a 12-MeV electron beam. The curve was obtained by calculating a dose image pixel-by-pixel from several multislice images processed on a Sun workstation. The depth dose plot was generated by considering this image a "virtual phantom" and averaging over an approximately 0.3 cm^3 volume

yet unresolved discrepancy in the build-up region. FeMRI dose images were generated, and the depth dose plot of the 12 MeV electron beam obtained by averaging over a volume comparable to a 0.1 cm^3 chamber is shown in Fig. 2.

Conclusions

The FeMRI system used for these dose profiles was determined to have a sensitivity of $0.0425 \, s^{-1} \, Gy^{-1}$, which appears adequate for determining radiation absorbed doses with an accuracy of 5% in the range of 10–50 Gy (Hazle et al. 1991). Improvements in dosimeter sensitivity or in relaxation time approximation could further refine the system's ability accurately to measure radiation absorbed dose and would increase the usefulness in determining three-dimensional absorbed dose distributions, particularly in regions of high spatial dose gradients. In the case of high dose gradients, the lack of sensitivity of this method may be compensated for by its significantly better spatial resolution and three-dimensional properties.

References

Appleby A, Christman EA, Leghrouz A (1987) Imaging of spatial radiation dose distribution in agarose gels using magnetic resonance. Med Phys 14: 382–384.

Fricke H, Hart EJ (1966) Radiation dosimetry. In: Attix FH, Roesch WC (eds) Academic, New York

Gore J, Kang YS, Schulz RJ (1984) Measurement of radiation dose distributions by nuclear magnetic resonance (NMR) imaging. Phys Med Biol 29: 1189–1197

Hazle JD, Hefner LF, Wilson L, Boyer AL (1991) Dose response characteristics of a ferrous sulfate doped gelatin system for determining radiation absorbed dose distributions by magnetic resonance imaging (FeMRI). Phys Med Biol 36: 1117–1125

Olsson LE, Petersson S, Ahlgren L, Mattson S (1989) Ferrous sulfate gels for date of absorbed dose determination using MRI technique: basic studies. Phys Med Biol 34: 43–52

Olsson LE, Fransson A, Ericsson A, Mattsson S (1990) MR imaging of absorbed dose distributions for radiotherapy using ferrous sulfate gels. Phys Med Biol 35: 1623–1632

Schulz RJ, deGuzman AF, Nguyen DB, Gore JC (1990) Dose-response curves for Fricke-infused gels as obtained by nuclear magnetic resonance. Phys Med Biol 35: 1611–1622

Correlation Between the Dose Calculated from Plan and the Dose Measured with Thermoluminescence Dosimetry in Radiotherapy

T. Kron, M. Schneider, and C. Amies

Introduction

The Department of Radiation Oncology of the Prince of Wales Hospital in Sydney is one of the major centres for radiotherapy in Australia. About 1600 patients are treated per year using four linear accelerators (Varian Clinac 4, Clinac 6, Clinac 10/18 and Clinac 1800), one superficial (Philips RT100) and one orthovoltage unit (Siemens Stabilipan). In addition to portal imaging for the check of patient positioning, thermoluminescence dosimeters (TLDs) are used in order to verify the treatment. The planning radiographers request TLD measurements to be done on approximately 100 patients per year. In their treatments about 200 TLD measurements are performed per year. This is the highest number of direct dose monitoring on patients in Australasia (Fox 1990).

The aim of this retrospective study was to identify the cases where TLD results were not in agreement with the dose expected from the treatment plan, and to determine the reasons for the discrepancies. This should lead to an improved TLD service, and it should help to recognise critical steps in the treatment planning procedure and find strategies to avoid such errors in the future.

Methods

Treatment planning is performed on a GE RT/Plan planning computer (version 3.32). It has a computed tomography (CT) option. CT scans are used for planning in about 30% of the patients. The system utilises two-dimensional algorithms for X-ray (Milan and Bentley 1974) and electron (Hogstrom et al. 1981) isodose calculations. Two methods of inhomogeneity corrections can be used for X-rays: (a) an equivalent path length correction and (b) a power law correction. For beam blocking a first-order correction is performed. For electron dose calculations fast and full scatter (two dimensional) correction

Prince of Wales Hospital, Department of Radiation Oncology, Cnr. High/Avoca Streets, Randwick NSW 2031, Australia

Advanced Radiation Therapy Tumor Response
Monitoring and Treatment Planning
Breit (Editor-in-Chief)
© Springer-Verlag, Berlin Heidelberg 1992

methods are available. An algorithm based on the work of Cunningham et al. (1972) is used for irregular field dose calculations.

TLD measurements were performed with Harshaw TLD100 LiF ribbons ($3.1 \times 3.1 \times 0.9$ mm^3). They were read in a manual TLD reader (Harshaw 2000A/2000B). Using two to four chips per measuring point and two standards irradiated immediately after the patient treatment, an accuracy of $\pm 5\%$ is obtained on a 95% confidence level. TLD measurements are done on patients (a) to determine the dose in difficult geometries or set-ups (e.g. head and neck), (b) to record the dose to critical organs (e.g. lens, scrotum) and (c) to monitor special treatments (e.g. total body irradiation, total skin electron rotation treatments). A more detailed description of the TLD measurements is given elsewhere (Kron et al. 1990).

TLD reports, patient treatment sheets and plans for the past 5 years (1986–1990) were investigated. The correlation between measured dose and the dose calculated and expected from the treatment plan was regarded as satisfactory if there was less than 10% difference between them. A difference greater than 10% for any measuring point qualified as a discrepancy. Cases were not included if the difference between measured and expected dose was smaller than 10 cGy, since many TLD measurements were aimed at determining the relatively small dose to shielded organs. A 10% difference in dose in these measurements is not of clinical significance. All discrepancies were divided into three groups:

1. Discrepancies due to errors made in the TLD determination or evaluation, such as misplacement of the chips or the use of the wrong standards.
2. Discrepancies due to mistakes made during the treatment set-up, such as wrong or insufficient shielding or bolus used and/or inadequate patient immobilisation.
3. Discrepancies due to the treatment planning and dose calculation procedure (discussed later in more detail).

The allocation of a case to more than one category was allowed.

Results

Table 1 lists the number of patients investigated with TLDs in the past 5 years (1986–1990). Also, the total number of TLD measurements which can be more than one per patient, is given. The table distinguishes between X-ray and electron treatments and compares the number of TLD measurements to the total number of treatments performed per year. About 60% of the patients had only one TLD measurement.

If there was a discrepancy between the measured and the expected dose, the TLD measurement was repeated. In cases where the discrepancy still persisted,

Table 1. Thermoluminescence dosimetry in the Prince of Wales Hospital between 1986 and 1990

	X-rays	Electrons	Total
Number of patients with TLDs	332	93	417
Number of TLD measurements	586	318	904
Number of treatments per year	23 000	5000	28 000
Percent of treatments with TLDs	0.5%	1.3%	0.7%

Table 2. Discrepancies between expected and measured dose between 1986 and 1990

	X-rays	Electrons	Total
Discrepancy due to TLD measurement	12	5	17 (18%)
Discrepancy due to treatment set up	14	15	29 (30%)
Discrepancy due to treatment planning	14	25	39 (41%)
Unclear reason for discrepancy	9	2	11 (11%)

the treatment plan and/or set-up was reviewed and changed. The TLD measurement was then repeated again. This practice and special treatments, such as total body irradiations, which were monitored with TLDs at each treatment day resulted in an average of more than two TLD measurements per patient.

For 79 patients (19% of all investigated ones) there was no satisfactory correlation between measured and expected dose. Nearly half of them (34) were treated with electrons. Table 2 shows the reasons for these discrepancies and lists the number of cases for the 5 years between 1986 and 1990. In Table 2 the allocation of a case to more than one category is possible. In 10% of cases, no allocation to one of the categories was possible using this retrospective analysis. In addition to problems arising from the TLD measurement itself and the patient set-up, nearly one-half of the discrepancies were caused by inadequate planning procedures. In particular, the following problem areas were identified:

- Small or irregularly shaped electron fields (8 cases); especially when treated in extended focus-to-skin distance or on curved surfaces.
- Oblique incidence of electrons (7 cases); in most of these cases the full scatter correction was not performed, and so hot spots were not revealed.
- Non-standard shielding (5 cases); e.g. small lens shield.
- Difficult patient geometries (11 cases); most problems of this category could have been avoided if a three-dimensional planning system had been used. Typical examples are: scatter from the third dimension was ignored, or the critical organ was not in the calculation plane.
- Others (8 cases).

Discussion and Conclusion

Even though only one in six treatments is performed with electrons, more than one-third of all TLD measurements were made in electron fields. This indicates the usefulness of TLDs as a surface/skin dosimeter, as well as a lack of confidence in electron treatment planning. This is reflected in Table 2 showing that 64% of all planning-related discrepancies occurred in electron fields. Also, the list of critical areas for planning reveals more uncertainties for electron treatment planning.

In most of the studied cases assessment of the delivered dose in vivo with TLDs proved to be a valuable verification of the patients treatment. In addition to the revelation of treatment errors, it can help to avoid mistakes in similar cases. The recognition of TLDs as a useful clinical verification tool is reflected in an increasing number of TLD requests in the Prince of Wales Hospital (Kron et al. 1990). Accordingly, the TLD reader has been upgraded recently to a automated system.

Since some of the detected discrepancies are a result of limitations of a two-dimensional planning system, we are also looking forward to purchasing a three-dimensional planning computer in the future. Both investments should help to improve patient radiotherapy treatment in the future.

References

Cunningham JR, Shrivastava PN, Wilkinson JM (1972) Program IRREG — calculation of dose from irregularly shaped radiation beams. Comput Programs Biomed 2: 192
Fox RA (1990) A survey of therapy physics workload in Australasia. Aust Eng Phys Sci Med 13: 42–44
Hogstrom KR, Mills MD, Almond PR (1981) Electron beam dose calculations. Phys Med Biol 26: 445–459
Kron T, Schmiedeberg D, Schneider M, Oliver L (1990) Thermoluminescence dosimetry in the Prince of Wales Hospital, Sydney. Aust Eng Phys Sci Med 13: 192–196
Milan J, Bentley RE (1974) Storage and manipulation of radiation dose data in a small digital computer. Br J Radiol 47: 115–121

Treatment Planning:
Display and Evaluation

Visualization of Treatment Plans Using Three-Dimensional Magnetic Resonance Imaging Data Sets*

C. Prüll[3], H. Kett[1], K. Pfändner[2], P. Held[1], and A. Breit[1]

Introduction

The optimization of physical treatment planning requires the deposition of an adequate homogeneous dose to the target volume while minimizing the dose distribution to the surrounding healthy tissue and critical organs. The complete three-dimensional anatomical information is necessary for the evaluation of the target volume as well as for the definition and control of the treatment plan.

Advantages of Three-Dimensional MRI in Radiation Therapy Planning

Because of the high soft-tissue contrast in magnetic resonance imaging (MRI), tumor and surrounding structures can be differentiated very well. This contrast can generally be enhanced even using the paramagnetic contrast agent Gd-DTPA. The three-dimensional technique allows acquisition of the whole volume of interest with high spatial resolution within a single data set. Voxel sizes of $1 \times 1 \times 1.5$ mm^3 or $1 \times 1 \times 1$ mm^3 are possible for the complete imaging of the head or neck. Depending on the spatial resolution and the repetition time (TR), the measurement time for a three-dimensional data set consisting of 128 partitions is between 10 and 20 min. Starting with a three-dimensional data set, slices with arbitrary position and orientation can be reconstructed.

Problems and Possible Solutions

Due to inhomogeneities of the external magnetic field or non-linearities of the magnetic field gradients, MR images are geometrically distorted. A complicated

[1] Institut für MR-Tomographie, Klinikum Passau, Leonhard-Paminger Str. 1, W-8390 Passau, FRG
[2] Klinikum Passau, Bischof-Piligrim Str. 1, 8390 Passau FRG
[3] Klinikum Regensburg, Institut für Röntgendiagnostik, Franz-Joseph-Strauß-Allee 11, 8400 Regensburg, FRG
* This research was supported in part by the German Bundesminister für Forschung und Technologie, grant 01 VF 8708.

Advanced Radiation Therapy Tumor Response
Monitoring and Treatment Planning
Breit (Editor-in-Chief)
© Springer-Verlag, Berlin Heidelberg 1992

algorithm can be used to correct these distortions. For most MRI units this correction is not necessary, especially for small fields of view (FOV). We have ignored the distortions in all cases because they were less than ± 0.5 cm for a FOV of 30 cm and less than ± 1 cm for a FOV of 50 cm.

In contrast to the Hounsfield units of computed tomography images, the signal intensities in MR images are not correlated to the absorption coefficients of different tissues. Therefore, the electron density must be entered manually. Instead of a voxel-by-voxel correction the inhomogeneity correction can be performed for contiguous regions such as lung or bone (Lukas et al. 1988). For the head and neck we assumed the electron density to be constant ($=1$) for the whole region. A three-dimensional MRI data set typically consists of 128 partitions. For this reason special display modes are required to review this large amount of information — the anatomical structures and the treatment plan.

We worked with two different computer systems. First, the images were prepared (see below) on an image analysis system (Mipron, Kontron). For the calculation of dose distribution a commercial treatment planning system (Meva-plan, Siemens) was used. The dose distribution was calculated for a slice in the plane of the central beam and for parallel slices. These "pseudo-3D" calculations were performed only for some slices within the volume of interest—typically for 10–15 slices; alternatively, we started with thicker slices generated by linear combination of the original slices. In both cases the dose distribution was transferred back to the image analysis system, and an interpolation algorithm provided the information for those slices for which no calculations had been performed. Further postprocessing and display were carried out on the image analysis system.

Display Techniques

The first step was to delineate the tumor or the target interactively in a series of parallel slices chosing the most suited orientation. All voxels belonging to the marked tumor or target were coded with red color. Using a color-coded overlay, this additional information can be displayed together with anatomical structures in the whole three-dimensional data set. Color-coding further allows the evaluation of the maximum tumor extension (tumor volume) or the target volume. This maximum extension can be projected on arbitrary slices and is displayed as a contour with orange or pink color. This display technique facilitates the exact definition of the beam parameters and the control of the dose distribution. Internal or artificial landmarks (small tubes filled with Gd-DTPA) can be used for a correct positioning of the irradiation fields. These landmarks can also be projected on arbitrary slices. Irradiation fields or regions of given dose intervals were coded in a similar way as the tumor and were marked with

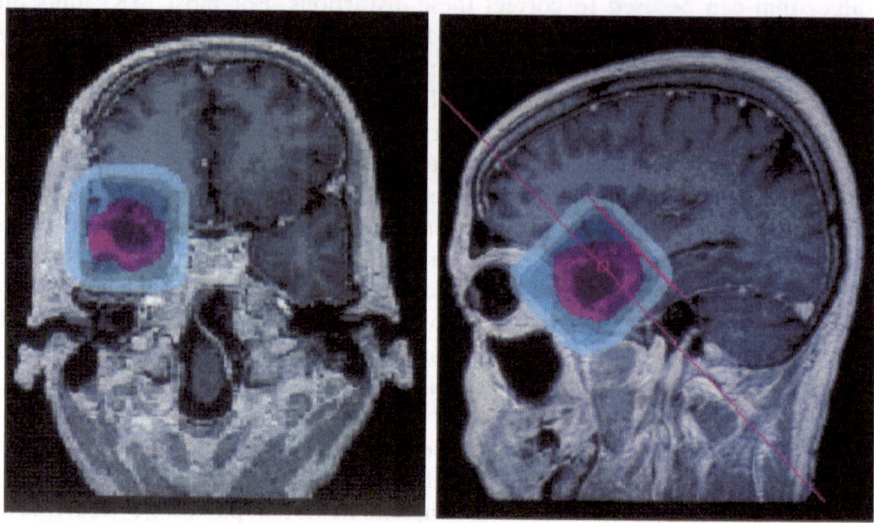

Fig. 1. Oblique coronal cut and sagittal slice with actual cutline. Color-coding of the tumor (*violet*) and the dose distribution (*dark blue*, regions containing the 90% isodose; *blue*, regions containing additionally the 80% isodose; *light blue*, regions containing additionally the 60% isodose)

blue color. The color of the tumor or target (red–violet) indicates whether it lies without or within a region of given dose intervals or irradiation fields.

Two different display modes — confirmed in diagnostic MRI — were used for visualization of the anatomical structures together with the treatment plan (Kneschaurek et al. 1990). Moving slice by slice in an arbitrary direction (Fig. 1) is suited for screening of the data as well as for detailed information. A cutline on a reference image (perpendicular to the reconstructed image) can also be displayed, indicating the actual slice position of the reconstructed image. For the main plane cuts (Fig. 2) three perpendicular slices through one point in the three-dimensional data set are displayed. Marked with a cross, the point of intersection can be defined either in the sagittal, coronal, or transverse image. The main plane cuts give a very distinct display of the irradiation fields or of the dose distribution together with anatomical information. Because the additional information, such as tumor or target and irradiation fields or regions of given dose intervals, are color coded, each of them can be switched on and off independently.

Conclusions

Optimization of a physical treatment plan can be achieved only on the basis of the complete three-dimensional information. Because of the excellent soft-tissue

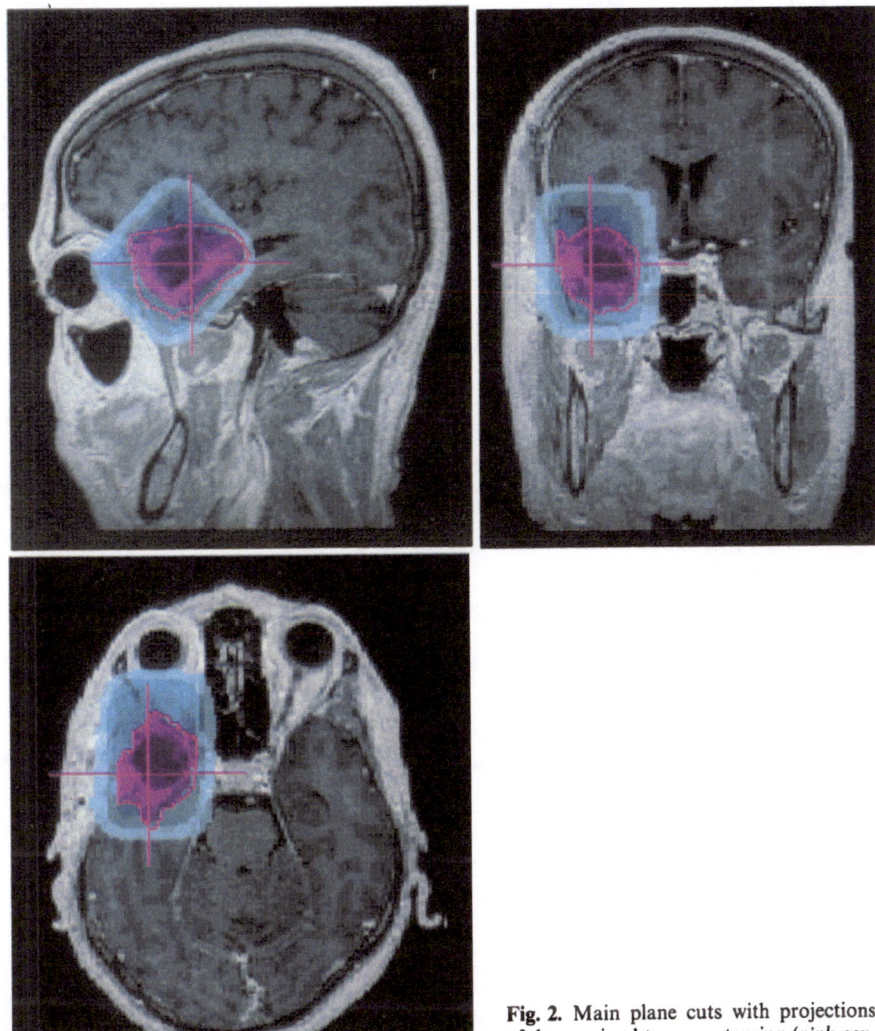

Fig. 2. Main plane cuts with projections of the maximal tumor extension (*pink contour*). (Color-coding, see Fig. 1)

contrast and the high spatial resolution three-dimensional MRI data sets are suited as the basis for radiation therapy planning. Using the three-dimensional technique display as well as threrapy planning on slices with arbitrary position and orientation is possible. With color-coding of the tumor or the target and of the irradiation fields or dose distribution this additional information can be visualized together with anatomical structures. Furthermore, this display technique allows the evaluation of the maximum tumor extension or target volume and its projection on arbitrary slices.

References

Kneschaurek P, Kett H, Prüll C, Breit A (1990) The value of MRI in the treatment planning in radiation therapy. In: Breit A (ed) ESO monographs, magnetic resonance in oncology. Springer, Berlin Heidelberg New York

Lukas P, Theurer G, Kneschaurek P (1988) Untersuchungen zur Genauigkeit einer MR-gestützten Bestrahlungsplanung im Vergleich zur CT-Planung. In: Österreichischer Röntgenkongreß, Graz 1988, book of abstracts, p 68

Experience with Magnetic Resonance Imaging Assisted Simulation (Integrating Sagittal and Coronal Imaging) in Tumors of the Head: A First Step to Conformation Radiotherapy

R. Pötter, B. Lenzen, L. Schneider, U. Haverkamp, and C. Al Dandashi

Introduction

In conformation radiotherapy the treatment volume is precisely adjusted to an irregular target and tumor volume (Tate et al. 1986). A precondition is a sophisticated treatment planning procedure with delineation of tumor, target, normal anatomy, and organs at risk in different planes. The delineation may be carried out in transverse planes and then reconstructed in coronal and sagittal or even arbitrary planes (beam's eye view; Goitein et al. 1983). An analogous procedure can also be used for dose distribution display. A different way is based on direct imaging of transverse, coronal, sagittal or even arbitrary planes. Magnetic resonance imaging (MRI) is a method which today renders this multiplanar imaging possible. As the majority of tumors are at present irradiated by parallel opposed and three or four orthogonal fields, a delineation of tumor, target and normal anatomy, and organs at risk in these planes is most important for clinical use. Treatment planning including the design of individual shielding blocks based on beam's eye view projections represents a first step to an adjustment of treatment to an irregular target volume and thus makes conformation radiotherapy clinically feasible (Pötter 1989).

Radiotherapy of tumors of the head is often performed using parallel opposed fields and three-field techniques with individual beam shaping (Chang and Hilal 1984; Karlsson and Brady 1987). A study was performed looking at the impact of MRI on clinical treatment planning in tumors of the head, in particular on the benefit of additional sagittal and coronal slice orientation from MRI for target delineation on lateral and anterior–posterior (AP) simulator radiographs.

Materials and Methods

The procedure for treatment planning with definition of target volume and organs at risk was (a) conventional computed tomography (CT) assisted

Klinik für Strahlentherapie, Radioonkologie, Westfälische Wilhelms-Universität Münster, Albert Schweitzer-Straße, 4400 Münster, FRG

Advanced Radiation Therapy Tumor Response Monitoring and Treatment Planning
Breit (Editor-in-Chief)
© Springer-Verlag, Berlin Heidelberg 1992

simulation: transverse CT planes and lateral or AP simulator radiographs; and
(b) MRI-assisted simulation: MR slices in transverse, coronal, and sagittal
orientation — the latter two superimposed on AP and lateral simulator
radiographs. In CT-assisted simulation information on the localization of tumor

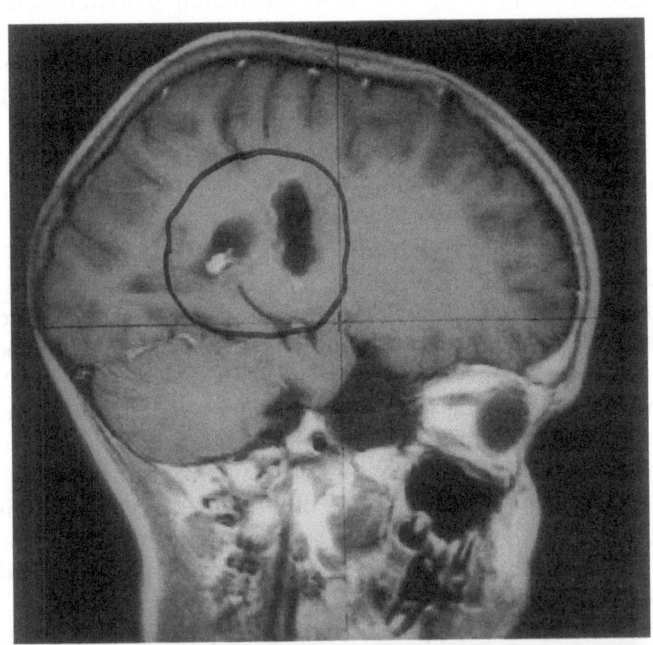

a

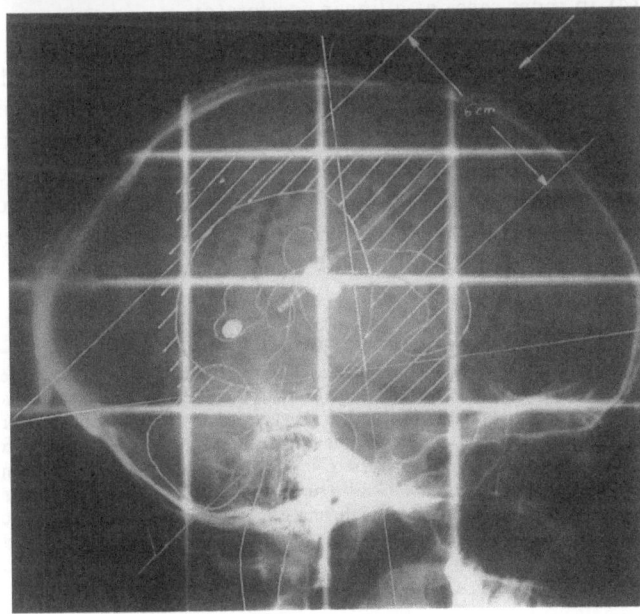

b

and target was "translated" mentally by the physician — based to varying degrees on reference structures — from transverse, parallel projected images onto the centrally projected sagittal and coronal X-ray images, the simulation films. This rather complicated "translation procedure" entails many uncertainties, in particular a considerable risk of mislocalization and over- or underestimation of the target. Rectangular open fields were common in brain tumors, additional standard blocking was used for tumors of the head near the base of the skull. In MRI-assisted simulation imaging information could be superimposed directly from coronal and sagittal MRI slices on lateral and AP simulation films based on the use of a subtrascope without interposing a poorly defined "translation procedure." Uncertainties in localization due to image information transfer were thus avoided. Individual shielding blocks were regularly used (Fig. 1).

Spin-echo sequences (T1- and T2-weighted) were obtained in 37 patients: 13 brain tumors and 24 tumors of the head. Imaging was performed with the patient in treatment position in 16 cases. Superimposition of sagittal and coronal MR images onto simulator radiographs was done at a subtrascope (Pötter 1989). As a reference frame anatomical landmarks were used which could be identified with both imaging methods: sella turcica, cribriform plate, frontal and sphenoid sinuses, vault of the neurocranium with subcutaneous fat, hard palate, and epipharyngeal space. The amount of geometric distortion in the MR images was up to 2–3 mm within a volume of $10 \times 10 \times 10$ cm (phantom measurements) (Pötter 1989). Compared to the size on MRI and taking the midsagittal plane as reference frame, distortions due to magnification and different projection averaged under 1 mm (Schneider 1991).

Radiotherapy was delivered from opposed lateral fields ($n = 23$) or in three-field technique ($n = 14$), in most cases at a linear accelerator.

The target definitions were compared to conventional CT-assisted simulation and MRI-assisted simulation and the number of changes were registered. A quantitative comparison was made for definitions of target in ten patients and for treatment volume in nine patients based on planimetric measurements on simulator radiographs (Pötter 1989; Pötter et al. 1991). For determination of the treatment volume the target areas as measured on the simulation films were multiplied by the irradiated distance along the central beam assuming parallel opposed fields.

Fig. 1a, b. MRI-assisted target volume definition (boost volume) using the subtrascope for image superimposition in an 8-year-old child with macroscopic residual disease after surgery for a primitive neuroectodermal tumor. **a** Sagittal MRI (T1, Gd-DTPA) demonstrating residual tumor with high signal intensity; *drawn line,* suspected area of potential residual disease. **b** Targets on lateral simulation film: from simulation based on transverse CT plane (*wire frame*) and simulation based on image superimposition from sagittal MRI (*blank area surrounded by hatched area within the wire frame*). Due to difficulties in translating the image information in CT-based simulation the target was chosen far too large, and target definition nearly missed the region of potential spread defined by sagittal MRI. Radiotherapy was performed by a three-field technique: two opposed lateral, one parietofrontal (*arrow* in **b**)

In considering the results, well-known geometric principles must be kept in mind: reducing an area (6 × 6 cm) by 1 cm in length and width (5 × 5 cm) leads to a reduction of 11 cm^2 (31%), conforming its shape to a circle (diameter 5 cm), even to a reduction of 16 cm^2 (44%; see Fig. 2).

Results

The additional information from sagittal and coronal images from MRI led to a change in the target definition in 82% of the investigated cases compared to the target definitions based on CT-assisted simulation alone. The largest differences were seen in tumors of the brain (95%) and tumors near the base of the skull (96%). When using coronal and sagittal planes from MRI, a reduction in the target was achieved in every case compared to conventional fluoroscopic simulation based on transverse planes from CT alone. Field length and width were reduced by 1–2 cm. The target was adjusted to the individual tumor volume and the region of potential spread. The resulting average reduction in brain tumors was 48.5 cm^2 (19–81 cm^2), in tumors of the head 19 cm^2 (10–30 cm^2), the average relative reduction in brain tumors was 55% and in tumors of the head 22%.

Due to uncertainties in localization, simulation based on transverse planes alone (CT-assisted) led to considerable overestimation of the target. Taking the visible tumor in MRI and adding a margin of 2 cm the mean target area gave 48 cm^2 (21–108 cm^2). In CT-assisted simulation the mean target area, however, was 95 cm^2 (60–140 cm^2) and in MRI-assisted simulation only 55 cm^2 (23–110 cm^2). This comparison demonstrates clearly that including the information from the additional sagittal or coronal plane avoided the overestimation of

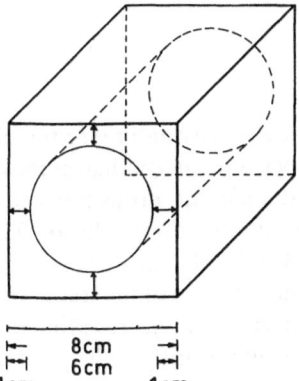

8cm
6cm
1cm   1cm

Fig. 2. Target reduction assessment: square area (8 × 8cm) reduced to a circle with a diameter of 6 cm [π/4 (6 × 6 cm)] leads to 64 and 28 cm^2, respectively. The target area is reduced by 36 cm^2 (56%). This reduction translates into volume reduction.

Table 1. Value of MRI-assisted treatment volume definition integrating sagittal planes into conventional fluoroscopic simulation (parallel opposed fields) in tumors of the head (patients no. 2–4) and of the brain (patients no. 5–10): quantitative comparison of treatment volume based on transverse planes (often open fields; CT-assisted) and additional sagittal planes (always individually shielded; MRI-assisted)

Patient no.	Diameter	Treatment volume		Reduction	
		CT-assisted simulation	MRI-assisted simulation	cm^3	%
2	15 cm	15 cm × 60 cm^2 (900 cm^3)	15 cm × 48 cm^2 (720 cm^3)	180	20
3	15 cm	15 cm × 140 cm^2 (2100 cm^3)	15 cm × 110 cm^2 (1650 cm^3)	450	21
4	10 cm	10 cm × 70 cm^2 (700 cm^3)	10 cm × 46 cm^2 (460 cm^3)	240	34
5	15 cm	15 cm × 100 cm^2 (1500 cm^3)	15 cm × 54 cm^2 (810 cm^3)	690	46
6	14 cm	14 cm × 88 cm^2 (1232 cm^3)	14 cm × 46 cm^2 (644 cm^3)	588	48
7	14 cm	14 cm × 77 cm^2 (1078 cm^3)	14 cm × 23 cm^2 (322 cm^3)	756	70
8	13 cm	13 cm × 135 cm^2 (1755 cm^3)	13 cm × 54 cm^2 (702 cm^3)	1053	60
9	9 cm	9 cm × 97 cm^2 (873 cm^3)	9 cm × 58 cm^2 (522 cm^3)	351	40
10	14 cm	14 cm × 36 cm^2 (504 cm^3)	14 cm × 17 cm^2 (238 cm^3)	266	53

target from uncertainty in localization when taking transverse planes alone; this led to a high degree of target conformation by MRI-assisted simulation (Pötter 1989).

Taking opposed lateral fields — comparing MRI-with CT-assisted simulation — the average reduction in treatment volume was 508 cm^3 on an absolute scale and 43% on a relative scale (Pötter 1989; Fig. 2, Table 1).

Conclusions

MRI-assisted fluoroscopic simulation makes possible a precise and reproducible integration of transverse, coronal, and sagittal planes. Geometric inaccuracies due to inhomogeneities of the magnetic field and different projections and magnifications are not of clinical importance in tumors of the head. The integrated use of three orthogonal planes from CT/MRI leads to a more adequate definition of the target in all three planes than the use of the transverse plane with additional sagittal and coronal X-ray projections alone, resulting in a change of target in 82%. The target volume can be significantly reduced. The treatment volume can consequently be adjusted to the target volume in a more appropriate manner by using individual shielding blocks for the different planes, resulting in a mean reduction in treatment volume for opposing lateral fields of 43%. The irradiation of organs at risk is reduced. Using a subtrascope, the MRI-assisted fluoroscopic simulation in tumors of the head represents a first step to making conformation radiotherapy feasible for clinical practice with little additional effort.

Acknowledgements. The authors would like to thank C. Rademacher and P. Fischer for assistance in performing the study and P. Mause and I. Liebe for help in preparing the manuscript.

References

Chang CH, Hilal SK (1984) Brain tumor localization: determination of extent and volume for radiation treatment. In: Levitt SH, du Tapley N (eds) Technological basis of radiation therapy: practical clinical applications. Lea and Febiger, Philadelphia, pp 172–192

Goitein M, Abrams M, Rowell D, Pollari H, Wiles J (1983) Multidimensional treatment planning. II. Beam's eye-view, back-projection and projection through CT sections. Int J Radiat Oncol Biol Phys 9: 789–797

Karlsson UL, Brady LW (1987) Primary Intracranial Neoplasms. In: Perez CA, Brady LW (eds) Principles and practice of radiation oncology. Lippincott, Philadelphia, pp 408–436

Pötter R (1989) Lokalisation mit Hilfe bildgebender Verfahren in der Strahlentherapie maligner Tumoren. Habilitationsschrift, University of Münster

Pötter R, Heil B, Schneider L, Lenzen H, Al-Dandashi C, Schnepper E (1992) Sagittal and coronal planes from MRI for treatment planning in tumors of brain, head and neck: MRI assisted simulation. Radiother Oncol 23: 127–130

Schneider L (1991) MRT-gestützte Simulation in der Planung der Strahlentherapie von Tumoren des Kopfes. Dissertationsschrift, University of Münster

Tate T, Brace JA, Morgan H, Skeggs DBL (1986) Conformation therapy: a method of improving the tumour treatment volume ratio. Clin Radiol 37: 267–271

Application of Computer Graphics in Three-Dimensional Radiotherapy Treatment Planning

G. Becker[1,2], J. Pross[1], R. Bendl[1], G. Mayer[1], R. Lohrum[1], and W. Schlegel[1]

Introduction

In the past few years radiotherapy treatment planning has made important advances with the aid of computers and three-dimensional medical imaging such as computer tomography (CT) and magnetic resonance imaging [10]. Recently the first three-dimensional treatment planning systems became available for clinical use [4–6]. With the availability of three-dimensional imaging devices the ability to make anatomical and pathological structures visible has been tremendously enhanced. The shape of a tumor or the surrounding healthy tissue can vary from section to section. However, the stereotactically guided and multileaf collimator aided conforming high-precision radiotherapy techniques make totally new demands on the planning systems. Thus at the German Cancer Research Center (DKFZ) the experience of three-dimensional treatment planning from more than 100 patients led to the development of a sophisticated computer graphic, which is described below.

Materials and Methods

Hardware. At the Department of Radiology and Pathophysiology of the DKFZ medical workstations (DEC VAX stations 3200 and 3520) are available. They are used in a local area VAX cluster with a DEC 3600 as node. Imaging data from CT, magnetic resonance imaging, and positron emission tomography were transferred directly to this network (Ethernet with DECNET protocol). As operating system VMS was used.

Software. The software was written in the programming language C into which existing FORTRAN routines for reading the patient files were integrated. The object-oriented user interface was constructed with the XWindows system and

[1] German Cancer Research Center, Im Neuenheimer Feld 280, 6900 Heidelberg, FRG
[2] Current address: Department of Radiotherapy, University Clinic for Radiology, Hoppe-Seyler-Str. 3, 7400 Tübingen, FRG

Advanced Radiation Therapy Tumor Response
Monitoring and Treatment Planning
Breit (Editor-in-Chief)
© Springer-Verlag, Berlin Heidelberg 1992

the DECWindows Toolkit. XWindows has been developed with Digital Equipment to construct a device-independent graphic–user interface. The three-dimensional reconstruction and presentation of contour lines is realized by means of the DEC PHIGS graphic system. DEC PHIGS conforms to the international PHIGS standard ISO 9592:1988/E, which is also device independent and promises good portability.

The interaction with the user is completely mouse driven. All user interface objects are mouse sensitive. Functions of the program can be started simply by clicking with the mouse on icons in a control panel or by selecting entries of pulldown menus. Dialogs with the user are handled with dialog boxes. A dialog box consists of interactive elements such as text entry fields, radioboxes, listboxes, and scaleboxes. The user has a good overview of all program functions and can fully concentrate on his work on the screen [3].

Results

Radiotherapy treatment planning consists of various independent steps. To optimize the computer assistance for the radiooncologist the optimum tool must be made available for every single working cycle.

Definition of Target Volumes and Organs at Risk. Careful execution of modern irradiation techniques, such as stereotactic radiosurgery, achieve an accuracy which is limited only by the resolution of the applied imaging techniques. This opens new dimensions in demands on the quality of the imaging and on the therapist. To meet these requirements and to shorten the time-consuming process, fast and user-friendly three-dimensional image segmentation and modeling tools were developed [7, 10]. The images are presented in three windows, of which the first shows the original transversal section. The other two are used for reconstructed sagittal and frontal views of the imaging data. Reference lines indicate the spatial position of a section in the other two corresponding views. They can also be used to select an interesting slice simply by moving the line with the mouse to the requested positions. This method allows the therapist to obtain a three-dimensional impression of the patient's anatomy. In a larger working window the user can select one of the three views for presentation. This window is used for outlining anatomic structures on the images. Small structures of interest can be enlarged to up to eight times their original size. By moving a rectangle on the image the area to be zoomed is selected interactively. A presentation with a high zoom factor can be smoothed by low-pass filtering. The contouring is performed with the mouse using a tomographic image as background. This can be done free-hand, by polygon, or by ellipse drawing. Unwanted lines can be deleted at any time. If it is necessary to keep a well-defined safe distance between tumor and target volume, the cursor can be changed in a circle with the specified distance. The use of circle and ellipse drawing function is extremely time shortening in the case of structures such as the eyes (Fig. 1).

Virtual Therapy Simulation. Complete three-dimensional outlining of the organs at risk and the target volume is necessary to provide the spatial information required for virtual radiotherapy planning. One must determine the irradiation technique that is the best compromise among closely matching the dose distribution to the contour of the target volume, achieving a homogeneous dose distribution over the target volume, and optimal protection of the organs at risk [2]. The user interface of the virtual therapy simulation consists of four windows: transversal sagittal, and frontal CT sections and the beam's eye view. Beam's eye view means the presentation of contours which outline the patients' anatomic structures in three dimensions as if viewed from the radiation source

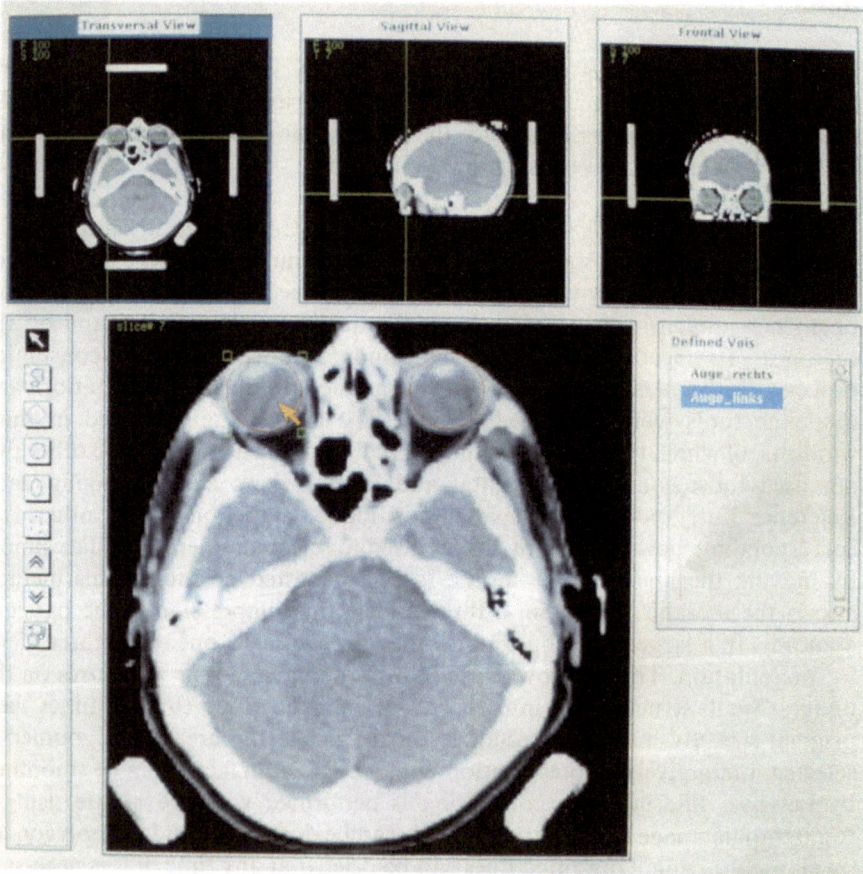

Fig. 1. Definition of target volume and organs at risk

along the central ray of the beam [8, 9, 11]. By means of buttons in a control panel or of the scales for gantry and couch positions, the therapist is able to rotate the contours in real time around the axes of the device. For better orientation the cross-sections of the irradiation field in the CT slices are shown in the CT windows. This tool allows the therapist to find the optimal irradiation direction quickly and easily. The shape and size of the irradiation field can also be determined in the beam's eye window (Fig. 2).

Display of Dose Distribution. After the virtual therapy simulation the irradiation dose is calculated. However, the presentation, evaluation, and selection of such spatial information as three-dimensional dose distribution is a great problem. In the clinical use the three-dimensional display of target volumes, organs at risk, and isodoses as shaded surfaces are helpful tools [1]. On the basis of this spatial presentation the therapist is able to recognize possible clinically relevant over-

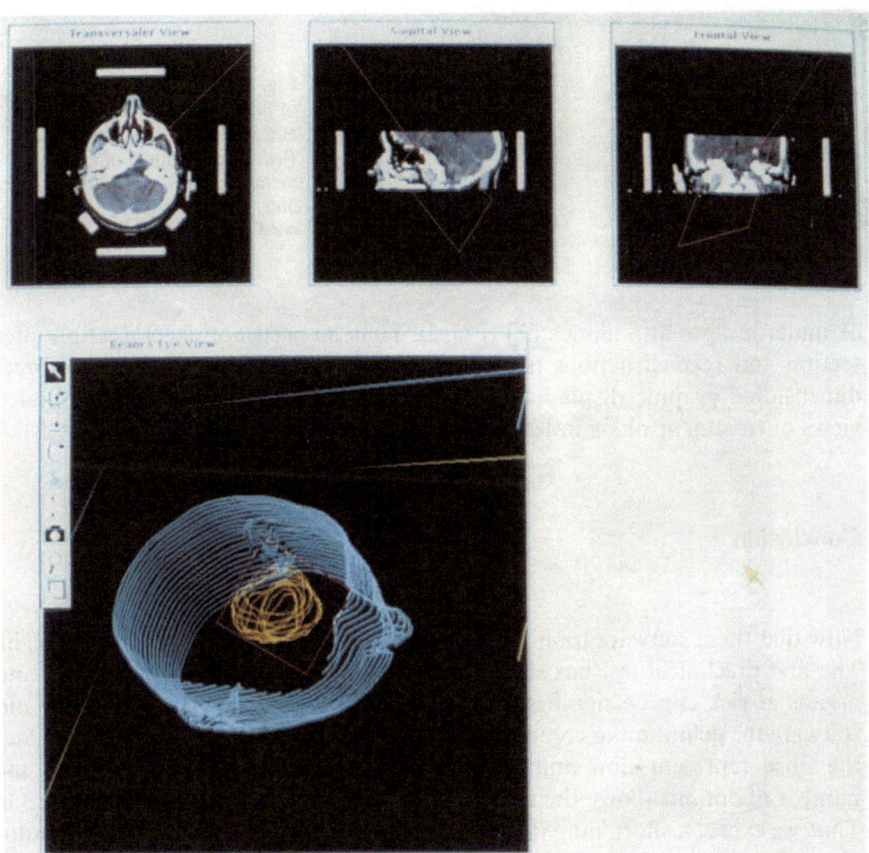

Fig. 2. Virtual therapy simulation

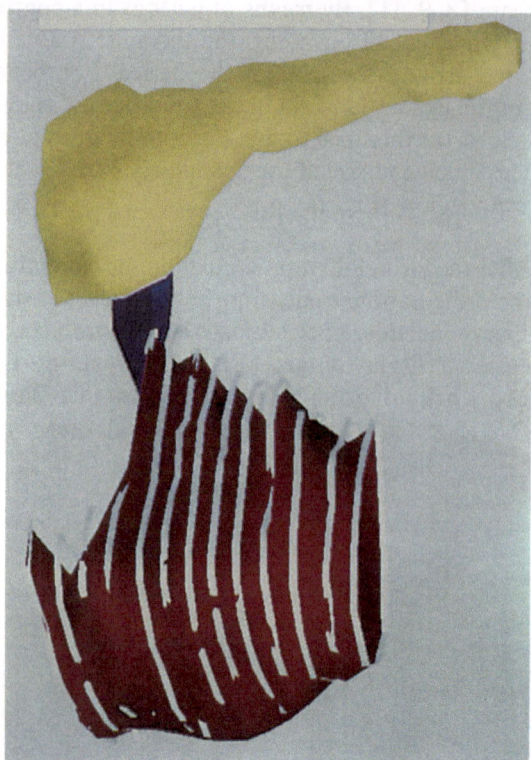

Fig. 3. Three-dimensional display of target volumes, organs at risk, and isodoses as shaded surfaces. *Red*, target volume of a meningioma; *white*, 80% isodose; *blue*, pituitary gland; *yellow* spinal cord and brain stem

or underdosages at a glance [2] (Fig. 3). Thus he need not check section after section and reconstructions (sagittal or frontal). With the help of this three-dimensional graphic display option it is possible to generate surface-shaded views of treatment plans in less than 2 s.

Conclusion

Now that these software tools have been developed, their clinical use can begin. The first preclinical test has shown that the time to define target volumes and organs at risk can be significantly reduced. Whereas in the past with the old software the definition of volumes of interest, the virtual therapy simulation, and the dose representation and evaluation required 3–4 h, depending on the number of optimizations, the new software allows this in only 1 or at most 3 h. Thus we expect a shortening in the interactive working time of the radiooncologist at the display by more than half. The reasons for this are: (a) the simple and quick man–machine interaction; (b) the mouse-driven system; (c) the software, which is not hierarchically structured; (d) the controlled menu and dialog box; (e) the buttons, scale, and list boxes; and (f) the almost real-time system. In addition, simultaneous representation of transversal, sagittal, and frontal sections and volumes of interest makes the spatial information considerably clearer for the therapist. Clinical use has shown that the conformation of the dose distribution on the target volume is possible only by means of the beam's eye view. Easy handling and almost real-time systems are prerequisites for the rapid spreading of three-dimensional treatment planning tools in radiotherapy.

References

1. Bauer-Kirpes B, Schlegel W, Boesecke R, Lorenz WJ (1987) Display of organs and isodoses as shaded 3D objects for 3D therapy planning. Int J Radiat Oncol Biol Phys 13: 135–140
2. Becker G, Lohrum R, Werner T, Bürkelbach J, Nemeth G, Boesecke R, Schlegel W, Lorenz WJ (1989) Presentation and evaluation of 3D dose distribution in radiotherapy planning. In: Lemke HU, Rhodes ML, Jaffe CC, Felix R (eds) Computer assisted radiology. Springer, Berlin Heidelberg New York, pp 254–261
3. Bendl R, Pross J, Schlegel W (1990) Application of computer graphics in 3D radiotherapy treatment planning: manual image segmentation and virtual therapy simulation. In: Dickhaus H, Leo T, Russo P (eds) Proceedings of the 3rd joint seminar on medical informatics and bioengineering, University of Ancona, Ancona, pp 20–32
4. Chin LM, Siddon RL, Svensson GK, Rose C (1985) Progress in 3-D treatment planning for photon beam therapy. Int J Radiat Oncol Biol Phys 11: 2011–2019
5. Chu JC, Richter MP, Sontag MR, Larson RD, Fong K, Bloch P (1987) Practice of 3-dimensional treatment planning at the Fox Chase Cancer Center, University of Pennsylvania. Radiother Oncol 8 (2): 137–143
6. Gademann G, Schlegel W, Becker G, Romahn J, Höver KH, Pastyr O, van Kaick G, Wannenmacher M (1990) High precision radiotherapy of head and neck tumors by means of an integrated stereotactic and 3D planning system. Int J Radiat Oncol Biol Phys 19 [Suppl 1]: 135
7. Goitein M, Abrams M (1983) Multi-dimensional treatment planning. I. Delineation of anatomy. Int J Radiat Oncol Biol Phys 9: 777–787
8. Goitein M, Abrams M, Powell D, Pollari H, Wills J (1983) Multi-dimensional treatment planning. II Beam's eye-view, back projection and projection through CT-sections. Int J Radiat Oncol Biol Phys 9: 789–797
9. Mohan R, Brewster J, Barest GD, Chui CS (1989) Computer graphics tools for radiation treatment planning. Comput Methods Programs Biomed 28: 157–170
10. Schlegel W (1990) Computer assisted radiation therapy planning. In: Höhne KH, Fuchs H, Pizer SM (eds) 3D imaging in medicine. Springer, Berlin Heidelberg New York, pp 399–410 (NATO ASI series, Vol F 60)
11. Sherouse GW, Mosher CE (1987) User interface issues in radiotherapy CAD software. In: Bruinvis IAD (ed) The use of computers in radiation therapy. North Holland, Amsterdam, pp 429–463

Treatment Management System: The Integrated Network Solution for Better Cancer Treatment

H. Dahlin, P. Ekström, and B. Högström

Introduction

The rapid development of computer-controlled medical equipment, especially in radiology and oncology, has increased the need for efficient computer networks. At various research centers and at major manufacturers various network solutions have been developed. Among these, the so-called American College of Radiology/National Electrical Manufacturers Association (ACR/NEMA) protocol for digital image transfer seems the most promising. For many years it has been thought that the ACR/NEMA standard would solve the general problem of how to transfer image data from one image-generating node to another regardless of the manufacturers of the equipments. Although the major suppliers have agreed upon the ACR/NEMA concept, very little has been done to make a commercial imaging network available and clinically useful. This is also the case with other medical data communication networks.

Radiation Oncology

The complexity of data processing in the medical area is most pronounced in radiation oncology. The radiation therapy patient information flow, illustrated by the Computer-Aided Radiation Therapy project [1] (Fig. 1), contains not only an enormous amount of digital images but also data describing the radiation beam characteristics, physical parameters, dose information, radiation beam set-up parameters, treatment data, etc. These data are absolutely necessary at different stages throughout the treatment course of each cancer patient. Unfortunately, the efficiency of today's information processing in radiation oncology is very poor, and this can result in many unnecessary mistreatments.

Helax, Box 1704, 751 47 Uppsala, Sweden

Advanced Radiation Therapy Tumor Response
Monitoring and Treatment Planning
Breit (Editor-in-Chief)
© Springer-Verlag, Berlin Heidelberg 1992

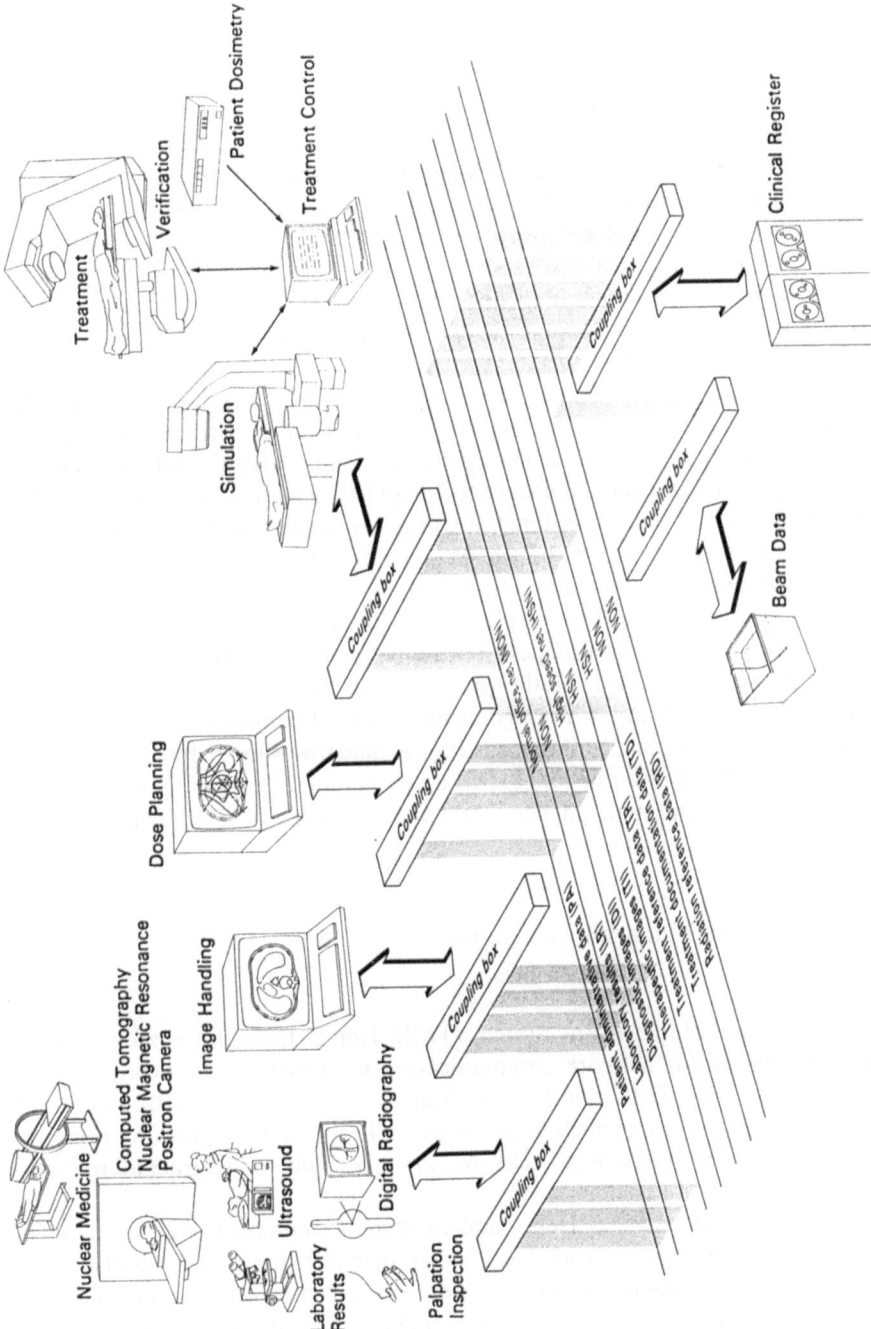

Fig. 1. Computer-aided radiation therapy (CART)

Export/Import Interpreter

To use a computer network in practice, whether set up as a standard serial line communication or Ethernet protocol, the specifications of the logical format must be fulfilled to all relevant levels for each application. Very often the attempt to establish a general protocol, such as the ACR/NEMA, results in practically useless solutions, as the protocol may be fulfilled but no relevant data are available — a situation that is especially critical when transferring image data from radiological equipments to oncology planning systems. The situation is even more critical if the geometric relationship between images is not fully described.

To overcome the problem it is necessary to define export/import rules based on an "agreement" between the import node and the export node on exactly what data are to be transferred. The agreement defines a request for import data; the most primitive form is a mutual agreement between the manufacturers of the different "nodes" resulting in functions/program codes enabling the requested data transfer (export/import) by use of a standard protocol.

The mutual agreement may result in a more general solution, a so-called export/import interpreter, which picks up or inserts data in the local database according to the prescribed request. The requests are based on the specifications of the parameters needed for the processing of the specific application. The request is sent as an input message using a general communication format as carrier. Acknowledgement of the message is made by similar functions on the export node. The transfer of data between export functions and import functions is thereby always optimal, independently of the complexity of the logical format.

The Treatment Management System

The Treatment Management System (TMS; Helax, Uppsala) is an oncology planning system for network communication according to the export/import rules (Fig. 2). The TMS database is designed using the MIMER relational binary database system, which is extremely well suited for integration programs for export/import functions, thereby making it possible to integrate all relevant oncology applications.

An agreement between Helax and Siemens Gammasonics in the United States has resulted in a Helax TMS image network interpreter based on the ACR/NEMA-SPI (Siemens network protocol for the picture archiving and communication system, PACS) which makes efficient image transfer from Siemens imaging equipment to the TMS planning system easy and safe. The Siemens-Helax network solution has been in clinical operation at four major radiation oncology centers in Sweden for over a year. The positive experience

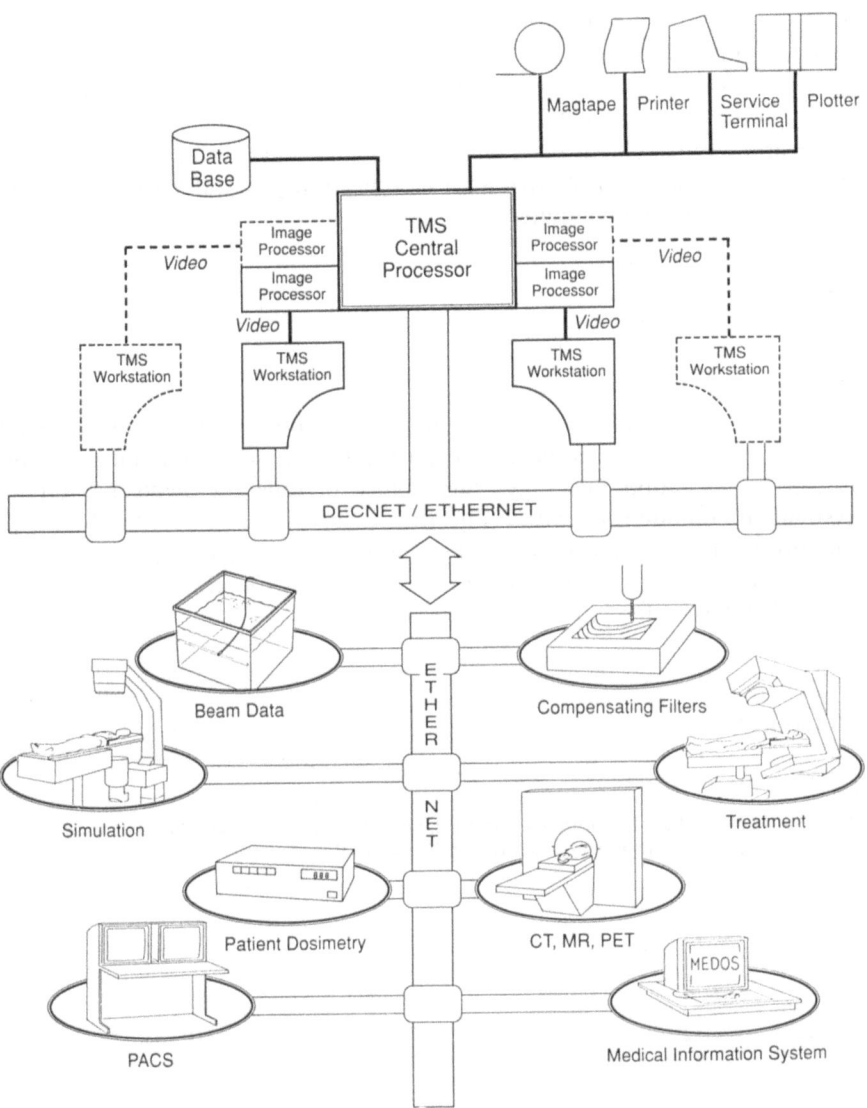

Fig. 2. Treatment Management System (TMS)

from these centers has also resulted in many new demands for improved use of computed tomography (CT) and magnetic resonance imaging (MRI) data for planning of radiation therapy. The enormous interest by clinicians in using CT and MRI data for target volume definition has opened new possibilities for three-dimensional treatment planning, which will result in better radiotherapy and more consistent and safe data handling. The TMS export/import interpreter will be further improved to allow for more complicated images, such as angiographies, to be used in three-dimensional reconstructions and image matching in radiotherapy.

The export/import interpreter is also used for other applications such as check and confirm, block and compensating filter constructions, multileaf collimator setting, etc. In these environments various network architecture are used for example PATHWORKS for merging TMS central VAX computers to clients with personal computers.

Conclusion

TMS is an example of a successful practical solution for using available general network protocols by supporting export/import requests for different applications in radiation oncology. The ability of different medical equipment systems to communicate with each other, achieved by standardized networks and protocols, must not result in a flow of nonsense data merely for the sake of communicating but should be used for the transport of relevant data, mutually specified between the import and export nodes.

Reference

1. Westerlund K (1988) The Scandinavian Program CART, Joint US-Scandinavian symposium on future directions of computer aided radiotherapy, AAPM, August 1988, San Antonio, Texas

Three-Dimensional Tumor Therapy Management

U. Quast[1], L. Glaeser[1], H. Dahlin[3], W. Sauerwein[2], and H. Sack[2]

Tumor Treatment

Optimal tumor treatment is the aim of radiooncology. To achieve the maximal probability of uncomplicated cure for tumors even at complex anatomical sites — such as head and neck tumors — or at later stages of disease, all treatment modalities, all experience in radiooncology, radiobiology, and medical physics as well as all possibilities of diagnostic imaging and modern radiotherapy must be considered. New technical developments can help in the spatial visualization of the complex topographical situation, and all physical knowledge must be included to optimize and realize the spatial distribution of the radiation absorbed dose that is really needed.

Tumor Radiotherapy

The increase in radiooncological understanding and the methodological and technical developments in the past decade have brought a large number of interesting tools for all steps of tumor therapy. However, up to now these have usually been separate tools, used independently without direct communication between them.

There are at least three levels of links between steps in radiooncology. The data input level deals with the collection of patient data, clinical, diagnostic, and localization data regarding physical and beam data, and includes all dialog information. The central level (Fig. 1) contains all steps of tumor treatment. This begins with the decision for tumor therapy and about a radiotherapy concept and is followed by the technical steps of positioning and fixation, of computed tomography, magnetic resonance imaging, positron emission tomography, ultrasound and X-ray localization in reproduceable treament position. The medical planning steps are: assignment of corresponding anatomical data, three-

---

[1] Department of Clinical Radiation Physics, University Hospital, 4300 Essen, FRG
[2] Department of Radiation Therapy, University Hospital, 4300 Essen, FRG
[3] Helax, Box 1704, 751 47 Uppsala, Sweden

Advanced Radiation Therapy Tumor Response
Monitoring and Treatment Planning
Breit (Editor-in-Chief)
© Springer-Verlag, Berlin Heidelberg 1992

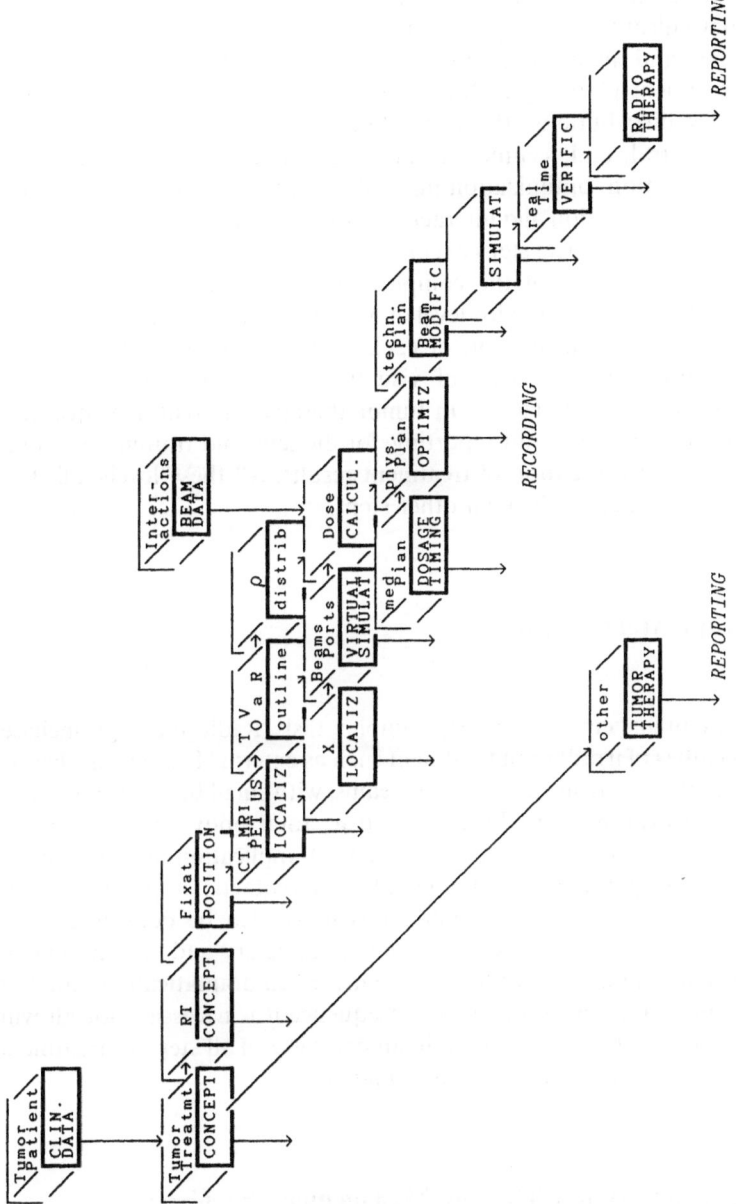

Fig. 1. Complexity of tumor radiotherapy

dimensional delineation of target volumes and organs at risk, visualization of the spatial anatomical-topographical relationship, possible radiation beams and entrance portals, and the prescription of dose, time, and fractionation. Physical irradiation treatment planning includes the generation of artifact-free spatial electron density distributions, the generation and selection of all physical, dosimetrical, spectral, and technical beam data, true three-dimensional dose distribution calculation, optimization and calculated beam modification, considering all types of radiation and interactions. Realization of the treatment plan needs to consider the technical steps of control of beam shapes and dose profiles, simulation and verification of the complete procedure, and finally the performance of radiotherapy. The third level of handling tumor treatment concerns quality control and documentation of each step of treatment planning and treatment. Essential are the steps of visualization and presentation of all information on the complex factors in tumor therapy for treatment decisions and optimization, recording, and reporting, for didactic and training purposes, and for research and evaluation of treatment results. All these levels, all these steps, are linked directly or through other steps.

Tumor Therapy Management

Tumor therapy management is a very complex task. Radiooncology includes different specialities of irradiation treatment such as external beam radiotherapy with X-ray, gamma, electron, and neutron beams, with small beam sizes (e.g., the treatment of the eye), or large beam sizes (e.g., total body irradiation), and brachyradiotherapy encompasses various types of application (e.g., intracavitary afterloading radiotherapy and interstitial stereotactic implantation). In addition, all other tumor therapy modalities must also be considered. The required number and precision of treatment parameters and the amount of diagnostic, physical, and technical data have increased dramatically in modern three-dimensional radiooncology. As a consequence it is necessary for all who are involved in tumor treatment to retain an overview of all steps of treatment. Optimal tumor therapy management is demanded.

Three-Dimensional Tumor Therapy Management, Archiving, and Communication System

The handling of so many different types of data almost in real time requires a very versatile data network, an effective treatment management, archiving, and communication system (e.g., Treatment Management System, TMS, of Helax).

Virtual Treatment Simulation. An effective new tool for radiooncology is virtual treatment simulation. This uses real-time handling of all three-dimensional imaging data and fast beam's eye view algorithms for visualization of the spatial anatomical relationship of beams and body, target volumes, and organs at risk. This essential tool of three-dimensional topographical treatment planning enables decisions about the number, shape, and incidene of beams and the delineation of beam portals. As a supplementary treatment planning tool virtual simulation assists in the delivery of the prescribed homogeneous distribution of dose to all target volumes under optimal sparing of organs at risk.

True Three-Dimensional Dose Distribution Optimization. True three-dimensional calculation of dose is demanded in the treatment of tumors at complex sites. Fast algorithms (e.g., those by Ahnesjö) enable one to consider all relevant interactions of the radiation beams with the body and with all beam-limiting devices or dose-modifying filters in consideration of the actual spectrum of radiation energy. The three-dimensional optimization procedure yields all values of relevant treatment parameters and enables direct treatment control, for instance, by multileaf collimators or dynamic treatment. Algorithms such as those for dose distribution optimization by inverse back projection (A. Brahme) will enable the calculation of the exact shape of dose-modifying filters regarding all physical influences.

On-Line Beam Shaping and Intensity Modification. Exact beam shaping and dose modification is possible by on-line control of shielding block mold shaping and filter mold cutting devices.

Radiooncological Network. In addition to medical and physical treatment planning as the central steps in tumor radiotherapy, tumor treatment management is essential. The handling of so much information related to a single treatment requires an effective and fast network for transfer, handling, and archiving of three-dimensional data, integrating the diagnostic picture archiving and communication network, linking all workstations for interactive medical, physical, and technical treatment planning, as well as all dedicated planning work stations such as for brachyradiotherapy, stereotactic treatment, n-therapy, or TBI, and providing for direct data communication with all tumor treatment modalities.

Data Presentation. The immense amount of three-dimensional information demands the integration of new tools for fast data selection and real-time, large-scale presentation and fast hard-copy documentation of related data for tumor treatment planning conferences, for education and for research.

Quality Assurance. Effective quality control of all steps and each link in this complex system of tumor therapy is demanded. This includes adequate acceptance tests after each modification of hardware or software and functional control of each device and procedure, especially of exact and safe data transfer, handling, and archiving.

Conclusion

This complete concept of radiooncology enables the collection, handling, transfer, documentation, visualization, and evaluation of all patient data, three-dimensional imaging data, physical data, treatment data, and treatment results, encompassing all steps in tumor therapy and integrating all tumor therapy modalities applied. Improvement in current tumor therapy results is possible only if true three-dimensional treatment planning and tumor therapy management is integrated at all radiooncological centers. Sufficient financial support for adequate installations and qualified staff is therefore essential. This comprehensive system of management, archiving, and communication of radiooncology data will help to improve therapeutic results and to increase our knowledge of tumor response and tissue tolerance.

New Perspectives for Three-Dimensional Radiosurgery Planning by Magnetic Resonance Angiography

H.-H. Ehricke[1] and L.R. Schad[2]

Introduction

Visualization and geometric evaluation of intracranial vascular anatomy is of vital importance for most stereotactic applications, such as needle biopsies, radioactive seed implantation, functional stereotaxy, and stereotactic radiosurgery. Recently, flow-compensated gradient-echo sequences have been introduced into clinical protocols for magnetic resonance imaging (MRI) and have shown great potential in the assessment of angiographic anatomy (Edelman et al. 1989; Marchal et al. 1990). Since it is now possible to use a single modality to image flowing as well as stationary tissue, new perspectives for stereotactic treatment planning have been opened up.

To evaluate the use of magnetic resonance angiography (MRA) for stereotactic treatment planning purposes the clinical example of radiosurgical treatment of cerebral angiomas has been chosen. Cerebral angiomas are congenital malformations which represent 5% of all intracranial tumors. These are caused by arteriovenous shunts and have a high risk of bleeding. Besides surgical extirpation and embolization, radiosurgery (Leksell 1951) is an alternative treatment technique which has shown good results (Leksell 1987; Souhami et al. 1990; Engenhart et al. 1990). By the use of moving field irradiation with multiple arcs, sharp dose fall-offs (from 90% to 10% in the order of centimeters) and spherical isodose surfaces are achieved independently of tissue densities (Hartmann et al. 1985; Podgorsak et al. 1989).

For the purpose of treatment planning we have developed a three-dimensional graphics workstation allowing the definition of target volumes and evaluation of treatment plans on the basis of MRA. Particular emphasis has been placed on the three-dimensional visualization aspect to provide physicians with a convenient and reliable planning tool. This has been realized by integration of concepts and algorithms from the field of three-dimensional computer graphics (Herman and Liu 1979; Ehricke and Laub 1990).

[1] MR-Engineering Group, Siemens Medical Systems, Henkestr. 127, 8520 Erlangen, FRG
[2] Department of Radiology and Pathophysiology, German Cancer Research Center, Im Neuenheimer Feld 280, 6900 Heidelberg, FRG

Advanced Radiation Therapy Tumor Response
Monitoring and Treatment Planning
Breit (Editor-in-Chief)
© Springer-Verlag, Berlin Heidelberg 1992

MRA Data Acquisition Under Stereotactic Conditions

Imaging was performed on a whole-body MRI system operating at 1.5 T field strength (Siemens Magnetom SP). To minimize flow voids, flow-compensated gradient-echo pulse sequences were used (Laub and Kaiser 1988; Ruggieri and Laub 1989). A three-dimensional fast imaging with steady precession sequence with 15° flip angle, 35-ms repetition time, and 7-ms echo time was used to assess venous and arterial anatomy with high contrast. Depending on the volume size to be imaged, from one to three overlaping datasets with 64 transaxial partitions were acquired with a slice thickness of 1.0 mm. A field of view of 265 mm was used. This gave an inplane resolution of about 1 mm. The localization system, which is based on the Riechert and Mundinger stereotactic head frame, included a wooden base ring fixed to the patient's head with an individually adaptable mask. Plastic tubes filled with a gadolinium solution were used as MRA markers. The tubes are imbedded into four plexiglas plates attached to the head ring. Since it was not possible to use a standard, circularly polarized head-coil with the MRA marker system, a special-purpose head-coil with a diameter of 300 mm was used.

Treatment Planning Workstation

Based on a standard HW configuration, a workstation system for radiosurgery treatment planning on an MRA basis has been developed. This allows the following functions to be performed:

- Stereotactic image registration
- Generation of vessel-tree views by maximum intensity projection (MIP)
- Definition of target volumes
- Calculation of target spheres
- Plan evaluation and optimization
- Three-dimensional plan visualization
- Printing of a planning protocol

If necessary, the acquired angiographic datasets may be corrected for spatial distortion using a distortion polynomial. This can be derived from a single phantom study with a phantom containing a rectangular grid of water-filled plastic tubes (Schmitt 1985; Schad et al. 1987).

For our scanner, in a phantom study with the aim of localizing in MRA datasets a predefined point within the stereotactic coordinate system (given by the crossing of two water-filled tubes), we found a deviation from the original coordinates of maximum 1.0 mm. This accuracy was tolerable for most cases of AVM radiosurgery, and therefore geometric correction was not necessary.

Fiducial markers are easily detectable in MRA slice images as a set of four point pairs. By an automatic registration of the fiducial marker system in the three-dimensional dataset transformation of image coordinates into stereotactic x, y, and z coordinates is possible.

Since it is very difficult to reconstruct mentally the anatomy of the vascular tree from a series of cross-sections, we have integrated MIP (Ehricke and Laub 1990) into the workstation system using an extremely speed-optimized projection algorithm. This allows generation of arbitrary views of the vascular tree. Exact definition of the target volume is a prerequisite for successful radiotherapy treatment. In radiosurgical angioma treatment the principal goal is to cover vessels to be occluded with high dose values while sparing surrounding tissue and vasculature. Angiographic projection images provide a good overview of vascular anatomy and permit delineation of vessels of interest. However, they fail to reveal the anatomy of adjacent stationary tissue such as vital brain structures. This information may be derived from the original slice images. Therefore one of the basic design concepts of the planning system has been to permit the simultaneous display of both projection and slice images.

Figure 1 demonstrates the setup of the image display field on the planning workstation. It is divided into four segments which, after selection of a patient study, are automatically filled with an original slice image and, transaxial, sagittal, and coronal main plane projections. When paging through the original dataset, the z position of the current slice is marked by a red orientation line in the sagittal and coronal projections. Zooming of a region of interest in a slice image is simultaneously performed on the projection images. This configuration provides the user with a means of easy orientation in three-dimensional space and permits simultaneous evaluation of stationary and flowing tissue. Target definition is carried out via mouse input either on a series of slice images or directly on projection images.

It has been demonstrated that for convergent beam irradiation with a single field the shape of high isodose surfaces may be considered spherical, and that tissue inhomogeneities do not influence the shape of relative dose distributions (Hartmann et al. 1985). After definition of a volume of interest the system automatically computes a treatment plan proposal by fitting it with a spherical volume. The sphere diameter allows selection of the collimator size. For smaller angiomas a single-field irradiation usually yields good treatment results. However, large angiomas with several feeding vessels must be treated with multiple fields. Therefore the system allows the combination of several fields for a treatment plan.

Three-dimensional visualization of a treatment plan is achieved by a cine-loop display showing the rotating vascular tree with color-coded target vessels (Fig. 2). For this purpose the target vasculature within a certain isodose region is determined by applying the MIP algorithm limited to the target volume. For every viewing angle the results of this targeted MIP are depicted into the already existing projection images by color coding. The aim of this display option is to

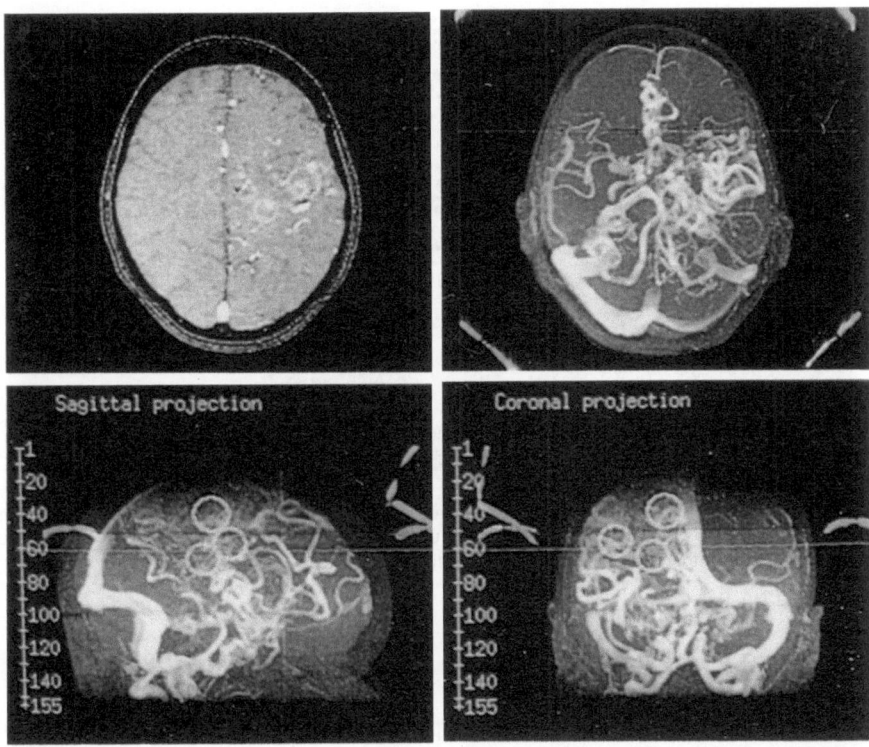

Fig. 1. Display configuration on our three-dimensional graphics workstation system. The display screen is divided into four segments showing a slice image from the original dataset (*upper left*) together with transaxial (*upper right*), sagittal (*lower left*), and coronal (*lower right*) main plane projections. In this case three targets were used in order to cause necrosis of arteriovenous shunts

facilitate the process of obtaining an idea of the three-dimensional spatial configuration of isodose surfaces and adjacent vasculature.

The planning process is completed by printing a treatment protocol containing field parameters such as stereotactic isocenter coordinates, collimator size, and average isocenter depth.

Results and Conclusions

Our planning approach has been evaluated by a clinical study with the goal of comparing it to a conventional method on the basis of X-ray angiography. With the conventional method irradiation parameters (isocenter coordinates, collimator size, average isocenter depth) are derived from pairs of frontal and lateral radiographic projections.

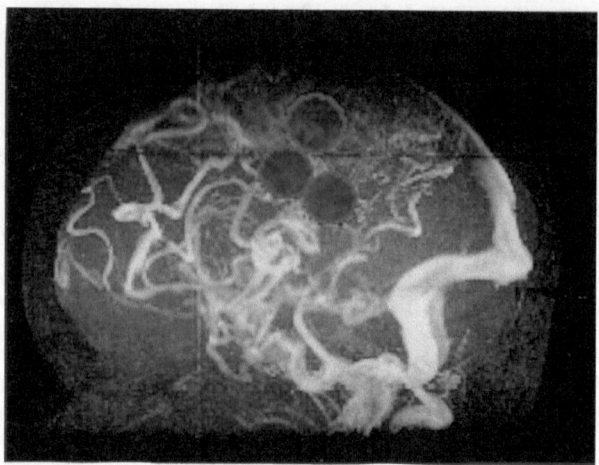

Fig. 2. Sample three-dimensional projection image from a cine-loop display showing the rotating vascular tree with color-coded target vasculature. This function allows easy plan evaluation by giving a spatial impression of target spheres and vasculature

The results show that the MRA approach possesses high clinical practicality and allows convenient and exact delineation of target vasculature due to the true three-dimensionality and the high vascular contrast of the image data. Conventional angiography may provide additional information with respect to the distinction between arterial and venous flow (hemodynamics).

We have demonstrated that for stereotactic radiosurgery geometric distortion of MRA datasets is not a handicap. For other stereotactic applications requiring a more precise coordinate localization, the use of our correction approach should allow similar results to be obtained.

Although with the MRA-based approach problems regarding the localization and treatment of very small lesions are encountered, the method has several significant advantages: (a) the possibility of providing vasculature and neuro-anatomic soft-tissue structures with a single modality; (b) true three-dimensionality of image data; and (c) noninvasiveness, easy follow-up.

In summary we conclude that stereotactic applications will certainly benefit from the introduction of MRA as an imaging modality for treatment planning. In this context the role of three-dimensional graphics workstations should not be underestimated. Only by making available to physicians easy-to-use and reliable planning tools is it possible to introduce new modalities and methods into clinical routine treatment planning. We are optimistic that improved availability of both MR scanners and planning workstation systems in the clinical routine environment will enhance the preoperative value of MRA in the near future.

References

Edelman R, Wentz KU, Mattle HP, O'Reilly G, Candia G, Liu C, Zhao B, Kjellberg RN, Davis KR (1989) Intracerebral arteriovenous malformations: evaluation with selective MR angiography and venography. Radiology 173: 831–837

Ehricke H-H, Laub G (1990) Integrated 3D display of brain anatomy and intracranial vasculature in MR imaging. J Comput Assist Tomogr 5: 846–852

Engenhart, R, Kimming BN, Höver K-H et al. (1990) Stereotactic single high dose radiation therapy of benign intracranial angiomas. Int J Radiat Oncol Biol Phys 19: 1021–1026

Hartmann GH, Schlegel W, Sturm V, Kober B, Pastyr O, Lorenz WJ (1985) Cerebral radiation surgery using moving field irradiation at a linear accelerator facility. Int J Radiat Oncol Biol Phys 11: 1185–1192

Herman GT, Liu HK (1979) Three-dimensional display of human organs from computed tomograms. Comput Graph Image Process 9: 1–21

Laub G, Kaiser W (1988) MR angiography with gradient motion refocussing. J Comput Assist Tomogr 12: 377–382

Leksell DG (1987) Stereotactic radiosurgery: present status and future trends. Neurol Res 9: 60–68

Leksell L (1951) The stereotaxic method and radiosurgery of the brain. Acta Chir Scand 102: 316–319

Marchal G, Bosmans H, Fraeyenhoven L, Wilms G, van Hecke P, Plets C, Baert AL (1990) Intracranial vascular lesions: optimization and clinical evaluation of three-dimensional time-of-flight MR angiograpy. Radiology 175: 443–448

Podgorsak EB, Pike GB, Olivier A, Pla M, Souhami L (1989) Radiosurgery with high energy photon beams: a comparison among techniques. Int J Radiat Oncol Biol Phys 16: 857–865

Ruggieri P, Laub G (1989) Intracranial circulation: pulse-sequence considerations in three-dimensional MR-angiography. Radiology 171: 785–779

Schad L, Lott S, Schmitt F, Sturn V, Lorenz WJ (1987) Correction of spatial distortion in MR imaging: a prerequisite for accurate stereotaxy. J Comput Assist Tomogr 3: 499–505

Schmitt F (1985) Correction of geometrical distortions in MR-images. In: Lemke HU, (ed) Computer assisted radiology. Springer, Berlin Heidelberg New York, pp 15–23

Souhami L, Olivier A, Podgorsak EB, Pla M, Pike B (1990) Radiosurgery of cerebral arteriovenous malformations with dynamic stereotactic irradiation. Int J Radiat Oncol Biol Phys 19: 775–782

Clinical and Experimental Observations Concerning Treatment Planning in Mantle Field Irradiation

D. Matthaei, M. Goltermann, K. Dieckmann, S. Sehlen,
G. Kaiser, V. Geppert, H. Kirschner, E. Dühmke, R.-P. Müller,
U. Rühl, N. Willich, and V. Diehl

Introduction

Clinically successful results with irradiation in Hodgkin's disease using shaped fields for supra- and infradiaphragmatic treatment were first reported by Kaplan. Since that time the large field technique has experienced wide variations concerning the shape of the fields, the fractionation, and the use of special absorbers [6]. Some of the geometric variants can be ascribed to different opinions concerning the "lymphatic organ," which is defined as the sum of the lymph node localizations in one field [5].

To perform quality assessment we examined a variety of different mantle field shapes over the past 3 years used by different centers in the German Hodgkin's Disease Study Group [8]. These were from patients with early stages of the disease, treated by radiotherapy alone [11]. Most of these fields were generally correct; however, minor deviations are reported here. To evaluate the planning performance of clinical radiotherapists, we sent films of one of our patients to 20 centers, asking for the design of a mantle field.

Materials and Methods

In the German Hodgkin's Lymphoma Study Group plain films and treatment planning materials from different centers were collected for patients in pathological stages I and II without certain risk factors who were treated by radiotherapy alone. The concise clinical and diagnostic material from these patients was tested by a panel. From 74 patients the results of "too small" or "too large" fields were reported for about 40 plannings, with variation due to the panelist. These were not counted as faults in the study. The distribution of these minor "mistakes" is given in Fig. 2. Unfortunately, the study's results are hardly comparable in terms of geometry. To attain digitally comparable results concerning mantle field borders, the films of an 18-year-old woman with a stage IIB

Klinik und Poliklinik für Strahlentherapie, Zentrum Radiologie, Universitätsklinik Göttingen, Robert-Koch-Straße 40, 3400 Göttingen, FRG

Advanced Radiation Therapy Tumor Response
Monitoring and Treatment Planning
Breit (Editor-in-Chief)
© Springer-Verlag, Berlin Heidelberg 1992

nodular sclerosis Hodgkin's disease without bulky disease were sent to 20 participating radiotherapists of the German Hodgkin's Disease Study Group. These colleagues were asked to design opposing mantle fields for this specific patient. We received differently designed mantle field volumes from 15 hospitals. Using a personal computer, the anterior and posterior fields were digitized and mounted on a matrix containing the borders of the heart, the lungs, claviculae, mandibulae, tenth thoracic vertebra, and the humeri. The results of these calculations are shown in Fig. 3.

Results and Discussion

One pair of collected mantle planning films is shown in Fig. 1. These images demonstrate a very individual solution, where a well-defined recommendation (Kaplan) was given for anatomical borders. Figure 2 summarizes the smaller mistakes for the different regions that have been criticized by the panelists. It is obvious that major deviations appear in the mediastinum, the lower parts of the axillae, and in the neck region. These minor deviations did not exclude the patients from the study. Twelve patients showed major deviations which are not included in Fig. 2. Figure 3 presents the anterior and posterior mantle shapes of 15 fields obtained in this study. The area covered by all fields demonstrates the smallest volume from the proposals of the clinical participants. This inner border outlines the volume which would have been irradiated safely by all institutions. The observation of clinical material here demonstrates that opinions concerning the shape of mantle fields show a similar variation as the daily port films, which has been reported recently [3, 10]. Our observations allow certain suggestions for the planning of mantle fields in accordance with the literature. Of course, these recommendations have not as yet been deduced from clinical treatment outcome.

Thus a block from posterior for the cervical spinal cord should be used if it does not obscure known lymphoma involvement. This block should touch the inner borders of the vertebral archs. A similar block, in our opinion, should not be used in anterior fields. The upper borders should encompass the mastoids and touch the floor of the mouth, to cover safely the upper cervical nodes. It is also important to treat the axillary and supra-/infraclavicular nodes without underdosage and to shield the upper outer part of the caput humeri to prevent shrinking of the joint capsule. Sparing the female breast may at least in parts require a special fixation technique. The lower border of the axilla normally (without involvement) matches the level of the base of the ninth thoracic vertebra. The lung at the thoracic side should be included for the diameter of two ribs (1.5 cm) at the top and should approach one-half the diameter of a rib (0.5 cm) at the bottom. The hili should be included with a 3 cm safety margin, and computed tomography planning is required [7]. The upper border of the

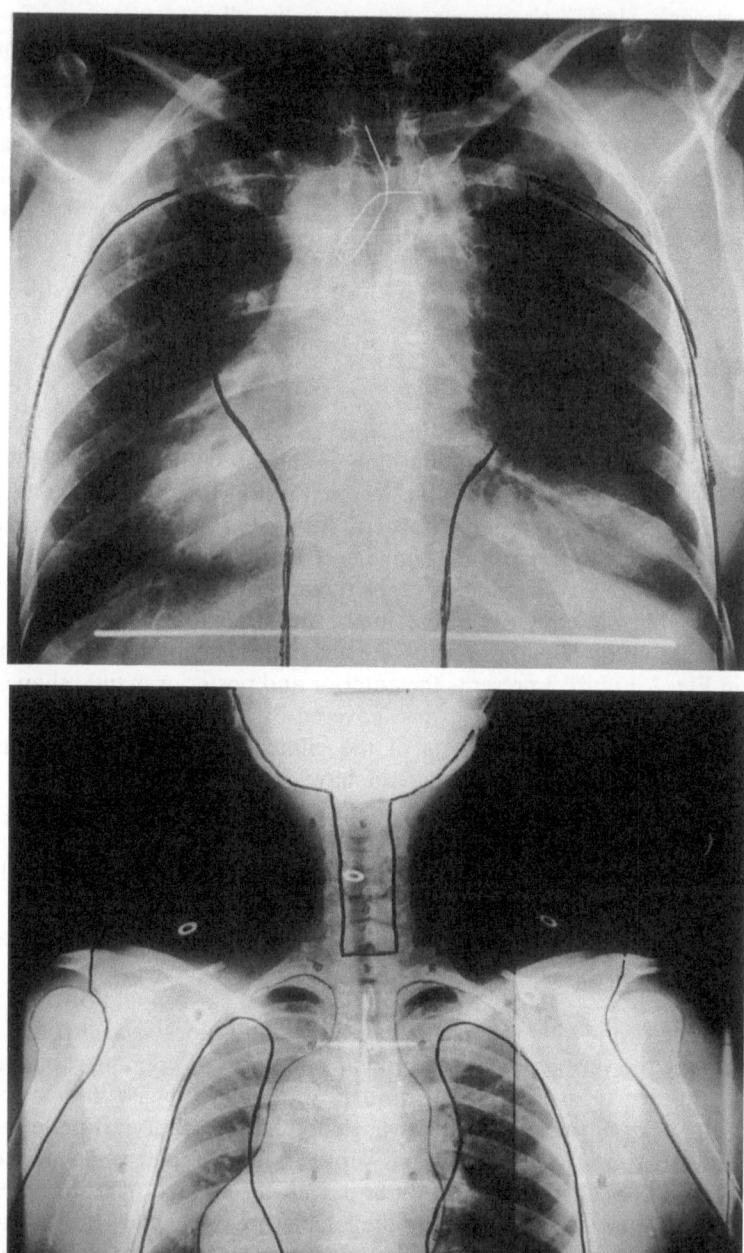

Fig. 1a, b. Two different examples of a planning film for mantle irradiation in prone position. Film **a** was criticized because of incomplete imaging (axillae) and unblocked cervical spinal cord. The film in **b** was accepted by the panel with minor restriction (the contours of the lungs are shown additionally)

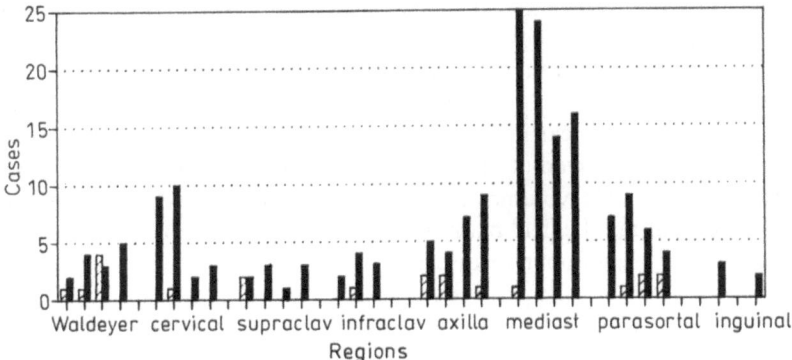

Fig. 2. After evaluation of clinical materials from 74 patients (X-rays, portals, planning documents), minor corrections were suggested for the different regions in the mantle fields by a panel of four members. Here the number of corrections is given for each anatomic region (infradiaphragmatic results included). *Black bars*, fields judged too small; *hatched bars*, fields considered too small

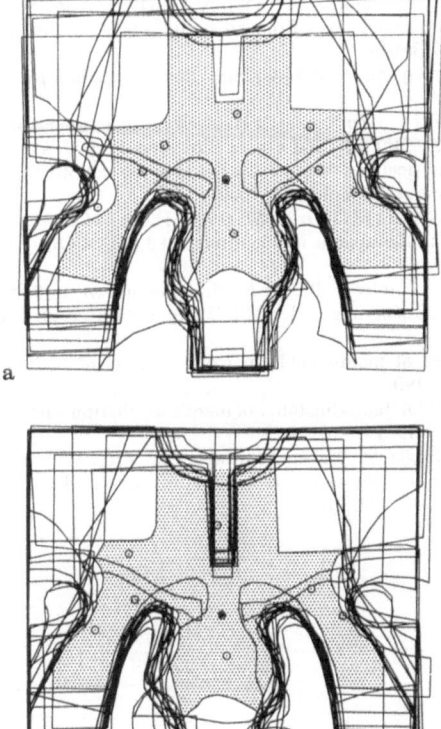

Fig. 3a, b. For the test patients from 15 hospitals a mantle field proposal was received from ventral and dorsal. Here the entire fields are depicted with a contour for the pulmo, claviculae, humeri, and tenth vertebra. The area covered by all proposed fields (*shaded*) obviously is rather small

lung blocks should approach the clavicular to 1.5 times the claviculae diameter from anterior and reach their lower margin from posterior [6]. The lower border should be at the base of tenth vertebra as the junction to a subdiaphragmatic radiotherapy.

Our results from clinical images and the literature suggest that opinions concerning mantle field irradiation differ. The panelists tended more to regard the planned mantle field volumes as too small than as too large. Therefore we recommend that mantle field planning be carried out generously so as not to miss subclinical or even apparent disease.

References

1. Bonadonna G, Valagussa B (1990) Influence of clinical trials on current treatment strategy for Hodgkin's disease. Int J Radiat Oncol Biol Phys 19: 209–218
2. Dühmke E, Brix F, Hebbinghaus D, Jensen JM (1986) Befundorientierte CT-gestützte Optimierung der Dosisverteilung mit Hilfe von individuellen Feldblenden und Kompensatoren. In: Frommhold W, Hübener K-H (eds) Computertomografie in der Strahlentherapie. Thieme, Stuttgart, pp 100–108
3. Graham ML, Cheng AY, Geer LY, Binns WR, Vannier MW, Wong JW (1991) A method to analyze 2-dimensional daily radiotherapy portal images from an online fiber-optic imaging system. Int J Radiat Oncol Biol Phys 20: 613–619
4. Hoppe RT (1988) The contemporary management of Hodgkin's disease. Radiology 169: 297–304
5. Hulshof M, Vanuytsel L, van den Bogaert W, van der Schueren E (1989) Localization errors in mantel-field irradiation for Hodgkin's disease. Int J Radiat Oncol Biol Phys 17: 679–683
6. Page V, Gardner A, Karzmark CJ (1970) Physical and dosimetric aspects of the radiotherapy of malignant lymphomas. I. The mantle technique. Radiology 96: 609–618
7. Rostock RA, Siegelman SS, Lenhard RE, Wharam MD, Order SE (1983) Thoracic CT scanning for mediastinal Hodgkin's disease: results and therapeutic implications. Int J Radiat Oncol Biol Phys 9: 1451–1457
8. Roth S, Dühmke E, Kirschner H, Willich N, Müller R, Bleher A, Pfreundschuh M, Löffler M, Diehl V (1990) Radiotherapeutische Qualitätssicherung in der BMFT-Studie Morbus Hodgkin (HD4). Strahlenther Onkol 166: 584–587
9. Svahn-Tapper G (1970) Dosimetric studies of mantle-fields in Co60 therapy of malignant lymphomas. Acta Radiol Ther Phys Biol 9: 190
10. Taylor BW, Mendenhall NP, Million RR (1990) Reproducibility of mantle irradiation with daily imaging films. Int J Radiat Oncol Biol Phys 19: 149–151
11. Tubiana M, Henry-Amar M, Hayat M, Burger M, Qasim M, Somers R, Sizoo W, van der Schueren E (1984) The EORTC treatment of early stages of Hodgkin's disease: the role of radiotherapy. Int J Radiat Oncol Biol Phys 10: 197–210

The Impact of Imaging Modalities on Patient Management: Quantitative Assessment Using Decision Analysis

C.F. Hess, H. Schmidberger, and M. Bamberg

Introduction

Modern imaging modalities such as ultrasound, computed tomography, and magnetic resonance imaging play an essential role in the diagnostic work-up strategy for a majority of cancer patients [2, 3]. However, relative little systematic work has focused on effective selection of diagnostic procedure, interpretation of results, and consideration of their therapeutic consequences [4–6]. The goals of our methodologic considerations were to assess quantitatively the clinical impact of these principal components of oncologic strategy. For this purpose specific tools of decision analysis — a set of mathematical rules for simplifying complex decisions — are discussed [5]. These are demonstrated by the implication of noninvasive diagnosis of splenic disease on patient management in Hodgkin's disease.

Methodologic Considerations

Measurement of Diagnostic Performance. For each imaging procedure traditional measures of diagnostic performance, such as sensitivity (SE; true-positive rate) and specificity (SP: true-negative rate), are strongly dependent on the specific choice of decision criteria [4, 5]. The tendency of an observer to overread or underread a test result greatly affects these measures. If quantitative decision criteria are used by an observer, the confidence in a positive or negative decision changes considerably with varying confidence thresholds (Fig. 1). Thus, a single pair of numbers representing SE and SP is not entirely adequate as a description of diagnostic performance. These limitations may be largely overcome by the construction of receiver operating characteristic (ROC) curves (Fig. 2). If the confidence threshold is varied over a wide range of repeated experiments, a variety of $(1 - SP, SE)$ pairs is generated which can be plotted as a set of points in a unique square. Similar curves may result from visual detection

Abteilung für Strahlentherapie, Radiologische Universitätsklinik, Hoppe-Seyler-Str.3, 7400 Tübingen, FRG

Advanced Radiation Therapy Tumor Response
Monitoring and Treatment Planning
Breit (Editor-in-Chief)
© Springer-Verlag, Berlin Heidelberg 1992

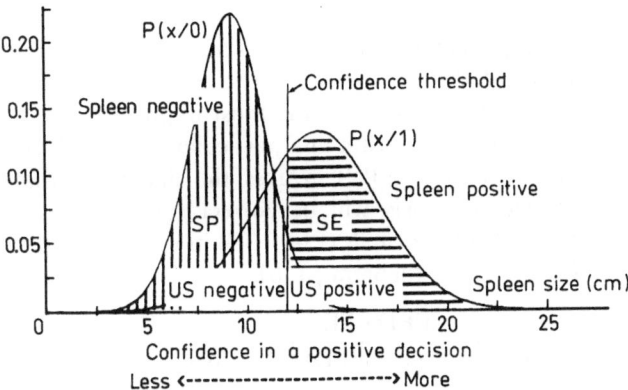

Fig. 1. Probability density distributions of the longitudinal diameter of the spleen, as measured by ultrasound, for two groups of patients with $[P(x/1)]$ and without $[P(x/0)]$ lymphomatous involvement of the spleen. A confidence threshold (*vertical line*) separates positive from negative decisions. Varying the threshold considerably influences the confidence in a positive or negative decision

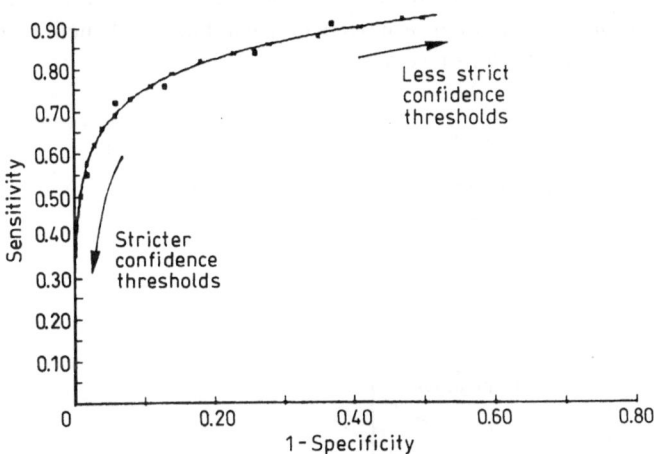

Fig. 2. ROC analysis of splenic size in Hodgkin's disease, as measured by ultrasound. Systematic variation of confidence thresholds generates a variety of (1 − SP, SE) pairs, which are plotted in a unique square

experiments [4]. Each ROC curve indicates the trade-offs between SE and SP that are available from a diagnosis system and thus enables a critical review of diagnostic data. The discrimination capacity of a particular imaging modality is expressed by the location of its ROC curve. The farther upward and farther to the left a curve is located, the better is the discrimination capacity.

Probability of Disease: Impact of Imaging Modality. ROC curves cannot be used to compare tests in a specific patient because they do not reflect the pretest probability PPD (prevalence) of disease (or of a specific finding). Posttest probabilities of disease or predictive values are the most important terms to assess quantitatively the impact of a test result in a particular patient. Positive (PPV) and negative predictive values (NPV) express the likelihood that a positive or negative radiologic diagnosis will be correct. They are greatly affected by the variable proportion of normals (1 − PPD) in each investigative series and can be calculated by Bayes' theorem [4–6]:

$$PPV = \frac{PPD * SE}{PPD * SE + (1 - PPD) * (1 - SP)}$$

$$NPV = \frac{(1 - PPD) * SP}{(1 - PPD) * SP + PPD * (1 - SE)}$$

For example, in an examination with 87% sensitivity and 90% specificity PPV ranges from 0.9 at 50% disease prevalence to 0.5 at 10% disease prevalence (Fig. 3). Under typical clinical conditions (PPD < 0.3) PPV is strongly dependent on PPD, while NPV is less variable and tends to be high. In general, tests have large effects when the PPD is intermediate, or when the test result does not confirm the clinical impression. Patients are particularly unlikely to benefit from testing when the PPD is very high or very low.

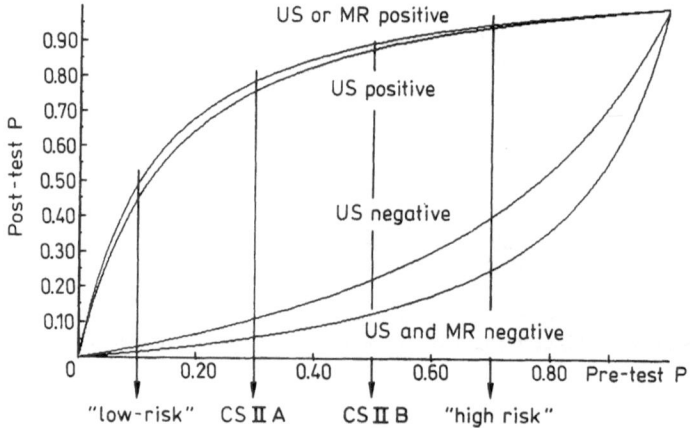

Fig. 3. Pretest and posttest probability (*P*) of splenic involvement in Hodgkin's disease, clinical stage (*CS*) I/II. Posttest P is strongly dependent on pretest P (low risk, CS I/II A, CS I/II B, high risk). In the positive case (PPV) the curve shows a steep increase for small pretest P and flattens with greater P; the opposite is true in the negative case (1 − NPV). As compared to ultrasound (*US*) measurement of splenic size alone (here: SP = 0.9, SE = 0.74; see Fig. 2) the additional consideration of magnetic resonance (*MR*) visualization of individual lymphomatous lesions (SE = 0.87, SP = 0.9) may be helpful in some clinical situations if both US and MRI examinations are negative. However, there is only minimal improvement in the positive case

Therapeutic Consequences of Test Results. Predictive values do not take into account the correct classification benefits and misclassification costs associated with the possible test results. For that purpose the oncologist must measure the likelihood that the result of a test will cause a patient management threshold to be exceeded [2, 4, 5]. These thresholds are determined by the expected "utilities" (survival, relapse-free survival, survival conditioned by treatment sequelae) of treatment alternatives in the case of correct and of incorrect diagnostic decision (Fig. 4) [5]. For each treatment modality and for each probability (P) of disease the expected utility EU(P) can be easily calculated as the weighted sum of EU(0) and EU(1): EU(P) = (1 − P) ∗ EU(0) + P ∗ EU(1), with EU(0) and EU(1) being the stage-determined expected utilities (e.g., cure rates in Hodgkin's disease with and without splenic involvement). For any value of P the treatment strategy with maximum EU(P) is the optimal one. In the example shown in Fig. 4, the management threshold for immediate radiotherapy (without using staging laparatomy) is P1 = 0.08. Figure 3 shows that probabilities of abdominal disease are less than 0.08 if there is a low clinical risk of abdominal disease (e.g., Hodgkin's disease with only mediastinal involvement [1]) *and* if the results of ultrasound examination of the spleen are negative. In all patients with Hodgkin's disease in clinical stage IIA (PPD = 0.3) laparatomy is indicated, since neither the management threshold for immediate radiotherapy nor the threshold for immediate chemotherapy (P2 = 0.80) is exceeded, regardless of the result of ultrasound examination. The additional use of magnetic resonance imaging may potentially obviate the need for laparatomy in the case of negative

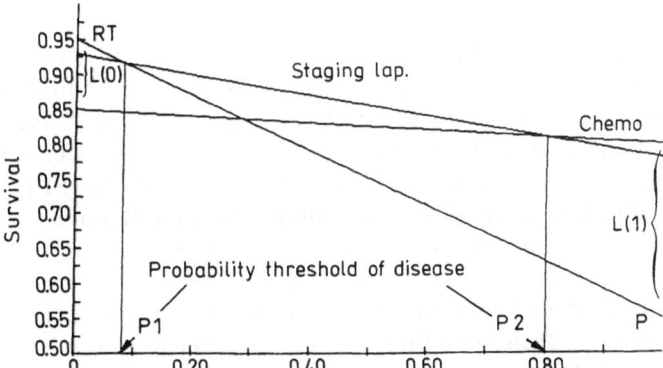

Fig. 4. Expected utility (EU; here, expected survival) for three different management strategies in Hodgkin's disease, CS I/II A (*MPA*-RT, immediate mantle and periaortic radiotherapy; *Chemo*, immediate multiagent chemotherapy; *Lap*, initial staging laparatomy, followed by MPA-RT if Lap is negative, or by Chemo if Lap is positive). For an individual patient with probability P of abdominal disease the "utility line" with maximum EU(P) represents the optimal treatment strategy. The utility lines for the management alternatives intersect at the management thresholds P1 = L(Lap)/L(1) and P2 = 1 − L(Lap)/L(0). L(0) and L(1) are the differences between the expected survival of RT and Chemo, in Hodgkin's disease pathologic stage PS I/II A and PS III A, respectively. In this example there is a mortality rate of L(LAP) = 2%

test results. However, thresholds P1 and P2 may vary considerably if the utilities of the treatment alternatives or the individual risk of laparatomy change.

Discussion

The capacity of current imaging techniques such as ultrasound, computed tomography, and magnetic resonance imaging in the staging process of malignant tumors has been well accepted. However, high technology advances in diagnostic capability, rather than making decisions simpler, have tended to increase the complexity of medical decision making. Overlapping indications for various diagnostic procedures, differences in their diagnostic efficiency, invasiveness, or risk, and high costs have made physicians aware of the need to consider the choice of procedure carefully [2–6]. In particular, the selection of diagnostic procedures, interpretation of results, and estimation of correct classification benefits and misclassification costs must be taken into account. Our analysis of these principal components of oncologic strategy reveals several aspects which may be unexpected for the unaware clinician.

Firstly, the tendency of the diagnostic physician to overread or to underread a specific test result greatly influences traditional measures of diagnostic performance such as SE and SP. Thus, a single pair of these terms is not entirely adequate to describe the capacity of an imaging test. This limitation may be largely overcome by the use of ROC analysis, a method which is based in mathematical decision theory and which was first developed in signal detection theory [4].

Secondly, the increment of diagnostic information yielded by a test result is considerably influenced by the PPD [6]. Patients are particularly unlikely to benefit from even highly accurate tests when the PPD is very high or very low. In contrast, the probability of disease may be greatly affected — even when the diagnostic capacity of the imaging modality is limited — if the PPD is intermediate, or if the test result does not confirm the clinical impression. Consequently, a thorough analysis of the pretest status is mandatory. In addition, since the posttest probability of one finding becomes the pre-test probability for the next, it is often more effective to perform tests sequentially rather than concurrently. When more than one test is considered, correlations between one test and another with respect to disease status must be taken into account.

Finally, the extent to which diagnosis needs to be pursued and refined depends primarily on the degree to which knowledge of it will influence patient prognosis and/or therapy [2, 3]. Consequently, the oncologist should estimate the probability thresholds of disease which must be exceeded for optimal therapeutic strategy. Using "utility analysis" it can easily be demonstrated how these thresholds may be determined by considering the stage-dependent rates of cure, relapse and sequelae for the available treatment modalities. In addition, the clinical impact of a suboptimal strategy may be quantitatively addressed.

Obviously, the issues and examples reported here are much simpler than most decision problems in oncologic practice. However, the methodologic considerations discussed may be helpful in the sense that they identify operative criteria for action. They should allow experts to discuss the decision-making process more precisely and identify areas of agreement and disagreement. The potential consequences of this analysis may be that fewer tests are performed, thereby decreasing morbidity, mortality, and hospital costs. In contrast to the general tendency of advanced medical technology to increase the cost of medical care, decision analysis may decrease it.

References

1. Aragon de la Cruz G, Cardenes H, Otero et al. (1989) Individual risk of abdominal disease in patients with stages I and II supradiaphragmatic Hodgkin's disease. Cancer 63: 1799–1803
2. Castellino RA (1988) Hodgkin disease: imaging studies and patient management. Radiology 169: 170–269
3. De Vita VT, Hellman S, Rosenberg SA (1989) Cancer. Principles and practice of oncology. Lippincott, Philadelphia
4. Gelfand DW, Ott DJ (1984) Methodologic considerations in comparing imaging methods. AJR 144: 1117–1121
5. Pauker SG, Kassirer JP (1987) Decision analysis. N Engl J Med 316: 250–258
6. Sox HC (1986) Probability theory in the use of diagnostic tests. An introduction to critical study of the literature. Ann Intern Med 104: 60–66

The Key to Evaluation of Cure Rate and Tissue Tolerance: Clear Dose Specification

U. Quast

The Dose Specification Dilemma

Curative radiotherapy of malignant diseases must provide maximal probability of uncomplicated cure. Cure rate and complication rate depend on many parameters. However, the parameters are often defined variously, determined differently, recorded nonuniformly, or reported incompletely, even as reported in clinical trials. The differences in dose values reported for the same treatment ($\pm$ 10%–20%) are larger than all dosimetrical and technical uncertainties together ($\pm$ 5%–10%) [1]. Thus, clear, comparable, and correct verbal, numerical, and graphic definition, determination, and description of the prescribed, planned, and performed radiotherapy treatment are crucial [1–4].

The Dualism of Treatment Optimization and Dose Specification

Combining the two tasks of radiotherapy — treatment optimization and dose specification — is the source of the dose specification dilemma. *Maximal probability of uncomplicated cure* requires a sufficiently high rate of tumor cell kill. Thus, depending on the concentration of tumor cells, a certain minimum dose is needed in each target volume. This minimum dose is a necessary condition for treatment plan optimization, but, not a sufficient condition, and thus — as a sole value — not suited for dose specification. *Treatment plan optimization* means chosing an irradiation technique and beam incidence, radiation quality and beam energy, field size, and dose weight which enable one to deliver a certain minimum dose to each target volume and to guarantee dose homogeneity. Dose specification must be representative for the biological effect in tumor cells and in organs at risk. As there is no simple measure for the biological effect which can be determined in vivo, the spatial and temporal distribution of absorbed dose is used as an approach.

Division of Clinical Radiation Physics, Department of Radiotherapy, Radiological Center, University Hospital, Hufelandstr. 55, 4300 Essen, FRG

Advanced Radiation Therapy Tumor Response Monitoring and Treatment Planning
Breit (Editor-in-Chief)
© Springer-Verlag, Berlin Heidelberg 1992

Target Volume Concept and Tolerance Dose Concept

In curative radiotherapy almost always two or more target volumes are involved, and the dose required as well as the dose tolerated is usually different for each target volume. This includes the following:

Target volume
    First-order: Demonstrated tumor plus subclinical disease
    Second- or third-order: Neighboring or distant tumor cell bearing tissue (e.g., lymphatic system)
    Oncological target volume: Tumor cell bearing tissue (including oncological uncertainties),
    Planning target volume: Tumer cell bearing tissue and safety margin (motion or organ-function displacements; position or alignment uncertainties, technical or dosimetrical uncertainties)
Dose specification point: Central in each target volume
    Reference points: Additional points for dose determination in complex or multiple target volumes and in organs at risk.

It is essential to provide for sufficient sparing of each neighboring vital organ at risk to maintain its organ function. For almost all organs this means that the part (V_{OaR}) irradiated with a dose lower than a tolerable level (D_{tol}) must be larger than the relative volume (V_{tol}) necessary to keep the vital function. There is one exception: in serial organ structures like the spinal cord *any* overdosage of any part of this organ at risk must be avoided.

Dose Specification

Specification of Dose to Target Volumes. The specified target absorbed dose assigned to a suitable point near the center of the target volume is taken as representative for the achieved spatial distribution of dose and thus for the biological effect on target cells.

Target absorbed dose
    Representative: Spatial distribution of total dose/Gy (and its distribution in time)
    Approximation: Dose at the dose specification point, at the center of each target volume, and the dose variance: $D_{TV,spec}$ ($D_{TV,min}$, $D_{TV, max}$)
Dose Specification Point
    Representative: For biological effect in the target volume
    Approximation: Point, representative for the spatial distribution of dose

Reproduceability: Described in terms of patient's anatomy, easy and accurate determination of dose

Requirements: Independent of treatment technique, insensitive to treatment uncertainties

Position: Central in each target volume, not at steep dose gradient

Suited for: Dose prescription and dose calculation, dose weighting and dose normalization, dose accumulation and dose reporting

Clear reporting of radiotherapy demands at least a triple of total dose values for each target volume. In addition, the minimum and maximum doses in the target volume are required to describe the dose variance, but neither is suitable for dose specification.

Dose Weighting and Normalization. There is only one method of beam weighting in accordance with the target volume concept: The weight should be the contribution of relative dose to the common dose specification point, all dose-modifying influences already taken into account. In complex or multiple target volumes additional reference points are needed for dose specification and beam weighting. One should be aware of the large discrepancies in dose distribution if other definitions are used for beam weighting. The beams should not be weighted to the maximum of each single beam because this is not relevant for the dose to the target volume. The absolute distribution of dose is relevant for biological effects. The relative distribution of dose — helpful for treatment planning — should always be normalized to the dose specification point (of first-order target volume).

Specification of Dose to Organs at Risk. The dose to organs at risk must be defined according to the tolerance dose concept:

Representative parameters: Spatial *and* temporal distribution of dose
Timing: Fractionation, OaR dose rate/Gy $\cdot$ min^{-1}
Dose distribution: $D_{OaR, frac}$/Gy, $D_{OaR,tot}$/Gy
Interactions: Time and dosage schedule of other treatment modalities
Reporting: $D_{max,frac}$, $D_{max,tot}$ V_{OaR} ($D_{max} < D_{tol}$) $> V_{tol}$.

Conclusion

A number of problems are discussed. The reasons for some confusions are shown. A common proposal for clear dose specification is given, in agreement with but extending the ICRU report [2] and its revised draft [3]. All radio-oncologists should be encouraged to follow these ICRU recommendations strictly.

References

1. Hendrickson FR (1988) Dose prescription dilemma. Int J Radiol Biol Phys 14: 595–596
2. ICRU (1978) Dose specification for reporting external beam therapy with photons and electrons. ICRU report 29
3. Landberg T et al (1991) ICRU report 50 (10. 1991) Prescribing, recording and reporting photon beam therapy, in press
4. Quast U, Glaeser L, Nocken A (1990) Precision in radiotherapy through clear dose specification. Proceedings of the 2nd European Mevatron-User's conference, Berlin, pp 247–260

Exact Planning of Surgical Interventions Based on Three-Dimensional Correlation Between Metastases and Liver Segments by Integration of Computed Tomography and Digital Subtraction Angiography Sequences

L. Köhler[1], N. Rilinger[2], A. Hewett[1], H. Niemann[2], and P. Jensch[1]

Introduction

An indispensable precondition to curative liver surgery is the exact topographic assignment of metastases to liver veins. Liver segments can thereby be identified and an assessment of operability achieved. This paper describes a computer-based front end for the three-dimensional combined presentation of results from computed tomography (CT) and digital subtraction angiography (DSA). Today there is a gap between the three-dimensional information requirements of surgeons and the various two-dimensional information modalities that di-agnositc procedures can supply. These modalities are brought together to form a spatial liver representation consisting of the transparent liver surface together with embedded metastases and veins. From this the surgeon can easily derive depictions from any viewpoint around the liver. The consideration of certain standards (UNIX, X Windows) gives portability to the system so that it can be used on a range of modern graphic workstations. Parallel algorithms and neural networks serve in reconstructing three-dimensional models of liver veins out of biplane angiographic images. CT sequences are used both to extract and to reconstruct the liver surface and to calculate the spatial extensions and locations of metastases. After identifying the main liver vein in CT and DSA images a normalization and fusion of the two image modalities is obtained.

Method

A variety of imaging tests for the evaluation of the liver is available. Which of these is the most sensitive for detection of focal hepatic lesions continues to be the subject of intense debate among investigators. Several studies have shown

[1] Angewandte Informatik, Universität Oldenburg, Fachbereich 10, Postfach 2503, 2900 Oldenburg, FRG
[2] Radiologie/Nuklearmedizin, Städtische Kliniken Oldenburg-Kreyenbrük, Dr. Eden Str. 10, 2900 Oldenburg, FRG

CT to be superior to ultrasound and radionuclide scintigraphy [1, 9]. To optimize surgical planning the surgeons must know which liver segments are involved by the disease. However, due to the complex liver anatomy and variations in the main liver veins, established imaging procedures such as CT can only approximately specify the liver segments. This may result in uncertainty regarding the surgical decision. Therefore it was the aim of this study to develop a computer-based fronted for the three-dimensional presentation of combined CT and DSA examinations to overcome this problem.

The study was performed in patients with known colorectal carcinoma and suspected liver metastases and who were potential candidates for curative partial hepatectomy.

CT scans were obtained on a Siemens Somatom DRH system with 4-mm sections at 4 to 8-mm intervals throughout the whole liver (Fig. 1). Immediately after CT we performed angiography during arterial portography with injection of contrast material through an angiographic catheter placed in the superior mesenteric artery. We used 60 ml Iohexol combined with 30 ml physiological saline solution so that we obtained a total volume of 90 ml. The liver was examined by fast scan mode. Contrast material was injected by using a computer-assisted application pump 20 s before scanning, and then continued throughout the rapid run. Directly after this procedure the patient was transferred to retrograde presentation of the hepatic veins using a special balloon catheter placed in the upper part of the inferior vena cava. The total amount of contrast material used for the angiographic procedures and CT examination was between 150 and 210 ml.

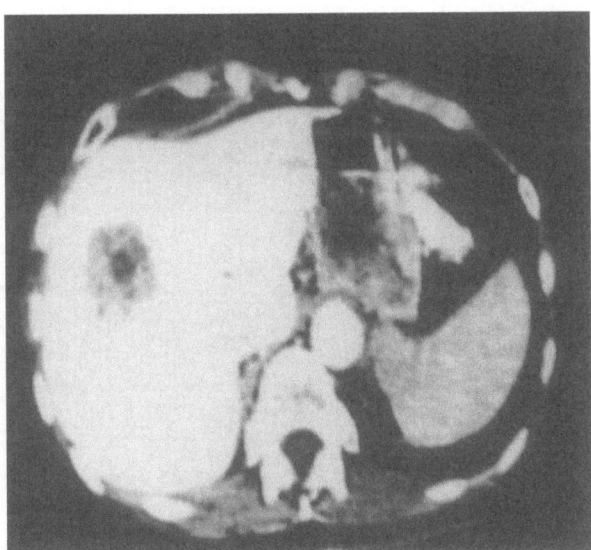

Fig. 1. CT slice showing the liver contour and a metastasis (artificial markers are added)

Image Processing

To be able to perform integrated imaging repetitively, we defined standards and processing facilities for each individual imaging system (CT, DSA). Both image modalities are described by labeled graphs. Angiograms are prestructured in an object-oriented and model-based way. Classification and measuring is performed by an adaptive matching and region-growing process. The center lines of vessels found in angiograms define a graph in which the nodes are the bifurcation points, and the edges reflect the course of the vessel branches. An associated list structure carries the coordinates, their diameter at certain fixpoints, and labels used for interrelating. CT data is treated as rigid bodies in a CAD-like way, where the homogeneity and isolation of regions of interest is one decisive factor. The connectivity between modality graphs is guided by a "rubber-band" approach, performing — with an appropriate metric and energy function — and elastic matching. The labeling and matching process is organized in the following way:

1. Evaluation of biplane angiograms, normalization, labeling of bifurcations, definition of reference points (DSA landmarks). The thinned vessels are used for three-dimensional reconstruction, applying CAD techniques and contextual knowledge where reconstruction is ambiguous. The three-dimensional branch model may be extended in space by using diameter information. This leads to a vessel tree within a DSA three-dimensional space.
2. Evaluation of CT data by contour-extraction and region-growing algorithms, normalization of regions in CT three-dimensional space, defining reference points (CT landmarks).

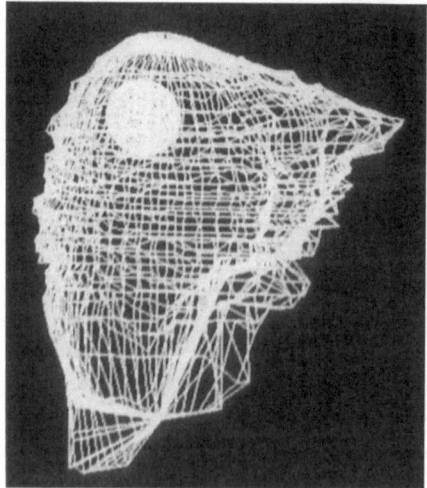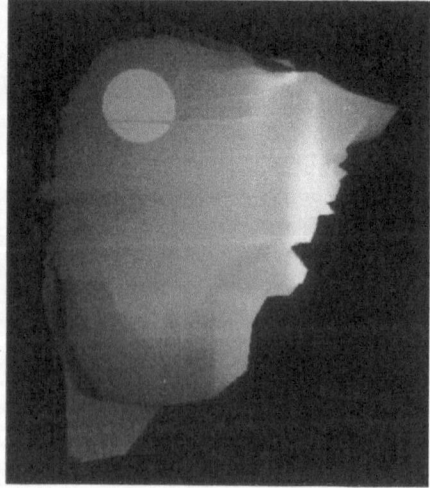

a
b

Fig. 2a, b. Liver surface with embedded metastasis (wire frame, artificially illuminated)

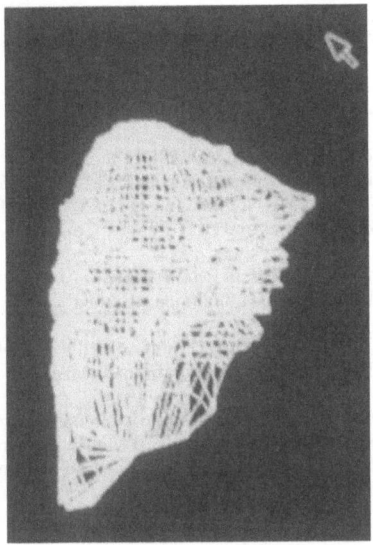

Fig. 3. Liver surface with embedded vessels (wire frame)

3. Matching of DSA and CT three-dimensional space using morphological information and reference points.

We have set up an environment to merge vessel trees, obtained from postprocessed biplane angiograms, with three-dimensional CT contours. The fusion of processed images results in innovative three-dimensional models (Figs. 2, 3), whose constituents may be depicted in different colors, at arbitrary angles, and annotated with information.

Conclusion

The fusion of all relevant information into a single object representation could facilitate surgical decisions. Different image modalities are interrelated in an object-oriented way. This approach for presenting diagnostic information can thus lead from an image-based diagnosis to an object-based one. Depictions from any viewpoint around the three-dimensional object help in assessing and interrelating pathological findings.

References

1. Alderson PO, Adams DF, McNeil BJ (1983) Computed tomography, ultrasound, and scintigraphy of the liver in patients with colon or breast carcinoma: a prospective comparison. Radiology 149: 225–230

2. Adson MA (1983) Cannon lecture: hepatic metastases in perspective. AJR 140: 695–700
3. Becker N, Frentzel-Beyme R, Wagner G (1984) Krebsatlas der Bundesrepublik Deutschland, 2nd edn. Springer, Berlin Heidelberg New York
4. Foster JH (1982) Treatment of metastatic cancer to liver. In: Devita VT Jr, Hellman S, Rosenberg SA (eds) Cancer: principles and practice of oncology. Lippincott, Philadelphia, pp 1553–1563
5. Jensch P, Niemann H (1990) Multimedia medical communication with ISDN technologies — early experiences. SPIE (Symposium Medical Imaging IV, Newport Beach Calif) 1234: 610–616
6. Jensch P, Köhler L, Schwanke J, Hewett A, Reil G-H, Rilinger N, Niemann H (1990) Extended coronary trees by neural network based fusion of DSA-sequences and ECT-images. Computers in cardiology, Sept 90, Computer Society
7. Köhler L, Schwanke J, Hewett A, Reil G-H, Niemann H, Jensch P (1990) Fusion von Bild-modalitäten zur verbesserten Diagnose für kardiochirurgische Maßnahmen. Biomed Techn 35: 286
8. Köhler L, Schwanke J, Hewett A, Reil G-H, Niemann H, Jensch P (1991) Integrated diagnosis by fusion of angiographic and scintigraphic scenes. 1st European conference on biomedical engineering, Nice, Febr 91
9. Rilinger N, Munz DL, Niemann H, Halbfa HJ (1990) I.a./i.v. immunoscintigraphy in comparison with i.a./i.v. contrast. CT using the Tc 99m labeled monoclonal antibody BW 431/26 in the detection of liver metastases, in nuclear medicine, quantitative analysis in imaging and function. Schattauer, Stuttgart, pp 556–560

Magentic Resonance Imaging Assisted Localization of Tumor and Applicator for Brachytherapy of Cancer of the Esophagus

F.J. Prott, R. Pötter, G. Kovacs, B. Lenzen, and U. Schaefer

Introduction

Despite major advantages in surgical and radiotherapeutic techniques, the survival of patients with esophagus cancer is extremely poor. For all therapeutic methods the 5-year survival rate is not more than 4%–6% [3]. Some investigations, especially Japanese, have shown better local control of esophageal cancer in association with intracavitary irradiation after external irradiation [3–6]. For an effective combination therapy (tele-brachytherapy) of esophageal cancer the exact delineation of the intra- and extra-esophageal tumor in relation to the neighboring structures is necessary.

Normally the size of the target is determined by endoscopy and barium swallow 1 day before treatment, in which the length for intracavitary irradiation is extended beyond the superior and inferior margins of the tumor by 2.5–4 cm [5]. For improved determination of target volume for brachytherapy magnetic resonance imaging (MRI) assisted treatment planning with a dummy applicator for esophageal brachytherapy has been used at our institution since October 1989. MRI makes possible the imaging of tumor and surrounding critical structures in any plane, in particular along the axis of the applicator.

Materials and Methods

Since October 1989, 21 patients with primary inoperable esophageal cancer or recurrence after surgery were examined by planning MRI of the thorax. In 12 of these patients a dummy applicator was inserted into the esophagus filled with diluted gadolinium DTPA (1:200). Nine patients did not receive this dummy device because of nearly complete esophagus stenosis. The outside diameter of the dummy applicator corresponds the applicator used for brachytherapy (diameter 4 mm). After the dummy applicator is introduced into the esophagus, MRI is performed parallel to the axis of the applicator in paracoronal and

Radioonkologie, Klinik und Poliklinik für Strahlentherapie, Westfälische Wilhelms-Universität Münster, Albert-Schweitzer-Str. 33, 4400 Münster, FRG

Advanced Radiation Therapy Tumor Response Monitoring and Treatment Planning
Breit (Editor-in-Chief)
© Springer-Verlag, Berlin Heidelberg 1992

parasagittal and different sagittal planes. Because of the high soft-tissue contrast in MRI and the very good delineation of the dummy, the tumor, target volume, critical structures, and even the dummy applicator are clearly demarcated (Figs. 1, 2).

After this procedure an X-ray film is made showing the dummy applicator and the swallowed barium. The next step is the electronic superimposition of the MR image and the X-ray film showing the dummy and the barium swallow together with the individual dose distributions, using the tracheal bifurcation as reference structure. The pretreatment procedure is carried out on the basis of the planning MR images. The procedure is completed by the help of a subtrascope, which allows images to be superimposed electronically onto the simulation film, showing the resulting MRI on simulation film on a screen. This method has also been used in several other anatomic regions (see Pötter et al., pp. 555, 631, 667, this volume) [7–9]. The tumor volume and critical structures can then be drawn from the MRI on the localization film. The target volume as defined on this film is the basis for the calculation of the individual dose distribution. On the day on which brachytherapy is performed the position of the esophageal treatment applicator is documented on X-ray film. This position should be compared with the pretreatment planning subtraction film showing the dummy, tumor volume,

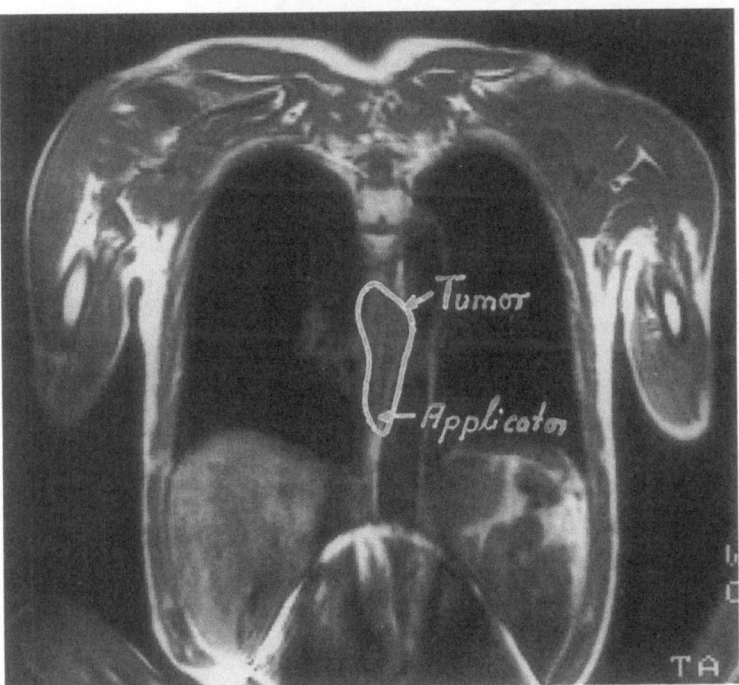

Fig. 1. Paracoronal MR image (T1-weighted) showing the esophagus, with the gadolinium DTPA marked dummy applicator and the well demarcated tumor

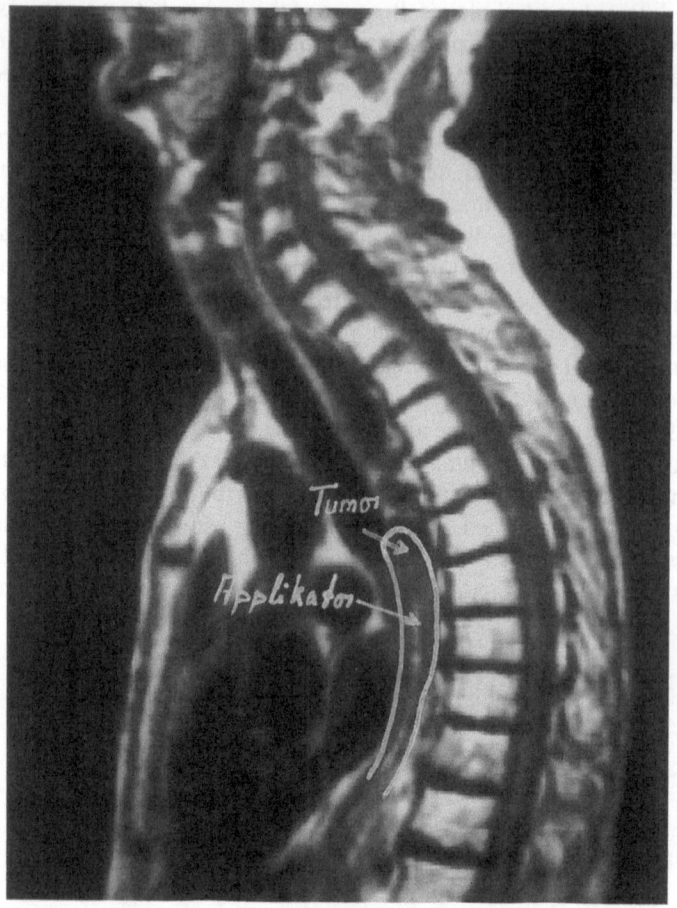

Fig. 2. Sagittal MR image (T1-weighted) showing the esophagus, gadolinium DTPA marked dummy applicator, and well-demarcated tumor. The critical organs such as heart, aorta, and spinal cord are precisely delineated

critical, radiosensitive structures, and individual dose distributions (Fig. 3). High dose rate intracavitary brachytherapy is carried out when individual tumor length, dose distributions, and reference points are prescribed according to the definition in MRI-assisted brachytherapy planning.

Results

The combination therapy (teletherapy followed by brachytherapy) is seen by many authors as a useful approach to local tumor control for quickly enabling

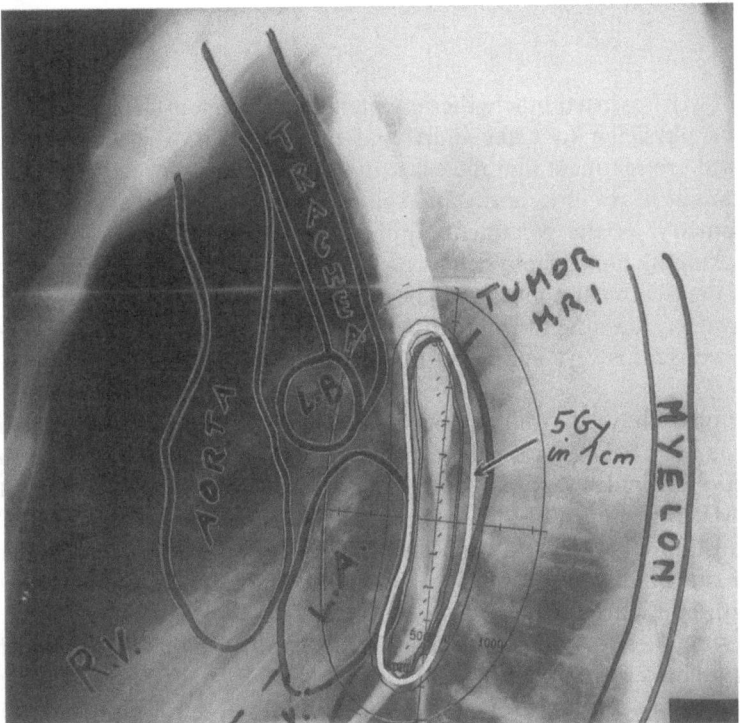

Fig. 3. Superimposition of MRI and simulation film, with delineation of superimposed dose distributions, tumor volume, and margins of critical organs. *LB*, left bronchus; *LA*, left atrium; *RV*, right ventricle

patients to eat and swallow again [1–3, 6]. This method allows one to see the margins of the esophageal tumor very clearly in any planes on MRI. The tumor length has been compared with the margins that one observes on X-ray film by barium swallowing.

Our examinations using MRI-assisted brachytherapy treatment planning show that the irradiated length is often too short when the irradiation is planned only by conventional X-ray radiographs. In these cases we extended the active irradiation length due to the margins that we had seen on MRI.

In MRI-assisted brachytherapy treatment planning, the amount of magnification and geometric inaccuracy is to be taken into account. As esophageal tumors are near the central axis of the X-ray projection and usually on MRI not further than 10 cm away from the center of the magnetic field, the geometric inaccuracy is only upto 2–3 mm. Other studies show similar results (see Pötter et al., pp. 555, 631, this volume) [7, 8].

All the 12 patients treated in this way (three of whom had almost completely occluding stenosis) were able to take food orally after the treatment.

Discussion

The value of MRI-assisted brachytherapy planning lies first in the ability that it provides the physician to make individual dose calculations, seeing on the superimposed pretreatment film the exact margins of the tumor as well as such critical organs as heart, lung, aorta, and spinal cord. The dummy applicator has similar geometry as the treatment applicator. By superimposing the pretreatment planning film the physician can compare the position of the dummy and that of the treatment applicator. The patient can be irradiated very quickly without any delay, because the pretreatment plan for brachytherapy has already been prepared. This is very important because patients are often in a very poor condition.

It was noted above that nine patients were unable to swallow the dummy applicator on MRI before the combined treatment; these patients were nevertheless planned in a similar way, because in the paracoronal and different sagittal planes on MRI, the lumen of the tumorous esophagus could be seen and by it the likely position of the dummy applicator. Therefore, the introduced brachytherapy treatment planning can also be carried out, defining the individual tumor length and margins of the critical organs.

This method therefore appears useful in patients with esophageal cancer who are to be irradiated by brachytherapy. It offers a precise method for delineating the tumor volume and the target volume. The result is a more accurate determination of dose in the target and in surrounding normal tissue in different planes than using the conventional treatment planning procedure. The procedure requires that T1-weighted MRI in paracoronal, parasagittal, and different sagittal planes be performed, and that barium swallow must be administered before the planning procedure begins. In the daily routine of our department there has been no delay for any patient planned in this way. The method entails an additional application without irradiation, with the advantage of a better defined target. This requires some 30 min of additional planning time for the staff.

References

1. Baader M, Dittler HJ, Ries G, Ultsch B, Lehr L, Siewert JR (1985) Endokavitäre Strahlentherapie in Afterloading-Technik bei malignen Stenosen des oberen Gastrointestialtraktes und der Gallenwege. Leber, Magen, Darm 15 (6): 247–255
2. Bergemann W, Heuer C, Tölle H, Schuhmacher W, Koch K (1986) Afterloading-Bestrahlung gastrointestinaler Tumoren. Med Klin 21: 672–675
3. Flores A, Nelems B, Evans K, Hay JH, Stoller J, Jackson SM (1989) Impact of new radiotherapy modalities on the surgical management of cancer esophagus and cardia. Int J Radiat Oncol Biol Phys 17: 937–944

4. Hishikawa Y, Taniguchi M, Kamikonya N, Tanaka S, Miura T (1988) External beam radiotherapy alone or combined with high dose rate intracavitary irradiation in the treatment of cancer: autopsy findings in 35 cases. Radiother Oncol 11: 223–227
5. Hishikawa Y, Kurisu K, Taniguchi M, Kamikonya N, Miura T (1989) Small superficial esophageal carcinoma treated with high-dose-rate intracavitary irradiation only. Radiology 172: 267–270
6. Hishikawa Y, Kamikonya N, Tanaka S, Miura T (1987) Radiotherapy of esophageal carcinoma: role of high-dose-rate intracavitary irradiation. Radiother Oncol 9:13–20
7. Pötter R, Heil B, Schneider L, Lenzen H, Al-Dandashi C, Schnepper E (1992) Magnetic resonance imaging in treatment planning of head and neck tumors including the brain: MRI-assisted simulation. Radiother Oncol 23: 127–130
8. Pötter R (1989) Lokalisation mit Hilfe bildgebender Verfahren in der Strahlentherapie maligner Tumoren. Habilitationsschrift, University of Münster
9. Pötter R, Kovacs G, Lenzen B, Prott FJ, Knocke TH, Haverkamp U (1989) Technique of MRI assisted treatment planning in intraluminal brachytherapy. Activ Selectr Brachyther J 5(3): 145–148

Treatment Planning:
Treatment Volume Definition
and Three-Dimensional
Treatment Planning

Individual Treatment Planning of Subdiaphragmatic Radiation Therapy Using Magnetic Resonance Tomography and Magnetic Resonance Angiography

M. Müller-Schimpfle[1], G. Layer[1], A. Köster[2], B. Kimmig[2], G. Brix[1], W. Semmler[1], and G. van Kaick

Introduction

The target volume in subdiaphragmatic radiation therapy of malignant lymphoma is commonly defined on plain X-ray simulation film [1]. Both correct inclusion of lymphatic tissue adjacent to blood vessels and the exclusion of radiosensitive organs are obligatory [7]. This is facilitated by a combination of several imaging techniques. Thus, imaging information as obtained by intravenous nephrogram, lymphogram, computed tomography, and ultrasound is transferred onto simulation film [3, 4]. Computed tomography and ultrasound, however, lack the possibility of direct image projection onto simulation film, which makes data transfer more difficult. For identification of the splenic pedicle, which shows marked anatomical variations in its vicinity to the left kidney, even surgical clipping or intravenous digital subtraction angiography is employed [6]. In clinical routine, however, the complete set of diagnostic information, which partly is obtained by invasive methods, is rarely available.

The aim of our study was to introduce magnetic resonance imaging (MRI) techniques for convenient and accurate treatment planning in subdiaphragmatic radiation therapy. For this, noninvasive visualization of the target volume (perivascular space including splenic pedicle, spleen, enlarged lymph nodes) and the radiosensitive kidneys was performed by MR tomography (MRT) and MR angiography (MRA).

Materials and Methods

MRI measurements were performed on a 1.5-T imager (Magnetom SP, Siemens, Erlangen, FRG) using a body coil. MRT used a breath-holding technique in expiration within a 14-s breath-holding period by a modified rapid acquisition

[1] Department of Radiology and Pathophysiology, German Cancer Research Center, Im Neuenheimer Feld 280, 6900 Heidelberg, FRG
[2] Department of Radiology/Radiotherapy, University Clinic for Radiology, University of Heidelberg, Im Neuenheimer Feld 400, 6900 Heidelberg, FRG

Advanced Radiation Therapy Tumor Response
Monitoring and Treatment Planning
Breit (Editor-in-Chief)
© Springer-Verlag, Berlin Heidelberg 1992

spin-echo (SE) technique (TR = 150 ms, TE = 10 ms; NEX = 1; matrix size 128 * 256; modified after [5]). To control patient positioning and to evaluate the body diameter acquisitions in axial and sagittal orientation were performed. Coronal slices were acquired for displaying the abdominal and retroperitoneal anatomy and, if present, the paraaortal lymphatic masses. Additionally, coronal MRA data acquisition in breath-holding technique was performed by using a sequential FLASH two-dimensional sequence in single-slice mode (TR = 30 ms, TE = 10 ms; flip angle = 30°, NEX = 1, matrix size = 256 * 256), breath-holding time being 10 s.

For three-dimensional reconstruction of the MR angiogram a maximum intensity projection (MIP) algorithm was used. An MR tomogram displaying the lumbar spine as well as spleen and kidneys in maximum diameter and the MIP-processed MR angiogram in frontal view were selected for further processing. The data sets of both tomogram and angiogram were matched and superimposed by a computer program. The program allowed reduction of the gray scale level and weighted addition of images, which could be processed within a given region of interest.

The superimposed image was magnified according to the geometry of the simulator unit, referring to the coronal plane through the center of the first lumbar vertebra. This was taken as the standard plane since it lies approximately in the center of the volume relevant for radiotherapy planning. Therefore, after identification on the sagittal slice and determining its position by grid calculation L1 was marked on the superimposed images for correct correlation with the simulation film. In two cases with prominent lymphatic masses additional coronal rapid SE images were acquired for better visualization of the enlarged lymph nodes. These images were then magnified referring to their position in anterior-posterior direction.

To quantify effects of positional error in MRI and X-ray simulation, phantom measurements were performed. The phantom consists of a water-filled cylinder 20 cm in radius and 13.7 cm in depth, which contains a rectangular grid of plastic rods spaced 2 cm apart. Measurements were performed in the MR imager using the above mentioned sequences as well as on the radiation therapy simulator under treatment planning conditions (source-to-object distance = 100 cm; source-to-film distance = 130 cm).

Localization errors due to projection of the superposition onto the simulation film were also assessed by comparing the contours of L1. Additionally, the contours of the kidneys, iliac crests, and psoas muscle were used, if clearly definable on the simulation film.

Subdiaphragmatic radiotherapy planning was performed in eight male and seven female patients suffering from malignant lymphoma, including three patients after diagnostic splenectomy and two with prominent lymphatic masses. Nine patients suffered from Hodgkin's disease and six from non-Hodgkin's lymphoma. The age of the patients ranged from 19 to 70 years (mean 46 years). Informed consent was given by all patients.

Results

Phantom measurements revealed that the positional error due to magnetic field inhomogeneities and gradient field nonlinearities was less than 4 mm at a radius of 14 cm (field size on simulation film).

On rapid SE images a good demarcation of kidney, spleen, liver and spine was achieved. On the image selected for superposition the left kidney and the spleen were displayed in maximum size in 14/15 cases. In one case the maximum diameter of the left kidney was underestimated by 1 cm and the diameter of the spleen by 1.5 cm. The right kidney was visualized in maximum size in 9/15 cases, while in six cases the diameter was up to 1 cm below maximum. A favorable contrast was achieved between vertebrae and intervertebral discs. The contours

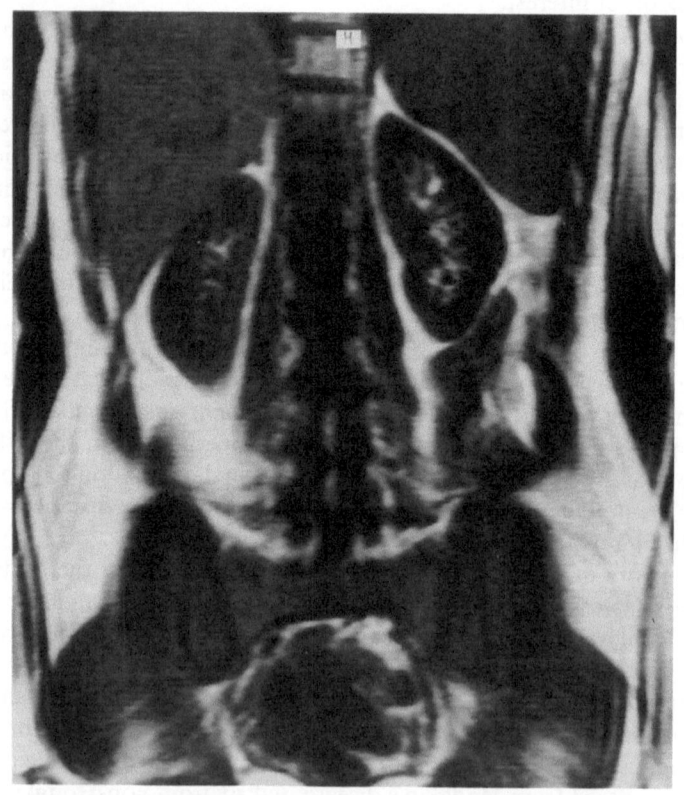

Fig. 1. Coronal rapid spin-echo image (SE 150/10) of a 28-year-old woman suffering from Hodgkin's disease. Note the favorable organ demarcation. Due to a marked lumbar lordosis L1 is visualized only by its dorsal contours

of L1 were identified in all cases, although in patients with a marked lumbar lordosis this vertebra was not displayed in maximum diameter (Fig. 1).

On MIP-processed MR angiograms in frontal view the main abdominal vessels necessary for treatment planning were displayed in all cases in sufficient quality, including particularly the splenic pedicle (Fig. 2). In three cases of splenectomized patients a more scattered signal was obtained from lienal vessels reflecting the diminished flow. Problems in delineation arose in the infrarenal part of the inferior vena cava, which showed markedly decreased flow signal in three cases and signal extinction in one case due to impression by a large paraaortal lymphatic mass.

Exact localization of vascular and organ anatomy was achieved on the superposition images. Vascular and organ anatomy fit together exactly in 14/15 cases. In one case the MRI examination had to be repeated because of incongruency of MRT and MRA, which resulted from patient movement during the examination. Also, the contours of L1 were still definable after superposition in 14/15 cases. In one case the position of L1 had to be marked by a box according to its position in coronal rapid SE images (Fig. 3).

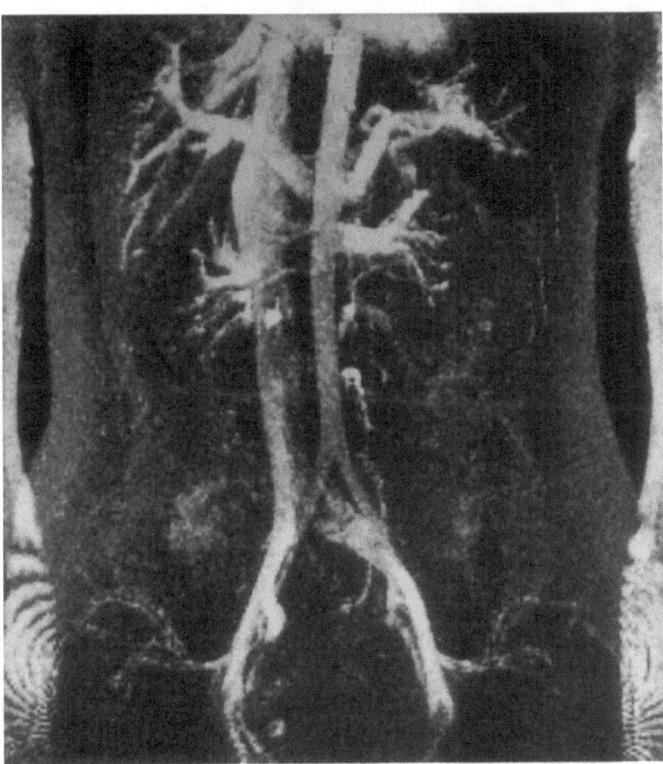

Fig. 2. MRA in coronal view after MIP processing. Note the excellent delineation of the splenic pedicle, with distinguishable lienal vein and lienal artery

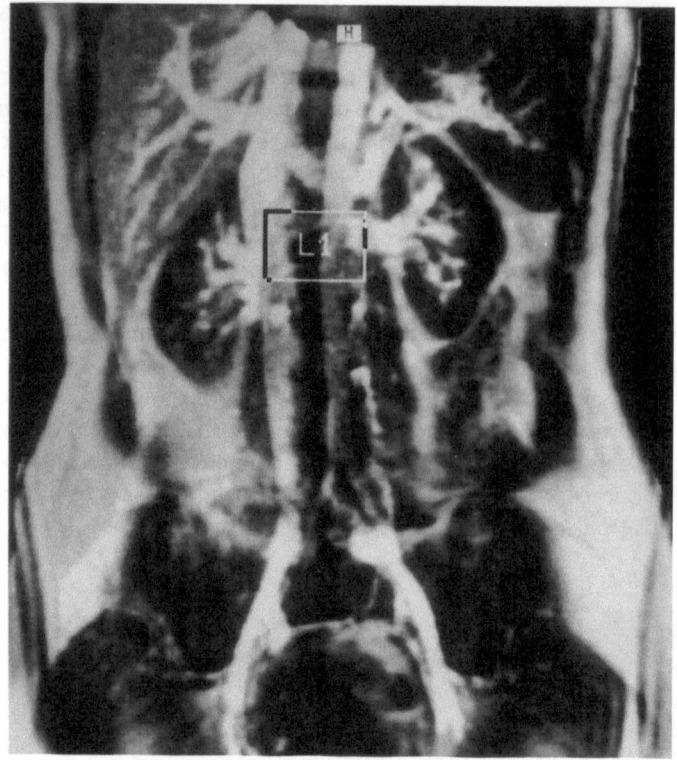

Fig. 3. Superposition of MRT and MRA. *Box*, first lumbar vertebra; this is placed on an anterior image after the contours of L1 in full extension. On the superposition image the same box is seen, thus representing accurately the position and contour of L1. Note the ability to localize the splenic pedicle in relation to the upper pole of the left kidney

After projecting the superposition onto simulation film the size of L1 differed less than 5 mm. In those cases in which the kidney contours were clearly identifiable on simulation film (5/15) the sizes differed within the same range.

Discussion

Until now individual field definition in subdiaphragmatic radiotherapy planning has required several more or less invasive methods (surgical clipping of splenic pedicle or intravenous digital subtraction angiography, intravenous nephrogram, lymphogram, computed tomography [3, 4, 6]. The information gathered by this variety of examinations can now be obtained by a single noninvasive MRI examination lasting about 30 min. It was demonstrated that spatial distortion of MRI methods is not a major problem in subdiaphragmatic radiotherapy planning. The relevant anatomical information needed for field definition can be visualized on a single coronal image. Magnification in correct scale according to simulator geometry makes possible direct projection of the MRI superposition onto the simulation film. And although most of the vessels are located anteriorly to the reference plane through L1, the lienal artery and vein as the most relevant vessels are located within and close to the coronal reference plane. The other vessels are useful particularly for control of organ-to-vessel congruency. In cases with prominent lymphatic masses localization errors are minimized by acquisition of additional coronal images which are magnified according to their anterior-posterior position. Thus localization errors due to the different projection techniques are kept within an acceptable range, as far as large field irradiation is concerned. Furthermore, the localization error as assessed by the contour of L1 has even decreased in the most recent cases.

Patient cooperation is crucial especially when using a breath-holding technique for achieving reproducible organ localization. Except for one case, compliance was not a problem, and the patients showed high motivation. In addition, slightly differing subdiaphragmatic anatomy due to differing diaphragma position on the single FLASH two-dimensional slices is equalized by the MIP algorithm.

In conclusion, we recommend this method for routine radiotherapy planning of malignant lymphoma patients because of acceptible costs, noninvasiveness, convenience, and accuracy.

References

1. Abbatucci JS, Quint R, Bloquel J, Roussel A, Urbatjel M (1976) Techniken der kurativen Teletherapie. Enke, Stuttgart
2. Edelman RR, Mattle HP, Atkinson DJ, Hoogewoud HM (1990) MR angiography. AJR 154: 937–946
3. Hoppe RT (1987) Treatment planning in the radiation therapy of Hodgkin's disease. Front Radiat Ther Onc 21: 270–287
4. Meyer JL (1987) Radiotherapy treatment planning for the non-Hodgkin's lymphomas. Front Radiat Ther Onc 21: 288–301
5. Mirowitz SA, Lee JKT, Brown JJ, Eilenberg SS, Heiken JP, Perman WH (1990) Rapid acquisition spin-echo (RASE) MR imaging: a new technique for reduction of artifacts and acquisition time. Radiology 175: 131–135
6. Pötter R, Sciuk J, Haverkamp U (1989) Digital subtraction angiography (iv DSA) in treatment planning of subdiaphragmatic Hodgkin's disease. Int J Radiat Oncol Biol Phys 17: 389–396
7. Wannenmacher M (1989) Strahlentherapie maligner Lymphome. Röntgen-Bl. 42, 31–33

Definition of Radiation Portals for Subdiaphragmal Nodal Disease: Magnetic Resonance Imaging and Plain Film Versus Three-Dimensional Computed Tomography

W. Reuschel, T. Auberger, M. Mayr, P. Lukas, W. Riedl, C. Hugo, P. Kneschaurek, and A. Breit

A basic problem in radiation therapy is definition of the exact target volume in adjuvant cases in which lymph nodes or the tumor bed are to be treated. In seminoma or Hodgkin's disease the lymph nodes adjacent to large vessels represent the target volume. The vessels serve as guidelines to mark and define the treatment volume if no lymphography has been performed. The individual localization of the vessels is defined by angiography or tomographic techniques such as computed tomography (CT) or magnetic resonance imaging (MRI). In the treatment of subdiaphragmal nodal disease we compared the radiation portals based on MRI and plain film with the portals obtained by three-dimensional CT treatment planning.

For treatment planning in the paraaortal, iliacal, or inguinal region we use conventional radiography (contrast renography) at a simulator facility together with MRI in coronal planes (T1-weighted, 8 to 10-mm slices). In these MR images organs of risk (e.g., kidneys) and vessels are defined and marked. With the aid of an optical projection system this information is transferred onto the simulation film. Osseous structures such as vertebral bodies and femoral heads serve for exact overlay between MRI and simulation film. With this information the irradiation portals are defined.

In 16 cases of abdominal lymph node irradiation the portals obtained using only plain radiography were compared with MRI-based plans. In four cases the kidneys could not be localized with plain radiography. In 3/16 cases the radiation portals had to be corrected according to the location of large vessels obtained from additional MRI information. MRI offers important additional information to the simulator radiographs and makes the contrast radiography of kidneys and vessels unnecessary. Problems with MRI-based treatment planning are distortion and the impossibility of using coronal MRI data within our planning system.

In selected cases we used CT for the definition of radiation portals to perform three-dimensional treatment planning. This is as follows. After definition and marking of craniocaudal field extension continuous CT investigation with a maximal slice distance of 20 mm is performed. The next step is the creation of a three-dimensional CT cube in the planning system (Siemens Mevaplan 10.1) and the selection of field size, orientation, and definition of

Institut für Strahlentherapie und Radiologische Onkologie, Technische Universität München, Klinikum rechts der Isar, Ismaninger Str. 15, 8000 Munich 80, FRG

Advanced Radiation Therapy Tumor Response
Monitoring and Treatment Planning
Breit (Editor-in-Chief)
© Springer-Verlag, Berlin Heidelberg 1992

individual blocks, assisted by beam's eye view. Finally, the radiation portals are transferred onto the patient at the simulator.

For multiplanar reconstruction it is necessary to indicate regions of interest (ROI) in each plane for the target volume (e.g., vessels) and organs of risk. The planning system allows one to select seven ROIs consisting of three sub-ROIs which must be marked point-by-point, creating a polygon. This procedure is very time consuming and should be performed by an experienced physician. The exact entering of these contours and the patient's outer contour is important for the definition of the radiation portals aided by the beam's eye view option, which is a convergent projection of all contours onto a plane which is perpendicular to the central axis of the beam. In this projection it is possible to select beam size collimator and gantry position and, finally, the position of individual blocks.

As a next step, it is easy to create a three-dimensional dose matrix and to display the dose distribution in each axial, coronal, sagittal, or an arbitrary oblique plane. The isodoses can be drawn as lines or as areas (color wash mode). As a further evaluative criterion dose-volume histograms can be calculated and displayed for all of the defined volumes of interest. This is especially important for comparison of the effect of different beam configurations on organs of risk. The transmission of selected portals onto the patient must be carried out by individual landmarks because it is still not possible to create a simulator radiograph by digital reconstruction.

In conclusion, the advantages of the MRI-based treatment planning are exact localization of vessels and critical organs with a noninvasive and fast method. However, this method is expensive and not always available. In contrast to a CT investigation, it provides no correlation between tissue description and radiation interaction. Furthermore, the distortion of MRI, especially at the periphery of the images, is still problematic. Consequently, it is always important to correlate coronal MRI with radiographs in the same projection. Most of the disadvantages of three-dimensional CT planning originate in the time-consuming and complicated handling of the planning system. One of the fundamental problems of three-dimensional CT planning is the impossibility of display and documentation of all the information obtained by three-dimensional calculation.

Especially in situations in which organs of risk are recessed, three-dimensional treatment planning offers helpful information and facilitates the definition of radiation portals. When handling is improved and calculation time reduced, it will certainly become a routine method in treatment planning whenever individual and sophisticated irradiation techniques are to be employed.

Experience with Digital Subtraction Angiography in Treatment Planning of Subdiaphragmatic Malignant Lymphoma

R. Pötter, J. Sciuk, and U. Haverkamp

Introduction

Intravenous digital subtraction angiography (DSA) was introduced into clinical treatment planning for subdiaphragmatic Hodgkin's disease at Münster University in December 1985. After a pilot phase in which basic conditions were investigated, it has been used continuously since in routine clinical treatment planning for all patients to be irradiated for subdiaphragmatic malignant lymphoma. The basic principles of the method and the first clinical experience were described by Pötter et al. (1989) and Sciuk et al. (1989). Intravenous DSA allows direct frontal imaging of lymph node bearing areas (vascular topography) corresponding to the beam's eye view in irradiation, which continues to be based on AP/PA treatment fields. Vascular topography (celiac trunk, abdominal artery, hepatic artery, splenic pedicle, iliac arteries) and the spleen can be delineated exactly; the vascular topography particularly of the splenic pedicle, the spleen, and hepatic arteries can be related accurately to the topography of the kidney, the main organ at risk in the upper abdomen.

The aim of this study was the evaluation of intravenous DSA in the treatment planning of subdiaphragmatic malignant lymphoma over a 5-year period (December 1985 to December 1990) in 135 patients by the quantitative assessment of 44 patients and by discussion of advantages and limitations when using this method in routine treatment planning.

Materials and Methods

Pötter et al. 1989 and Pötter 1989 have described in detail the principles of diagnostic DSA and its modification for so-called treatment planning DSA and those of the subtrascope and its modified use for treatment planning in radiotherapy — in particular for accurate definition of target volume and organs at risk (Fig. 1).

Klinik für Strahlentherapie, Radioonkologie, Westfälische Wilhelms-Universität Münster, Albert Schweitzer-Str. 33, 4400 Münster, FRG

Advanced Radiation Therapy Tumor Response
Monitoring and Treatment Planning
Breit (Editor-in-Chief)
© Springer-Verlag, Berlin Heidelberg 1992

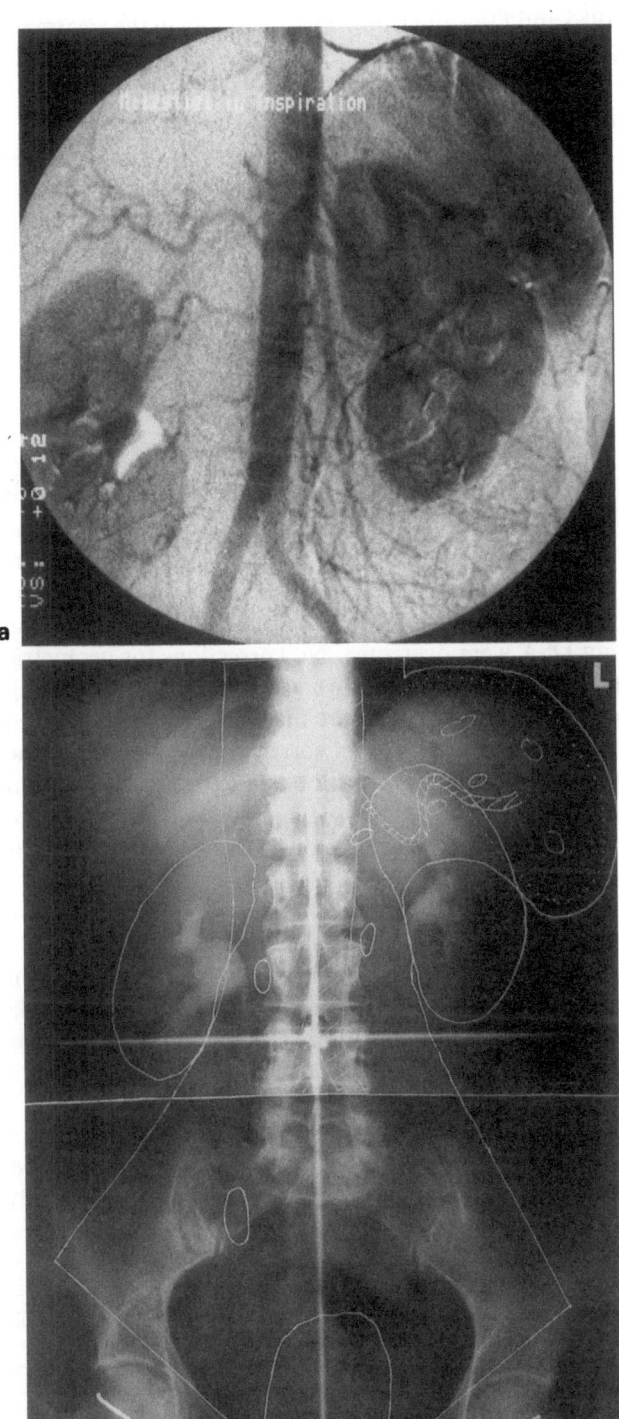

Between December 1985 and December 1987 DSA was used in the treatment planning of subdiaphragmatic malignant lymphoma in 49 patients, Hodgkin's disease in 38, and non-Hodgkin lymphoma in 11. Of these, 21 patients presented with indication of subdiaphragmatic disease, one patient stage I, 25 stage II, 18 stage III, and 5 stage IV. Radiotherapy was performed at a linear accelerator (10 MV) using opposed AP/PA fields with individually focused shielding blocks, including the splenic pedicle in every case, the porta hepatis in cases of involvement, and the spleen after clinical staging alone (Hoppe 1987; Wannenmacher et al. 1978).

Results

Performance data on intravenous DSA for treatment planning corresponded to those described previously (Pötter et al. 1989). Concerning the use of the subtrascope, different physicians (mostly residents) performed the image super-imposition and target volume definition, which took a mean of 20 min. The difficulties that were met in the beginning of the study in delineation of the spine on the treatment planning DSA were overcome. No corrections for geometric distortions due to shifting of the central axis were carried out in designing paraaortic fields. Corrections of up to 0.6 cm were included when planning an "inverted Y" or an "abdominal bath." In cases of correction, the volume of the left kidney to be irradiated increased slightly (Pötter 1989). From phantom investigations, distortions in radial direction up to 4 mm due to the bent surface of the image intensifier of the DSA were measured, but not corrected for (Pötter 1989).

For the assessment of imaging data the same criteria as described elsewhere (Pötter et al. 1989) were applied. The imaging accuracy for all sites (total of 207 judgements) was excellent in 160 (77.3%), reasonable in 34 (16.4%), and poor in 13 (6.3%) cases. As simultaneous imaging of the spine is mandatory — the spine serving as reference structure for superimposition — imaging accuracy was defined according to the same criteria for the spine: the majority of the 14 judgements (total 41) which were classified as "reasonable" ($n = 7$) or "poor" ($n = 7$) were found in the beginning of the study and were due to inadequate postprocessing for the needs of treatment planning DSA. The celiac trunk and the course of the splenic artery could be defined in each case (44/44), which is most important for adequate target volume definition. In 4 of 33 evaluable cases

Fig. 1. a Treatment planning DSA imaging vessels, kidney, spleen, and spine (inspiration). b Simulation film in AP projection after superimposition of vascular topography and spleen from treatment planning DSA (inspiration). Definition of target and treatment volume (with individually focused shielding blocks) based on delineation of the individual lymph node bearing area around the splenic artery and of the spleen in relation to the kidney (subdiaphragmatic disease with lymph nodes in the paraaortic and parailiac region and along the splenic artery and nodular involvement in the spleen)

(12%) imaging was regarded as "poor" for delineation of the spleen. In most cases this was due to insufficient imaging of the late parenchymatous phase, which is necessary for delineation of the margins of the spleen, in some cases because of lack of imaging the entire spleen.

The origin of the splenic pedicle and the hepatic artery in relation to the spine was at the level of T12/L1 in 36/44 cases (82%), the origin of the hepatic artery at the same level in 27/38 (71%) cases. The course of the splenic artery as to the left kidney was in 36 cases projected within or above the upper third (82%) and in 8 cases between the upper and middle thirds or within the middle third (Fig. 2b). As to the course of the hepatic artery 28/38 (74%) cases projected above the right kidney, 7 (18%) within the upper third, and 3 (8%) within the middle third (Fig. 2a). Topography of the spleen revealed 11/23 (48%) in close contact to the craniolateral margin of the left kidney, 8/23 (35%) with a gap of 1–2 cm between kidney and spleen, and 4/23 (17%) with the spleen overlapping the craniolateral margin of the left kidney by 1–2 cm (Fig. 2c). As to different respiratory phases there was no change with inspiration in the origin of the splenic artery at the celiac trunk (at the spine) but an increasing change with inspiration toward the direction of the spleen (away from the spine) up to the height of one vertebra. Nevertheless, there was no indication of a significant change when looking at vascular topography and the position of the spleen in

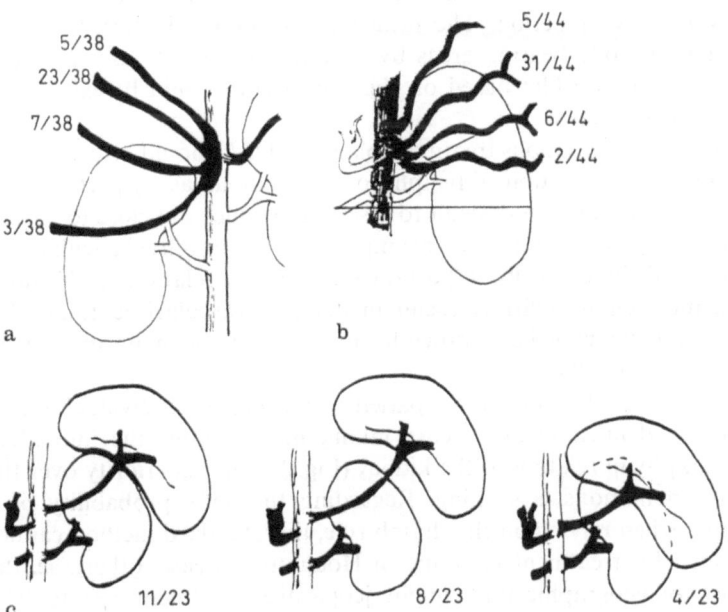

Fig. 2a–c. Topography of vessels in the upper abdomen and of the spleen in relation to the kidney based on findings from intravenous DSA in frontal projection. **a** Hepatic artery and right kidney. **b** Splenic artery and left kidney. **c** Spleen and left kidney

relation to the position of the kidney in different respiratory phases (Pötter 1989).

The accuracy in target volume definition was defined according to the same criteria described elsewhere (Pötter et al. 1989) and was compared to the so-called thumb rule (including upper third) and the earlier method described by Abbatucci et al. (including L1) (1976). Evaluating the thumb rule from radioon-cological criteria for target and treatment volume definition, the target was completely missed in 2 cases (4%) and on the field margin in 20 cases (41%), meaning a 45% probability of a geographic miss. The thumb rule thus often underestimates the target and the volume of the left kidney which is to be included. Compared to the target definition described by Abbatucci et al. (1976), which included the target with a rather wide margin in every case, DSA-assisted individual target volume definition and beam shaping led to a significant reduction in target volume and consequently in irradiation of the kidney in 26/44 cases (59%); the amount of reduction varied from 15% to > 25%.

Discussion

Intravenous DSA for treatment planning of subdiaphragmatic malignant lymphoma has proven to be a clinically feasible method on the basis of our experience over a 5-year period. The principal advantages in target volume definition of lymph node bearing areas by superimposition of vascular topography on the simulation film based on the subtrascope could be extensively used within clinical practice.

For certain clinical situations treatment planning DSA should be considered for defining the precise location of lymph node bearing areas, in particular in regions in which topography is difficult to assess, and which are close to organs at risk. In malignant lymphoma, for example, this is the infraclavicular and axillary region with its clinically important topographic relation to the lung. Furthermore, intravenous DSA is useful in imaging vascularized tumor for treatment planning, which is best known from arteriovenous malformations in the brain (Peters et al. 1986).

As the detailed evaluation of 44 patients showed, an individual target volume could be defined in every case taking into account the individual vascular topography in relation to the kidney (Fig. 1). The superiority over the usual standard definitions is striking. Regarding the 45% probability of a geographic miss when relying on the thumb rule, this standard method cannot be recommended for treatment planning in Hodgkin's disease; otherwise, the significant risk of geographic miss might jeopardize treatment results. The standard splenic pedicle-paraaortic fields shown in the literature, according to our results, do not always adequately cover the whole region of the splenic pedicle, in particular in those cases where its extent is rather small (see Hoppe

1987). On the other hand, by this method the area of the kidney to be included in the treatment volume can be defined accurately and — compared to the standard definition "including L1" — it can often be reduced (59%) by highly individualized kidney blocking (Pötter et al. 1989). In our experience, there is a wide variety in vascular topography (Fig. 2) which must be taken into account for target definition, in addition to data from cross-sectional imaging and pathological data from laparotomy.

The policy of field matching at the bottom of T9 proved to be advantageous in the majority of patients, leaving a wide margin between celiac region (T12/L1) — rather often involved — and matching area with the known uncertainties in radiation dose distribution. Only in certain clinical situations (e.g., slim patients) was this matching policy not feasible.

As to the quality of imaging, it could be used for the needs of treatment planning in the majority of cases (94%). Nevertheless, in routine performance of treatment planning DSA, there is a tendency not to include simultaneous imaging of the spine in the usual postprocessing familiar to the philosophy for DSA in diagnostic departments. As discussed elsewhere (Pötter et al. 1989), regular communication between the diagnostic radiologist and the radiation oncologist is a precondition for the successful integration of treatment planning DSA into the program of diagnostic DSA.

Whereas imaging of vascular topography was always at least reasonable, some limitations in imaging the spleen must be taken into account (poor delineation in 12%).

Although imaging by DSA meets many needs of treatment planning, it must be noted that with magnetic resonance imaging a method is now available which makes delineation of lymph node bearing area (vessels) *and* tumor (lymphoma) possible by direct coronal imaging, and which might be integrated into conventional treatment planning (Pötter et al., this volume) or even combined with magnetic resonance angiography (Müller-Schimpfle et al., this volume). The promising capabilities of magnetic resonance imaging should be compared with the proven value of treatment planning DSA for malignant lymphoma in a prospective clinical trial.

References

Abbatucci JS, Quint R, Bloquel J, Roussel A, Urbatjel M (1976) Techniken der kurativen Teletherapie. Enke, Stuttgart

Hoppe RT (1987) Treatment planning in the radiation therapy of Hodgkin's disease. In: Vaeth JM, Meyer J (eds) Treatment planning in the radiation therapy of cancer. Karger, Basel, pp 270–287

Peters TM, Clark JA, Olivier A, Marchand EP, Mawko G, Dieumegarde M, Muresan LV, Ethier R (1986) Integrated stereotaxic imaging with CT, MR imaging, and digital subtraction angiography. Radiology 161: 821–826

Pötter R (1989) Lokalisation mit Hilfe bildgebender Verfahren in der Strahlentherapie maligner Tumoren. Habilitationsschrift, University of Münster

Pötter R, Sciuk J, Haverkamp U (1989) Digital subtraction angiography (IV DSA) in treatment planning of subdiaphragmatic Hodgkin's disease. Int J Radiat Oncol Biol Phys 17: 389–396

Sciuk J, Pötter R, Haverkamp U, Krings W (1989) Digitale Subtraktionsangiographie (i.V. DSA) zur infradiaphragmalen Bestrahlung beim malignen Lymphom. Radiologe 29: 85–88

Wannenmacher M, Slanina J, Kuphal K, Bruggmoser G (1978). Gegenwärtiger Stand der Großfeldtechnik unter Megavoltbedingungen bei der Strahlentherapie der Hodgkin'schen Erkrankung. Grundlagen, Durchführung, Nebenwirkungen. Radiologe 18: 371–387

Technique of Magnetic Resonance Imaging Assisted Simulation Based on Direct Coronal Imaging for Treatment Planning of Supradiaphragmatic Malignant Lymphoma

R. Pötter, F.J. Prott, C. Jaiser, U. Stöber, and D. Westrick

Introduction

In radiotherapy of malignant lymphoma radiotherapy has been delivered using opposed AP/PA large fields on linear accelerators for more than 20 years (Hoppe 1987; Wannenmacher et al. 1978). A basic precondition for treatment planning has always been the adequate localization of lymphoma, lymph node bearing areas, and organs at risk, which may have to be shielded by individual blocking. The procedure of localization is performed based on clinical, pathological, and imaging information. As imaging technology has evolved dramatically during the past two decades with the introduction of computed tomography (CT), ultrasound, digital subtraction angiography, and magnetic resonance imaging (MRI), the role of imaging has changed — becoming the most important tool in the localization procedure for malignant lymphoma nowadays. Nevertheless, the most widespread basic procedure for treatment planning in malignant lymphoma remains fluoroscopic imaging on the therapy simulator (Hoppe 1987; Timothy et al. 1989; Wannenmacher et al. 1978). Tumor, target volume, and organs at risk are defined on the X-ray simulation film based on information about the localization of tumor and target which must be "translated" from transverse cross-sectional, parallel projected imaging (mostly CT) onto the centrally projected coronal X-ray images, the simulation films. This rather complicated translation procedure entails many uncertainties, in particular a considerable risk of mislocalization.

As MRI is available today with its capability of direct cross-sectional coronal imaging lymphoma and lymph node bearing areas corresponding to the X-ray simulation film, MRI may be regarded as the imaging method of choice for localization in treatment planning of malignant lymphoma (Timothy et al. 1987). Using a subtrascope for direct imaging superimposition (Pötter et al. 1989; Pötter 1989) the complete information from different slices of MRI can be used directly for target definition on the simulation film, resulting in a comprehensive target definition in the beam's eye view without uncertainties in localization (Pötter et al. 1992).

Klinik für Strahlentherapie, Radioonkologie, Westfälische Wilhelms-Universität Münster, Albert-Schweitzer-Str. 33, 4400 Münster, FRG

Advanced Radiation Therapy Tumor Response
Monitoring and Treatment Planning
Breit (Editor-in-Chief)
© Springer-Verlag, Berlin Heidelberg 1992

The aim of this study was to describe the procedure of using the information from coronal MRI by superimposition at a subtrascope directly for the definition of target volume and organs at risk on the simulation film in the conventional way of fluoroscopic simulation in supradiaphragmatic malignant lymphoma.

Materials and Methods

Treatment planning for infra- and supradiaghragmatic radiotherapy was performed in 22 patients using this method of MRI-assisted simulation. T1-weighted coronal spin-echo sequences were obtained on a 1.5-T Magnet with patients in supine position with deep inspiration. A centered grid was superimposed on each image of interest, including the slices with anatomical landmarks for superimposition. The X-ray simulation film was exposed in a way that bifurcation of trachea and the bodies of the thoracic vertebrae could be precisely delineated.

At the subtrascope coronal MRI and simulation X-ray film were superimposed electronically, and the resulting image — MRI on simulation film — was visualized on the screen. With a zoom lens images could be magnified as much as necessary, i.e., as certain anatomical landmarks on specific MRI slices fitted to those on the simulation film: spine with thoracic vertebrae and bifurcation of trachea. The position of these anatomical landmarks is constant; in particular, it does not vary with breathing. The grid was then drawn from the reference MRI onto the simulation film under monitor control and served as a reference frame for superimposing other paracoronal MRI slices onto the simulation film (Pötter 1989; Pötter et al. 1991).

The resulting superimposed image could be displayed on the screen continuously, emphasizing either the MRI, the simulation film, or combining both, and could be documented by a multiformat camera (Pötter 1989). All information of interest could be drawn directly and precisely from any other paracoronal MRI of interest (Fig. 1) on the simulation film: malignant lymphoma at any location (mediastinum, hilum of the lung, paracardiac, cardiophrenic, paravertebral, cervical, supraclavicular, infraclavicular, axillary), lymph node bearing areas by delineating the vessels (e.g., sublavian and axillary vessels, common carotid arteries), and organs at risk (Fig. 2). Based on these drawings on the simulation film the individual target and the shape of shielding blocks were defined (Fig. 2), and individually focused beam shaping blocks were constructed in the conventional way.

This procedure of superimposition taking several coronal MRI slices for supradiaphragmatic treatment planning in malignant lymphoma took about 45 min per patient, depending heavily on imaging quality of the simulation film, in particular with regard to the delineation of anatomical landmarks.

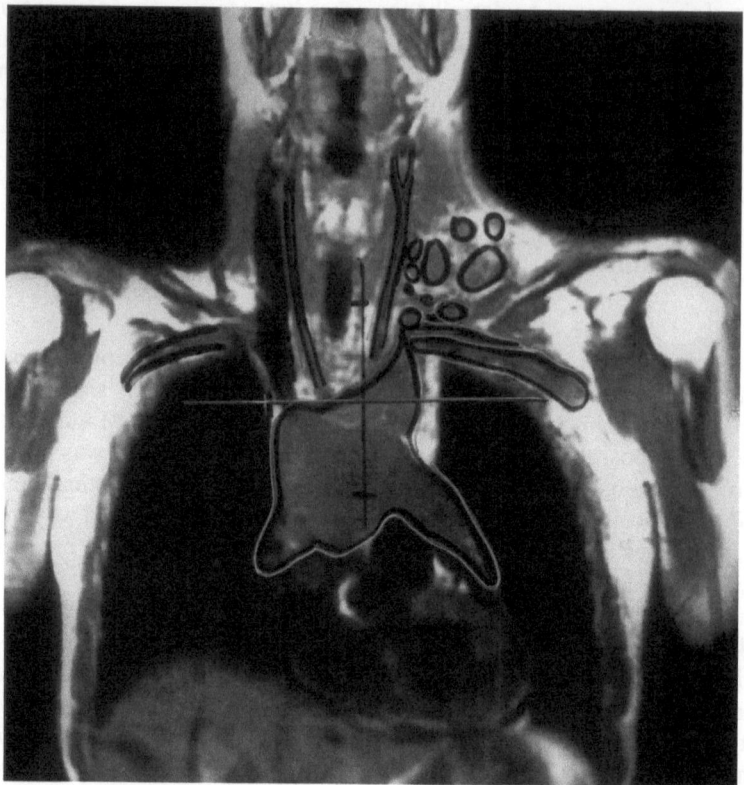

Fig. 1. Coronal MRI (T1-weighted) of a 42-year-old patient with Hodgkin's disease in the mediastinum (*large mass*), in the paracardiac and pulmonary hilar region, inlet of the thorax, low cervical, left supraclavicular and infraclavicular region with tumor along the subclavian vein leading to thrombosis confirmed by phlebography. Delineation of anatomic structures to be superimposed on the simulation film. Superimposition of a grid from the coronal MRI reference plane (bifurcation of the trachea) on other coronal planes of interest making precise superimposition of anatomy and pathology from different coronal planes on the simulation film possible

Geometrical Considerations

The geometrical distortions due to inhomogeneities of the main magnetic field and spatial nonlinearity of the field gradients were within 2–3 mm in a volume of 10 cm around the center of the magnetic field. At our magnet (1.5 Tesla) in coronal spin-echo sequences they rose up to a maximum of 4–6 mm toward the edges of a volume measuring $30 \times 30 \times 30$ cm (Pötter 1989). Consequently, no significant inaccuracies had to be taken into account for structures in the mediastinum or inlet of the thorax, whereas slight inaccuracies might be met in the cervical, supra-/infraclavicular, or axillary region.

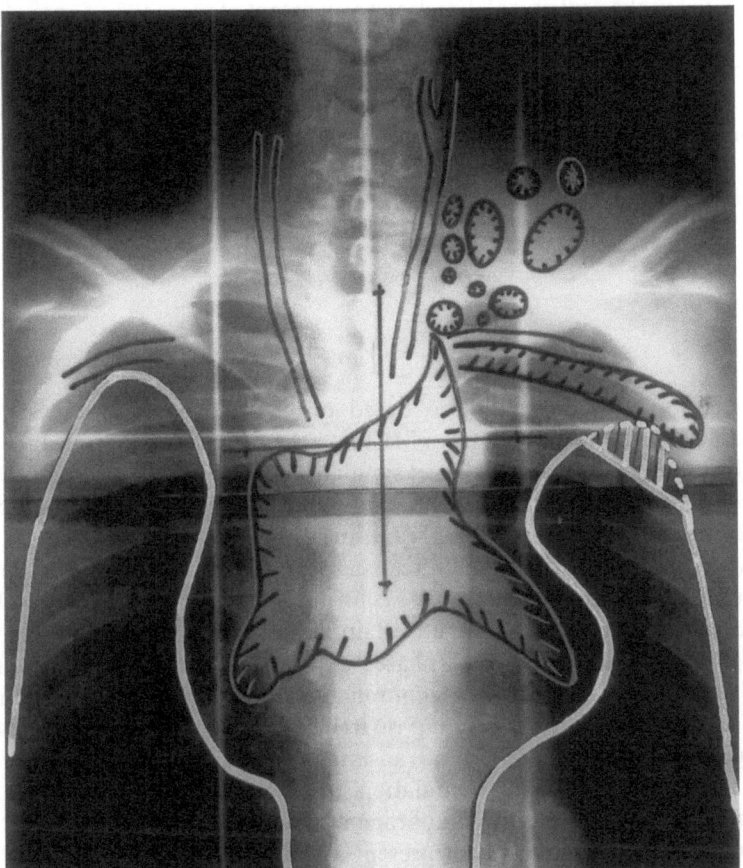

Fig. 2. Coronal X-ray simulation film (AP projection) with drawn delineation of lymphoma in the mediastinum, paracardiac, pulmonary hilar, left low cervical, supraclavicular and infraclavicular regions after precise superimposition of different coronal MRI slices at the subtrascope. Topography of the left subclavian vein related to topography of the left lung was confirmed by phlebography. No geometrical correction had to be carried out. Adjustment of the left lung block (reduction at the craniolateral margin) to the individual pathology had to be performed as well as adjustment of the top of the right lung block to the individual anatomy

The geometrical distortions due to different conditions of projection (central versus parallel projection) increase with the distance of the structures to be superimposed from the center of the X-ray beam and from the reference MRI slice. For mediastinal structures inaccuracies were neglected. In the cervical, supra-infraclavicular and axillary regions, however, the centripetally directed deviations increased to more than 5 mm, considering the conditions which are relevant for clinical use: borders between lymph node bearing areas and areas to be shielded because of their radiovulnerability (lung), i.e., 10 cm distance from the central beam, 5 cm from the MRI reference slice (bifurcation of the trachea; Westrick 1992). In the intraclavicular/axillary region these deviations were partly corrected in the centrifugal direction to an extent of more than 5 mm after having precisely superimposed structures onto the simulation films not considering these inaccuracies.

Nevertheless, in the thoracic region some basic uncertainties in precise localization remain to be taken into account in clinical treatment planning, in particular because of the considerably varying topography due mainly to the different phases of the respiratory cycle.

Conclusions

MRI-assisted fluoroscopic simulation based on the use of the subtrascope integrates different coronal planes from MRI into the conventional procedure of X-ray localization. Quality of imaging of simulation films is the crucial point for superimposition with regard to delineation of reference structures. Geometrical inaccuracies due to different projection and magnification must be taken into account when superimposing structures, in particular in the axillary and infraclavicular region. Corrections in the centrifugal direction may have to be carried out to a certain degree. Basic uncertainties in localization due mainly to the varying topography in different phases of the respiratory cycle must be considered carefully. An adequate definition of target volume and shielding blocks based on direct coronal imaging (MRI) is possible without taking into account significant uncertainties from translating information from transverse imaging (CT) onto coronal X-ray simulation films.

In treatment planning of supradiaphragmatic malignant lymphoma, MRI-assisted fluoroscopic simulation is at present a clinically feasible method with considerably additional effort leading to greater confidence in a rationally defined target, in particular in the inlet of the thorax, in the infraclavicular and axillary region, areas poorly imaged on X-ray films.

Acknowledgements. The authors would like to thank C. Rademacher and S. Köster for assistance in performing the study and P. Mause and I. Liebe for help with preparing the manuscript.

References

Hoppe RT (1987) Treatment planning in the radiation therapy of Hodgkin's disease. In: Vaeth JM, Meyer J (eds) Treatment planning in the radiation therapy of cancer. Karger, Basel, pp 270–287
Pötter R (1989) Lokalisation mit Hilfe bildgebender Verfahren in der Strahlentherapie maligner Tumoren. Habilitationsschrift, University of Münster
Pötter R, Sciuk J, Haverkamp U (1989) Digital subtraction angiography (IV DSA) in treatment planning of subdiaphragmatic Hodgkin's disease. Int J Radiat Oncol Biol Phys 17: 389–396

Pötter R, Heil B, Schneider L, Lenzen H, Al-Dandashi C, Schnepper E (1992) Sagittal and coronal planes from MRI for treatment planning in tumors of brain, head and neck: MRI assisted simulation. Radiother Oncol 23: 127–130

Timothy AR, Van Dyk J, Sutcliffe SB (1987) Radiation therapy for Hodgkin's disease. In: Selby P, McElwain TJ (eds) Hodgkin's disease. Blackwell, Oxford, pp 181–249

Wannenmacher M, Slanina J, Kuphal K, Bruggmoser G (1978) Gegenwärtiger Stand der Großfeldtechnik unter Megavoltbedingungen bei der Strahlentherapie der Hodgkin'schen Erkrankung. Grundlagen, Durchführung, Nebenwirkungen. Radiologe 18: 371–387

Westrick D (1992) MRT-gestützte Simulation in der Planung der Strahlentherapie von malignen Lymphomen. Dissertation, University of Münster

Improved Treatment Planning in Three Dimensions for Breast Cancer

L. Wittgren[1], Å. Arwidi[2], and T. Knöös[1]

Introduction

We present here a radiation treatment technique for breast cancer patients who have involvement of the lymph nodes, and who have been treated previously with conservative surgery including axillary resection. The clinical target volume (CTV) consists of the breast parenchyma and the lymph nodes in the axilla and the supraclavicular and the infraclavicular fossae. The planning target volume (PTV) includes this volume and appropriate margins (Wambersie et al. 1989). There are several problems in treating this rather large, irregularly shaped volume. Furthermore, the body contour varies, and the organs at risk — lung, spinal cord, and opposite breast — are located nearby. The whole target volume is given an absorbed dose of 54 Gy, as specified by ICRU (1978).

Methods

A large number of slices (approximately 30), with 1-cm spacing, covering the whole target volume are acquired using computed tomography (CT). This is necessary for an appropriate geometric description of the planning volume and the organs at risk and as the basis for dose calculations. The three-dimensional electron density distribution is calculated from the Hounsfield numbers (Knöös et al. 1986b). For these patients the radiation technique is fixed. The target volume is divided into two parts in the craniocaudal direction (approximately 3–4 cm below the apex of the lung). Four 6-MV fields with a common isocenter (placed in the intersection) are used. The fields are opposed two-by-two and generated using asymmetric collimator settings in this direction (Fig. 1). All four fields are closely conformed to the target volume using a beam's eye view facility in the planning system. Beam's eye view pictures (in the right scale) are used to manufacture polygonally shaped, nondivergent, individually shaped lead blocks, and another set of these are used at the simulator to check the actual shielding.

[1] Department of Radiation Physics, Lund University, Malmö Allmänna Sjukhus, 214 01 Malmö, Sweden
[2] Department of Oncology, Lund University, Malmö Allmänna Sjukhus, 214 01 Malmö, Sweden

Advanced Radiation Therapy Tumor Response
Monitoring and Treatment Planning
Breit (Editor-in-Chief)
© Springer-Verlag, Berlin Heidelberg 1992

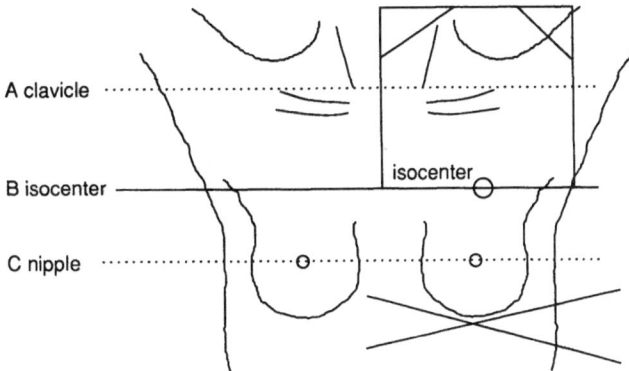

Fig. 1. Schematic view of the field arrangement

The relative dose distribution is optimized varying the gantry rotation, wedge filters, field shape, and relative weight for each field. The variation, in dose should be as low as possible, and the dose should not be less than 95% in any point. The gantry rotation is chosen so that the two upper fields do not irradiate the spinal cord, and so that the two lower fields avoid unnecessary irradiation of the opposite breast. It is also of great importance to minimize the absorbed dose to the lung. The resulting dose distribution is normalized according to the ICRU (1978) at a point in the middle of the breast parenchyma.

The three-dimensional dose calculations make use of a convolution algorithm based on pencil-beam energy deposition kernels. These kernels were calculated by superimposition of monoenergetic kernels generated by Monte Carlo simulations for each photon beam energy. The algorithm handles irregularly shaped fields and beam modifiers (Ahnesjö 1991). These calculations are implemented in a treatment planning system (TMS-Radix, Helax, Uppsala, Sweden).

Evaluation of the dose plan used conventional cross-sectional dose distributions, dose-volume histograms, and descriptive statistics for the target volume and the organs at risk. The criteria for acceptance was a dose distribution as homogeneous as possible, with no unnecessary irradiation of the lung or the spinal cord.

Results and Discussion

The resulting dose plans are presented as two-dimensional cross-sectional distributions in Fig. 2. The complete three-dimensional volumes are evaluated using dose-volume histograms for the target volume and the lung (Fig. 3).

Fig. 2. Cross-sectional dose distributions. **A** At the At the clavicle. **B** At the isocenter. **C** At the nipple. The isodose shown are: 50%, 85%, 90%, 95%, 100%, 105%, 110%, 115%, and 120%

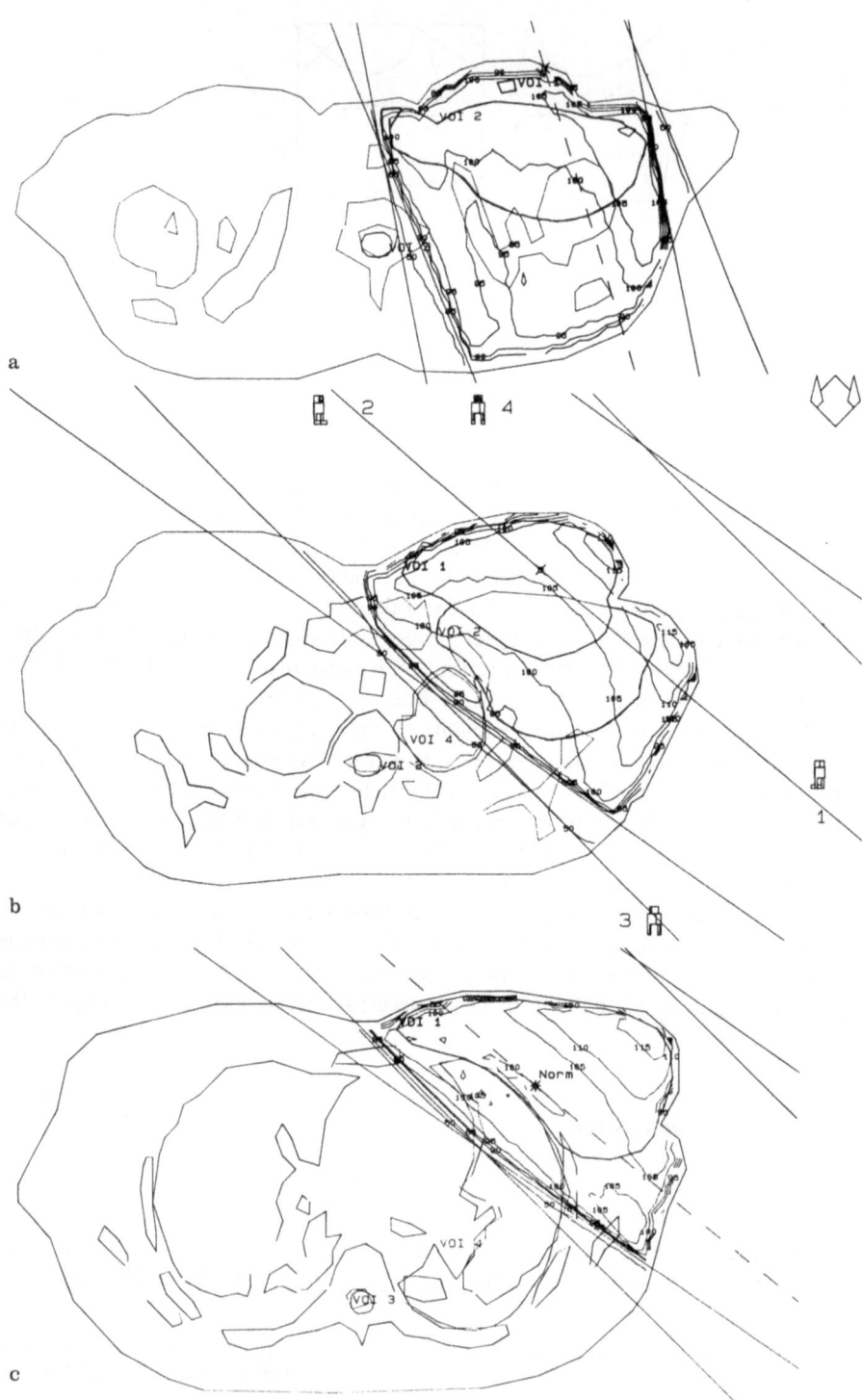

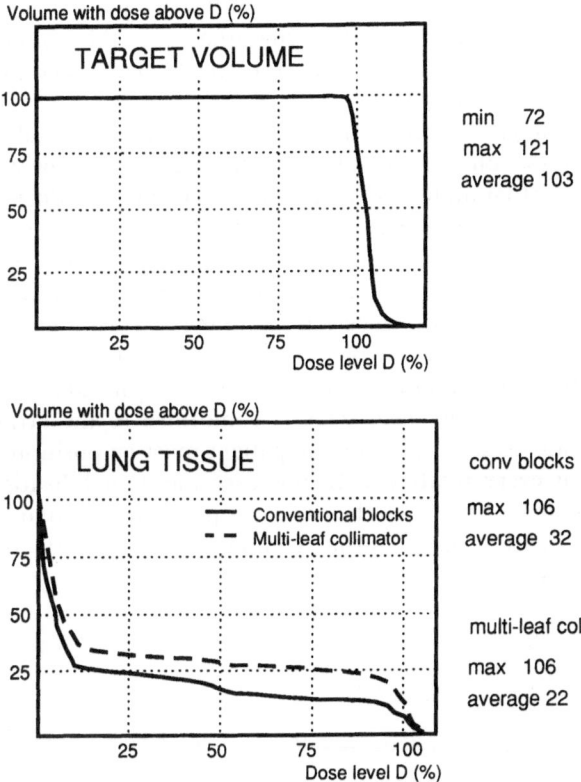

Fig. 3. Dose-volume histograms for the target volume and the lung

The absorbed dose showed variations inside the target of 70%–120%, with an average dose of 103%. The standard deviation for the whole target volume was 4%. The low dose contribution derived from few points at which the PTV was drawn close the skin. These dose values have no clinical relevance since the CTV remains at the same depth relative to the skin surface. The high dose values are found at areas situated in the lateral part of the breast. The dose calculation algorithm used a limited scatter mode, therefore the absorbed dose was overestimated in these parts. Similar results have been shown for other dose planning systems (Knöös et al. 1986a; van Bree et al. 1990). Thus, the actual variation in absorbed dose in the target was probably less than that registered by the treatment planning system.

The treatment of these patients was given with a fairly homogeneous dose distribution, while keeping the unwanted irradiation of the lung at an acceptable level. Approximately 70% of the lung received an absorbed dose less than 25 Gy, which is the upper level at which no late complications are expected to occur (Bentel et al. 1982).

An over- or underdosage in the intersection between the two pairs of fields can be avoided if the dose distribution is further smoothed over this volume. This is done by positioning the intersection level 1 cm caudad every 2nd treatment using the asymmetric collimator.

The use of a multileaf collimator for reduction of the treated volume resulted in a lower absorbed dose to the lung without affecting the target dose. This was shown in the dose-volume histogram for the lung (Fig. 3). The average dose to the lung was reduced by a factor of 30%. The amount of the lung which received a dose of 27 Gy (50% of the target absorbed dose) was reduced by 40%. The dose distribution inside the target volume was not affected by the multileaf collimator; however, the total absorbed dose may be increased without any complications in the lung. Further studies of this will be carried out in our hospital at the end of 1991, after a multileaf collimator has been installed.

To make use of all these facilities, fields closely conformed to the target volume, and a more accurate dose calculation, the patient must be positioned with very high accuracy at every treatment. In this case the immobilization device is a polyurethane foam cast in which the patient is positioned with arms on top of the head. This cast is used during computed tomography, the simulation process, and at every treatment.

Conclusions

The improvements in treatment planning using a three-dimensional system are:

- Three-dimensional volumetric description of the target and the organs at risk
- Three-dimensional description of the beam geometry
- Field shaping in beam's eye view resulting in treated volumes which are closely conformed to the target volume
- Three-dimensional dose calculation, which in the near future will be further improved using the collapsed cone convolution algorithm (Ahnesjö 1991), including better scatter modeling.

Particularly for this group of breast cancer patients, this radiation technique provides a homogeneous dose distribution while keeping the irradiation of the lung, spinal cord, and opposite breast an acceptably low level.

References

Ahnesjö A (1991) Dose calculation methods in photon beam therapy using energy deposition kernels, PhD thesis, University of Stockholm
Bentel GC, Nelson C H, Noell KT, Treatment planning and dose calculation in radiation oncology. Pergamon, New York

IRCU (1978) International commission on radiation units and measurements (ICRU), no 29: dose specifications for reporting external beam therapy with photons and electrons. Bethesda, Maryland,

Knöös T, Ahlgren L, Nilsson M (1986a) Comparison of measured and calculated absorbed doses from tangential irradiation of the breast, Radiother Oncol, 7, 81–88

Knöös T, Nilsson M, Ahlgren L (1986b) A method for conversion of Hounsfield number to electron density and prediction of macroscopic pair production cross-sections. Radiother Oncol 5: 337–345

van Bree NAM, van Battum LJ, Huizenga H, Mijnheer B (1990) Accuracy of tangential breast treatment in two commercial treatment planning systems. In: Proc 10th international conference on the use of computers in radiation therapy (ICCR). Lucknow, India, pp 274–277

Wambersie A, Landberg T, Johansson KA, Dobbs J, Gérard JP, Sentenac I (1989) Dose prescription and specification in external radiotherapy: evaluation of ICRU report 29 and new trends. ICRU News 2: 25–27

Three-Dimensional Treatment Planning
for Fast Neutrons

R. Schmidt[1], T. Schiemann[2], K.H. Höhne[2], and K.-H. Hübener[1]

Introduction

Based on differences in the energy deposition in biological matter, fast neutrons show a benefit for the radiotherapy of several tumors compared to photons [1]. The use of neutrons in radiotherapy involves treatment planning of at least the same quality as that for photons. The Mevaplan (Siemens) treatment planning system was adapted for the simulation of neutron dose distributions. The multiplanar reconstruction option of the system enables the coplanar calculation of three-dimensional dose distributions. The statistical evaluation is useful for discussing and comparing the different treatment plans. To improve the visualization of the treatment plans the topographic and dosimetric data were evaluated by the volume visualization system Voxel-Man. The treatment plans can be displayed in different types of views using the full spectrum of available rendering methods.

The small volume irradiation of a prostatic carcinoma was chosen as an example. The visualization clearly demonstrates the differences of four alternative dose calculations.

Materials and Methods

Neutron beams administered in radiotherapy are always contaminated with photons. As neutrons and photons have a considerably different relative biological effectiveness, the two types of radiation must be calculated in a treatment planning system [2]. Several modifications in the Mevaplan system had to be made for neutron treatment planning [3].

The multiplanar reconstruction option is used to calculate the total dose distribution in up to 40 coplanar computed tomography (CT) slices. In each of these slices the target and the organs at risk are encircled and are stored as

[1] Abteilung Strahlentherapie, Radiologische Klinik, Universitätskrankenhaus Eppendorf, Martinistr. 52, 2000 Hamburg 20, FRG
[2] Institut für Mathematik und Datenverarbeitung in der Medizin, Universitätskrankenhaus Eppendorf, Martinistr. 52, 2000 Hamburg 20, FRG

Advanced Radiation Therapy Tumor Response
Monitoring and Treatment Planning
Breit (Editor-in-Chief)
© Springer-Verlag, Berlin Heidelberg 1992

volumes of interest (VOIs). The beam's-eye view (BEV) technique was used to create irregularly shaped beams individually adapted to the corresponding projection of the target.

A quantitative evaluation of the three-dimensional treatment plans was performed by use of dose-volume histograms. Furthermore, the relative volume of the VOIs with a dose above a certain dose level was calculated and was available as dose-limit tables.

The CT and dose data can be reconstructed in any plane, but a three-dimensional visualization of these data is not possible with the Mevaplan system. Therefore further handling of the data in a volume visualization system was performed. The dose data were transferred together with the CT data and a matrix containing the VOIs to the Voxel-Man system via magtape.

Voxel-Man is an interactive system for rendering medical volume data, based on a data structure of volume elements (voxels) [4]. Two-dimensional projections of the data volumes are calculated by scanning the volumes with a ray-casting algorithm from the desired direction of view. Voxel-Man delivers a set of various rendering methods, such as differently shading algorithms, arbitrary cuts, transparency, and many possibilities for colored display of surfaces [5, 6]. Before rendering, some preprocessing steps must be applied to the data volumes. The original CT volume is compressed to a dynamic range of 256 gray values. To achieve cubic volume elements (isotropic data volumes), a linear interpolation of the intensity values between the original slices is performed, because in Mevaplan the distance between two slices is usually greater than the pixel distance within the slices. Additionally, a scaling must be applied to each slice of the dose volume, as the matrix for dose calculation is smaller than the matrix of the CT slices.

For the results shown here the bone was segmented from the CT data volume by thresholding. The surface normals were calculated from gray level gradients.

For three-dimensional rendering of the dose volume the z-buffer shading was used to obtain the impression of dose "clouds".

Results

The use of DT neutrons in radiotherapy requires complex treatment planning [7]. The treatment of a prostatic carcinoma is simulated as an example. The target volume includes the prostate, the seminal vesicles, and a 2-cm security margin [8].

Treatment plans resulting from two-dimensional planning were compared with three-dimensional treatment plans. For the two-dimensional planning the outlines of the target in numerous CT slices were projected to the central plane. In this plane the region of interest encompassed these projections. A standard

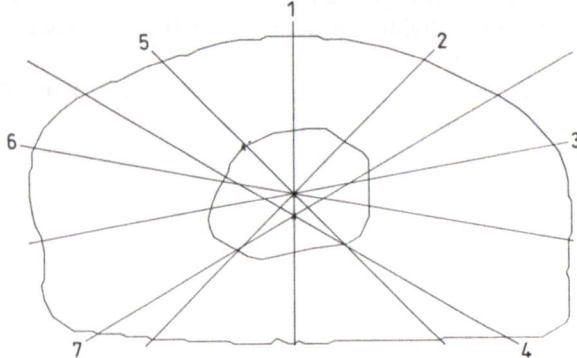

Fig. 1. Standard two-dimensional neutron treatment technique of a prostatic carcinoma

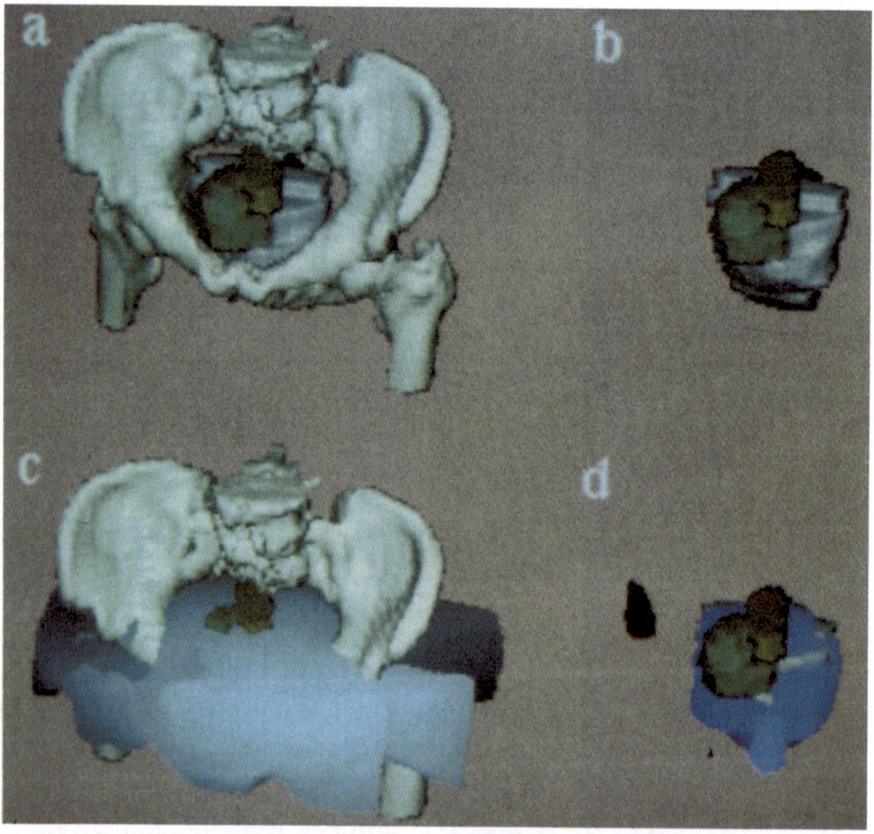

Fig. 2a–d. Examples of the interactive volume visualization of a three-dimensional treatment plan with fast neutrons. **a** Bone structures with VOIs. **b** VOIs: organs at risk *green*, bladder, *yellow* rectum, and target (*white*, prostate with seminal vesicles). **c** Bone and VOIs with 50% dose volume. **d** VOIs with 90% dose volume

technique with seven fixed isocentric neutron beams was applied (Fig. 1). For further three-dimensional evaluation this treatment plan was transferred to the multiplanar calculation so that the three-dimensional information of the original two-dimensional plan was available. The normalization of the total dose distributions was performed so that the minimum target dose in the central plane was 100% for each treatment plan.

For comparison the same CT data were used for the three-dimensional treatment plan. The arrangement of the neutron beams was adapted from the two-dimensional standard plan. The BEV was used to place nonfocused blocks into the fields to avoid irradiation of sensitive structures. These blocks were made of 12-cm-thick plates of stainless steel.

From outlining the target and the organs at risk on a series of coplanar CT scans, the VOIs can be displayed as three-dimensional structures, either together with anatomical structures (Fig. 2a) or without (Fig. 2b). Omitting the bony structure gives a better view of the VOIs. The dose distribution is displayed as dose volumes. A dose volume of a certain percentage includes all regions in which the dose is greater than or equal to this threshold. In Fig. 2c the 50% dose volume is displayed. To avoid some regions of the VOIs being hidden by the bone, omitting of the bone again gives a better view of the dose and VOIs (Fig. 2d). The Voxel-Man system is not only used to display dose and anatomical

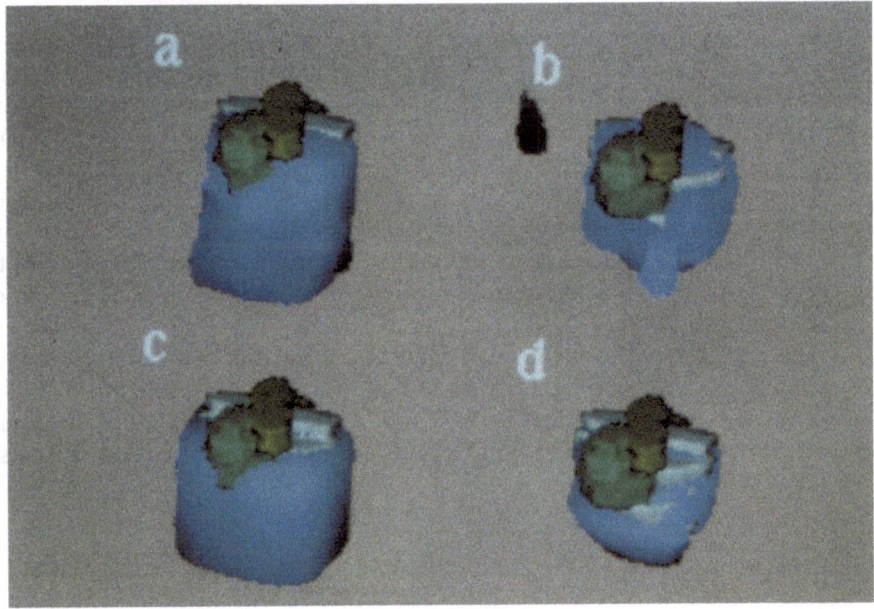

Fig. 3a–d. Examples of the interactive comparison of four treatment plans. **a** Seven fixed neutron fields, derived from two-dimensional standard. **b** Seven fixed neutron fields with blocks. **c** Five fixed X-ray fields, derived from two-dimensional standard. **d** Five fixed X-ray fields with irregularly shaped absorbers

structures but is also able to change these structures dynamically. Thus the displayed dose value can be changed continuously. This helps to monitor the concentration of the dose at the target. Anatomical stuctures can be added or hidden. The view can be rotated around any axis. This dynamic display is a powerful tool to display any desired dose value in three dimensions and to examine the dose distribution together with any desirable anatomical support.

Furthermore, the two neutron plans (Fig. 3a, b) were compared with two photon plans (Fig. 3c, d). One of these, again, is a standard two-dimensional plan with five fixed isocentric treatment fields with 16 MV X-rays (Fig. 3c). For the three-dimensional photon plan individually shaped, focused blocks were also used, with the BEV option for contouring the absorption filters. (Fig. 3d). The same features described can be used simultaneously with all four treatment plans so that the full spectrum of the visualization is used for comparison. Here the same representation as in Fig. 2d is chosen: rendering the VOIs together with the 90% dose volume.

In the three-dimensional photon plan the reference isodose is shaped very closely to the structure of the target. As this comparison is based on pure physical dose distributions only, the possible biological benefit of radiations with different LET must be taken into account as well.

Discussion

Three-dimensional treatment planning was used to simulate neutron dose distributions. The BEV and dose-volume histograms proved useful tools for optimizing and comparing dose distributions. The volume visualization system Voxel-Man was used to display the VOIs and the dose distributions dynamically in three-dimensional views.

The process of dynamically changing the anatomical display and the dose volumes gives a complete impression of the three-dimensional dose distribution. In contrast to dose-volume histograms that analyze the quality of dose given to target and organs at risk, the Voxel-Man system easily helps to locate regions of under- and overdosage.

This system is particularly suitable for the comparison of different treatment techniques even when different types of radiation are used. Here 14 MeV DT neutrons were compared to 16 MV X-rays. Although the quality of the X-ray dose distribution was superior to DT neutrons, the biological benefit must also be taken into account.

References

1. Schmitt G, Wambersie A (1990) Review of the clinical results of fast neutron therapy. Radiother Oncol 17: 47–56

2. Schmidt R, Heß A (1987) Computer assisted measurements for neutron therapy planning. In: Bruinvis IAD , van der Giessen PH, van Kleffens HJ, Wittkämper FW (eds) Proceedings of the 9th international conference on the use of computers in radiation therapy, Scheveningen, the Netherlands, 22–25 June, pp 421–424
3. Schmidt R, Thom E (1990) Neutron dose planning with the Mevaplan system. Strahlenther Onkol 166: 301–305
4. Höhne KH, Bomans M, Pommert A, Riemer M, Schiers C, Tiede U, Wiebecke G (1990) 3D-visualization of tomographic volume data using the generalized voxel-model. Visual Comput 6: 28–36
5. Höhne KH, Bomans M, Pommert A, Riemer M, Tiede U, Wiebecke G (1990) Rendering tomographic volume data: adequacy of methods for different modalities and organs. In: Höhne KH et al. (eds) 3D-imaging in medicine: algorithms, systems, applications. Springer, Berlin Heidelberg New York, pp 197–215 (NATO ASI series F: computer and systems sciences, Vol 60)
6. Tiede U, Höhne KH, Bomans M, Pommert A, Riemer M, Wiebecke G (1990) Investigation of medical 3D-rendering algorithms. IEEE Comput Graph Appl 10(2): 41–53
7. Franke HD, Schmidt R (1985) Clinical results with fast neutrons (DT, 14 MeV). Radiat Med 3: 151–160
8. Pilepich MV, Prasad SC, Perez CA (1982) Computed tomography in definitive radiotherapy of prostatic carcinoma. II. Definition of target volume. Int J Radiat Oncol Biol Phys 8: 235–240

Comparison of Dose Distributions With and Without Multileaf Collimator for the Treatment of Esophageal Carcinoma

J. Bauer, N. Hodapp, and H. Frommhold

Introduction

One of the major problems in external beam radiotherapy is achieving maximum protection of nonenvolved tissue. One way to do this is to use multileaf collimators, which have come into common use during recent years. At the Department of Radiotherapy in Freiburg we have also developed a multileaf collimator as an accessory system to a linear accelerator. A few cases, especially of esophageal carcinoma, have been treated with its help. In contrast to most multileaf collimators reported in the literature, which can be used only for fixed fields, our collimator is able to change the field shape continually during gantry rotation. Due to the small number of treated patients we still lack satisfying statistical results to verify the effectiveness of our multileaf collimator treatment. Therefore we apply decision criteria from the literature for comparison of treatment plans using multileaf collimated radiotherapy with those of conventional treatment techniques.

Materials and Methods

The Multileaf Collimator. As noted above, our multileaf collimator is capable of continuous field shaping during rotational therapy [1, 2]. The multileaf collimator, which is a separate system, can be mounted on the linear accelerator like a tray holder (Fig. 1). Each leaf of the collimator is driven mechanically by individually prepared disks. The transfer of the individual field shape from the therapy planning computer to the collimator has been carried out up to now with a special milling machine using target volume disks as stencils. We are now preparing to shorten this procedure by introducing a direct transfer of the target volume data to a CNC milling machine. The maximum possible enveloping cylinder has a diameter of 12 cm and a length of 20.8 cm. On each side of the collimator are 13 leafs with a width of 1.6 cm at the isocenter. The maximum

Abteilung Strahlentherapie, Universitätsklinik Hugstetterstraße 55, 7800 Freiburg, FRG

Advanced Radiation Therapy Tumor Response
Monitoring and Treatment Planning
Breit (Editor-in-Chief)
© Springer-Verlag, Berlin Heidelberg 1992

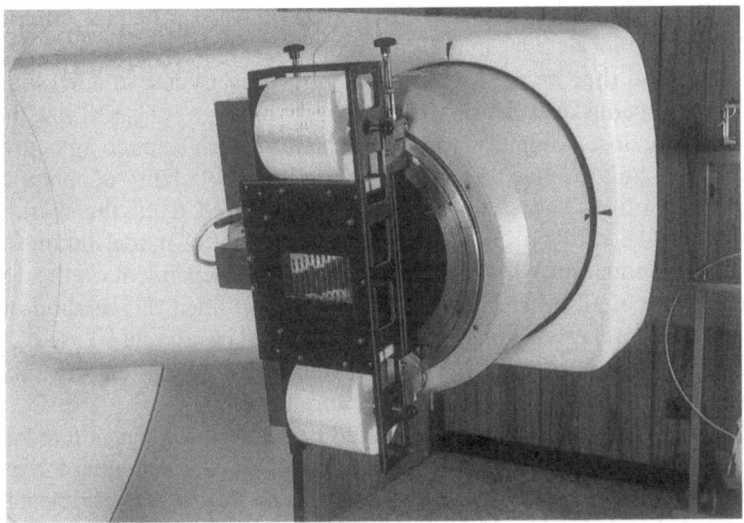

Fig. 1. Multileaf collimator at the treatment head of a Philips SL 75/20

travel of the leaves is about two-thirds of the maximum lateral width. The leaves diverge in longitudinal but not in lateral field direction.

Treatment Planning. For treatment planning and dose calculation we used a Siemens Evados treatment planning system with the software version Tele 9.4 D. The target volume was outlined in all computed tomography slices, which were taken 1.6 cm apart, depending on the width of the leaves. All outlines were projected onto one plane to obtain the diameter of the enveloping cylinder and its center as the location of the rotational axis. Continuous rotation with the multileaf collimator was approximated by overlaying the maximum number of ten fixed fields each supplied with the portal shape of the collimator at that position as an irregular field. For all relevant computed tomography slices the dose distribution was calculated, and, if necessary, the shape of the irregular field was modified.

Comparison of Treatment Plan Quality. For comparison of the treatment plan the dose-volume histogram of the whole target volume, several organs at risk, and the total volume minus the target volume was calculated (FORTRAN program was kindly provided by Dr. Killig, Siemens, Erlangen). With these dose-volume histograms we used two models for the evaluation of probabilities for tumor control and the risk of complications for several organs at risk. We recognize that the evaluation of probabilities using such models is still under discussion, and the experimental data which are the basis of the parameters of the models are rare and perhaps not reliable; nevertheless, we think that a comparison by sequencing the probability values may be a helpful criterion although the probability values may be inaccurate.

The first method that we used was that described by Lyman and Wolbarst [3]. For inhomogeneous dose delivery to the target volume or organ at risk they describe a stepwise dose-volume histogram reduction which leads to an equivalent dose for the whole volume and the corresponding probability of complication or tumor control. The second method was derived from the work of Schultheis et al. [4], who proposed an integral probability model taking the probability of escaping injury for each partial volume as dependent on the dose but not on the fate of all other partial volumes. We modified this method in a way that the same dose-volume histograms as in the first case could be used. For the dependence of the dose-effect relationship the logistic equation was taken with parameters D_{50} and k for specific late complications [4–6].

One of four esophageal carcinomas situated near the cardia which had been treated using our multileaf collimator was taken as an example for our comparison. Several factors suggest this situation as an advantageous object for the application of a multileaf collimator: (a) the lateral extension of the target volume changes rapidly along the longitudinal direction of the patient; (b) the centers of the target volume cross-sections do not lie on one axis; and (c) several organs at risk, such as spinal cord, heart, and lungs, are near the target volume. For the treatment of esophageal carcinoma several conventional techniques have been described. Due to restrictions by organs at risk it is often necessary to combine these to reach sufficient doses at the target volume. Our comparison is restricted to a few techniques which have been used in Freiburg: (a) Dorsoventral opposed fields with individual shielding blocks; the application of this technique is restricted by the tolerance of the spinal cord. (b) Oblique anterior wedge fields. Their disadvantage is a fairly high dose to the lungs. (c) Rotation of 300°. If the field is too long, there will be problems with the spinal cord. (d) Combination of a and b, weighted 1:1. (e) Combination of a and c, weighted 1:1. (f) Computed tomography planned multileaf collimator shaped treatment over 300° rotation. The dose-volume relationship was calculated for the target volume, lung, and spinal cord. The tumor control and complication probabilities refer to a dose of 60 GY.

Results

The dose-volume relationship (Fig. 2) for the target volume shows that a satisfying dose delivery is not possible, even for the combination of conventional treatment techniques. Better results are achieved with the multileaf arc technique. These are achieved with comparable or better results for the surrounding organs at risk. Similar results are obtained when calculating tumor control and complication probabilities (Table 1). These models differ only in their values for

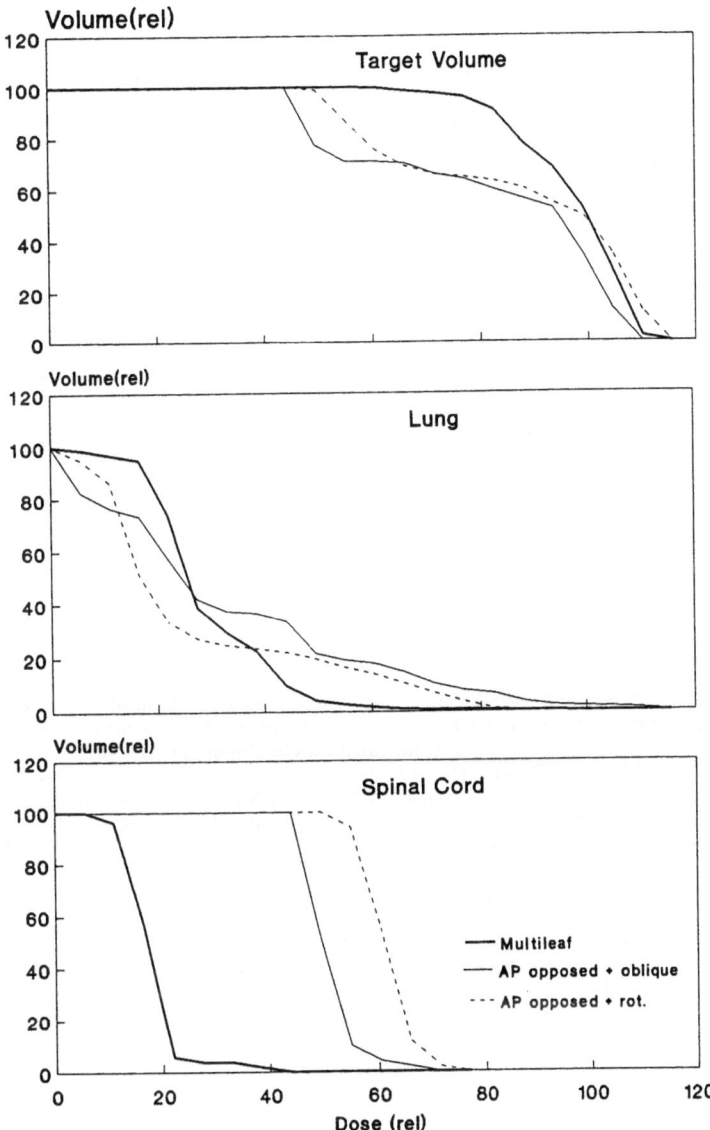

Fig. 2. Dose-volume histograms for three volumes of interest and three irradiation techniques

the lungs. Although these values may not be taken as a prediction of true tumor control or complication due to the reasons mentioned above, it should be possible to use such models to concentrate the information of the dose-volume histograms to have a simpler criterion for the judgement of new irradiation techniques such as the multileaf collimation.

Table 1. Tumor control and complication probabilities

Treatment technique	Lyman and Wolbarst [3]			Schultheiss et al. [4]		
	Target volume	Lung	Spinal cord	Target volume	Lung	Spinal cord
AP opposed	24	27	95	24	42	96
Oblique anterior	10	29	<1	11	38	<1
Rotation	20	3	<1	22	3	<1
AP opposed + oblique	18	31	<1	20	43	<1
AP opposed + rotation	28	19	<1	30	24	1
Multileaf collimator	36	1	<1	38	1	<1

References

1. Hodapp N, Nanko N, Neher A (1988) Ein mechanisch gesteuerter Multileafkollimator als Zusatzeinrichtung für die Therapie mit hochenergetischen Photonen. Medizinische Physik. Proc 19th Wiss Tagung der Deutschen Gesellschaft für Medizinische Physik, pp 178–182
2. Hodapp N, Nanko N, Slanina J, Neher A (1989) A low cost multileaf collimator as an accessory system for linear accelerators. Proc 6th Varian European Users Meeting, pp 114–116
3. Lyman JT, Wolbarst AB (1987) Optimisation of radiation therapy. III: A method of assessing complication probabilities from dose-volume histrograms. Int J Radiat Oncol Biol Phys 13: 103–109
4. Schultheiss TE, Orton CG, Peck B (1983) Models in radiotherapy: volume effect. Med Phys 10: 410–415
5. Diethelm L (1979) Die Strahlentherapie des Oesophaguscarcinoms. Radiologe 19: 245
6. Rubin P, Casarett G (1972) A direction for clinical radiation pathology. The tolerance dose. Front Radiat Ther Oncol 6: 1–16

Advantages of Three-Dimensional Treatment Planning Compared to Conventional Computed Tomography Planning for Radiotherapy of the Whole Liver

K. Sommer, W.-P. Brockmann, T. Wiegel, R. Schmidt, D. Entzian, A. Krüll, and K.-H. Hübener

Introduction

Radiotherapy of the whole liver in patients with colorectal cancer may be employed for progressive and disseminated hepatic metastases and in patients suffering from pain due to these metastases. Whole-liver radiotherapy seems a promising approach as well for improving the prognosis of patients with solitary liver metastases after a complete surgical resection. Conventional computed tomography (CT) planning for the liver does not include adaptation of the field shape to the irregular contour of the liver and thus causes side effects in the adjacent organs. To quantify the reduction of radiation in the adjacent organs, three-dimensional treatment planning with irregularly shaped fields has been compared to conventional CT planning for the liver.

Methods and Materials

In six patients with colorectal carcinomas and whole-liver irradiation conventional CT planning of the liver was performed, transferring the maximum liver extent to the reference plane. For the same patients three-dimensional treatment planning using irregularly shaped fields was performed using the Mevaplan-MPR software package for three-dimensional dose calculation (Siemens). This planning system can accomodate the entire information content of 40 CT slices. From a minimum of 5 cm above and 5 cm below the liver coplanar CT slices with a slice thickness of 8 mm were obtained. These data were then transferred into the Mevaplan format. Liver, kidneys, small intestine, and spinal cord were entered as volumes of interest (VOIs). Each VOI consists of several regions of interest (ROIs) which are defined manually via a resistor board as continuous contours in the CT images. Two rectangular, nearly opposing portals were used for the calculation of the conventional CT plan. The irregularly shaped fields were developed using the beam's eye view (BEV) of the software package, which

Abteilung für Strahlentherapie, Radiologische Klinik, Universitätskrankenhaus Eppendorf, Martinistr. 52. 2000 Hamburg 20, FRG

Advanced Radiation Therapy Tumor Response
Monitoring and Treatment Planning
Breit (Editor-in-Chief)
© Springer-Verlag, Berlin Heidelberg 1992

is used for field geometry optimization by visual exclusion of areas not within the target volume. To obtain a reliable statistical figure for the evaluation of the dose applied to the liver, right kidney, small intestine, and spinal cord, dose-limit histograms were calculated. These show the relative volume of each organ (VOI) within the reference isodose, i.e., the percentage of each organ receiving the prescribed dose.

Results

Figure 1 shows a sagittal slice reconstruction through liver and right kidney of a conventional treatment plan with two opposing rectangular portals. The right kidney is almost completely within the reference isodose. Figure 2 shows a corresponding sagittal slice reconstruction for the same patient of a three-dimensionally optimized treatment plan with two irregularly shaped fields constructed with the aid of the BEV (Fig. 3). For this treatment plan only a fraction of the superior pole of the right kidney lies within the reference isodose. To quantify the differences between the two treatment plans for all patients, dose-limit histograms were calculated. Figure 4 shows the mean values for all patients, comparing the modalities. The dose administered to the liver varied only minimally (96% versus 97% within the reference isodose). The most

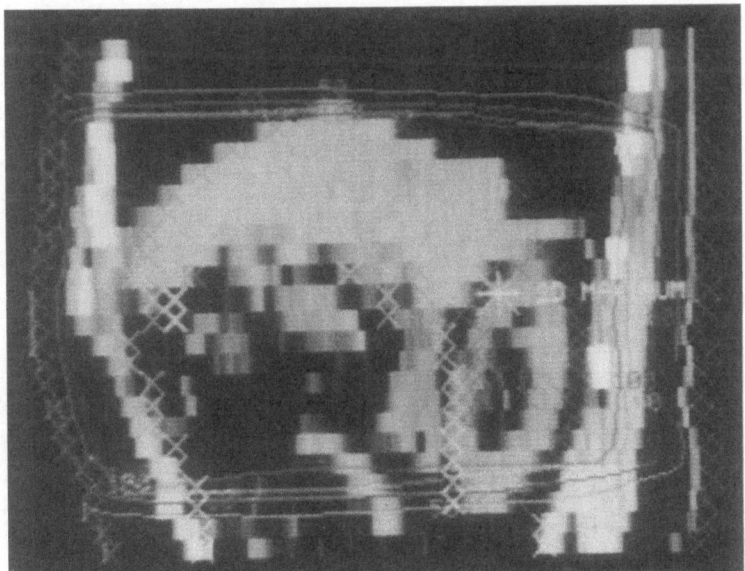

Fig. 1. Sagittal slice reconstruction through liver and right kidney for a conventional treatment plan with two opposing rectangular portals

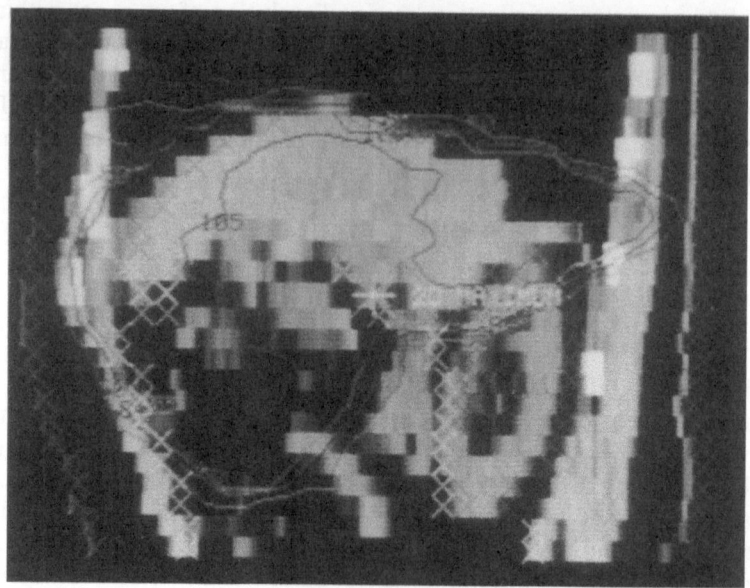

Fig. 2. Sagittal slice reconstruction through liver and right kidney for a three-dimensionally optimized treatment plan with two opposing irregularly shaped portals

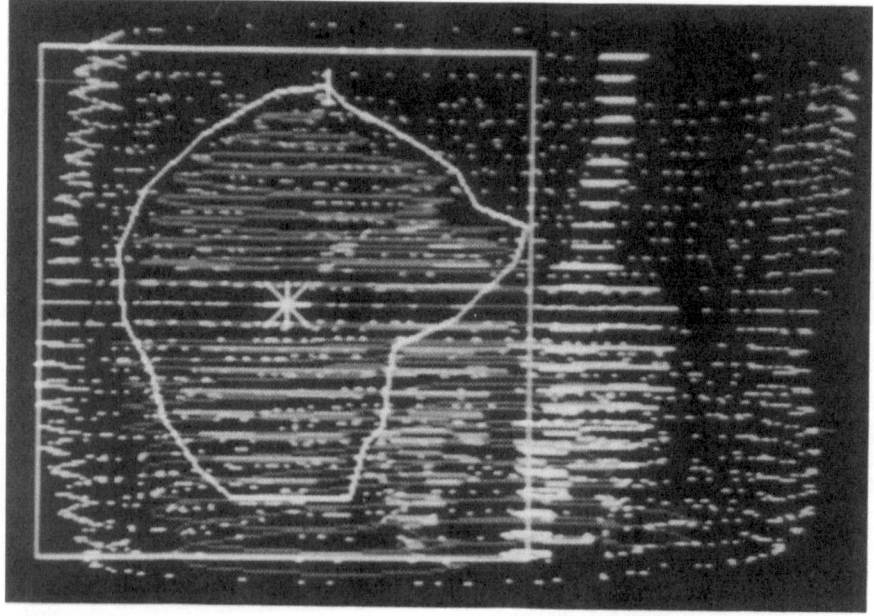

Fig. 3. Beam's eye view for field 1 of the three-dimensional treatment plan with irregularly shaped portals

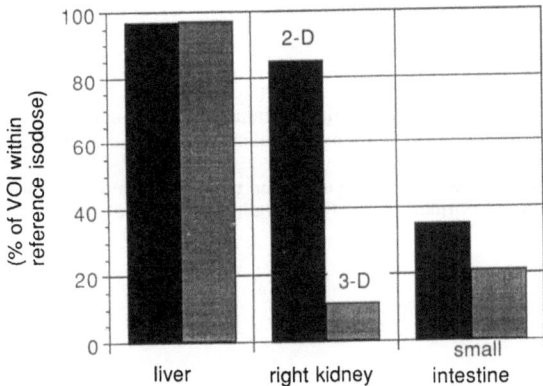

Fig. 4. Dose-limit histogram showing the mean values for all the examined patients, comparing conventional treatment plans with three-dimensional treatment plan with irregularly shaped portals

dramatic change was observed for the right kidney. With conventional CT planning 85% of this organ was located within the reference isodose, compared to only 11% with three-dimensionally optimized irregularly shaped fields. The volume of small intestine within the reference isodose was reduced from 35% to 21%. Spinal cord and left kidney received almost no radiation with either form of treatment plan.

Discussion

Three-dimensionally optimized treatment plans for the whole liver effectively spare the adjacent organs from radiation. This is especially the case for the right kidney (85% versus 11% within the reference isodose). Radiation tolerance for the kidney has been assessed in several publications. Dewit et al. found a reduction of the glomerular filtration rate (GFR) to 30%–40% after 5 years for human kidneys irradiated totally with 40 Gy in 5.5 weeks. Irradiation of the superior pole of human kidneys with 40 Gy in 4 weeks resulted in a GFR of 75% –80% after 5 years (Dewit et al. 1990). For canine kidneys Markoe et al. reported a GFR of 60%–80% after 3 months following irradiation of the whole kidney with 25 Gy (Markoe et al. 1989).

In conclusion, three-dimensional treatment planning of the whole liver with irregularly shaped portals effectively spares the right kidney from radiation, which is especially important in patients with impaired renal function or unilateral right kidney function.

Acknowledgement. This publication contains crucial parts of the doctoral thesis of D. Entzian.

References

Dewit L, Anninga JK, Hoefnagel CA et al. (1990) Radiation injury in the human kidney: a prospective analysis using specific scintigraphic and biochemical endpoints. Int J Radiat Oncol Biol Phys 19: 977–983

Markoe AM, Brady LW, Swartz C et al. (1989) Radiation effects on renal function. In: Vaeth JM, Meyer JL (eds) Radiation tolerance of normal tissues. Front Radiat Ther Oncol 23: 310–322

The Münster Experience with Magnetic Resonance Imaging Assisted Treatment Planning Used for High Dose Rate Afterloading Therapy of Gynecological and Nasopharyngeal Cancer

G. Kovacs*, R. Pötter, F.J. Prott, B. Lenzen, and T.H. Knocke

Introduction

The need for complex technology in radiation oncology has been demonstrated at many sites in tumorous disease [1, 2]. Some publications concerning quality assurance have shown that treatment planning plays a very important role in the optimization of therapy results. The technique of magnetic resonance imaging (MRI) assisted treatment planning has been initiated for teletherapy at the University of Münster [3, 4]; this was described in its modification for treatment planning in brachytherapy [5]. The method has been used in daily routine since July 1989. Taking advantage of MRI integrated into treatment planning, we used an asymmetric balloon applicator for the therapy of small lateral residual disease of nasopharynx cancer after external beam therapy. To define the target volume in different planes for brachytherapy of gynecological cancer in relation to the applicator, tumor, and region of potential spread, we used MRI in the routine treatment planning for cancer of the uterus and vagina using a special dummy applicator.

The initial experiences and possible trends for the future are presented here.

Methods and Results

Treatment planning in brachytherapy is generally based on conventional AP and lateral radiograph imaging applicator and, to a limited extent, tumor region and normal tissue mostly in the AP and lateral directions. The X-ray localization film represents the basis for the calculation of dose distribution. The aim of this study was to individualize the definition of target volume in brachytherapy of gynecological and nasopharyngeal cancer by using MRI with its multiplanar imaging capacity, its high soft-tissue contrast, and its special advantages for treatment planning in brachytherapy [5].

Radioonkologie, Klinik und Poliklinik für Strahlentherapie, Westfälische Wilhelms-Universität Münster, Albert-Schweitzer-Str. 33, 4400 Münster, FRG
* Klinik für Strahlentherapie (Radioonkologie) des Klinikums der CAU zu Kiel, Arnold-Heller-Str. 9, 2300 Kiel, FRG

Advanced Radiation Therapy Tumor Response
Monitoring and Treatment Planning
Breit (Editor-in-Chief)
© Springer-Verlag, Berlin Heidelberg 1992

The dummy device has a similar geometry to that of the treatment applicator; it is not ferromagnetic and is filled with diluted Gd-DTPA. The dummy device is placed in treatment position, and MR images are obtained in applicator orientation. The method allows the viewing of dummy applicator, tumor, and critical structures in different planes. The freely chosen sequences are used for target volume definition and for calculation of dose distribution around the applicator within the target and at organs of risk. Before treatment with the active source the positions of the treatment applicator and the dummy device must be checked. If they are identical, the pretreatment planning can start on the basis of slices in which the dummy applicator is visible. This control is most precise when using the substrascope for image superimposition [3–5].

The thickness of the MRI slices used for treatment planning of brachytherapy was 7.0 mm (pelvis) and 5.0 mm (nasopharynx) in each investigated case. As a basis for dose calculations for nasophyaryngeal boost therapy we used T1-weighted sagittal and axial slices with or without intravenous Gd—DTPA. For gynecological tumors the chosen sequences were: T1, T2 in sagittal and applicator-related paraaxial and paracoronal slices. The MRI-based treatment planning helped to minimize the target area in the nasopharyngeal cube. For this reason we used an asymmetric or symmetric balloon applicator, fixed in the nasopharynx for the treatment time and a dummy for the planning procedure (Figs. 1, 2). The distance between tumor and iridium source is short, while healthy tissue that is not to be irradiated is pushed away by the balloon from the area of high dose (> 10 mm distance from the active source).

We treated four patients with advanced nasopharyngeal cancer by combined external beam (60 Gy) plus local afterloading boost (2 × 5 Gy, once per week) with the transnasal technique. The follow-up was carried out with one exception by MRI. There was no residual disease after therapy. While the follow-up has been short (16, 14, 6, 4 months), up to now we have not seen evidence of recurrence. For the treatment planning of gynecological cancer we put a dummy

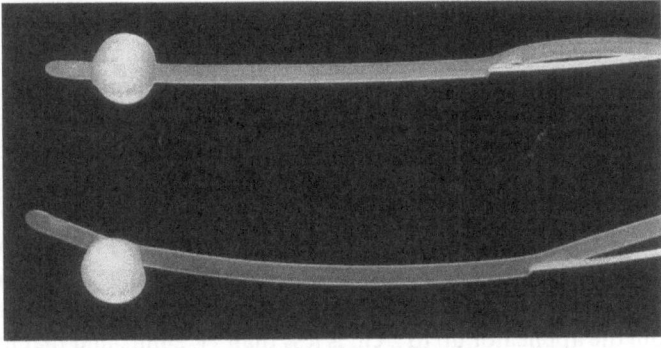

Fig. 1. The symmetric and asymmetric balloon applicator for use in minimal target volume irradiation of nasopharyngeal cancer

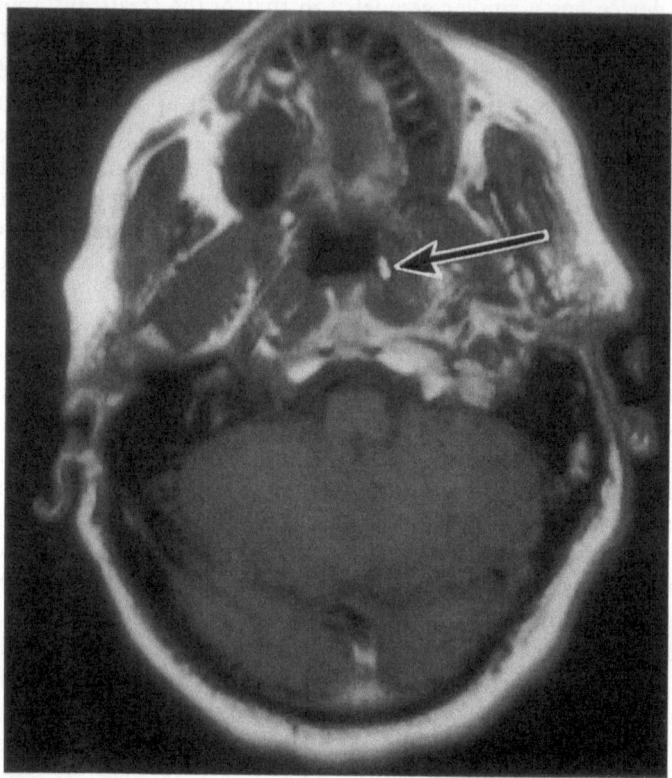

Fig. 2. Axial T1 slice (intravenous Gd-DTPA) showing laterally fixed asymmetric balloon applicator (*arrow*)

applicator into the vagina (5 patients) or the cervix and corpus uteri (11 patients). As side effect of the MRI-based treatment planning there was one perforation without any clinical symptoms.

The geometric distortion of our 1.5-T Magnetom MRI facility was investigated by a special phantom using spin-echo sequences. Within the center of the magnetic field — the region of interest in the images for gynecological and nasopharyngeal brachytherapy — this deviation was below 1 mm [4]. When directly superimposing objects with their true size from MR images onto radiographs, the amount of magnification due to beam divergence and the geometric inaccuracy due to decentral imaging must be taken into account.

If the deviation for 1 cm distance from the reference slice is $\pm 1\%$, and the distance between X-ray source and applicator is 115–125 cm (applicator plane as reference, 120 cm), the deviation for the small pelvis (active length under 10 cm, distance from the applicator up to 2 cm is less than ± 2 mm, and that for the nasopharyngeal region (active length up to 3 cm, distance from the applicator up to 2 cm) is less than ± 1 mm [4].

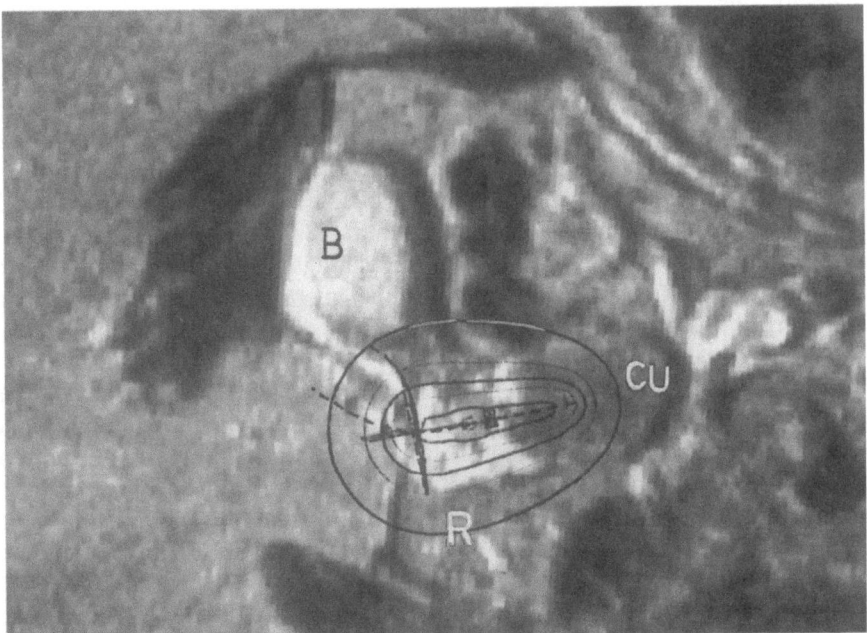

Fig. 3. T2-weighted sagittal plane of a junctional adenocarcinoma with superimposed dose calculation. *B*, Bladder; *R*, rectum; *CU*, corpus uteri

Discussion

The planning procedure integrating MRI — using (para-)coronal (para-)sagittal and transversed planes with a Gd-DTPA applicator — has the advantage of precise target volume definition in these planes along the axis of the applicator and of determination of dose within this target taking into account the critical dose at radiosensitive structures (for example, rectum and bladder in gynecological cancer, brain in nasopharyngeal cancer).

Using the MRI-based pretreatment planning, we found clinically evident advantages in cancers of the corpus-cervix junction area (Fig. 3). This type of tumor is adenocarcinoma, sometimes with larger corpus uteri and clinically normal portio. The length of the uterus probe and the result of the fractionated abrasio could suggest a corpus adenocarcinoma with its usual position in the fundus uteri. On the T2 sagittal sequences the tumor location can be clearly demonstrated, resulting in an adequate definition of target volume and dose distribution.

In one case MRI showed that instead of primary vaginal squamous cell cancer the patient had an advanced squamous cell cancer of the corpus and cervix uteri with a vaginal metastasis.

Conclusions

1. For the boost brachytherapy of nasopharyngeal tumors, MRI integrating transverse, coronal, and sagittal planes gives adequate information for definition of the individual target volume in relation to the position of the applicator.

2. For gynecological cancer the target volume can be adequately defined in different planes, imaging the applicator, tumor, area of potential spread, rectum, and bladder wall. This offers particular advantages in treatment planning for irregular targets, for the combination of different brachytherapy methods (e.g., intracorporal + intracervical + vaginal), and in specific tumor locations (e.g., junctional area).

3. MRI-assisted localization means for the patient an additional administration without radiation before the performance of brachytherapy but additional safety for a more clearly defined dose in the target and radiosensitive structures.

4. Investigation is necessary for evaluating the amount of change in target volume definition and dose distribution within the target which may be observed by adding multiplanar MRI to conventional fluoroscopy or computed tomography assisted treatment planning.

5. Further investigations are required to establish the role of MRI-assisted treatment planning in the individual combination of external beam radiotherapy and brachytherapy for gynecological cancer.

References

1. Brickner TJ (1990) Carcinoma of the cervix. Patterns of care study newsletter. American College of Radiology 1990–91, 1
2. Hanks GE, Henning DF, Kramer S (1983) Patterns of care outcome studies: results of the national practice in cancer of the cervix. Cancer 51 (5): 959–967
3. Pötter R, Heil B, Schneider L, Lenzen H, Al-Dandashi C, Schnepper E (1990) Sagittal and coronal planes from MRI for treatment planning in tumors of brain, head and neck: MRI assisted simulation. Radiother Oncol (in press)
4. Pötter R (1989) Lokalisation mit Hilfe bildgebender Verfahren in der Strahlentherapie maligner Tumoren. Habilitationschrift, University of Münster
5. Pötter R, Kovacs G, Lenzen B, Prott FJ, Knocke TH, Haverkamp U (1990) Technique of MRI assisted treatment planning in intraluminal Brachytherapy. Activ Selectr Brachyther J 5(3): 145–148
6. Wang CC (1983) Radiation therapy for head and neck neoplasms. Bright, Boston, p 207

Impact of Magnetic Resonance Imaging Assisted Simulation on Target, Treatment, and Irradiation Volume in Treatment Planning of Prostate Cancer

R. Pötter, M. Kelker, F.J. Prott, and B. Lenzen

Introduction

In magnetic resonance imaging (MRI) assisted treatment planning it is possible to define the individual target and organs at risk precisely and reproducibly in any plane of interest, in particular in sagittal, coronal, oblique, and arbitrary planes [2, 6]. Prostate cancer is usually irradiated by multiple fields, often by fixed orthogonal AP and lateral fields [1]. In conventional computer tomography (CT) assisted fluoroscopic simulation the target volume and organs at risk are defined in transverse planes based on high soft-tissue contrast [4, 5] and in AP, lateral, and oblique X-ray projections based on low soft-tissue contrast, except using contrast media for bladder and rectum [1].

Materials and Methods

In MRI-assisted fluoroscopic simulation tumor (prostate), target volume, and organs at risk (rectum, bladder) were superimposed electronically from coronal and sagittal planes (MRI) onto AP and lateral simulator radiographs (SR) using a subtrascope [6, 7] with adjustment of magnification. The superimposition was based on bony anatomical landmarks: acetabula, femoral heads, and outer contour of iliac bones in the AP projection (coronal plane); symphysis ossis pubis, os sacrum vertebral bodies L4/L5 in the lateral projection (sagittal plane). The choice of the bony landmarks was determined by the possibility of delineation in both imaging modalities and the possibility of localization within the plane of the prostate (reference plane). Taking the plane from MRI as reference plane, geometric inaccuracy due to magnification is $\leq 1\%$ per centimeter distance from the reference plane [3].

MRI was carried out using spin-echo sequences (T1, T2) with the patient in supine position analogous to the treatment position. Radiotherapy was performed by a four-field technique (AP/PA, lateral, 10-MV linear accelerator)

Klinik und Poliklinik für Strahlentherapie, Radioonkologie, Westfälische Wilhelms-Universität Münster, Albert Schweitzer-Str. 33, 4400 Münster, FRG

Advanced Radiation Therapy Tumor Response
Monitoring and Treatment Planning
Breit (Editor-in-Chief)
© Springer-Verlag, Berlin Heidelberg 1992

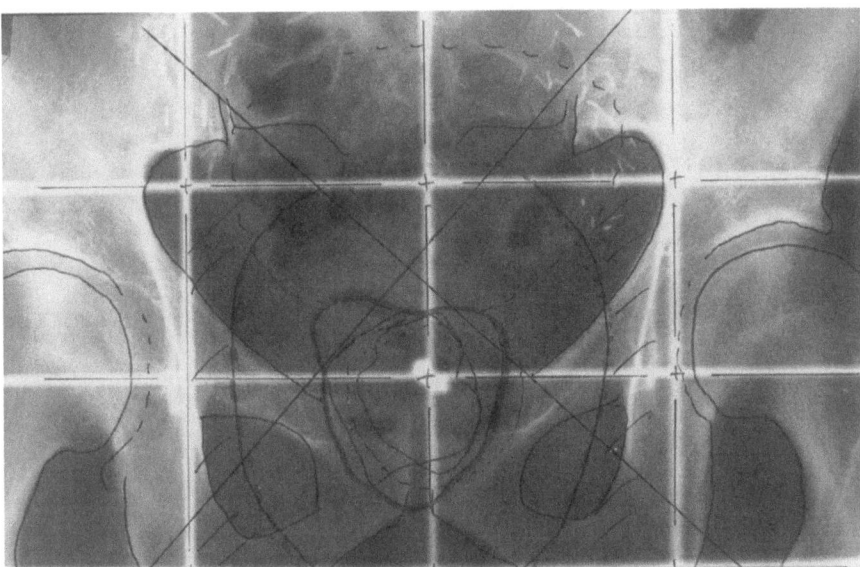

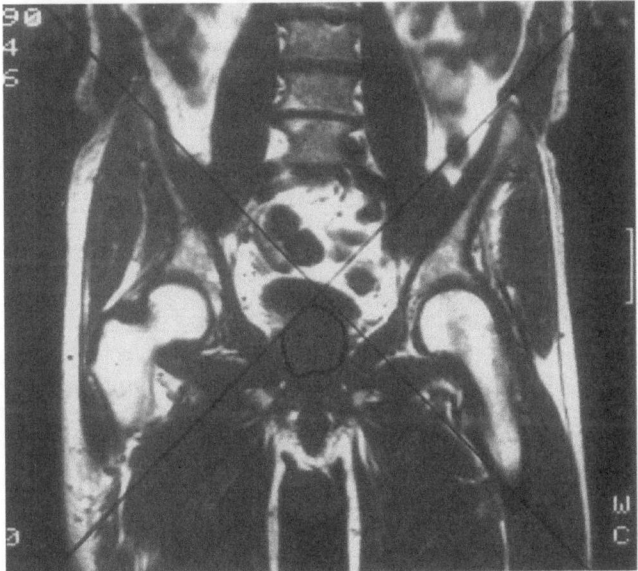

a

Fig. 1a, b. Target and treatment volume in treatment planning of prostate cancer (T1, G1, N0, M0) based on delineation of prostate, seminal vesicle, and organs at risk by superimposition of MRI and simulation films. **a** Coronal MRI and anteriorposterior simulation film. **b** Sagittal MRI and lateral simulation film (including seminal vesicle). Change in target and treatment volume (adequacy, reduction) using coronal and sagittal planes (MRI) (dotted line) compared to using transverse planes (CT) and AP and lateral simulation films (wire frame)

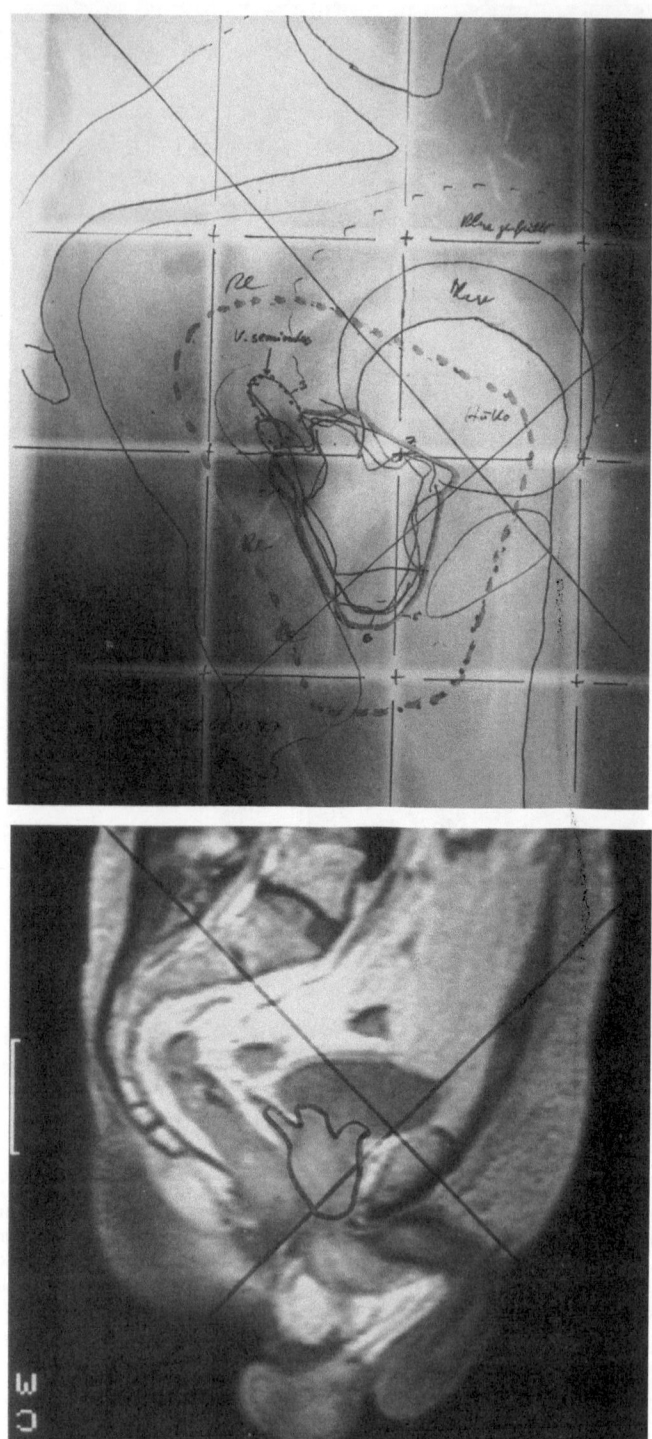

Fig. 1b.

based on transverse CT planes and computed dose calculations. Additional individual shielding blocks were designed on the basis of MRI-assisted target volume definitions in coronal and sagittal planes.

CT- and MRI-assisted simulation was performed for nine patients with prostate adenocarcinoma after clinical and surgical staging (T1/T2, GI/II, N0, M0). Target volumes were regional lymph nodes including the prostate (true pelvis), prostate alone (in part including the seminal vesicles) with a safety margin of 1–2 cm (planning volume) [1, 4, 5]. In CT-assisted simulation the target was defined as individually shaped in transverse planes and by standard rectangular open fields in AP and lateral projections. In MRI-assisted simulation the target was defined as individually shaped in transverse planes and in

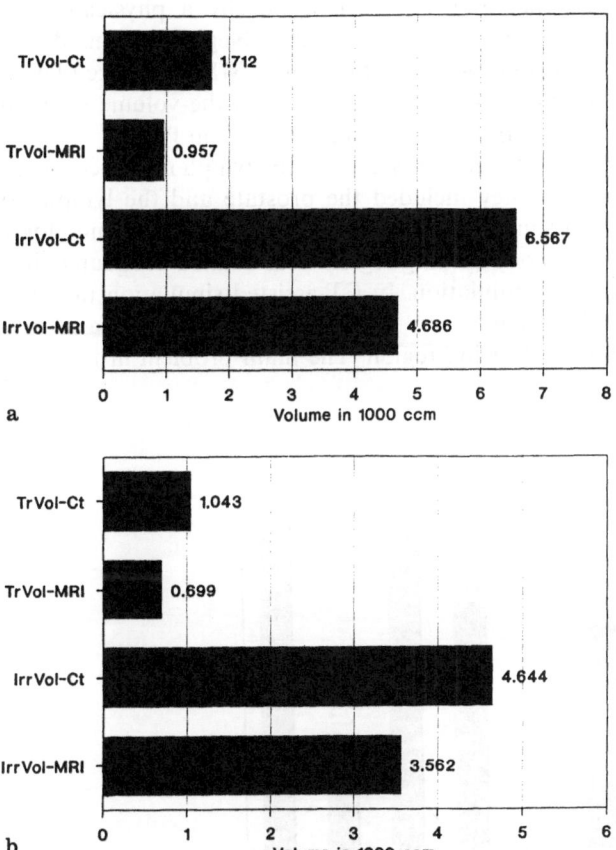

Fig. 2a, b. Mean values for treatment volume (90% isodose) and irradiation volume (50%–60% including isodose) for localized prostate cancer ($n = 9$). Comparison of fluoroscopic simulation based on transverse planes from CT (rectangular open fields) and fluoroscopic simulation based on additional coronal and sagittal planes from MRI (with individual shielding blocks). **a** Target: regional lymph nodes including the prostate (true pelvis). **b** Target: prostate (safety margin of 1–2 cm)

coronal and sagittal orientations. Target, treatment volume (90% isodose), and irradiation volume (50%–60% including isodose) were defined for CT- and MRI-assisted simulation independently and compared (Fig. 1).

The anatomical adequacy of target definition was judged using as criterion the definition in transverse (CT), coronal (MRI/SR), and sagittal (MRI/SR) planes. The quantitative comparison was based on planimetric measurements on AP and lateral SR [3].

Results

The procedure of superimposition was carried out by a physician at the subtrascope mean within 30 min for one patient. Neglecting the different magnification factors in different planes and taking as MRI reference plane the midplane of the prostate, the geometrical distortion in the volume of interest ($5 \times 5 \times 5$ cm) due to magnification was only up to 1.25 mm [3].

Target volume definitions for the prostate and the lymph node bearing area were defined as adequate if they included the prostate and the lymph node bearing area with a safety margin of about 1.5 cm. Target volumes for the prostate and for the lymph node bearing region were defined adequately in 9/9 patients using MRI-assisted simulation. In CT-assisted simulation target volumes were defined inadequately in 4/9 patients for the prostate and in 2/9 patients for the lymph node bearing region. The main problem in inadequate

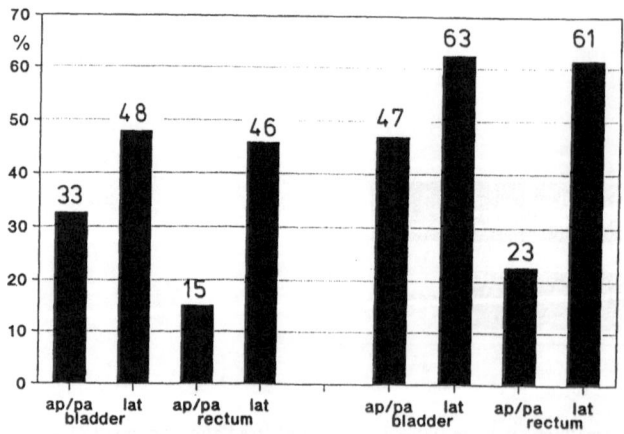

Fig. 3. Mean values of relative reduction in radiation dose (90% isodose) of bladder and rectum in localized prostate cancer ($n = 9$). Comparison of fluoroscopic simulation based on transverse planes from CT (rectangular fields) and fluoroscopic simulation based on additional coronal and sagittal planes from MRI (with individual shielding blocks). *Left*, true pelvis; *right*, prostate

definitions was the lack of precise delineation of the caudal border of the target (bottom of the prostate).

Based on a four-field box technique the mean reduction in treatment volume comparing MRI- to CT-assisted simulation was 44% for the lymph node bearing area and 33% for the prostate (Fig. 2; compare results in [8]). The irradiation volume was reduced on average by 29% and 23%, respectively (Fig. 2; compare results in [8]). Volumes of urinary bladder and rectum within the treatment volume were reduced on average by 47% (from 33% to 63%) and 36% (from 15% to 61%) comparing MRI- to CT-assisted simulation (Fig. 3; compare results in [8]). The main reductions were found in the lateral projections.

Conclusions

MRI-assisted fluoroscopic simulation integrates precisely and reproducibly transverse, coronal, and sagittal planes in treatment planning of prostate cancer. Geometrical inaccuracies due to different projection and magnification are of minimal importance. An adequate anatomical definition of target volume was achieved in all planes, whereas based on transverse planes and lateral and AP X-ray projections definition was inadequate in 6/18 targets. MRI-assisted fluoroscopic simulation resulted in a significant reduction (one-third) in treatment and irradiation volume and in irradiation of critical organs (bladder, rectum). The use of a subtrascope MRI-assisted simulation in prostate cancer is a clinically feasible method leading to conformation therapy that entails only little additional effort.

Acknowledgements. The authors would like to thank C. Rademacher and S. Köster for assistance in performing the study and P. Mause and I. Liebe for help with preparing the manuscript.

References

1. Bagshaw MA (1984) A technique for external beam irradiation of carcinoma of the prostate. In: Lewitt SH, du Tapley N (eds) Technological basis for radiation therapy. Lea and Febiger, Philadelphia, pp 244–270
2. Hricak H, Williams RD, Spring DB, Moon KL, Hedgcock MW, Watson RA, Crooks LE (1983) Anatomy and pathology of the male pelvis by magnetic resonance imaging. AJR 141: 1101–1110
3. Kelker M (1992) MRT-gestützte Simulation in der Planung der Strahlentherapie von Beckentumoren. Dissertationsschrift, University of Münster
4. Pilepich MV, Perez CA, Prasad S (1980) Computed tomography in definitive radiotherapy of prostatic carcinoma. Int J Radiat Oncol Biol Phys 6: 923–926

5. Pilepich MV, Prasad S, Perez CA (1982) Computed tomography in definitive radiotherapy of prostatic carcinoma. II. definition of target volume. Int J Radiat Oncol Biol Phys 8: 235–240
6. Pötter R (1989) Lokalisation mit Hilfe bildgebender Verfahren in der Strahlentherapie maligner Tumoren. Habilitationsschrift. University of Münster
7. Pötter R, Heil B, Schneider L, Lenzen H, Al-Dandashi C, Schnepper E (1992) Sagittal and coronal planes from MRI for treatment planning in tumors of brain, head and neck: MRI assisted simulation. Radiother Oncol 23: 127–130
8. TenHaken RK, Perez-Tamago C, Tesser RJ, McShan DL, Fraass BA, Lichter AS (1989) Boost treatment of the prostate using shaped, fixed fields. Int J Radiat Oncol Biol Phys 16: 193–200

Multiple Myeloma: Comparative Imaging Assessment

Introduction

Because the risk is so relevant to the risk of involving calcaneus bone lesion in patients with multiple myeloma. Bone lesions are usually confirmed or determined solely on plain radiography to infiltration of myeloma cells. Magnetic resonance imaging (MRI) is now known for excellent depiction of bone marrow in multiple myeloma. Studies on plain films are not new of bone. It has been that accounts for correlation with the increased comparable in bone. Comparison of MRI in configuration in the more increases in extension by (MRI) in different hematologic malignant disorders have been published recently (Hopper et al. 1988). The study presented here compared results of plain films and MRI in patients with multiple myeloma.

Patients and Methods

A total of 25 patients with multiple myeloma were studied prospectively by MRI at 1.5 T. Each examination made of elevated of art was used in combination with a spin-echo phase gradient. Sequence repetition time, TR, 400 ms; echo time, TE, 22 ms; 90°; A three-plate thickness 5 mm. Semiquantitative equal Gaussian was performed before and after intravenous administration of 0.1 mmol/kg gadolinium-DTPA per location body weight. Using the back and body regions. Post-DTPA enhanced examined all diffuse marrow spine, pelvis, and femora bones were imaged in the same total. Plain films acquired within 5 days of the MRI examination were available in all patients and complete tomography (in 17 scans in which lesions were detected on MRI scans were available in 6). Plain films were evaluated by an independent observer. Multiple myeloma was...

Multiple Myeloma: Treatment Planning Assisted by Magnetic Resonance Imaging

N. Hosten[1], W. Schörner[1], C. Zwicker[1], A. Kirsch[2], D. Huhn[2], and R. Felix[1]

Introduction

Radiation therapy is an effective way of treating osteolytic bone lesions in patients with multiple myeloma. Plain films are usually employed to detect osteolytic changes secondary to infiltrates of myeloma cells. Magnetic resonance imaging (MRI) is now known for excellent depiction of bone marrow (Vogler and Murphy 1988). Unlike on plain films, it is not bone or loss of bone mass that accounts for contrast in MRI but the cellular compounds. A higher sensitivity of MRI in detecting marrow lesions may therefore be expected. Results of MRI in different hematologic disorders have been published recently (Döhner et al. 1989). The study presented here compares results of plain films and MRI in patients with multiple myeloma.

Patients and Methods

A total of 25 patients with multiple myeloma were studied prospectively by MRI at 0.5 T. A body coil with a field of view of 52 cm was used in combination with an opposed-phase gradient-echo sequence (repetition time, TR, 400 ms; echo time, TE, 22 ms; 90°; 13 slices; slice thickness 5 mm; 3-mm interslice gap). Imaging was performed before and after intravenous administration of 0.1 mmol gadolinium-DTPA per kilogram body weight. Using the body coil and gadolinium-DTPA enhanced coronal MR images, lumbar spine, pelvis, and femoral bones were imaged in 6.25 min. Alternatively, imaging of thoracic spine and rips was carried out in the same time. Plain films acquired within 3 days of the MRI examination were available in all patients and computed tomography (CT) scans of areas in which lesions were detected on MRI scans were available in 7. Plain films were evaluated by an independent observer. Multiple myeloma was

[1] Department of Radiology, Klinikum Rudolf Virchow/Charlottenburg, Spandauer Damm 130, W-1000 Berlin 19, FRG
[2] Department of Internal Medicine, Klinikum Rudolf Virchow/Charlottenburg, Spandauer Damm 130, W-1000 Berlin 19, FRG

Advanced Radiation Therapy Tumor Response
Monitoring and Treatment Planning
Breit (Editor-in-Chief)
© Springer-Verlag, Berlin Heidelberg 1992

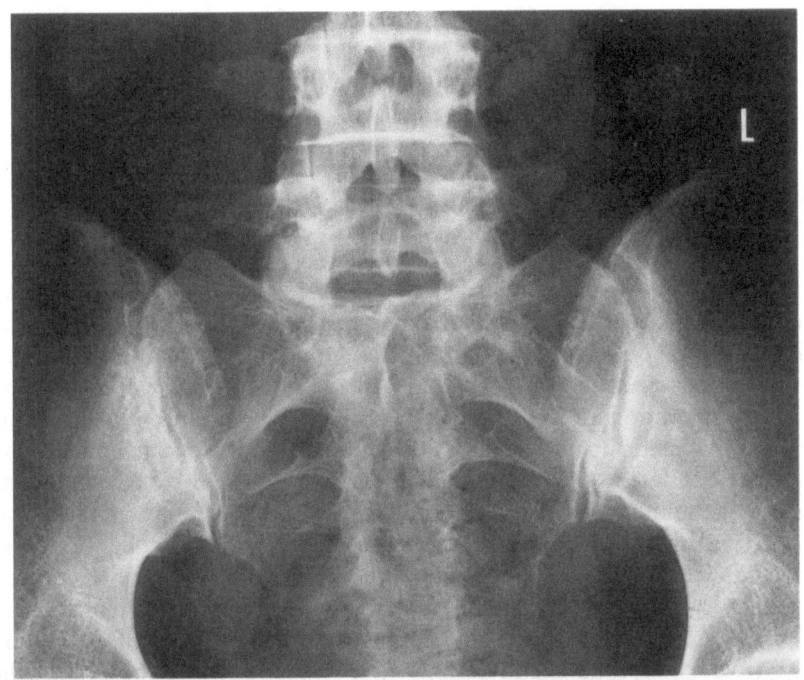

a

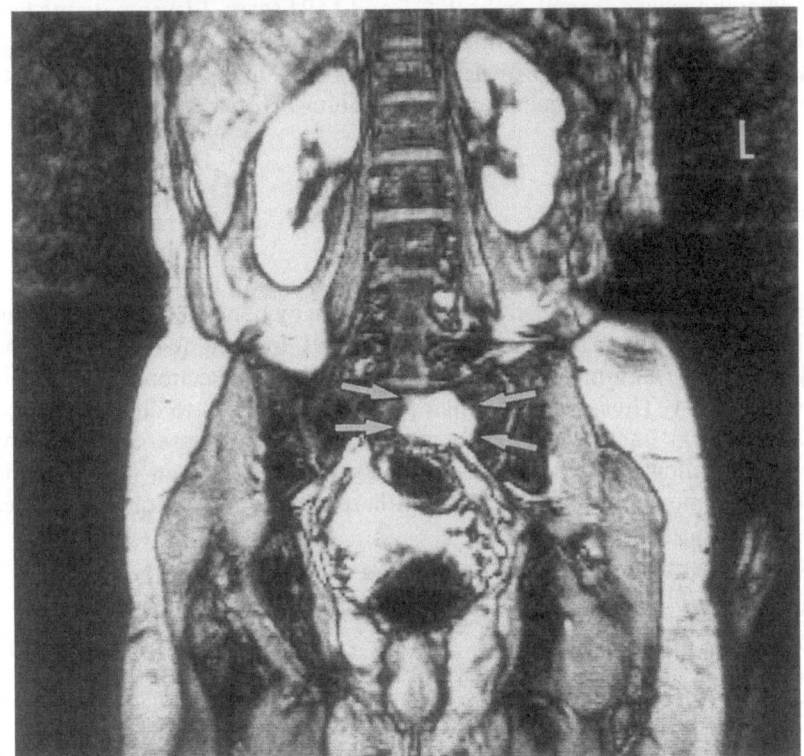

b

diagnosed when more than 15% plasma cells were found in iliac crest biopsy, and when monoclonal proteins were detected in either serum or urine. Stage I myeloma was diagnosed in two patients, stage II in one, and stage III in 22.

Results

Plain films detected large osteolyses in two patients; small osteolyses were found in seven. Eight patients had diffuse demineralization of the lumbar spine; one had diffuse demineralization of the pelvis. Red blood marrow had close to zero signal on opposed-phase gradient-echo MR images. Focal lesions of high signal intensity were found in 12 patients. Large lesions that pervaded cortical bone were seen in five patients and small lesions confined to trabecular bone in ten. All large lesions were seen on both plain and gadolinium-DTPA enhanced images, but gadolinium-DTPA enhanced images detected more small lesions than plain MR images (59 versus 35; see Fig. 1). Open biopsy was performed in one large pelvic lesion seen on both plain films and opposed-phase MR images: histologically, infiltration of bone marrow by a conglomeration of plasma cells was seen. CT scans demonstrated osteolytic destruction of bone corresponding to large (two cases) and small lesions (five cases) detected by MRI; the surrounding bone was normal on both CT and MRI scans. Eleven patients had normal signal loss inside lumbar vertebrae, indicating presence of noninfiltrated red marrow as in normals. Fourteen patients had high signal of vertebral marrow with slight enhancement after gadolinium-DTPA.

Discussion

Accurate diagnosis of multiple myeloma is possible by bone marrow biopsy and detection of monoclonal proteins (Bergsagel 1989). Imaging is required as the focally destructive nature of multiple myeloma makes detection of osteolytic changes necessary. Thus, radiation therapy may be initiated to alleviate symptoms and prevent fracture of long bones or vertebral collapse. Scintigraphy, which usually allows an easy-to-perform survey of the skeleton in metastatic disease, was demonstrated early to have little sensitivity in detecting osteolyses

---

Fig. 1a, b. Improved sensitivity of Gd-DTPA enhanced MRI compared to plain film study (in a 62-year-old patient with stage III multiple myeloma; lower back pain; no treatment at time of images). a Plain film of pelvis demonstrates some structural changes of the sacrum. No definite osteolysis. b Coronal MR image (GE, TR 400 ms; TE 22 ms; postcontrast). Large bone marrow infiltrate (*arrows*) in the sacrum is clearly discernible from surrounding low-signal marrow. (b, with permission of Georg Thieme Verlag, Stuttgart)

caused by myeloma (Wahner et al. 1980). As a result, plain film surveys of the whole skeleton are necessary. These are time consuming and have drawbacks in sensitivity (pelvis) and specificity (demonstration of demineralization only in involved vertebrae). MRI was demonstrated to show bone marrow infiltrates in multiple myeloma patients that were not visible on plain films (Frühwald et al. 1988). However, comparable to CT (Helms and Genant 1982) the clinical use of MRI was limited by the necessary use of a surface coil that allowed for imaging of a small section of the body only (vertebral column in the study quoted).

Opposed-phase images exploit chemical-shift effects as a contrast parameter in addition to influence of T1 and T2 relaxation times. Voxels that contain equal amounts of fat (fat cells in bone marrow) and water protons (hemopoietic cells in marrow) give no signal as a result of the signal negation resulting from opposed phases of fat and water spins. TE of the opposed-phase gradient-echo sequence used in this study was set at a value that resulted in signal loss in red marrow; myeloma infiltrates with their higher cellularity underwent no signal loss and were thus distinguishable from surrounding normal marrow by very high signal intensity. An additional increase in signal intensity was a result of gadolinium-DTPA enhancement. The high difference in signal intensity of normal marrow and myeloma infiltrates made screening with a large field of view possible. As a result, lesions verified by CT but not detectable on plain films were demonstrated by MRI using the approach described. In addition, MRI demonstrated diffuse signal alterations of lumbar spine marrow in a number of patients. In our opinion, this holds potential for demonstration of diffuse involvement of the spine, a form of myeloma that is hardly, if ever, demonstrable by any other noninvasive method.

References

Bergsagel DE (1989) Plasma cell myeloma. In: Williams WJ (ed) Hematology. McGraw-Hill, New York

Döhner K, Gluckel F, Knauf W et al. (1989) Magnetic resonance imaging of bone marrow in lymphoproliferative disorders: correlation with bone marrow biopsy. Br J Haematol 73: 12–17

Frühwald FXJ, Tscholakoff D, Schwaighofer B et al. (1988) Magnetic resonance imaging of the lower vertebral column in patients with multiple myeloma. Invest Radiol 23: 193–199

Helms CA, Genant HK (1982) Computed tomography in the early detection of skeletal involvement with multiple myeloma. JAMA 248: 2886–2887

Vogler JB, Murphy WA (1988) Bone marrow imaging. Radiology 168: 679–693

Wahner HW, Kyle RA, Beabout JW (1980) Scintigraphic evaluation of the skeleton in multiple myeloma. Mayo Clin Proc 55: 739–746

Comparison of Three-Dimensional to Two-Dimensional Treatment Planning for Radiotherapy of Localized Prostatic Carcinoma

T. Wiegel, R. Schmidt, R. Schwarz, A. Krüll, K. Sommer, and K.-H. Hübener

Introduction

Primary high-dose percutaneous radiation of the prostatic and periprostatic region is used in cases of prostatic carcinoma stages A1–B1 if operative therapy is not possible. Randomized prospective studies have shown in these stages the missing benefit of elective irradiation of the lymphatic drainage of the small pelvis [12]. The inclusion of the seminal vesicles and a margin seems necessary because the seminal vesicles are involved in up to 25% of cases of clinical stage B2 [3]. This must also be carried out after radical prostatectomy in case of a microscopic tumor rest or infiltration of the seminal vesicles. In these two special cases a reduced total radiation dose is administered [2]. Involvement of the organs at risk — rectum and urinary bladder — is the dose-limiting factor. Administering a dose of more than 70 Gr, the probability of radiogenic side effects increases dramatically [9, 12]. In up to 35% of patients complications such as severe proctitis or cystitis are seen. Using three-dimensional treatment planning, a relief of the organs at risk seems possible by using irregular shaped fields.

The aim of this study was to quantify the advantage of three-dimensional treatment planning over conventional treatment planning in the therapy of localized prostatic carcinoma.

Materials and Methods

For ten patients a two- and a three-dimensional radiation plan was established. The irradiation field contains the prostate, the seminal vesicles, and a surrounding margin of 2 cm. The aim of the radiation planning was to optimize the radiation plan with both methods. The reference isodose was fixed in these plans at comparable levels. The probable advantage of three-dimensional treatment

Abteilung für Strahlentherapie, Radiologische Klinik, Universitätskrankenhaus Eppendorf, Martinistr. 52, 2000 Hamburg 20, FRG

Advanced Radiation Therapy Tumor Response
Monitoring and Treatment Planning
Breit (Editor-in-Chief)
© Springer-Verlag, Berlin Heidelberg 1992

planning could thus be determined as objectively as possible. The Mevaplan system was used for treatment planning. Dosage distribution was calculated for 40 coplanar computed tomography (CT) scans of 8 mm. Rectum and urinary bladder were marked as organs at risk; the target was encircled, and all were defined as volumes of interest (VOIs). Using beam's eye view (BEV), irregularly

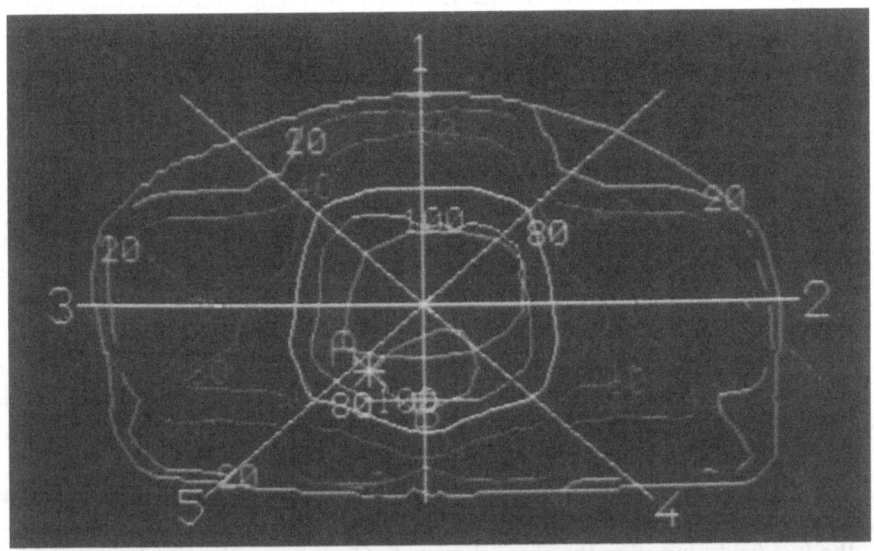

a

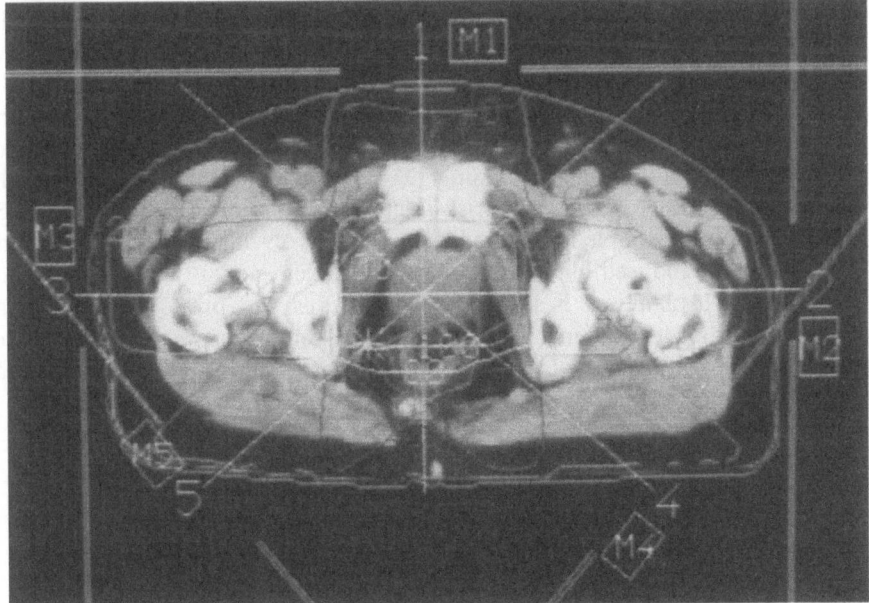

b

Fig. 1a, b. Five-field plans for radiation of the prostate. **a** Two-dimensional. **b** Three-dimensional

shaped fields were constructed. The dosage distribution was shown by transversal, coronar, and sagittal reconstructions. Quantitative elaboration of the two- and three-dimensional radiation plans was done in the form of dose-volume histograms (DVH). We also calculated the VOI with defined dose administration of target and organs at risk. With this technique the volume involvement of rectum and urinary bladder were determined, according to the tumor-encompassing reference isodose. For all ten patients DVHs with two-dimensional and three-dimensional treatment planning were established for the prostate, the complete urinary bladder, and the rectum up to the sigma.

Results

Treatment plans resulting from the two-dimensional planning were compared to three-dimensional treatment plans. For the two-dimensional planning standard techniques were applied. For further three-dimensional evaluation these treatment plans were transferred to the multiplanar calculation so that the three-dimensional information of the original two-dimensional plans was available. For comparison the same CT data were used for three-dimensional treatment planning. In all ten patients five fixed fields were used. These had different sizes and were individually weighted. In some cases the two dorsal fields had a deeper isocenter than the lateral and ventral fields. Two patients received an additional rotation technique treatment plan for comparison with the five-field plan. For the three-dimensional planning the five-field technique was generally used. Each of these fields was irregularly shaped using individually molded absorbers. The shape of these absorbers was determined by the BEV.

A typical example of a conventional five-field plan is shown in Fig. 1a and a typical three-dimensional plan in Fig. 1b. Figure 2a shows the corresponding sagittal two-dimensional reconstruction and Fig. 2b this reconstruction for three-dimensional treatment planning. DVHs show the volume reduction of the radiogenically related organs at risk (rectum and urinary bladder). Figure 3a shows a typical example for the reduced rectal involvement (patient no. 1) and Fig. 3b for the reduced bladder involvement (patient no. 6). The dose administered for both plannings is shown in these figures. The proportion of volume reduction in all ten patients calculated for the tumor encompassing reference isodose is shown in Table 1. Median reduction for the rectum was 19% (range 9.5%–36.6%) and that for the urinary bladder 29% (range 15.7%–47.8%).

Discussion

Localized prostate cancer may be cured either by radiation therapy or by radical prostatectomy with equivalent results [2, 12]. In case of nearly equivalent results

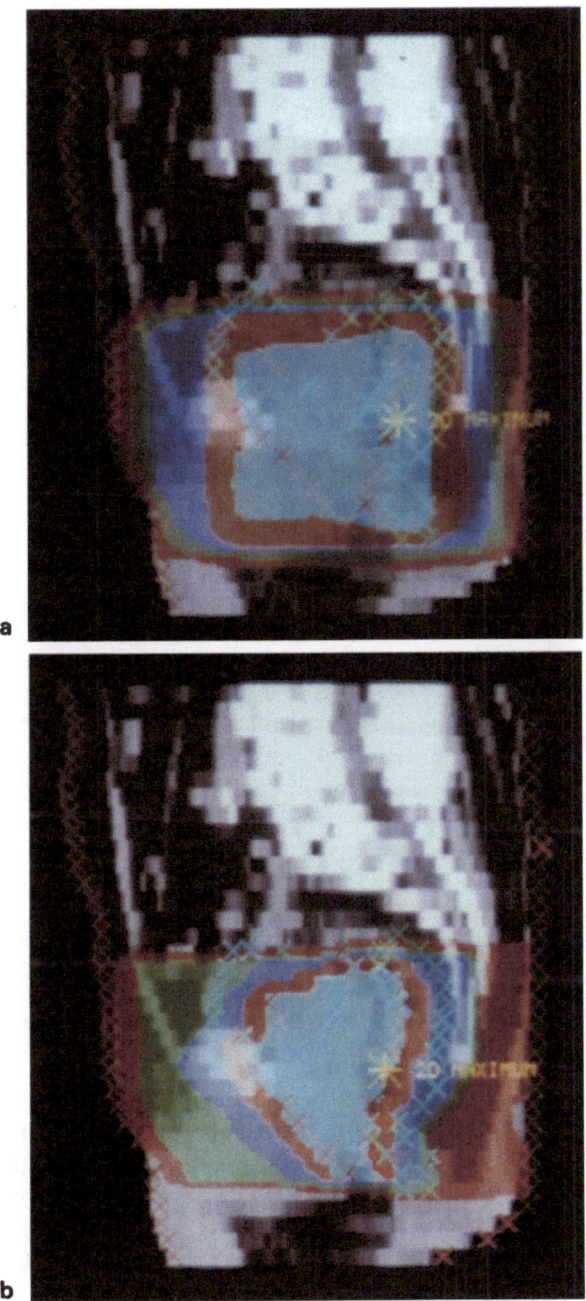

Fig. 2a, b. Sagittal reconstruction of planning for the five-field plan. **a** Two-dimensional. **b** Three-dimensional

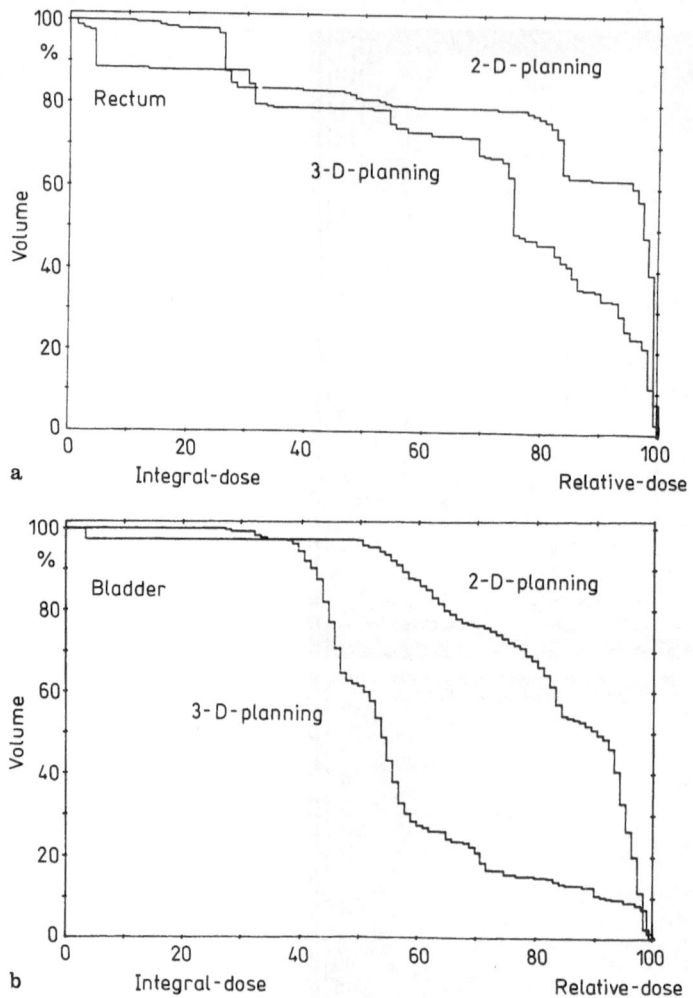

Fig. 3a, b. Dose-volume histograms for two- and three-dimensional treatment planning. **a** Rectum. **b** Urinary bladder

comparison of side effects of these therapeutic approaches becomes important. Important side effects of radical prostatectomy are impotence, incontinence, and death [2]. On the other hand, proctitis and cystitis, up to severe forms, are complications of high-dose percutaneous radiation therapy [9]. With doses higher than about 66 Gy the incidence and intensity of radiation-related side effects increase strongly [9, 12].

Since CT-based planning came into use, studies have shown its benefit for prostate cancer. Pilepich and coworkers have shown that 12%–24% of patients received inadequate radiation therapy without CT information. Dose deviation for the prostate in these cases ranged from 3% to 10% [5, 6]. Using a standard

Table 1. Volume reduction of the tumor-encompassing reference isodose in organs at risk

Patient no.	2-D/3-D	Reference isodose		Volume reduction	
		2-D	3-D	Rectum (%)	Bladder (%)
1	5-F-P	95.1	94.8	36.6	15.7
2	5-F-P	96.0	96.0	32.7	47.8
3	5-F-P	94.5	97.0	28.9	33.9
4	5-F-P	93.6	95.0	20.4	32.4
5	5-F-P	94.5	93.8	19.9	23.7
6	5-F-P	95.0	94.4	17.9	17.6
7	5-F-P	93.8	94.0	16.6	22.0
8	5-F-P	89.5	91.5	15.7	38.4
9	5-F-P	94.7	95.2	9.8	35.6
10	5-F-P	95.0	93.0	9.5	17.3
3	Rotation/5-F-P	78.8	97.0	20.4	54.6
5	Rotation/5-F-P	79.7	93.8	4.8	21.9

5-F-P, Five-field plan.

irradiation volume of $8 \times 8 \times 8$ cm^3, Asbell showed differences between this volume and the prostate volume of 18%–25% [1].

Recently published reports demonstrate the advantage of BEV for treatment planning in prostatic cancer [4, 9, 11]. Low and coworkers reported that BEV-directed treatment planning provides volumetric and topographic information to the radiation oncologist that has not been available until now. Using BEV shows the possibility of genuinely individual treatment planning [4]. Ten Haken et al. compared dosimetry of six-field BEV-blocked plans with unblocked four-field plans, using surrounding margins of only 5 mm. They found that on average the DVHs for the conformational four-field plan show substantially more irradiated tissue of rectum and urinary bladder compared with the six-field technique [11]. We therefore used five-field planning technique to reduce irradiation of normal tissue in standard treatment planning.

Our study shows that the reduced volume encompassed by the reference isodose is reduced by 19% for the rectum and 28% for the bladder. This minor volume involvement may or may not result in a decreased incidence of proctitis or cystitis, but it can be expected that overall injury to the rectum and bladder will decrease. Consequently, it seems possible to raise the dose for improving local control of higher stages of prostate cancer since local control in stages C and D1 today seems unsatisfactory. Sandler et al. reported on a prospective study in patients with stage C prostatic cancer [7]. They administered 45–50 Gy with a four-field technique to the pelvis and an additional boost up to 76 Gy planned with six fields, all planning three-dimensional using BEV. The average follow-up was 16.5 months. Of these patients 77% had an actuarial freedom from complications, and no high-grade toxicity occurred. In contrast, Smit et al. reported an expected 60% 2-year risk for moderate to severe rectal side effects [9].

The expected benefit of three-dimensional planning for irradiation in localized prostate cancer in stages A–B2 is even higher. Prospective studies must verify this expectation, but three-dimensional planning using BEV for localized prostatic cancer seems a promising way to reduce acute and late radiation-related proctitis and cystitis.

References

1. Asbell SA, Schlager B, Baker AS (1980) Revision of treatment planning for carcinoma of the prostate. Int J Radiat Oncol Biol Phys 6: 861–865
2. Hanks GE (1989) The prostate. In: Moss WT, Cox JD (eds) Radiation oncology, 6th edn. Mosby, St Louis, pp 501–504
3. Lange PH, Narayan P (1983) Understaging and undergrading of prostate cancer: argument for postoperative radiation as adjuvant therapy. Urology 21: 113–118
4. Low NN, Vijayakumar S, Rosenberg I, Rubin S, Virudachalam R, Spelbring D, Chen GT (1990) Beams eye view based prostate treatment planning: is it useful? Int J Radiat Oncol Biol Phys 19: 759–768
5. Pilepich MV, Perez CA, Prasad S (1980) Computed tomography in definitive radiotherapy of prostate carcinoma. Int J Radiat Oncol Biol Phys 6: 923–926
6. Pilepich MV, Prasad SC, Perez CA (1982) Computed tomography in definitive radiotherapy of prostatic carcinoma. II. Definition of target volume. Int J Radiat Oncol Biol Phys 8: 235–240
7. Sandler H, Perez-Tamayo C, Lichter A (1990) Dose escalation in the treatment of stage C (T3) prostate cancer: report on the rectal toxicity observed in a prospective series using a conformational external beam technique (abstract). ESTRO 9th annual meeting, Montecatini, Italy, p 329
8. Serago CG, Lewin AA, Houdek PB, Schwade JG, Abitbol AA (1989) Multiplanar arc boost radiation therapy for protate cancer. Radiology 172: 561–564
9. Smit WG, Helle PA, van Putten WL, Wijnmaalen AJ, Seldenrath JJ, van der Werf-Messing BH (1990) Late radiation damage in prostate cancer patients treated by high dose external radiotherapy in relation to rectal dose. Int J Radiat Oncol Biol Phys 18: 23–29
10. Soffen ME, Hanks GE, Hwang CC, Chu JC (1990) Conformal static field therapy for low volume low grade prostate cancer with rigid immobilization. Int J Radiat Oncol Biol Phys 20: 141–146
11. Ten Haken RK, Perez tymayo C, Tesser RJ, Mcshan DL, Fraass BA, Lichter AS (1989) Boost treatment of the prostate using shaped fixed fields. Int J Radiat Oncol Biol Phys 16: 193–200
12. Zagars GK, von Eschenbach AC, Johnson DE, Oswald MJ (1988) The role of radiation therapy in stages A2 and B adenocarcinoma of the prostate. Int J Radiat Oncol Biol Phys 14: 701–709

Evaluation of Target Volume by Computed Tomography in the Irradiation of Lung Cancer

T. Feyerabend[1], R. Schmitt[2], E. Richter[1], and W. Bohndorf[3]

Introduction

Determination of target volume in the irradiation of malignant tumors is a major aspect of radiotherapy. This may be achieved by conventional X-ray simulator methods or with the help of computed tomography (CT). The role of CT here has been investigated in various studies since Emami et al. [2] published their results in 1978. However, these studies include various tumor sites, are based on small patient numbers, and usually do not provide clear criteria for defining the role of CT. Therefore we studied CT examinations and X-ray simulator films in 133 patients with lung cancer to evaluate the role of CT in the determination of target volume.

Patients and Methods

A total of 434 CT examinations were analyzed from 133 patients (121 men, 12 women) with histologically confirmed bronchogenic carcinoma (22/133 with small-cell lung cancer). Of these, 90% were diagnosed in an advanced stage of disease (stage III, 106; stage IV, 16). There were 96 patients with centrally located tumors and 37 with peripheral tumors. All patients received radiotherapy, with a mean dose of 70 Gy isocentrically in non-small-cell lung cancer and 58 Gy in small-cell lung cancer. CT examinations (slice increment, 9 mm; intravenous contrast medium in most cases) were performed before, during, and up to 6 years after radiotherapy. The target volume was defined as the region of the primary and of hilar and mediastinal lymph node compartments with a safety margin of 1.5 cm. This target volume was determined by conventional X-ray films and compared with the target volume determined by CT. For this comparison the diagnostic value of CT was determined by a special evaluation

[1] Department of Radiation Oncology and Nuclear Medicine, Ratzeburger Allec 160, 2400-Lübeck, FRG
[2] Department of Diagnostic Radiology, Krumenauerstraße 25, 8070-Ingolstadt, FRG
[3] Department of Radiation Oncology, Josef-Schneider-Str. 11, 8700-Würzburg, FRG

Advanced Radiation Therapy Tumor Response
Monitoring and Treatment Planning
Breit (Editor-in-Chief)
© Springer-Verlag, Berlin Heidelberg 1992

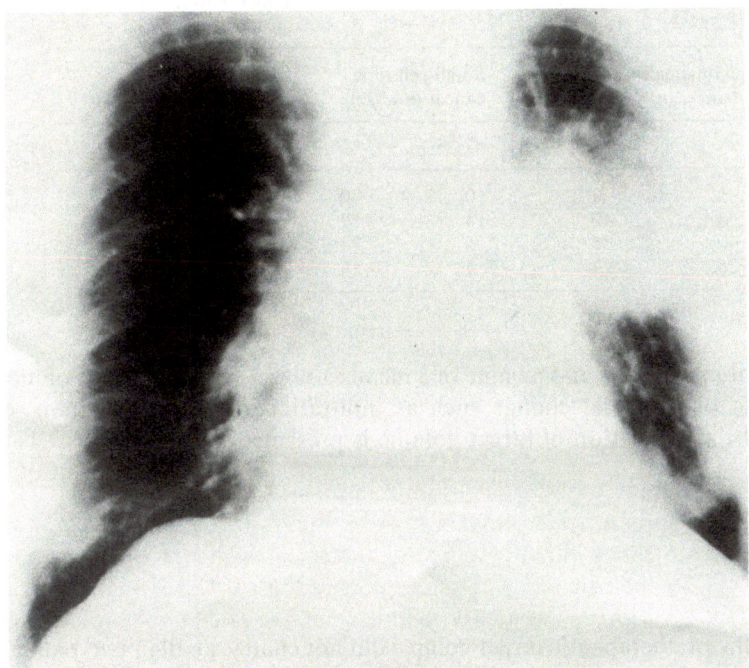

a

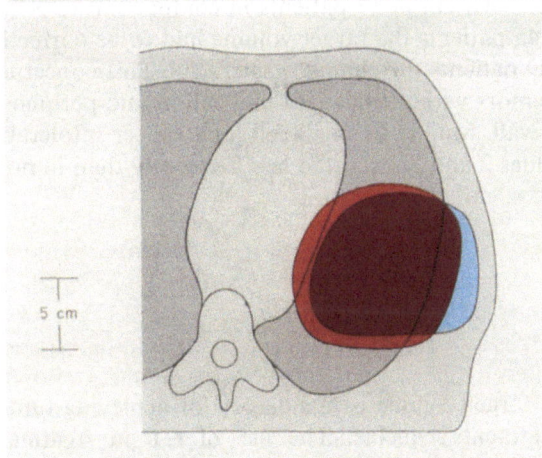

b

Fig. 1a, b. A 63-year old patient with inoperable peripheral lung cancer was referred to the radiotherapy unit because of hemoptysis. **a** Posteroanterior plain film of the chest. **b** Comparison of the target volumes defined by X-ray simulator (*red*) and CT (*blue*). The maximum difference in target volumes is < 2.5 cm, but only CT reveals the infiltration of the thoracic wall. The latter represents a crucial change of the target volume (score 3)

score indicating the degree of change of the target volume: score 0, no change; score 1, change of less than 1 cm; score 2, change of 1–2.5 cm; score 3, change of more than 2.5 cm or crucial change. The score includes dislocation in any direction, enlargement or reduction; for example, a value of 0 means no change

Table 1. Results of evaluation score for comparing target volume by CT to X-ray simulator films

Score	Non-small-cell lung cancer ($n = 111$)		Small-cell lung cancer ($n = 22$)		Total ($n = 133$)	
	n	%	n	%	n	%
0	2	2	0	0	2	1
1	44	40	13	59	57	43
2	40	36	5	23	45	34
3	25	22	4	18	29	22

in target volume on CT, and a value of 3 means a target volume change of more than 2.5 cm or a crucial change such as infiltration of the pericardium. An example of the evaluation of target volume is presented in Fig. 1.

Results

Using CT the pretherapeutic target volume did not change at all in two patients, and it changed by a maximum of 1 cm in 57 patients in comparison to X-ray simulator films (Table 1). In 45 patients the target volume had to be corrected for more than 1 cm, and in 29 patients the change was crucial. This concerned especially centrally located tumors with mediastinal infiltration and peripheral tumors infiltrating the chest wall. Mainly in small-cell lung cancer intolerable changes in target volume (values 2 and 3) occurred less frequently than in non-small-cell lung cancer.

Discussion

Correct determination of the target volume is mandatory for achieving tumor control and minimizing treatment sequelae. The use of CT in treatment planning has increased since Emami et al. [2] showed its superiority to the conventional X-ray simulator method. Munzenrider et al. [5] evaluated 75 patients, among them 10 patients with lung cancer. Conventional planning was sufficient in 53% ($n = 40$) and insufficient in 20% ($n = 15$); the target volume was slightly changed by CT in 27%. According to Seydel et al. [7], CT information was crucial in 11 out of 23 analyzed patients, thus changing the target volume in 26% of the patients. Van Houtte et al. [8] reported on 45 postoperatively irradiated patients with lung cancer. Conventional and CT methods planning were compared on the basis of the different tumor doses, which varied between 5% and 20%. The sufficient determination of target volume was not at issue in this study. Dobbs et al. [1] reported a 30% benefit (28/94 patients with lung cancer) by CT treatment planning. All of these data are based upon the subjective opinion of the responsible radiotherapist. Ragan et al. [6] presented a method to quantify the value of CT by inhomogeneity factors and "local efficiency factors".

Our study of 133 patients with lung cancer sought an easy approach to the evaluation of CT-defined target volumes by a special score. This study showed that conventional treatment planning methods were decisively inferior to CT in more than 50% of cases. This was especially the case in centrally located tumors, tumors with infiltration of the chest wall, and in the evaluation of mediastinal lymph nodes [3]. The latter may be achieved as well by magnetic resonance imaging [4], which, according to Weiss et al. [9], has the advantage of differentiating between tumor nucleus and obstructive atelectasis or retention pneumonia if a multiecho technique is used.

In conclusion, our experience shows CT to be indispensable for the correct definition of the target volume, at least in lung cancer.

References

1. Dobbs J, Husband JE (1984) Computed tomography for radiotherapy planning. Appl Radiol 13: 51–60
2. Emami B, Melo A, Carter BL, Munzenrider JE, Piro AJ (1978) Value of computed tomography in radiotherapy of lung cancer. AJR 131: 63–67
3. Khan A, Gersten KC, Garvey J, Khan FA, Steinberg H (1985) Oblique hilar tomography, computed tomography, and mediastinoscopy for prethoracotomy staging of bronchogenic carcinoma. Radiology 156: 295–298
4. Levitt RG, Glazer HS, Roper CL, Lee JKT, Murphy WA (1985) Magnetic resonance imaging of mediastinal and hilar masses: comparison with CT. AJR 145: 9–14
5. Munzenrider JE, Pilepich M, Rene-Ferrero JB, Tschakarova J, Carter BL (1977) Use of body scanner in radiotherapy treatment planning. Cancer 40: 170–179
6. Ragan DF, Perez CA (1978) Efficacy of CT-assisted two-dimensional treatment planning: analysis of 45 patients. AJR 131: 75–79
7. Seydel HG, Kutcher GJ, Steiner RM, Mohiuddin M, Goldberg B (1980) Computed tomography in planning radiation therapy for bronchogenic carcinoma. Int J Radiat Oncol Biol Phys 6: 601–606
8. Van Houtte P, Piron A, Lustman-Maréchal J, Osteaux M, Henry J (1978) Computed axial tomography (CAT) contribution for dosimetry and treatment evaluation in lung cancer. Int J Radiat Oncol Biol Phys 6: 995–1000
9. Weiss T, Loddenkemper R, Bittner R, Husen-Weiss E, Kaiser D, Felix R (1987) Kernspintomographie intrathorakaler Tumoren. Fortschr Roentgenstr 147: 486–492

Portal Imaging

Verification of Patient Positioning During Radiotherapy Using an Integrated Megavoltage Imaging System*

J. Gildersleve[1], W. Swindell[2], P. Evans[2], E. Morton[2], C. Rawlings[1], and D. Dearnaley[1]

In order to maximise local tumour control probability whilst minimising the risk of damage to adjacent normal tissue, it is necessary to ensure that the irradiation portal, at each treatment fraction, corresponds to that defined as ideal at the time of simulation in terms of size, shape and positioning. The ultimate check of the entire planning and treatment procedure is to verify that the radiation beam accurately covers the treatment volume on each occasion that treatment is delivered. A number of investigators have developed megavoltage imaging systems with the intention of obtaining a transmission image of the irradiation portal with a convenience and image quality superior to that obtainable with film [1–4].

We have developed an integrated megavoltage imaging system, comprising a frame store from which digitised simulator images can be obtained and a scanning detector with associated image display, analysis and comparison facilities. This system has been in clinical operation for approximately 9 months, and approximately 2000 portal images have been obtained [5]. This system has been used to obtain measurements of day-to-day positioning variability (random error) for radical irradiation of the brain, head and neck, abdomen and pelvis, using standard Royal Marsden Hospital immobilisation and set-up techniques. No modification of the treatment procedure was necessary for the scans to be performed.

Measurements are made by assigning a given portal image (typically day 1) as a reference image. The image to be measured and the reference image are displayed in rapid succession as a movie [6]. Rigid attachment of the detector to the gantry obviates the need for prior field edge realignment. Differences in position of anatomical structures between the two images are perceived by the eye as rapid movement. We then shift the position of the measurement image relative to the reference image by an iterative process of translation and rotation until the anatomical structures are seen as stationary between the two images.

Positioning variability is then calculated as the extent of movement of visible structures within the treatment portal with respect to the mean daily position.

[1] Department of Radiotherapy, Institute of Cancer Research and Royal Marsden Hospital, Sutton, Surrey SM2 5PT, UK
[2] Department of Physics, Institute of Cancer Research and Royal Marsden Hospital, Sutton, Surrey SM2 5PT, UK
* This research was supported by the Cancer Research Campaign.

Advanced Radiation Therapy Tumor Response
Monitoring and Treatment Planning
Breit (Editor-in-Chief)
© Springer-Verlag, Berlin Heidelberg 1992

This is achieved by choosing an arbitrary image as reference and calculating the difference in anatomical position in the X and Y directions between the measurement and reference images. The average value of this difference is then calculated to determine the mean daily position. This mean value is then subtracted from each difference measurement to give the daily variation from the mean value. The standard deviation of the difference measurement for each parameter is then determined, and the results expressed as $\pm$ two standard deviations from the mean daily position. We have made a preliminary analysis of 446 patient set-ups, and the results of the observations are as follows:

Pelvis
    Anterior/posterior fields (178 observations)
        $\pm$ 2.7 mm lateral displacement
        $\pm$ 4.3 mm cranio-caudal displacement
    Lateral fields (40 observations)
        $\pm$ 5.4 mm antero-posterior displacement
        $\pm$ 5.0 mm cranio-caudal displacement
Abdominal nodes
    Anterior/posterior fields (110 observations)
        $\pm$ 3.7 mm lateral displacement
        $\pm$ 5.6 mm cranio-caudal displacement
Brain/head and neck (in fixation shell)
    Lateral fields (118 observations)
        $\pm$ 2.2 mm cranio-caudal displacement
        $\pm$ 3.1 mm antero-posterior displacement

These and ongoing positioning studies should enable definition of treatment margins for different sites and treatment techniques which will avoid the risk of target volume miss due to random set-up variation. We are presently addressing the problem of systematic error (repeated at each treatment fraction), by analysing simulator-to-machine variation, using the simulator check image as reference. The results presented here do not take systematic error into account, and must not therefore be regarded as recommendations for margins which are adequate in daily practice. A knowledge of the extent of systematic and random errors for given sites of treatment and set-up techniques will enable individual institutions to rationalise treatment volume margins, thus avoiding unnecessary irradiation of adjacent normal tissues.

In conclusion, we have used a megavoltage imaging system to measure random variation in daily patient positioning during radiotherapy. In our Institute, more than 95% of treatments are within $\pm$ 6 mm of the daily mean for pelvic and abdominal nodal treatment and within 3.5 mm for brain/head and neck treatments where a fixation shell is used.

References

1. Meertens H, van Herk M, Bijhold J, Bartelink H (1990) First clinical experience with a newly developed electronic portal imaging device. Int J Radiat Oncol Biol Phys 18: 1173–1181
2. Leong J (1986) Use of digital fluoroscopy as an on-line verification device in radiation therapy. Phys Med Biol 31: 985–992
3. Munro P, Rawlinson J, Fenster A (1990) A digital fluoroscopic imaging device for radiotherapy localisation. Int J Radiat Oncol Biol Phys 18: 641–649
4. Visser A, Huizenga H, Althof V, Swaneburg B (1990) Performance of a prototype fluoroscopic radiotherapy imaging system. Int J Radiat Oncol Biol Phys 18: 43–50
5. Gildersleve J, Swindell W, Morton E, Evans P, Dearnaley D (1991) Preliminary clinical performance of a scanning detector for rapid portal imaging (to be published)
6. Reinstein L, Shalev S, Leszczynski K, Cosby S, Meek A (1988) Megavoltage movies. Int J Radiat Oncol Biol Phys 15: 200–201

A Multilayer Detector for Verification of Cobalt-60 Treatment Fields

H. Schüller[1], P. Barwig[1], A. Badura[2], H.J. Besch[2], D. Bornstein[2],
J. Dangendorf[2], A. Sack[2], and A.H. Walenta[2]

The collaboration between the Radiological Clinic at the University of Bonn and the Physics Department at the University of Siegen has led to the development of a new imaging detector for portal verification of cobalt-60 radiation. All methods so far used, for example, films, xeroradiography, image intensifier, and liquid ionization detector, have the disadvantage of not being able to suppress scattered radiation. Our aim was to construct a device that can distinguish between primary and secondary radiation and at the same time produce high-resolution images.

Material and Methods

To meet the above requirements a new detector system has been developed (Fig. 1). The detector system is a line device and consists of four layers of multiwire proportional chambers. Each chamber contains 16 anode wires (diameter 50 μm) at distances of 1 mm. Between these there are 15 potential wires (diameter 200 μm). The chambers are filled with isobutane at atmospheric pressure. Chambers 1 and 2 are separated by a converter foil (thickness 500 μm) and chambers 3 and 4 by an absorber layer (thickness 2 mm). Unscattered photons pass through the first chamber, and in the converter foil a compton electron is created. The direction of such an electron is straight ahead or almost so. This electron now passes through chambers 2 and 3 and causes ionization. In the absorber layer it loses energy but still reaches chamber 4.

Scattered photons of lower energy produce low-energy electrons which are stopped in the absorber layer, and these may show a different direction. Electrons are accepted as counts coming from primary radiation in the case of signal coincidence of chambers 2, 3, and 4. All other combinations of signals suggest a different origin of the electron and are rejected. Chamber 1 is a veto chamber because it suggests the primary existence of an electron and not a photon, which is to be rejected in any case. Monte Carlo studies following trajectories from the source through the object into the detector were conducted to determine the parameters of the system.

[1] Radiologische Klinik, Universität Bonn, 5300 Bonn-Venusberg, FRG
[2] Fachbereich Physik, Universität Siegen, 5900 Siegen, FRG

Advanced Radiation Therapy Tumor Response
Monitoring and Treatment Planning
Breit (Editor-in-Chief)
© Springer-Verlag, Berlin Heidelberg 1992

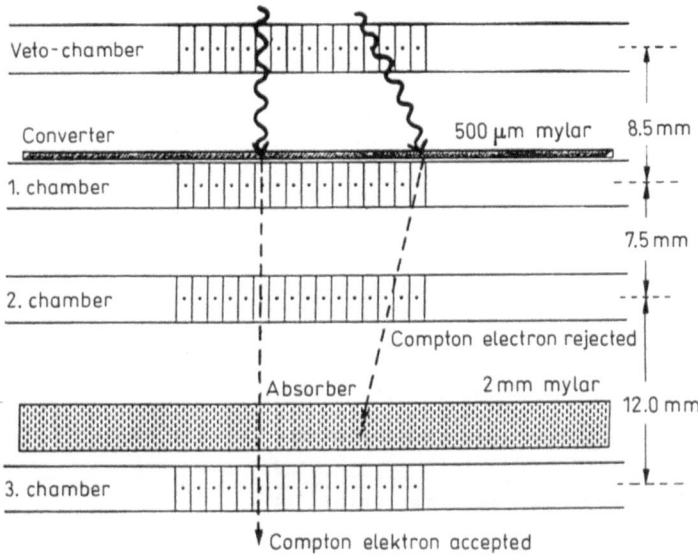

Fig. 1. Detector system

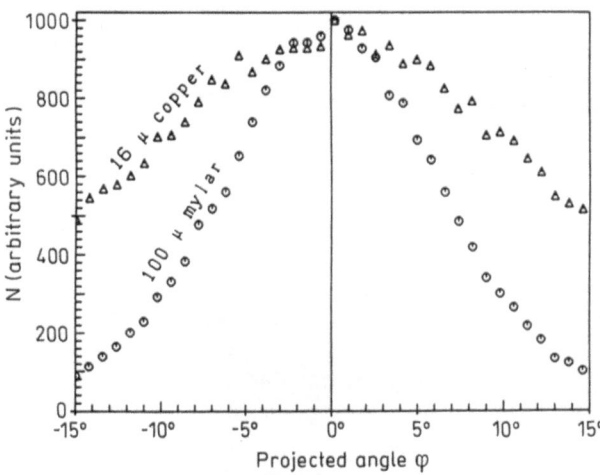

Fig. 2. Angle distribution of a 1 MeV electron point beam (Monte Carlo simulation)

Results

Materials with a low electron number are most suitable for the converter foil. An equal number of compton electrons are generated by 16 μm copper foil and 100 μm mylar foil. These differ, however, in the distribution of the projected

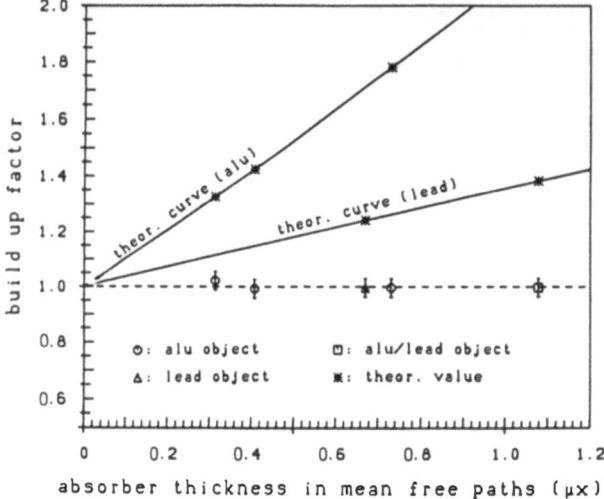

Fig. 3. Calculated and measured build-up factor of different aluminum and lead objects

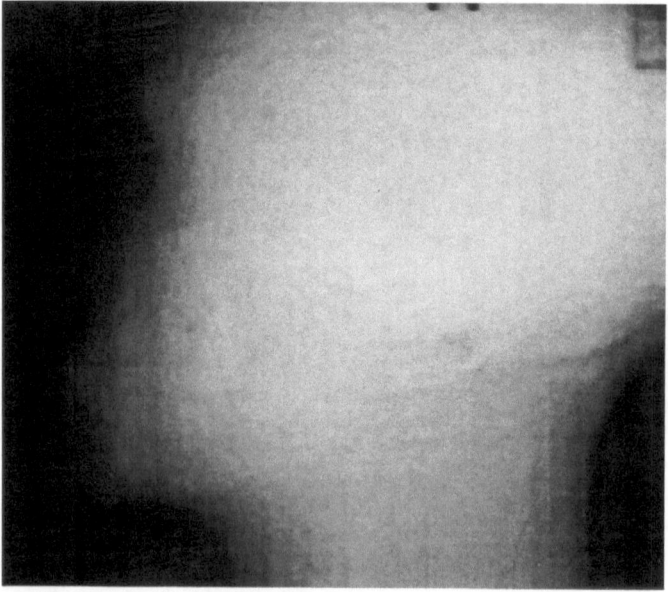

Fig. 4. Image of a head phantom

angle (Fig. 2). The disadvantage of copper is the wide scattering of electrons. Mylar foil creates almost only "one-direction" electrons.

The suppression of scattered radiation was measured with our standard therapeutic source using different absorbers. Without scatter rejection the measured intensity depends on the primary radiation intensity, the linear absorption coefficient μ, the photon energy, E, and the electron number Z [1, 2]:

$$I(x) = B(\mu x, E, Z) \, \text{lo} \exp(-\mu x)$$

B is the so-called build-up factor indicating the increasing number of photons caused by scattering. Any imaging device which can completely suppress scattered radiation will show a direct correlation between $I(x)$ and $\text{lo} \exp(-\mu x)$, which means that the build-up factor B equals 1. Figure 3 shows the theoretically calculated build-up factors of aluminum and lead objects of various thickness; the actually measured build-up factors equaled 1. The results suggest that the device is able to eliminate scattered radiation completely.

Finally, we conducted a test with a human skull phantom. The image in Fig. 4 is a reconstruction of many 16 * 1 mm stripes. The result is an image which clearly shows the contours of the skull and its homogeneous structure, except for the pneumatized mastoid cells.

Conclusions

Our new detector seems to be superior to most methods of portal verification in cobalt therapy because of its ability to suppress scattered radiation. Further enlargement of the active area and higher spatial resolution by smaller distances between the wires are aims for the future.

References

1. Aglinzew KK (1961) Dosimetrie ionisierender Strahlung. VEB Deutscher Verlag der Wissenschaften, Berlin
2. Profio AE (1979) Radiation shielding and dosimetry. Wiley, New York

Experimental Investigations on In Vivo Dosimetry Using Portal Imaging for Magna Field Irradiation

H. Kirschner[1], I. Awad[2], and E. Dühmke[1]

Introduction

We present the results of investigations aimed at testing control of mainly the midplane dose distribution, but also at other planes in the patient during magna field irradiation of irregular and compensated fields in the area of the chest and the abdomen. This method does not use dosimeter manipulation and therefore lacks shadows from the build-up layer of the dosimeters on the skin of the patient, and it is quite independent of any algorithm of treatment planning.

Methods

The setup for conducting measurements is presented in Fig. 1. The dosimeters are small condenser chambers. The small air-filled part of the condenser chamber is seen on the port film when exposing the port film in the cassettes for photon portals (^{60}Co, 5–42 MV), as described in Table 1 [1]. The thermo-luminescence dosimeter is not seen on the port film here. Light-protected films between selected slices of an Alderson phantom are calibrated by the condenser chambers in the adherent slice to obtain a dose in the Alderson phantom at any point of the irradiated volume. The condenser chambers are seen on the film. In the same procedure the port film is calibrated by the condenser chambers in the dosimeter array above the port film cassette. The films serve as an interpolating medium of the dose distribution and not as a dosimeter.

The dose $D(a)$ in the Alderson phantom is determined along a fanline for $a = 0.50$, the midplane dose, and for $a = 0.25$ and $a = 0.75$. Where the fanline meets the dosimeter array, the exit dose D_2 is evaluated by measurement with the Alderson phantom. In the same geometric arrangement but without the

[1] Department of Radiation Therapy, University of Göttingen, TL 190, Robert-Koch-Str. 40, 3400 Göttingen, FRG
[2] University of Mansoura, Radiotherapy Department, Faculty of Medicine, ET Mansoura, Egypt

Advanced Radiation Therapy Tumor Response
Monitoring and Treatment Planning
Breit (Editor-in-Chief)
© Springer-Verlag, Berlin Heidelberg 1992

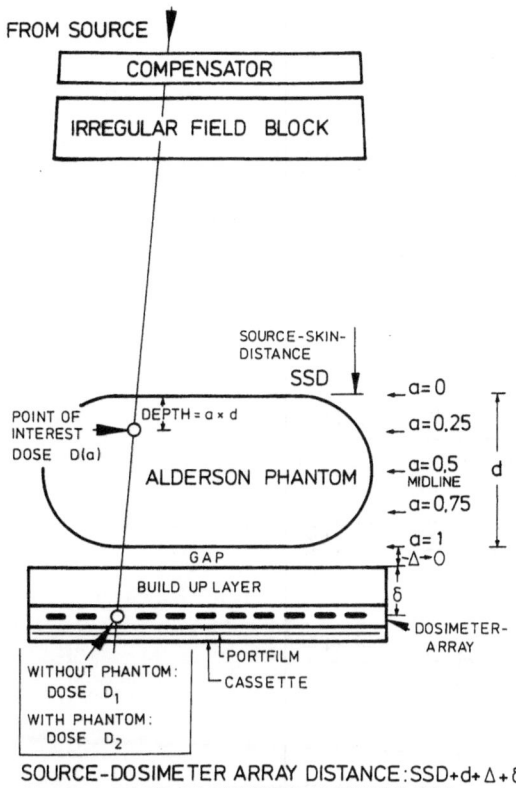

Fig. 1. Arrangement of measurements

Table 1. Cassettes for photon portals (^{60}Co, 5–42 MV). (From [1])

Cassettes	Aluminium	Steel	Tungsten
In front of film	2 mm Al	2 mm stainless steel	2 mm W
Behind film	2 mm Al	Black foam + 0.1 mm UV absorber + 3 mm Makrolon (plastic) + 4 mm aluminium, but no lead on the rear cassette wall	(As "Steel")
Area of application	^{60}Co	^{60}Co, 5–16 MV	16–42 MV
Mass of cassette for port films, 35 × 43 cm	2.5 kg	5.5 kg	9.0 kg

Films: Kodak XV-2, Du Pont DOT-1

Table 2. Adjustment Factor (K) for various regions (SSD, 80–150 cm; $n = 15$)

	a = 0.25			a = 0.50 (midline)			a = 0.75		
	^{60}Co	8 MV	16 MV	^{60}Co	8 MV	16 MV	^{60}Co	8 MV	16 MV
1. Open field, abdomen	1.08 ± 3.3%	1.06 ± 5.5%	1.15 ± 4.1%	1.10 ± 3.4%	1.08 ± 2.2%	1.11 ± 4.0%	1.08 ± 4.4%	1.08 ± 4.8%	1.11 ± 5.4%
2. Open field, chest lung + mediastinum	1.05 ± 2.3%	1.06 ± 4.1%	1.08 ± 4.1%	1.08 ± 4.7%	1.08 ± 3.9%	1.11 ± 4.8%	1.10 ± 4.6%	1.10 ± 4.0%	1.10 ± 5.5%
3. Irregular field, abdomen	1.05 ± 3.6%	1.11 ± 3.9%	–	1.10 ± 3.4%	1.11 ± 2.6%	–	1.16 ± 3.2%	1.10 ± 3.8%	–
4. Mantle field, chest	1.10 ± 6.5%	1.14 ± 2.9%	1.14 ± 2.3%	1.14 ± 4.0%	1.17 ± 5.3%	1.13 ± 1.8%	1.18 ± 2.0%	1.14 ± 6.2%	1.12 ± 2.9%
5. Compensator, abdomen	1.10 ± 3.2%	1.17 ± 3.8%	1.14 ± 2.6%	1.11 ± 3.6%	1.15 ± 7.7%	1.13 ± 2.9%	1.10 ± 6.3%	–	1.13 ± 4.9%
6. Homogeneous phantom, 18 cm PMMA open field	–	–	–	1.14	1.13	1.14	–	–	–
Mean 1–5	1.08	1.11	1.13	1.11	1.12	1.12	1.12	1.10	1.11
7. Gap Δ = 12 cm, open field, abdomen, compare with 1	1.13 ± 3.7%	1.13 ± 3.7%	1.14 ± 4.5%	1.28 ± 3.1%	1.22 ± 4.9%	1.32 ± 3.1%	1.62 ± 4.8%	1.22 ± 5.8%	1.24 ± 4.2%

PMMA, polymethyl methacrylate

Alderson phantom, the dose D_1 is evaluated instead of the entrance dose:

$$D(a) = K(a, \ldots) \cdot D_1 \cdot \underbrace{\left(\frac{D_2}{D_1}\right)^a}_{\substack{\text{absorption}}} \cdot \underbrace{\left(\frac{\text{SSD} + d + \Delta + \delta}{\text{SSD} + a \cdot d}\right)^2}_{\substack{\text{distance correction}}}$$

$$\underbrace{}_{\substack{\text{adjustment} \\ \text{factor}}}$$

The adjustment factor K is derived from measurements of $D(a)$, D_1, and D_2. All other values in the formula are explained in Fig. 1. K is evaluated for a variety of examples.

Results

Examples of the adjustment factor K are given in Table 2. K depends weakly on the photon quality, on a, and on the transmission D_2/D_1. K depends somewhat more on the gap width Δ. Therefore the gap should be kept as small as possible. When the scattered radiation produced in the patient is kept away from the dosimeter array by a sandwich of 3 mm Makrolon on the top plus 2 mm aluminium and 2 mm steel instead of the build-up layer in Fig. 1, the SD in Table 2 is reduced. The sandwich would prevent the patient from the back-scattered radiation of the steel plate and the dosimeter array.

If the accepted accuracy is SD = $\pm$ 8% in calculating $D(a)$ from D_1 and D_2, only one K factor is needed per photon quality as long as the inhomogeneities are symmetrically distributed around the midline. For SD = $\pm$ 5% different K factors for $a = 0.25$, $a = 0.50$, and $a = 0.75$ are needed, and the influence of the inhomogeneities over all from the air-filled areas must be determined. For SD =3% the dependence of the K factor on the transmission D_2/D_1 is to be added, and a table of K factors is used, possibly supported by CT and treatment planning.

In agreement with Leunens et al. [2], it is insufficient to determine $D(a)$ by a single measurement of the exit dose D_2. A second measurement is needed to subtract the entrance dose, here by the measurement of D_1.

We are continuing the development of the dosimeter arrays. We would prefer a solution with a direct conversion from dose to computer reading and suitable for instant imaging, perhaps in accordance with Meertens et al. [3] and van Herk et al. [4]. The K factor must be related to the dosimeter array used.

References

1. Kirschner H. Busch M, Dühmke E (1990) Verifikationsaufnahmen in der Megavolttherapie mit den Aluminium-, Stahl- und Wolfram-Kassetten. In: Harder D (ed) Gemeinsame Jahrestagung 1990. Strahlenschutz im medizinischen Bereich und an Beschleunigern. TÜV Rheinland, Cologne, p 182

2. Leunens G, van Damm J, Dutreix A, van der Schueren E (1990) Quality assurance in radiotherapy by in vivo dosimetry. 2. Determination of the target absorbed dose. Radiother Oncol 19:
   73–87
3. Meertens H, van Herk M, Bijhold J, Bartelink H (1990) First clinical experience with a newly
   developed electronic portal imaging device. Int J Radiat Oncol Biol Phys 18: 1173–1181
4. van Herk M, Meertens H (1988) A matrix ionisation chamber imaging device for on-line patient
   setup verification during radiotherapy. Radiother Oncol 11: 369–378

Field Shaping Using a Beam's Eye View Facility and an Accurate Port Film Positioning Unit

T. Knöös, N.-E. Augustsson, and M. Nilsson

Introduction

The use of a beam's eye view tool (BEV) for field shaping during dose planning gives the opportunity to create treatment plans with treated volumes which conform closely to target volumes. The rate of complication is either decreased or kept at the same level depending on the changes made in the target dose. A decrease may result if the target dose is maintained. However, the use of smaller treated volumes requires greater accuracy in their administration. An accurate port film technique for verification of position must therefore be available to detect discrepancies between planned and actual beam position.

This study presents the clinical use of a BEV facility and a means for achieving high accuracy in the verification of treatment.

Methods

Patients who are intended for curative radiotherapy undergo computed tomography (CT) covering the whole volume including margins with transversal slices positioned every centimeter. Most patients are positioned in an immobilizing cast made of polyurethane foam, with their arms over the head in a fairly comfortable position. The outer dimensions of the cast are less than the aperture of the CT scanner. All CT data are entered into the treatment planning system (TMS-Radix, Helax, Uppsala, Sweden) using floppy disks. The attenuation data are transferred to electron density terms according to Knöös et al. (1986). The radiotherapist outlines the clinical (CTV) and the planning target volume(s) (PTV) as defined by Wambersie et al. (1989), organs at risk, and anatomical landmarks. Most patients are grouped according to their diagnosis and target volume. A preferred technique exists for each group. The beam orientation is selected, and the optimization of each field starts. This is done mainly in the BEV utility, where beam size, position, and shape, collimator, gantry and table

Department of Radiation Physics, Lund University, Malmö Allmänna Sjukhus 214 01, Sweden

Advanced Radiation Therapy Tumor Response
Monitoring and Treatment Planning
Breit (Editor-in-Chief)
© Springer-Verlag, Berlin Heidelberg 1992

rotation, etc. can be modified. The dose calculations are made using a convolution method based on polyenergetic pencil beams compiled from Monte Carlo
generated data for monoenergetic photons (Ahnesjö 1991). The output from the
planning system consists of dose distributions of the conventional cross-
sectional type together with dose volume histograms (DVH) for up to four
different volumes (volumes of interest, VOI) including the planning target

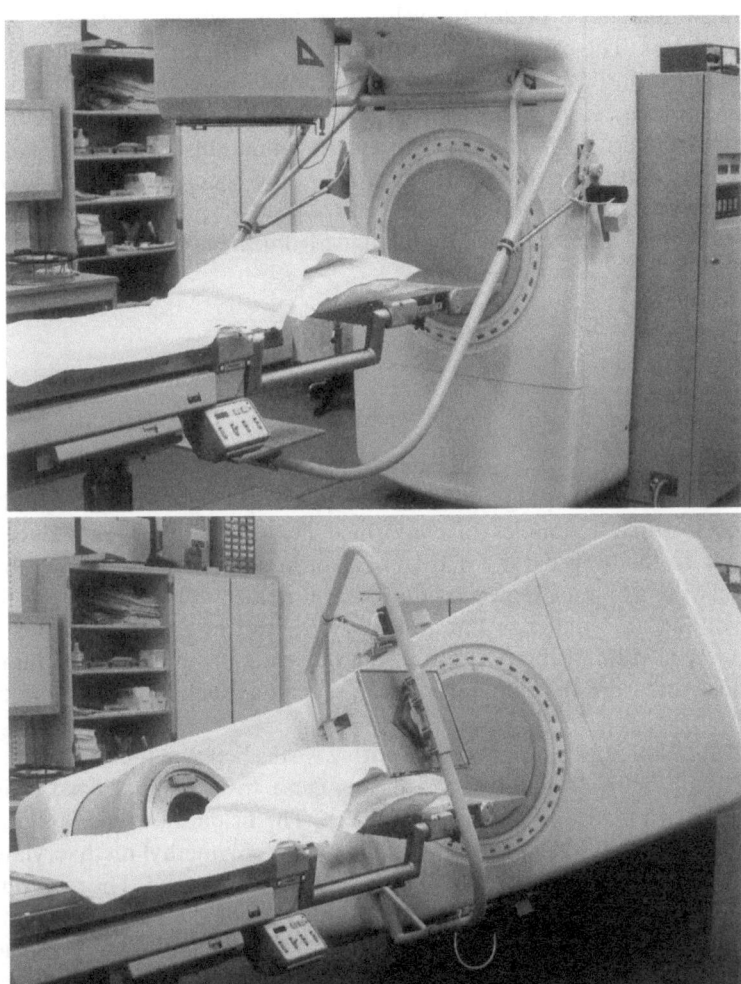

Fig. 1. The U-shaped cassette holder mounted on the gantry. This allows port films to be taken at
any gantry rotation (upper, 0°; lower, 270°). The holder is remote-controlled, and cassettes are
positioned using magnets. The focus film plane is always the same, and the cassette is normal to the
radiation beam axis

volume. The field shape together with the VOIs are projected to a user-selected image plane and plotted on paper. The most common projections are (a) the plane of the shadow tray for production of shadow blocks, (b) the film plane used during simulation, and (c) the film plane for port films. The patient position and the field shapes determined during the dose planning are verified on the simulator.

The treatment is executed with port films taken at the first treatment and thereafter at changes and once a week. The port film cassette is positioned using magnets on a remote-controlled U-shaped cassette holder (Fig. 1) mounted on the gantry. The holder is a product developed in-house which is available for various accelerators. The cassette holder rotates with the gantry; thus the port films are always exposed perpendicular to the radiation beam axis, independently of the gantry position. The holder is very rigid and a motor protection terminates immediately if something obstructs the holder during its movement. The port film cassette is either in the beam for the whole treatment or is retracted after a certain absorbed dose has been collected by a diode positioned behind the cassette. The retraction can be made from the console.

Results and Discussion

The use of BEV for field shaping and the technique for port films are intimately related to each other. Examples of conformed fields resulting in a reduced absorbed dose to the lung tissue for treatment of breast cancer are shown by Wittgren et al. (this volume). However, the closer a treated volume conforms to the target volume, the higher is the accuracy required in patient and beam positioning. Verification of the position of the radiation beam using port films must exclude errors from the actual port film procedures such as positioning of the cassette.

In Fig. 2, a pair of port films are shown with 2 weeks between the treatments. The chosen field enters from 110° and passes close to the spinal cord. The positions of the two fields are in close agreement. The fields shown are shaped using individual shadow blocks mounted tightly on a polymethyl methacrylate (PMMA) plate (5 mm thick) positioned in the shadow tray holder. The printout from the TMS-Radix formed the basis for the cutting of these blocks. Comparisons between the schematics and the port films have shown that the production and mounting of the shadow blocks on the shadow tray plate are with high precision.

A drawback using the cassette holder is the limited table rotation, which is reduced from $\pm 95°$ down to $\pm 25°$ when the gantry is at $0°$. This may cause problems when noncoplanar field arrangements are used.

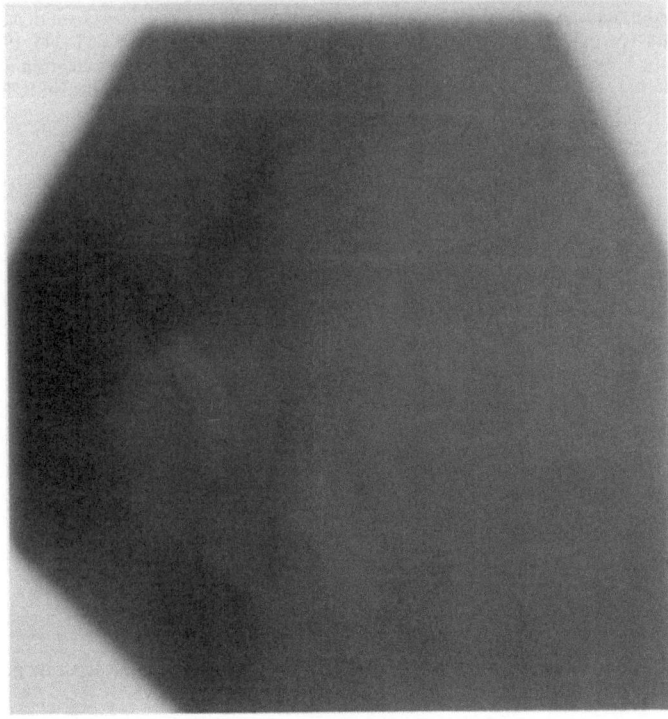

Conclusion

The use of the BEV utility together with the output from TMS-Radix has increased the agreement between the planned and the actual field shape. The transfer of block data to the final shadow blocks are much better using the TMS-Radix produced data. Work is in progress to install an automatic cutting device which will be connected via a network directly to the TMS-Radix system enabling the direct access of cutting information.

An increased use of more conformed field shapes will probably result in a decrease in complication frequency, for example, with fewer patients suffering radiation-induced pneumonitis when treated for thoracic diseases.

The cassette holder for port films has allowed the use of massive blocking for field shaping due to its accurate positioning of the cassette. Therefore, the port films may be used with certainty as very accurate detectors for the patient/beam orientation.

References

Ahnesjö A, Dose calculation methods in photon beam therapy using energy deposition kernels, PhD Thesis, Stockholm University, 1991

Knöös T, Nilsson M, Ahlgren L, A method for conversion of Hounsfield number to electron density and prediction of macroscopic pair production cross-sections, Radiother Oncol, 5, 337–345, 1986

Wambersie A, Landberg T, Johansson KA, Dobbs J, Gérard JP, Sentenac I, Dose prescription and specification in external radiotherapy: evaluation of ICRU report 29 and new trends, In: ICRU NEWS, Bethesda, Maryland, USA, 2, 25–27, 1989

Fig. 2. A pair of port films taken with 2 weeks between the treatments. The use of the accurate port film holder allows comparisons to be made from treatment to treatment

In Vitro Methods
and Animal Studies

The Respiratory Burst of Neutrophils:
A Prognostic Parameter in Head and Neck Cancer?

W. Kaffenberger[1], B.P.E. Clasen[2], and D. van Beuningen[1]

Phagocytic cells, such as neutrophilic and eosinophilic granulocytes and mono-cytes/macrophages, are cells "born to kill." The metabolic process by which these cells perform this function is the so-called respiratory or oxidative burst (RB). During this metabolic event, which is unique to phagocytes and which requires energy and oxygen, the cells produce a variety of cytotoxic oxygen species. An enzyme unique to phagocytes, the NADPH or, more correctly, the RB oxidase transfers one electron at the expense of NADPH to an oxygen molecule to produce the superoxide anion. This product dismutases sponta-neously or in the presence of superoxide dismutase to hydrogen peroxide. Hydrogen peroxide then serves as the parent product for a variety of other highly reactive oxygen metabolites which those who deal with ionizing radiation know very well, such as the hydroxyl radical, hypochlorous acid, and chlor-amines — all reagents that one would include in putting together a very effective disinfectant solution. Released into the phagosome, these products together with enzymes kill the engulfed bacteria.

Therefore, the RB of phagocytes is an important process in the orchestra of the unspecific immune response, which also includes the possibility that we are not only talking about a microbicidal but also about a tumoricidal effectiveness of this reaction. What we see in some tumors are large infiltrations with phagocytes, which means that these cells are involved in the tumor disease. Orchestrated by cytokines, phagocytes exert cytostatic and cytotoxic effects on tumor cells. It is assumed that the phagocyte-mediated killing of tumor cells is the same as the bactericidal activity, namely the RB activity. The tissue damaging effects of these products in a variety of clinical settings such as sepsis, shock, ischemia, and reperfusion are mentioned parenthetically.

As we are very interested in the immune consequences of ionizing radiation injury in man with the focus on functional immunological changes, we are studying — among other parameters — the RB function of neutrophils in patients who suffer from advanced squamous cell carcinomas of the head and neck, in close cooperation with the ENT department of the University Hospital "rechts der Isar" at the Technical University in Munich. The patients are being

[1] Institute of Radiobiology, Federal Armed Forces Medical Academy, Neuherbergstrasse 11, 8000 Munich 45, FRG
[2] ENT Department, University Hospital "rechts der Isar", Technical University Munich, Ismaninger Straße 22, 8000 Munich 80, FRG

Advanced Radiation Therapy Tumor Response
Monitoring and Treatment Planning
Breit (Editor-in-Chief)
© Springer-Verlag, Berlin Heidelberg 1992

treated with two courses of a combined modality regimen of radio-chemotherapy, separated by an interval of 2–3 weeks. The RB response of isolated
granulocytes is being analyzed by flow cytometry, where the increase in
fluorescence intensity of the fluorochrome-loaded cells serves as a measure for
the amount of hydrogen peroxide produced. In vitro an appropriate soluble
stimulus instead of the engulfed bacteria to induce the reaction can be the
phorbol ester PMA which directly activates the protein kinase C.

With regard to the in vivo regulation we can envisage that the RB is
orchestrated by cytokines such as granulocyte or granulocyte-macrophage
colony-stimulating factors, i.e., those of myelopoiesis. We recently found in
irradiated patients from the Chernobyl reactor accident that there is also a
positive correlation between the serum levels of the hormone prolactin and the
RB activity of granulocytes (Fig. 1). Seen in the light of a recent publication
(Larsen et al. 1990), we can also think of prolactin as a cytokine. This paper
showed a 20%–30% homology between human interleukin (IL) receptors for
IL-2, IL-3, IL-4, IL-7 and granulocyte colony-stimulating factor and the
prolactin receptor of the rat and the rabbit.

Individual patients enter the treatment with individual levels of RB activity
and respond differently to therapy. The following are three examples of patient
reactions. Prior to therapy and during the first course, patient A (Fig. 2) was
highly hyperreactive with regard to the RB response of his neutrophils. He
started with a threefold higher response than our controls. The response then
declined to values below the range of our controls and remained there through-

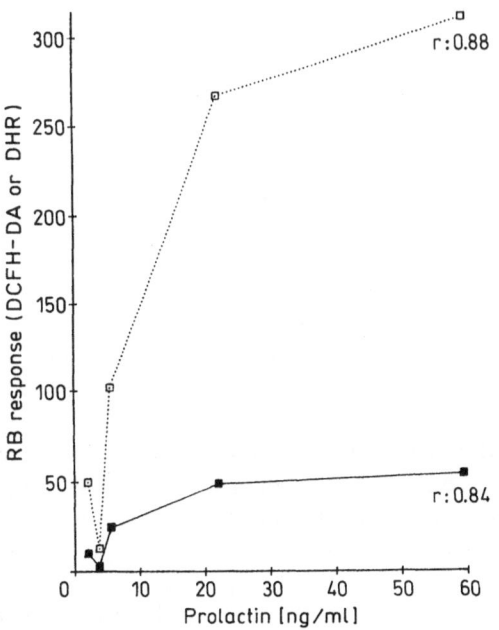

Fig. 1. Serum prolactin and
respiratory burst activity of
granulocytes in five irradiated
patients from the Chernobyl reactor
accident. *DCFH* (■ - - - ■), dichloro-
fluorescein diacetate; *DHR* (□ - - - □),
dihydrorhodamine. Both
fluorochromes are used to measure
respiratory burst activity separately

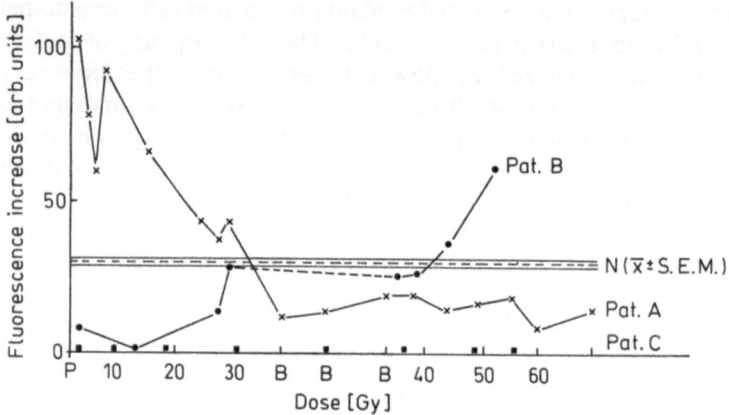

Fig. 2. Individual respiratory burst reactions in three patients during radiotherapy

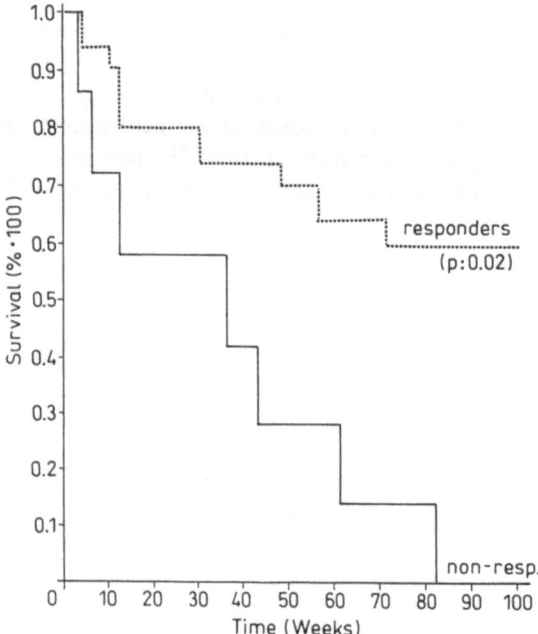

Fig. 3. Survival of responders and nonresponders after therapy

out therapy. We first considered a negative, immunosuppressive effect of therapy; however, thinking positive, one could also interpret the result in the light of a very good response of the tumor to the treatment and a relatively long relapse-free period as an indication for a therapeutically reduced burden on the neutrophils and their RB function. Patient B entered therapy as a low responder, showed increasing responsiveness during treatment, and exceeded the normal range at the end. Seen in the light of the next observation, we would also like to interpret this result as a positive effect. Patient C is an example from a subgroup of seven patients who exhibited no response throughout the period of treatment. Such nonresponse to in vitro. stimulus of the RB reaction is known from the literature in the case of the various forms of chronic granulomatous disease, seen mostly in children, as these patients suffer from very severe and recurrent bacterial and fungal infections and therefore very often reach only adolescence. To our knowledge such a defect has not been reported for tumor patients.

When we compared the survival time after therapy of our nonresponders with survival in the majority of patients who responded more or less normally, we found a significant difference: 82 weeks after the end of therapy all non-responders had died while 60% of normal responders were still alive (Fig. 3). We regard this correlation as the result of a disturbance in important parts of the immune surveillance, for which the nonresponse of granulocytes in the RB reaction is an obvious expression.

We are now conducting a study to confirm this interesting result and hopefully to extent it to other tumor entities. Its confirmation would enable us to offer the clinician a relatively easily measurable immunological parameter for use as a "predictive parameter" in planning the treatment of his patients, in other words, in individualizing their treatment. Nonresponsiveness of granulocytes to PMA stimulus of the RB reaction before or during treatment could indicate a very poor prognosis

References

Larsen A, Davis T, Curtis BM, Gimpel S, Sims JE, Cosman D, Park L, Sorenson E, March CJ, Smith CA (1990) Expression cloning of a human granulocyte colony-stimulating factor receptor: a structural mosaic of hematopoietin receptor, immunoglobulin, and fibronectin domains. J Exp Med 172: 1559–1570

Clinical Experiences with Cancer Diagnosis Based on the Measurement of Redox Potentials

D. Hamann and H. Heinrich

Introduction

Some 60 years ago Waterman (1933) reported an interesting observation. He irradiated serum samples steadily by X-rays for 60 min that had been obtained from patients suffering from malignant tumors. During the treatment he followed the oxidation reduction level in the serum samples and found generally a clear positive shift in values.

These examinations were not continued, and the findings have not been elucidated. We took up the results again and carried out further examinations of the redox behavior in serum samples of patients and healthy persons. For this purpose we developed a modified measuring method (see Heinrich and Hamann, this volume).

Materials

The first group that we examined comprised 100 patients with clinically verified primary malignant tumor or metastasis. The patients were not selected according to a specific criterion and thus represented a random distribution of 15 different malignant tumor types regarding both organ and histology. The examinations of blood serum redox behavior were carried out over 4 years resulting, and there have now been more than 2000 measurements. Among these were cases of solid carcinomas of different organ localizations as well as systemic diseases, osteogenic sarcoms, sarcomas of the soft tissues, and malignant melanomas. For comparison we determined the potentials in serum samples from 250 healthy blood donors (blood bank, Rostock); to date, we have the results of more than 500 such measurements. To examine the whole diagnostic spectrum of redox behavior eight serum samples (volume 0.5 ml are required.

Clinic of Radiology, University of Rostock, Department of Radiotherapy and Oncology, Südring 75, 2500 Rostock 6, FRG

Advanced Radiation Therapy Tumor Response
Monitoring and Treatment Planning
Breit (Editor-in-Chief)
© Springer-Verlag, Berlin Heidelberg 1992

Results

The difference in the alteration of redox potentials after irradiation in the sera of healthy persons and of tumor patients was highly significant. Figure 1 shows the mean values and the standard deviation of the redox potentials for 2000 tumor sera and for 250 blood donor sera after irradiation by X-rays with increasing doses of 10, 20, and 30 Gy. Figure 1 also demonstrates that there is no simple linear association between the behavior of redox potentials and radiation dosage. The graphs show roughly in mirror image the form of saturation curves. Analysis of the single results of the tumor patients revealed differences that explain the relatively high standard deviation.

Serum samples from patients suffering from expanded tumors (T3, T4) showed only a slight increase (about 15 mV) in redox values after irradiation, although the initial values already showed considerably high potentials. In contrast, in fast-growing tumors and cases of multiple metastases the initial values were clearly lower, and after irradiation the potentials showed a considerable increase, an average of 40 mV. In the sera of patients with brain tumors

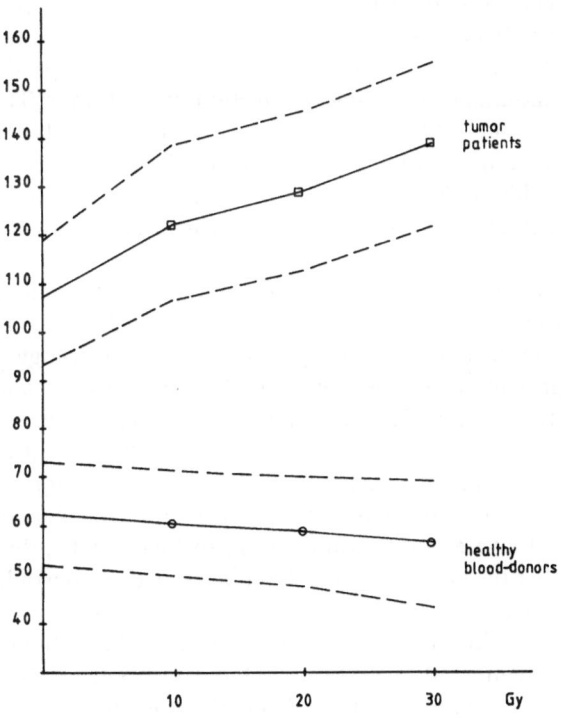

Fig. 1. Behavior of redox potentials in serum samples from tumor patients ($n = 2000$) and healthy blood donors ($n = 250$) after irradiation by X-rays (doses: 10, 20, and 30 Gy)

or peripheral bronchial carcinoma, as relatively slowly proliferating malignant cancers, the initial potentials were only moderately increased. Irradiation by X-rays caused an average increase of 20 mV.

We also examined the behavior of redox values after the tumor had been removed radically. For this purpose we determined the redox potentials in serum samples from ten patients with gynecological carcinoma (T1, and T2). The redox values were followed-up both preoperatively and after surgical removal of the tumor at 7- to 10-day intervals. Between 2 and 4 weeks after operation the redox potentials begin to drop again. By then the relatively slow tendency to decrease in redox values to a normal level was verified in more than 500 controls. The serum samples of all patients in the control group showed lack of effect upon redox potentials after irradiation, i.e., compared with the blanks in the irradiated samples only slight differences in the redox values were observed. In comparison to patients who experienced no recurrence after therapy over a long period (3 months), the tumor patients showed potentials on average 20–30 mV higher in blood serum samples.

It is worth mentioning that the lack of effect in serum redox potentials has continued now for several years in 93% of cases. Follow-up of patients at increasingly long intervals of 6 weeks to 1 year provided no essentially new findings regarding the problem of early cancer diagnosis. In only 21 of the control patients was a behavior of redox values observed in the serum samples resembling that in the tumor patients. At the same time, 15 of these showed the first metastases or recurrences. The other six patients showed tumor-specific characteristics 6 weeks to 3 months before clinical detection of the tumor. The prospect of early recognition is much more likely in the case of precancers. Up to now we have examined serum samples from only ten patients with undifferentiated leukoplakia or polymorphic adenoma. In two of these we found tumor characteristics in the serum samples 6 weeks and 3 months, respectively, before histology verified malignancy.

A group of 120 patients who were to be treated by conization were examined because of cytologically suspect findings. The results allowed a direct comparison between our values and histological findings. In the case of histological diagnosis of an invasively growing cancer we also found in our serum examination a tumor-characteristic reaction. Patients diagnosed with carcinoma in situ generally showed no positive results upon serum analysis. In the sera of 15 patients we detected tumor-characteristic behavior although the histological findings allowed no conclusion regarding an invasive growth. Our colleague for histological diagnoses was not aware of our examinations or their results; thus the question remains of whether the symptoms of a slight invasive growth would have been observed in these cases.

To assess the value of the redox diagnostic method in the field of tumor aftercare we examined 148 patients and carried out 200 measurements of their serum redox potentials. Of these, 138 had been treated earlier for carcinoma of the thyroid gland. Without our knowledge, ten had been dismissed with only benign thyroid disease.

In parallel with the determination of redox potentials both scintigraphic controls and measurements to provide verification of defined markers were carried out in the Department of Nuclear Medicine of our Clinic. We considered the correct diagnosis to be that based upon the results of these findings, and the results of all other examinations were then compared with these. We found here a correspondence to the findings by determination of redox potentials in 85% of cases. In 7.5% of patients the tumor was identified in the absence of positive results by the redox measurement method. The other 7.5% of patients showed a serum redox behavior characteristic of tumor, but no cancer was found by the methods of nuclear medicine.

The method of the redox measurement thus seems to provide positive indication of malignant cancer only when the tumor cells proliferate. We sought to confirm this by examination of ten pregnant women in the 16th–20th weeks of pregnancy. The findings were completely unnoteworthy. Patients suffering from hyperthyreosis, in spite of the accelerated metabolic turnover, showed no tumor-specific redox alterations upon serum analysis. In a further group of patients (carcinoma of basal cells, benign tumors, and progressive chronic polyarthritis) no alteration in serum redox potentials resembling tumor-specific ones were observed. However, examinations of patients suffering from severe inflammatory diseases, leading to considerable cellular destruction or extensive destruction of tissue, showed interesting results (abscessing pneumonia or endomyocarditis). Figure 2 presents the results of these examinations. In spite of

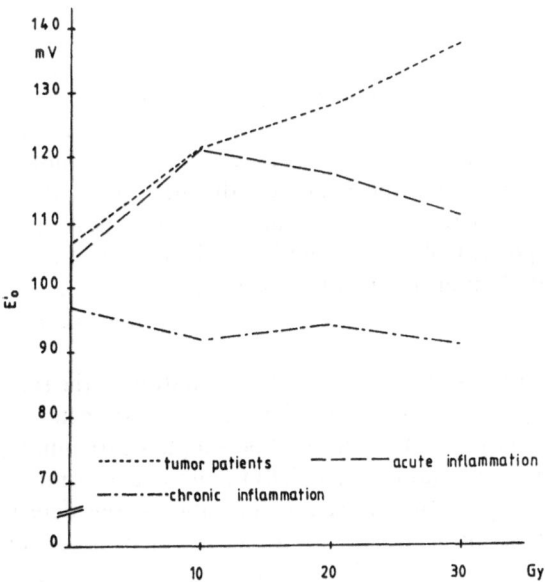

Fig. 2. Redox behavior of serum samples from patients suffering from acute and from chronic inflammation, compared with tumor serum values

Table 1. Diagnostic table based on oxidation reduction behavior in serum samples

Diagnostic criteria	Healthy donors	Tumor patients	Virus infections[a]	Bacterial infections[a]
Positive increase after irradiation	− −	+ + +	− (−)	+ + (+)
ATP test	+ + + +	+	+ + +	+ +
Action of caffeine	+ +	− −	(+/ −)	+
GTP	− −	+ +	+	−
FAD$^+$	+ + + +	(+)	+ + +	+ +
Injury index (Sign)	+	−	−	+

+ , Increasing positive potentials; − , decreasing positive potentials.
[a] Inflammations included.

the divergence at the endpoint in values for serum redox potentials, in particular cases the results allowed no unambiguous conclusions. Here, the use of additional biochemical parameters proved necessary to establish the diagnosis with certainty. In this way further differentiation of the diagnosis is possible, as summarized in Table 1. (For further information on those examinations, see Heinrich and Hamann, this volume).

Discussion and Conclusions

The method described here is well suited for distinguishing unambiguously between healthy persons and those bearing a malignant tumor. The diagnosis by means of this method is based upon examination of the serum, which shows the redox behavior either of a healthy person or that characteristic of a tumor. No conclusions are possible regarding organ specificity. On the other hand, there is an obvious correlation with the current state of a tumor concerning its extent and the speed of its cellular growth. We also found a slight tendency toward normalization of redox potentials after treatment of the malignant tumor. Thus, early findings cannot be expected concerning an initial or a lasting success of therapy.

However, controlling the progression of tumors, determination of the serum redox properties provides early information about the occurrence of metastases or recurrences, and by systematic application the method supplies early findings regarding the risk of malignant tumor (at least partially) some weeks or months before clinical evidence is available. In the case of precancers, the detected tumor-like redox behavior in serum samples may be interpreted as an early indication of a beginning malignancy and allows a much earlier beginning of therapy. When special differential diagnostic decisions are required (for example, in cases not verified by histological examination around a focus in the lungs), the determination of the redox potentials allows one to assess the dignity of the findings.

In follow-up examinations for comparison of findings in patients with carcinomas of the thyroid gland after treatment, we took the results of the nuclear medicine as providing the correct diagnosis. We calculated an 85% coincidence between the two sets of correct findings. We considered 7.5% of our cases to be suspect, in contrast to the findings of nuclear medicine. Some weeks earlier these patients had been treated by radioiodine therapy. The false negative conclusion should therefore be relativized and formulated as follows: "at present no indication of invasive tumor growth." The remaining cases (7.5%) can be considered as false positives. Taking into consideration the different possibilities for interpretation, the method thus gives results with a sensitivity of more than 90%. The characteristic behavior of the redox properties in the tumor serum samples after irradiation, according to our results, may be attributed neither to an intensification of the metabolic turnover nor to the high speed of the processes of cellular proliferation and growth. Many of our findings point to the following conclusion: invasive growth of the tumor leads to the destruction of healthy cells and tissues and therefore to the release of cellular enzymes and other substances such as constituents of the biomembranes, decisively influencing the redox level and behavior in the serum samples. Seen in this light it is comprehensible that not all cases of severe inflammatory diseases, which bring about a strong cellular breakdown, can be distinguished from the tumor-specific redox behavior in serum samples.

Reference

Waterman N (1933) Über Änderungen des Redox-Potentials in Serum durch Röntgenbestrahlung. Z Krebsforsch 38: 301–311

Demonstration of Early Tumor Reactions by Measurement of Glucose-6-Phosphate Isomerase Activity in the Serum of Irradiated Patients

M. Below, C. Gärtner, D. Tunak, and K.-H. Dallüge

Introduction

Quick evaluation of the efficacy of irradiation treatment still presents problems; this is especially the case with radiosensitizers, combined irradiation and chemotherapy, hyperthermia, hyperfractionation, and radiation with a high linear energy transfer. Our tests were aimed at finding a method to determine the effect of irradiation on a tumor in vivo at the beginning of treatment. We sought to detect the oncoradiogenic enzyme peak of aldolase [2], i.e., an increase in the serum enzyme level 16–19 h after initial irradiation of patients with bronchial or esophageal carcinoma; we examined the activity of glucose-6-phosphate isomerase (GPI; EC 5.3.1.9), an enzyme better suited for clinical laboratory routine, in patients with tumors of various localizations. The enzyme GPI, found in the cytoplasm, is omnipresent in nature and is also contained in human tissue in varying concentrations. Enzyme activity is particularly high in muscular and hepatic tissue and in malignant tumors. The normal range of serum enzyme activity is $0.3–3.0\ \mu mol\,l^{-1}\,s^{-1}$. Prior to the examination proper, the activity of GPI and creatine kinase (CK) in the serum of 16 healthy subjects was measured at hourly intervals over a period of 24 h. No pathological enzyme activity or significant changes in enzyme activity were observed throughout this period, and preanalytical factors such as food intake or physical activity were found to have no effect. The test was repeated in six patients with malignant tumors; also in this group we found no significant changes in GPI activity in the serum over a period of 24 h, and only higher mean values and greater dispersion were noted.

The patients were then irradiated with single doses of 2 or 5 Gy in the region of the tumor and the regional lymphatic drainage system, and GPI and CK activity were measured at 60-min intervals over a period of 24 h. Increases in GPI activity (referred to below as GPI peaks) were observed in all patients (Fig. 1). CK activity remained within the range of normal throughout the test.

An hourly measurement of GPI and CK activity in the serum after initial radiation with single doses of 2 Gy was also carried out in a control group of

Oncology Clinic and Outpatient Department, Medical School Charité, Humbold University, Schumannstr. 20/21, Berlin 1040, FRG

Advanced Radiation Therapy Tumor Response
Monitoring and Treatment Planning
Breit (Editor-in-Chief)

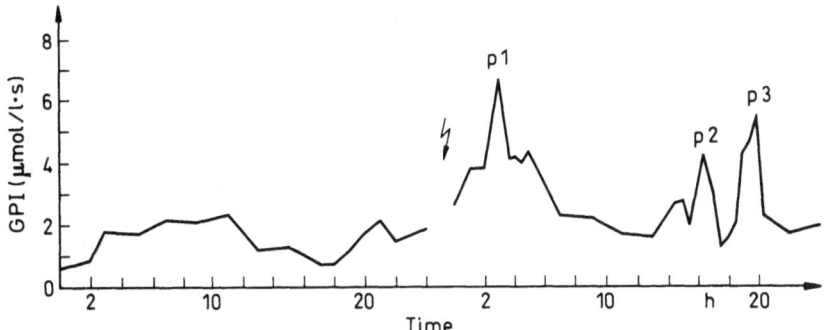

Fig. 1. Carcinoma of the breast T4N2M0 (56-year-old woman). Serum GPI activity before and after irradiation of the left breast and axilla with 2 Gy

four patients who had undergone a radical tumor operation (three with semi-noma, one with pharyngeal carcinoma) and two patients suffering from chronic inflammatory diseases in the pharyngeal region. Comparably reproducible changes in GPI and CK activity did not occur in any of these patients. These results encouraged us to start tests on a larger group of patients.

Materials and Methods

Tests were performed on 158 patients (aged 28–95 years, mean 62.3) with variously located carcinomas (Table 1). The majority of these cases were T3 or T4 tumors without distant metastases. Tumor volumes were determined with the help of computed tomography (CT) cross-sections; in cases of bad delimit-ation we used additional techniques such as chest X-ray on two planes (bron-chial carcinoma), contrast-media radiography (esophageal carcinoma), and palpation (cervical carcinoma).

All patients were irradiated with isocentrically corresponding cobalt-60 fields or at the 9-MeV linear accelerator with single doses of 1.8–5 Gy. The fields covered the primary tumor and regional lymphatic drainage system. Following initial irradiation blood was taken from a peripheral vein at hourly intervals (half-hourly intervals at hours 2–6 and hours 15–20) over a period of 24 h, using a technique which caused little discomfort to the patients. No restrictions were imposed on the patients with regard to diet or physical activity. Intramuscular injections were not allowed in the 12 h preceding or during the examination period. The blood samples were made to coagulate at room temperature and centrifuged for 5 min at 4000 rpm 2–3 h after sampling. Following this, 1 ml serum was pipetted into a plastic tube which was kept at a temperature of 4°C until the end of the test.

Table 1. Patient data ($n = 158$)

	n	Mean tumor volume (ml)
Bronchial carcinoma	69	70.7 ± 37.1 (11–180)
ENT carcinoma	42	15.5 ± 9.2 (9–42)
Cervical carcinoma	27	114 ± 56.4 (14–523)
Esophageal carcinoma	20	38.1 ± 19.9 (21–84)
N0	38	
N1	85	
N2	35	
Squamous cell carcinoma G1	38	
Squamous cell carcinoma G2	44	
Squamous cell carcinoma G3	26	
Undifferentiated carcinoma	13	
Small-cell carcinoma	16	
Glandular carcinoma	6	

GPI activity was measured at the Institute of Pathological and Clinical Biochemistry attached to the Charité Hospital according to the method developed by Bueding and McKinnon [1] using the Multistat III automatic laboratory device. CK and total protein concentration were determined in line with laboratory regulations issued in the German Democratic Republic in 1983. If the absolute quantity of enzyme released (e.g., from a tumor) is to be deduced from an increase in enzyme activity, which is proportional to enzyme concentration, the size of the distribution area — in this case, the plasma volume — must be known. This was calculated on the basis of height and body weight in line with the formulae set out in the Geigy book of tables [12]. According to the latter, the normal average plasma volume is 2.46 l for men and 2.13 l for women (mean values of 302 healthy subjects, ± 9.7%). All measurements of enzyme activity were standardized according to the following formula:

$$GPI_{corr} = GPI_{m} \cdot PLV_{pat} / PLV_{norm}$$

GPI_{corr} = corrected enzyme activity, GPI_{m} = measured enzyme activity, PLV_{pat} = individual plasma volume, and PLV_{norm} = standard plasma volume. An enzyme peak was defined as a rise in enzyme activity of at least 40% above the mean enzyme activity, the rise and the drop in the curve each being demonstrated by at least two measurements. The lower limit of 40% follows from the analytical and preanalytical error and from the average fluctuations in enzyme activity around the mean of the individual subject over a period of 24 h.

Results

Pretherapeutic GPI activity was in the range from 0.5–8.1 μmol l^{-1} s^{-1} and showed a pathological increase in 26% of patients with bronchial carcinoma (cervical carcinoma 22%, ENT carcinoma 16%, esophageal carcinoma 5%). There was a significant correlation between enzyme activity in the serum and tumor volume ($p < 0.025$); the incidence of GPI activity of more than $3 \, \mu mol \, l^{-1} s^{-1}$ was significantly higher among patients with a cervical carcinoma of more than 150 ml in volume. Due to its low sensitivity (18% in our case), the method of GPI measurement is not suitable for the detection of malignant diseases, however.

An average of 2.45 GPI peaks was observed in our 158 patients over a period of 24 h. In 73% of the patients (119/158), the first enzyme peak occurred on average 5.1 ± 0.8 h (3–7 h) after irradiation. On irradiation with single doses of ≤ 2 Gy, there was a significant correlation between the height of the enzyme peak and the tumor volume ($p < 0.025$) which was no longer demonstrable when the single doses were higher. In patients with lymph node metastases and on irradiation with single doses of 5 Gy, the first enzyme peak occurred significantly later than in those without lymph node metastases and on irradiation with doses of 1.8–2 Gy. A second enzyme activity peak was noted in 149 patients (94%) between the 16th and the 19th h after irradiation (mean 17.4 ± 0.9 h). No correlation was found between the times at which the GPI peaks occurred, on the one hand, and the tumor volume, degree of tumor differentiation, existence of regional metastases, or irradiation dose, on the other. A significant correlation between the height of the second GPI peak and the tumor volume existed independently of the site of the tumor (bronchial carcinoma, $p < 0.0001\%$; esophageal carcinoma, $p < 0.025$; ENT carcinoma, $p < 0.01$; cervical carcinoma, $p < 0.005$).

Significant increases in CK activity were noted in none of the patients. The correlation between the degree of tumor differentiation and the height of the

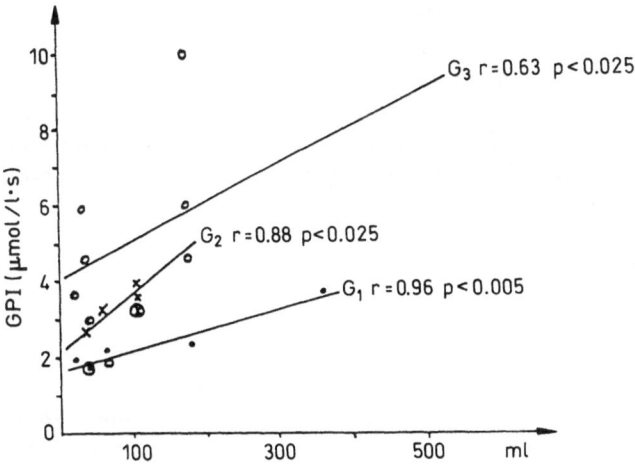

Fig. 2. Correlation between tumor volume and height of the oncoradiogenic GPI peak depending on the degree of tumor differentiation after initial irradiation with 2 Gy in 20 patients with cervical carcinoma

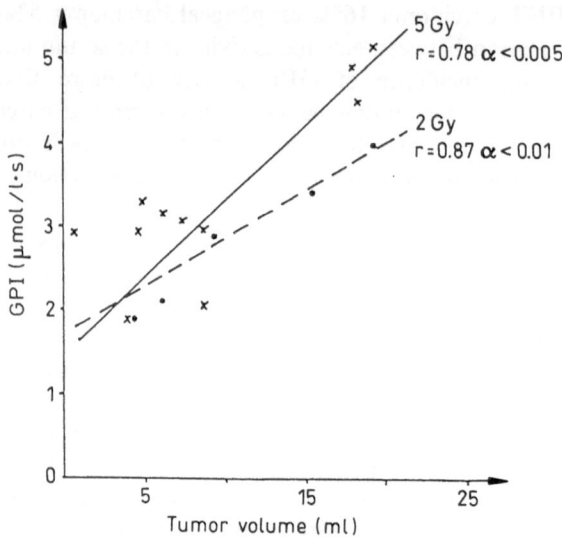

Fig. 3. Correlation between tumor volume and height of the oncoradiogenic GPI peak depending on tumor volume and irradiation dose in 17 patients with lingual carcinoma after initial irradiation

second GPI peak (referred to below as the oncoradiogenic GPI peak because it was closely related to the tumor volume) was examined in 20 patients with cervical carcinoma, 33 with bronchial carcinoma, and 10 with pharyngeal carcinoma. The tumor volume and irradiation dose being equal, patients with undifferentiated squamous cell carcinoma had higher oncoradiogenic GPI peaks than patients with medium-degree and well-differentiated carcinomas (Fig. 2). The correlation between the irradiation dose and the height of the oncoradiogenic peak was examined in 54 patients with bronchial carcinoma, 19 with esophageal carcinoma, and 19 with lingual carcinoma. Patients irradiated with single doses of 5 Gy had higher GPI peaks than those irradiated with single doses of 1.8–2 Gy (Fig. 3). A third enzyme activity peak occurred in 117 patients (74%) between 19.5 and 22.5 h after irradiation. Its incidence was significantly higher among patients with regional lymph node metastases, both in the group as a whole and in subgroups selected according to tumor site.

Discussion

At the cellular level, the release of cellular enzymes is attributed to the destruction of membrane structures [3, 4, 11] or changes in cell membrane permeability [5, 6, 10, 13]. In 73% of our patients a peak-shaped increase in GPI activity occurred 3–7 h after initial irradiation. On irradiation with small single doses it was mainly the tumor cells, being more sensitive to radiation and having a limited repair capacity, which reacted by releasing GPI between 2 and 7 h after irradiation. Since no significant correlation between the tumor volume and the height of the first GPI peak was found with higher single doses of radiation, we assume that as irradiation doses become higher, normal tissue also reacts increasingly by releasing GPI 3–7 h after irradiation.

The changes in the permeability of the cell membrane were of a temporary nature in most cases [7]. In functional terms, this is shown by the fact that the functional disorder of the membrane was reversed 6–8 h after the influence of the harmful noxa [8]. In cells that have a limited repair capacity the damage to the membrane caused by irradiation, which became manifest after 3–6 h, may be irreversible so that enzyme continues to be released. It seems that this release is not a continuous process but occurs in stages. About 10–12 h after the first GPI peak, a renewed enzyme release was noted in 94% of the patients.

In our view the correlation with the tumor volume, which showed an even higher significance when the series was divided according to the degree of tumor differentiation, suggests that the oncoradiogenic GPI peak is caused by the irradiation-induced enzyme release from tumor cells, and that — in contrast to what happens at the first enzyme peak — a reaction of the normal tissue no longer plays an essential part in it. We believe that at the time of the oncoradiogenic peak the normal cells, being more efficient at repair, have already overcome the irradiation damage so that the permeability of their membranes is no longer increased.

Kärcher [5] found initial increases in lactic and malic dehydrogenase activity in the serum after irradiation of radiation-sensitive tumors with doses of 8 Gy, a reaction which was not demonstrable in patients with relatively radiation-resistant tumors. In his opinion, these increases were attributable to the fact that the cells of highly differentiated tumors contain a greater number of cell organelles, in particular mitochondria, which help to compensate irradiation damage by releasing organelle-specific enzymes (adenosine triphosphatase, catalase). This view is confirmed by the results of our examinations, which show that enzyme release is higher the less differentiated the tumor is.

In anaplastic carcinomas the regional blood flow — in relation to tumor volume — is only about half that is highly differentiated tumors [9]. This may affect the transportation of cellular enzymes, and in view of these differences in blood circulation the absolute quantity of enzyme released by irradiation may be even larger in poorly differentiated tumors. On irradiation of tumors which are identical as to site, volume, histological features, and degree of differentiation, the height of the oncoradiogenic enzyme peak depends on the single dose applied. The increase in enzyme release (in relation to tumor volume) induced by administration of a high single irradiation dose is higher the greater the tumor volume is. In the case of small tumors, irradiation with low single doses is likely to affect a relatively large proportion of cells which are going through a sensitive stage in the cellular cycle, so that the percentage increase in the effect of irradiation caused by administration of a large single dose is lower than with large tumors.

Measurement of the oncoradiogenic enzyme peak of GPI allows a quantitative in vivo assessment of the effect of irradiation on a tumor immediately after the beginning of treatment. This in turn makes it possible to assess sensitivity to irradiation on an individual basis and to draw comparisons between various modifications of treatment which play an increasing role in clinical oncology (combined irradiation and chemotherapy, hyperthermia, hyperfractionation, administration of radiation qualities with high relative efficacy).

References

1. Bueding E, McKinnon IA (1955) Studies of the phosphoglucose isomerase of schistoma mansoni. J Bio Chem 215: 507
2. Dallüge K-H (1981) RBW-Bestimmung von Tumoren durch Serumaldolase? Radiobiol Radiother 22(3): 253–255
3. Hagen U (1962) Über die Entstehung der Thymusatrophie nach Röntgenbestrahlung. III. Über die Strahlenaktivierung von Fermenten. Strahlentherapie 117: 201–207
4. Harris RJC (1961) The initial effects of ionizing radiation on cells. Academic, London
5. Kärcher KH, Becker J (1962) Biochemische Verlaufskontrolle strahlenbehandelter Patienten. Radiologe 2: 304–309
6. Kärcher KH (1970) Enzymaktivitäten in strahlenbiologischem Experiment und radiologischer Klinik. Gerber GB (ed) Biochemisch nachweisbare Strahlenwirkungen und deren Beziehung zur Strahlentherapie. Thieme, Stuttgart
7. Köteles GJ (1982) Radiation effects on cell membranes. Radiat Environ Biophys 21: 1–18
8. Kröner H, Staib W (1967) Energiestoffwechsel und Serumenzyme. Z Klin Chem 5: 89
9. Mantyla MJ, Toivanen JT, Pitkänen MA et al. (1982) Radiation-induced changes in regional blood-flow in human tumors. Int J Radiat Oncol 8: 1711–1717
10. Rode I, Horvath M (1978) Changes of blood components on in vitro and in vivo irradiation in cancer therapy. Strahlentherapie 154: 559–563
11. Wills ED, Wilkinson AE (1966) Release of enzymes from lysosomes by irradiation and relation of lipid peroxide formation to enzyme release. Biochem J 99: 657–666
12. Ciba-Geigy (ed) (1979) Wissenschaftliche Tabellen Geigy Physikalische Chemie Blut-Humangenetik-Stoffwechsel von Xenobiotika. Ciba-Geigy, Basel
13. Yau TM (1981) Alterations in the structure and function of the mammalian cell membrane after exposure to ionizing radiation. Scanning electr Microsc 4: 47–54

Sequential Computed Radiographs of the Thorax in an Experimental Animal Study

E.M. Lang[1] and U. Krüger[2]

Introduction

At the Institute of Biophysics and Radiobiology in Hamburg experiments concerning palliative lung irradiation of artificial lung metastases of R1H rhabdomyosarcoma of the rat were performed. Fractionated lung irradiation with various doses was administered to the animals starting at defined stages of macroscopic metastatic development. Due to the biological scatter in metastatic development there was a need to monitor metastatic growth by sequential radiographs to determine the start of treatment for the various treatment groups. The aim of this study was to investigate computed radiography versus conventional X-ray imaging concerning their performance in detecting small metastases.

Material and Methods

The experiments were performed using the rhabdomyosarcoma R1H–WAG/Rij-rat tumor-host system. Artificial lung metastases were induced by injecting about 10^5 clonogenic tumor cells into the metatarsal vein of male rats weighing 220–250 g. Sequential chest radiographs for every rat were taken at least once a week. Metastatic growth was monitored using a four-stage scoring system. The dataset is based on the sequential chest radiographs of nine animals. A total of 170 radiographs entered the analysis. The incidence of metastases was checked by postmortem section at the end of experiments.

The images were taken by conventional radiography and computed radiography technique, as described by Tateno et al. (1984) (Philips Computed Radiography System with high-resolution luminescence screen). All images were performed with the Philips medical veterinary machine with 65 kV, 7.5 mA, focus–film distance 100 cm, and exposure time 0.12–0.16 s. For the conventional

[1] Department of Radiology, University of Hamburg, FRG
[2] Institute of Biophysics and Radiobiology, University of Hamburg, FRG

Advanced Radiation Therapy Tumor Response
Monitoring and Treatment Planning
Breit (Editor-in-Chief)
© Springer-Verlag, Berlin Heidelberg 1992

radiographs an Agfa Ortho GS film with high-resolution screen and daylight developing system were used.

The rats were anesthetized by isoflurane (4% Forene, Abbot, in 96% oxygen). The anesthesia lasted for about 3–4 min, so there was enough time to take the conventional and the digital chest radiographs directly one after another. As the lateral chest view consists mostly of the shade of the heart, only the posterior-anterior view was performed. A plexiglass stair was placed beside the animals as densitometric reference. A quality control was performed by measurements of two steps of the densitometric reference (step 3, 12 mm; step 5, 32 mm, plexiglass) which covered the same range of optical density as the rat thorax.

All images were examined by three independent investigators. A four-stage scoring system was used: stage 0, no metastases, normal appearance of the lung, heart, great vessels, and diaphragma: stage 1, one or two visible metastases not exceeding 5 mm in diameter; stage 2, metastases over 5 mm in diameter but less than half of the size of the lung; stage 3, more than 50% of the lung filled with metastases.

Results

Figure 1 gives the time intervals between induction of metastases and first diagnosis of status 1 or status 2 for both radiological techniques as seen by the three independent examiners. The vertical lines indicate the median values for all examiners. The median time interval between induction of metastases and diagnosis of stage 1 was 51 days if the conventional radiographs are scored.

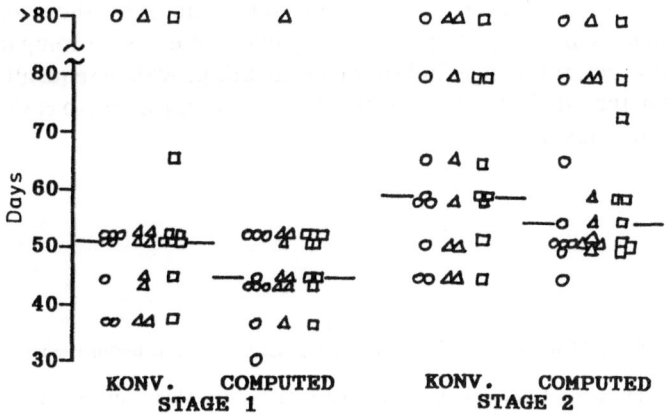

Fig. 1. Time of first diagnosis of status 1 or status 2: number of days after injection of tumor cells. Conventional versus computed radiography

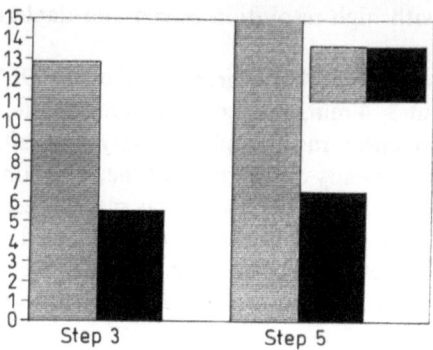

Fig. 2. Standard deviation of optical density values for steps 3 and 5 of the densitometric reference. *Gray bars*, conventional radiography; *black bars*, computed radiography

Using digital radiographs, stage 1 was seen already after 45 days. The stage 2 metastases became detectable after 58 days with conventional radiography and after 55 days using digital radiography. In this experiment digital radiography gave a diagnostic benefit of 6 days in detecting stage 1 metastases and a benefit of 3 days in detecting metastases of stage 2.

Discussion

Figure 2 shows the standard deviation of the optical density values for the conventional images versus digital images for step 3 and step 5 of the densitometric reference. The standard deviation for digital radiographs is lower than for conventional radiographs. This indicates a higher constancy of the digital images.

In this experiment the sequences of radiographs were examined without any other clues. The higher constancy of optical density makes it easier to compare and evaluate small structural changes indicating metastatic growth in sequential chest radiographs of the rat. This gives a diagnostic advantage leading to earlier detection of lung metastases.

References

Tateno Y, Iinuma T, Takano M (eds) (1984) Computed radiography. Springer, Berlin Heidelberg New York

Rufer HR (1958) Die Thoraxinnenmaße und die Zwerchfellgröße bei der Albinoratte in verschiedenen Lebensaltern. Morphol Jahrb V (99): 314–343

Tumor Necrosis Factor α Effects Studied in a Mouse Model Using Contrast-Enhanced Magnetic Resonance Imaging

K.P. Aicher[1,2], J.W. Dupon[1], S.L. Aukerman[3], D.L. White[1], and R.C. Brasch[1]

Introduction

Tumor necrosis factor α (TNF) is a polypeptide with many functions in biological systems [1]. It is produced by activated macrophages and stimulates macrophages, polynuclear neutrophilic leukocytes, and eosinophiles either to kill cells or to attach cells to the endothelium causing changes that lead to a remarkable antitumor effect, i.e., "tumor necrosis." The antitumor effect of TNF involves tumor vascular changes, and the efficacy is probably not caused directly by cell cytotoxity [2]. After TNF administration one can observe hemorrhage and thrombosis within the tumors [3]. Meth-A induced fibrosarcomas are known to respond to TNF treatment. The most commonly used model to study TNF effects is this tumor type implanted in mice.

We describe here our attempt to image in vivo the changes within the tumor associated with the administration of TNF using contrast-enhanced magnetic resonance imaging (MRI). MRI has shown considerable utility in the identification and characterization of Meth-A fibrosarcoma, as demonstrated recently [4]. The time-dependent increase in signal intensity after the administration of the macromolecular contrast agent albumin-(Gd-DTPA) into the tumorous tissue was attributed to the abnormal capillary permeability of tumor vessels. TNF targets tumor vessels. The question addressed was: Does TNF change tumor capillary permeability, and can this be demonstrated with by imaging means in vivo?

Materials and Methods

In 18 BALB/c mice Meth-A induced fibrosarcoma cells were implanted and grown to a size of 500 mm³. Prior to imaging in a group of ten mice 150 μg/kg TNF was administered intravenously as a bolus. TNF was provided by Cetus

[1] Contrast Media Laboratory, Department of Radiology, University of California, San Francisco, CA 94143-0628, USA
[2] Department of Radiology, University of Tübingen, Hoppe-Seyler-Str. 3, 7400 Tübingen, FRG
[3] Cetus Corporation, Emmeryville, CA 94608, USA

Advanced Radiation Therapy Tumor Response
Monitoring and Treatment Planning
Breit (Editor-in-Chief)
© Springer-Verlag, Berlin Heidelberg 1992

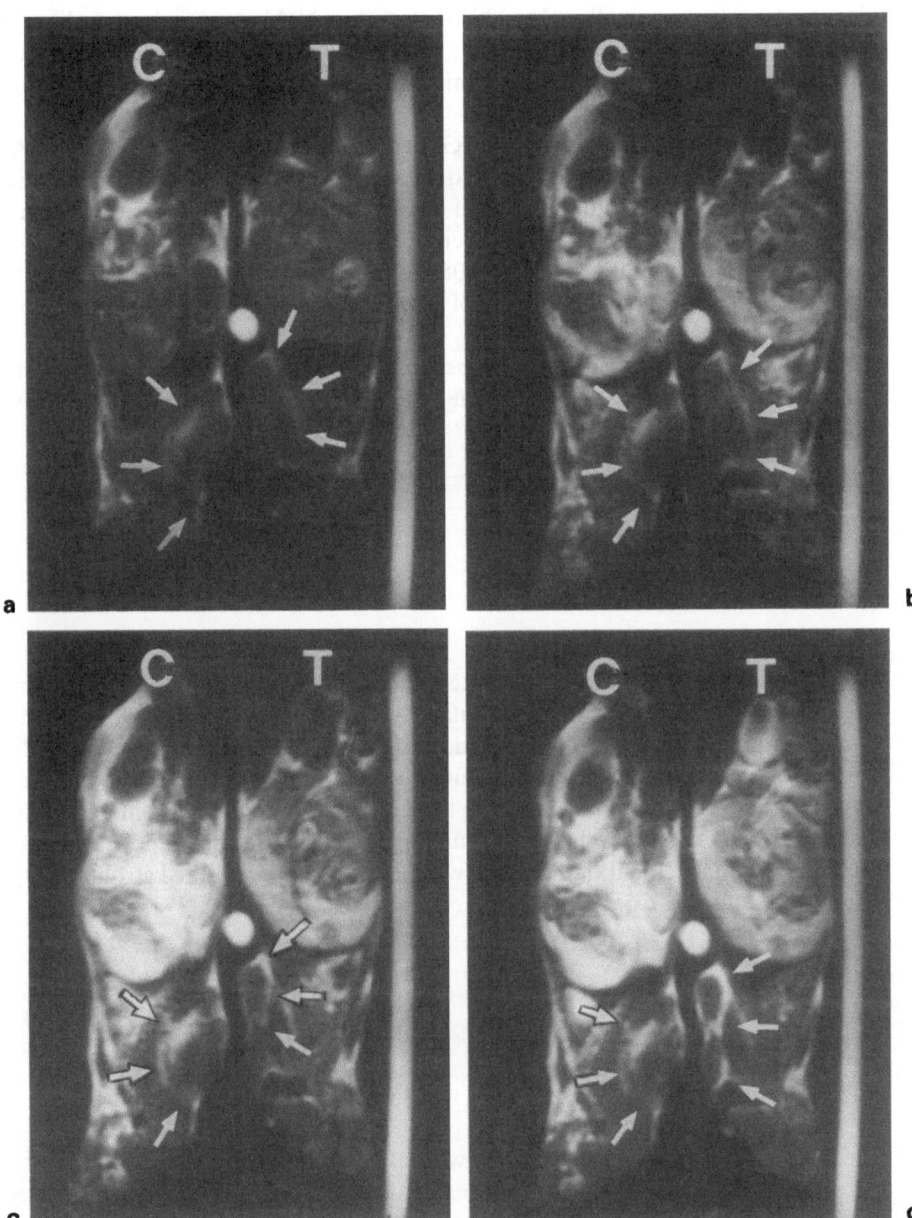

Fig. 1a–d. Sequential coronal SE images (TR 310/TE 15 ms) of a pair of tumor-bearing mice following the administration of albumin-(Gd-DTPA): *T*, TNF-treated mouse; *C*, untreated control. The precontrast image (**a**) as a baseline is compared with a 5-min (**b**), 15-min (**c**), and 60-min postcontrast (**d**) image. The enhancement is at nearly constant level in normal tissue between 5 and 60 min postcontrast. The tumors (*arrows*), however, show an increase over time, most evident in the vascularized rim portion. There is an obvious difference between control and TNF-treated tumor, with a stronger enhancement indicating an increased vascular permeability due to TNF treatment making tumor vessels more "leaky" for macromolecules such as albumin-(Gd-DTPA)

Corporation (Emmeryville, CA, USA). It was a highly purified recombinant human TNF from *Escherichia coli* and had a specific activity of 2.4×10^7 units/mg (i.e., 7.2×10^4 units of TNF/mouse). Eight control mice received saline solution instead of TNF.

Imaging was performed at 2 T (General Electrics, Freemont, CA, USA) employing T1-weighted spin-echo sequences (TR/TE: 310/15 ms) before and serially over 1 h after administration of the macromolecular contrast agent albumin-(Gd-DTPA). The contrast agent was injected intravenously in a dose of 160 mg/kg, corresponding a dose of 0.084 mmol Gd/kg. Intensity measurements were performed in different regions of interest, and the contrast enhancement over time was calculated.

All mice were injected with Evans blue (50 mg/kg), and 20 min later the animals were sacrificed. Evans blue staining was compared to contrast enhancement in the images.

Results

Tumor enhancement of the TNF-treated mice using a macromolecular contrast agent was significantly greater particularly in the vascularized periphery of the tumor compared to the saline-treated controls (59% versus 40%; Fig. 1). In normal tissue, including brain and muscle, no significant difference was observed in the TNF-treated mice versus the untreated animals. The enhancement remained at a constant level over the imaging period in the non-tumorous tissue. The in vivo enhancement pattern that was observed corresponded strongly with Evans blue staining ex vivo.

Conclusions

The different enhancement pattern between TNF-treated and untreated tumors are attributed to TNF-induced chances in tumor capillary integrity. The data indicate that early TNF effects on tumors include an increased capillary permeability for macromolecules. TNF seems to make certain tumors "leaky" and maybe more sensitive for other antitumor drugs or treatments.

We conclude that contrast-enhanced MRI using a macromolecular agent such as albumin-(Gd-DTPA) as a marker for capillary integrity may prove clinically useful for monitoring tumor response not only to TNF but also to other anticancer therapies.

References

1. Beutler B, Cerami A (1988) The common mediator of shock, cachexia, and tumor necrosis. Adv Immunol 42: 213–231
2. Watanabe N, Niitsu Y, Umeno H et al. (1988) Toxic effect of tumor necrosis factor on tumor vasculature in mice. Cancer Res 48: 2179–2183
3. Nawroth P, Handly D, Matsueda G et al. (1988) Tumor necrosis factor/cachexin-induced intravascular fibrin formation in Meth A fibrosarcomas. J Exp Med 168: 637–647
4. Wikström MG, Moseley ME, White DL et al. (1989) Contrast-enhanced MRI of tumor: comparison of Gd-DTPA and a macromolecular agent. Invest Radiol 24: 609–615

The Oxidation Reduction Potential:
A New Criterion for Cancer Diagnosis

H. Heinrich and D. Hamann

Introduction

Blood serum samples from tumor patients show striking disturbances in the oxidation reduction properties. As early as about 1930 examinations of the redox behavior in blood serum led to this conclusion (Roffo 1925, 1929, 1930; Roffo and Rivarola 1925; Gandolfo and Encina 1930; Gandolfo 1932; Waterman 1933; Kollath 1938). From these early results the conclusion was drawn that the differences in redox properties between sera of healthy blood donors and those of patients suffering from a malignant tumor possibly reflect basic properties connected with the pathophysiological state of the patient. We took up again the redox examinations with a measuring procedure modified for our need.

We examined the influence of X-rays and of several biocatalysts on the oxidation reduction power of the serum samples. On this basis we developed an analytical method for the examination of serum redox properties. Our experience with more than 2000 patients and 500 healthy blood donors shows this method to be routinely applicable for the diagnosis of cancer and other diseases.

Materials and Methods

The measurement of redox potentials is performed in a standardized volume of 0.5 ml blood serum. The venous blood (10 ml) is taken without adding any substances. For the characteristics of our patients, healthy donors, and analyzed subgroups see Hamann and Heinrich (this volume).

After centrifugation of the blood samples (10 min, 2500 rpm) the serum was pipetted off, frozen, and stored at $-22°C$. The potentials were measured in serum samples when thawed by the following simple method. An insulated shiny wire of platinum (0.625 mm in diameter) as conducting electrode is fixed to a support parallel to a glass capillary. On its top end the capillary is dilated. The

Clinic of Radiology, University of Rostock, Department of Radiotherapy and Oncology, Südring 75, 2500 Rostock 6, FRG

Advanced Radiation Therapy Tumor Response
Monitoring and Treatment Planning
Breit (Editor-in-Chief)
© Springer-Verlag, Berlin Heidelberg 1992

reference electrode can be inserted variably into the capillary, and the contact can be interrupted easily at any time. The capillary is filled with sodium chloride solution (0.9%) forming an electrolyte bridge. Both the shiny electrode of platinum and the reference electrode are connected by a flex with a digital voltmeter due to its low inertia of display. After every measuring step the mobile arrangement of capillary and platinum electrode is washed at its contact with the serum samples. In this way, the zero point of the potential results before every measuring step.

In all our examinations we used a saturated calomel electrode with an inherent potential of $+ 237$ mV (at 25°C) compared with the hydrogen electrode. The biochemical examinations were made after addition to the serum samples of the biocatalysts adenosine triphosphate (ATP), guanosine triphosphate (GTP), or flavin-adenosine dinucleotide as disodium salt (5 mg per sample at a time) and caffeine (50 µg per sample).

Results

After irradiation of serum samples by X-rays with various doses (10, 20, and 30 Gy) the summary redox potentials behave in quite different ways: the tumor serum potentials show an increasing tendency, whereas the potentials of donor serum samples drop progressively. Furthermore, the redox behavior in sera of patients with bacterial infections or malaria interferes with that in tumor sera (see Fig. 1). For unequivocal diagnostic results, because of this interference we examined the redox behavior after addition to the serum samples of selected biocatalysts. Initial trials led to the conclusion that both ATP and GTP cause a characteristic increase in the level of serum potentials.

Figure 2 shows the in vitro effect of ATP on the serum redox potentials (Heinrich and Hamann 1990). Further examination of the ATP reaction revealed that the actual effective substances may be cyclic adenosine monophosphate (3, 5-cAMP) and cyclic guanosine monophosphate (cGMP). When 3, 5-cAMP is used, the same values are measured as those with ATP, and after addition to the serum samples of caffeine as inhibitor of the 3, 5-cAMP phosphodiesterase enzyme the values are further increased. Upon the findings with ATP, GTP, and ATP plus caffeine we calculated a further diagnostic parameter: the cellular injury index. In our experience, this index reflects the degree of cellular destruction, of the destruction or impairment of cellular entities due to the disease (infiltrative growth, parasitical or virus infections etc.). The cellular injury index (CII) is calculated as follows:

$$ CII = \frac{E'_{0ATP} + \text{caffeine}}{E'_{0GTP}} - \frac{E'_{0GTP}}{E'_{0ATP} + \text{caffeine}} \cdot 1000 $$

where E'_0 is the redox potential at pH $= 7.4$ and 20 °C.

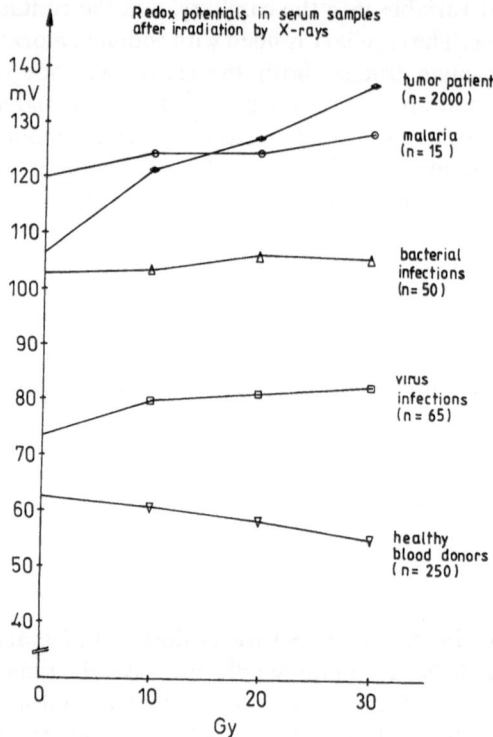

Fig. 1. Comparison of redox behavior in serum samples from healthy blood donors and from patients with tumor, bacterial, and virus infections. Irradiation by X-rays, doses: 10,20, and 30 Gy

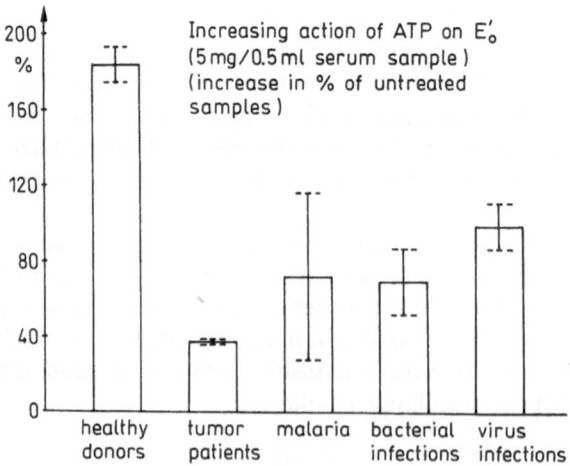

Fig. 2. Effect of ATP (5 mg/0.5 ml) on the redox potential in serum samples of healthy blood donors and those of patients with tumor, malaria, bacterial, and virus infections. (See also Heinrich and Hamann 1990)

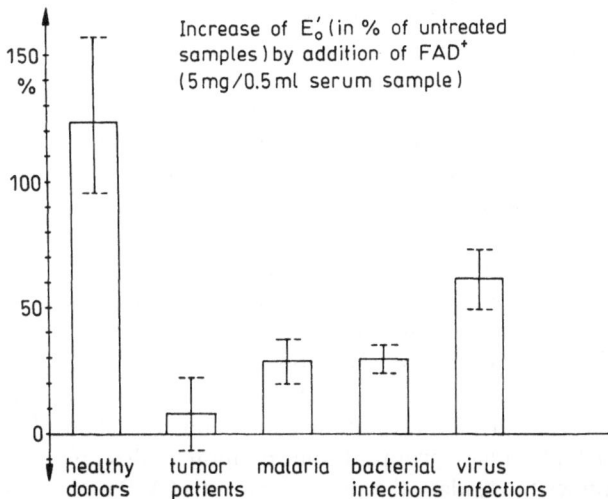

Fig. 3. Increase in redox potentials after addition of FAD^+ (5 mg/0.5 ml) to serum samples of healthy blood donors and to those of patients with tumor, malaria, and bacterial and virus infections

At high degrees of cellular destruction or impairment (e.g., in an acute fit of malaria) the index shows strongly negative values. In the case of bacterial disease this is not the case (Heinrich and Hamann, manuscript in preparation). Waravdekar and Powers (see Graffi and Bielka 1957) observed that the transfer of hydrogen of the biochemical substrates is substantially disturbed in malignant disease; these authors examined the action of serum NAD^+ and $NADP^+$. To our knowledge, there has been no reported examination of the action of FMN^+ or FAD^+ coenzymes in this context. The many flavin-mediated metabolic steps may also be disturbed, depending on the kind of the disease. Figure 3 shows the results of the in vitro addition of FAD^+ to serum samples of healthy blood donors and patients suffering from malignant, bacterial, virus, or parasitical diseases. In tumor serum samples there is often no increase in redox potential after addition of FAD^+, and there may even be a decrease. The administration of FAD^+ therefore serves as a further test parameter for the differential diagnosis of tumor disease.

Discussion and Conclusions

The method presented here is easily applicable for the routine clinical measurement of redox potentials in serum samples. The blood serum test consists of two main parts: (a) analysis of the biophysical behavior of the serum samples and (b) analysis of the action of defined biochemical catalysts. The physical exertion of influence on serum properties by irradiation with increasing doses of ionizing rays leads to the initiation of radical chain mechanisms. The behavior of the resulting redox potential reflects the pathophysiologically relevant properties of body fluids regarding the power of redox buffering capacity (poising action) and of the radical scavenging properties. At the very last, in the case of a malignant tumor the poising action and the radical scavenging ability, protecting the physiological metabolic regulation, obviously became disturbed and quickly exhausted (seen in the increase in redox level after irradiation of the samples). In comparison to this, the redox analysis of serum samples from patients suffering from malaria ($n = 15$) or bacterial infections (encephalitis, gastroenteritis, pneumococcal meningitis, etc.; $n = 50$) leads to similar results.

In the case of malignant diseases we recommend the analysis of redox potentials in serum samples after the addition of 5 mg ATP, GTP, or FAD^+ for differential diagnosis. This biochemical analysis provides supplementary diagnostic knowledge. In our experience the addition to serum samples of ATP, ATP plus caffeine, and GTP gives information concerning the state of the metabolism of energy-rich phosphate groups. In our opinion, it also reflects the power of the serum samples to regulate the proportions of cAMP and cGMP and hence to regulate the redox conditions, etc. (Cutler 1984; Pryor 1984; del Maestro 1984; Cornwell and Morisaki 1984; Torrielli and Dianzani 1984). This view is supported by the finding of differences in the action of the caffeine inhibitor on the 3, 5-cAMP phosphodiesterase enzyme; in tumor sera caffeine shows a slight inhibitory effect on the potentials after addition of ATP compared with the findings in serum samples of healthy donors. When GTP is used, the reaction reflected in the alteration of the redox potentials is reversed; in tumor sera the potentials often increase much more than those in donor sera. The proportions also proved correct with other cell-destroying diseases (e.g., malaria, virus, bacterial inflammations). In view of this relationship one should calculate the injury factor — the cellular injury index — reflecting the stage of cellular injury in the disease. In healthy cells the concentration of cAMP exceeds that of cGMP. In the case of any membrane injury the level of cGMP rises above that of cAMP. The serum redox behavior in tumor sera after the addition of FAD^+ also shows a profound imbalance in the redox buffering capacity. Compared to the redox conditions in healthy donor sera, FAD^+ in the case of infections shows lower levels of increased positive potentials but a very different behavior than in tumor serum.

Our experiences thus show this analysis of serum redox potentials to be of substantial clinical relevance. The value of this method has been confirmed repeatedly by screening and blind trials and in comparison to histological diagnoses.

References

Cornwell DG, Morisaki N (1984) Fatty acid paradoxes in the control of cell proliferation: prostaglandins, lipid peroxides, and cooxidation reactions. In: Pryor WA (ed) Free radicals in biology, Academic, New York, pp 95–148

Cutler RG (1984) Antioxidants, aging, and longevity. In: Pryor WA (ed) Free radicals in biology, vol VI. Academic, New york, pp 371–428

Del Maestro RF (1984) Free radical injury during inflammation. In: Armstrong D, Sohal RS, Cutler RG, Slater TF (eds) Free radicals in molecular biology, aging and disease. Raven, New York, pp 87–102

Gandolfo A (1932) Die Roffo'sche Krebsreaktion. Z Krebsforsch 37: 448–460

Gandolfo A, Encina A (1930) Der diagnostische Wert der Roffo'schen Reaktion. Sitzungsber. Med. Kongr. (Montevideo) 6: 58–71

Graffi A, Bielka H (eds) (1959) Probleme der Biologie, vol 6: Probleme der experimentellen Krebsforschung. Geest and Portig, Leipzig, p 378

Heinrich H, Hamann D (1990) Veränderungen des Redoxpotentials in Serumproben unter Einfluß von Adenosintriphosphat (ATP). Radiobiol Radiother (Berl) 31: 239–242

Kollath W (1938) Redoxpotentiale, Zellstoffwechsel und Krankheitsforschung. Ergeb Hyg Bakteriol Immunitaetsforsch Exp Ther 21: 269–337

Pryor WA (1984) Free radicals in autoxidation and in aging. In: Armstrong D, Sohal RS, Cutler RG, Slater TF (eds) Free radicals in molecular biology, aging and disease. Raven, New York, pp 13–41

Roffo AH (1925) Die Neutralrotreaktion bei normalen und Krebsseren. Bol Med Exp 2: 791–796

Roffo AH (1929) El azul de metileno en los cultivos de los tejidos normales y neoplásicos in vitro. Bol Med Exp 6: 67–85

Roffo AH (1930) La sensibilización del azul de metileno y su acción inhibidora sobre el crecimiento de los tejidos cultivados "in vitro." Bol Med Exp 7: 950–969

Roffo AH, Rivarola J (1925) Die Neutralrotreaktion beim Krebs: ihr diagnostischer Wert. Bol Med Exp 2: 709–714

Torrielli MV, Dianzani MU (1984) Free radicals in inflammatory disease. In: Armstrong D, Sohal RS, Cutler RG, Slater TF (eds) Free radicals in molecular biology, aging and disease. Raven, New York, pp 355–379

Waterman N (1933) Über Änderungen des Redox-Potentials im Serum durch Röntgenbestrahlung. Z. Krebsforsch 38: 301–311

Code Comparison and Verification for Patient-Specific Three-Dimensional Treatment Planning in Regional Hyperthermia*

P. Wust, J. Nadobny, H. Fähling, A. Jordan, and R. Felix

Introduction

A new generation of annular-phased-array systems has been in clinical use since 1988 (BSD-2000, BSD Medical Corp., Salt Lake City, Utah). The power deposition pattern inside the body is generated by four antenna pairs in a ring applicator of 60 cm diameter, with variation in phases/amplitudes of channels, frequency (70–110 MHz), and patient position possible. In principle, the treatment system is able to match the specific absorption rate (SAR) to an individual tumor case. However, for further development of radiofrequency hyperthermia technology, an improvement in planning and phantom techniques is required.

Clinical Considerations

The time-temperature curves of 15 patients (about 70 regional hyperthermia sessions) were analyzed. Temperature (T) measurements inside the tumor were performed in closed-end catheters implanted under computed tomography (CT) guide or fluoroscopy and documented in every case by CT. From the initial slope (after switching on of power) and final slope (after switching off of power) the local SAR value Q is deduced and related to the achieved temperature in the specified point. A diagram of intratumoral (steady-state) temperatures versus local SARs gives a rough classification of tumors in the three categories of easy-to-heat (low perfusion), intermediate, and difficult-to-heat (high effective thermal wash-out) tumors. It turns out that effective heat loss (mainly determined by perfusion) is only one predictor for achievement of therapeutic temperatures $\geq 42°C$ in the tumor. Further information is obtained if the intratumoral T values are correlated with normalized SAR values $q\ (=Q/P)$ and the tolerated power level (P). Clearly, T may be enhanced by increasing q as well as P, which was demonstrated in several patients.

Strahlenklinik und Poliklinik des Klinikum Rudolf Virchow, Freie Universität Berlin, Augustenburger Platz 1, 1000 Berlin 65, FRG
* This work was supported by the Deutsche Krebshilfe, Bonn, FRG (grant M6/90/Fe6).

Advanced Radiation Therapy Tumor Response
Monitoring and Treatment Planning
Breit (Editor-in-Chief)
© Springer-Verlag, Berlin Heidelberg 1992

The normalized SAR q depends mainly on anatomical topography (for example, it is considerably reduced for central tumors in large cross-sections) and is in our experience also biased by the conductivity of the tumor (for example, recurrent rectal cancer tends to have a lower conductivity because it often grows in an extensive preirradiated fibrotic tissue matrix). Treatment parameters such as phases/amplitudes, frequency, and patient positioning in the ring (especially in the direction of patient axis) evidently have some influence on q (Wust et al. 1991a). In fact, our clinical experience shows variations in q during a single heat session (by changing from one standard configuration to the other) as well as for different heat sessions of the same patient, whereby a qualitative correlation between local SAR qP and T for the same tumor became apparent. However, it is unclear at present what improvement is actually possible by patient-specific planning (and optimization) of SAR distribution.

On the other hand, T or Q is also determined by the total power (P) which is tolerated by the patient. A large range of applied power levels were seen clinically, which can even compensate for a low q in cases of unfavorable anatomy. Power levels above 1000 W (with the BSD-2000) entail an additional risk of tissue damage and should be administered with great care. Concerning the most frequent power range of 500–1000 W, the level is often (> 50%) limited by local discomfort of the patient at several sites, sometimes evidently outside the central treatment area and closer to the applicator edge. These power-limiting pain sensations may be caused by electrical phenomena at tissue interfaces, possibly to reduce or even circumvent by controlled manipulation of power deposition patterns.

In conclusion, both strategies of enhancing Q in the tumor (via q or P) ultimately require three-dimensional calculations of E fields for realistic treatment situations.

Numerical Methods

Several methods have been used for E field calculations regarding hyperthermia problems: those of finite difference time domain (FDTD; Sullivan 1990), finite integration theory (FIT; Weiland 1984, 1986), volume surface integral equation (VSIE; Wust et al. 1991b), finite element (FE), and hybrid methods (Paulsen et al. 1988). For further information see Paulsen 1990.

Nowadays, difference methods are favored for three-dimensional calculation of E fields in large inhomogeneous domains mainly because of their efficiency with regard to the calculation time and storage need, which results from sparse matrix algebra. Two finite-difference codes exist: the FIT code (T. Weiland, Technische Hochschule Darmstadt, FRG) and the FDTD code (D. Sullivan, Radiation Oncology, Stanford, USA). A VSIE code has been developed by Nadobny and Wust (Konrad-Zuse-Zentrum, Berlin, FRG), which in the present version is not comparable to finite-difference codes regarding efficiency but deals very carefully with E fields at electrical boundaries, explicitly considering topography of interfaces as well as validity of boundary conditions.

Code Comparison: VSIE Versus FIT. The comparison was performed for a specific test case: a layered cylinder (inner ring lossy medium with $\varepsilon_r = 78$, $\sigma = 0.55$ S/m, outer ring with deionised water $\varepsilon_r = 78$), embedded in air and illumin-ated by a transversely or axially polarized plane wave (90 MHz). This test case is extensively discussed by Wust et al. (1992). Briefly, a satisfactory agreement between the two codes is obtained around the central plane. However, toward the top/bottom of the cylinder, large perpendicular components occur at sharp electrical boundaries, causing increased polarization charges. In such critical regions slightly enhanced E fields are calculated by the VSIE method, which seems to be more adequate by physical reasons. Furthermore, it is probable that discomfort during regional hyperthermia is caused at least occasionally by similar boundary phenomena ("three-dimensional phenomena") and is therefore better predicted by the VSIE method. We note that further improvement in descretization and interpolation at interfaces (specifically at corners and edges) with the FIT code might yield fair agreement even at such steep and sharp boundaries.

Code Comparison: VSIE Versus FDTD. The FDTD method has been verified by Sullivan (1991) in an elliptical phantom (so-called CDRH phantom) of major axis 31 cm, minor axis 21 cm, and a fat equivalent ring of 2 cm thickness. Good agreement was obtained for 70–90 MHz, deviations occur at 100–110 MHz. For further clarification, a simultaneous code comparison and experimental code verification was performed for an elliptical phantom of major axis 37 cm, minor axis 23 cm, $\varepsilon_r = 78$, $\sigma = 0.55$ S/m, and length 50 cm in a SIGMA-60 applicator of 60 cm diameter. In the VSIE method, a cosine current distribution on antennas has been assumed, which has been measured in good approximation by loop antennas via H field (Wust et al. 1991b). In principle, the careful processing of interfaces by the VSIE code enables an inclusion of antennas as metal components into the problem.

A visualization of SAR distributions has been performed by a light-emitting diode (LED) phantom of same dimensions with a thin Lucite wall (3 mm) and an adjustable (in z direction)LED array, filled with salt water of 3 g NaCl/l (according to $\sigma = 0.55$ S/m at room temperature; Schneider and vanDijk 1991; Wust et al. 1990). Not even a qualitative agreement was obtained between calculations of both codes (see Fig. 1) and the LED visualization (Fig. 2, for 80 MHz). The measurements show for lower frequencies of 70–80 MHz a considerable SAR load at lateral sides and a SAR sparing at top and bottom of the phantom. Note that the LED phantom has an extended major axis in comparison to the CDRH phantom. The lateral load decreases for 90 MHz, which seems to be a suitable frequency for this specific phantom, and increases again slightly for 100 MHz. The SAR behavior along the whole frequency range

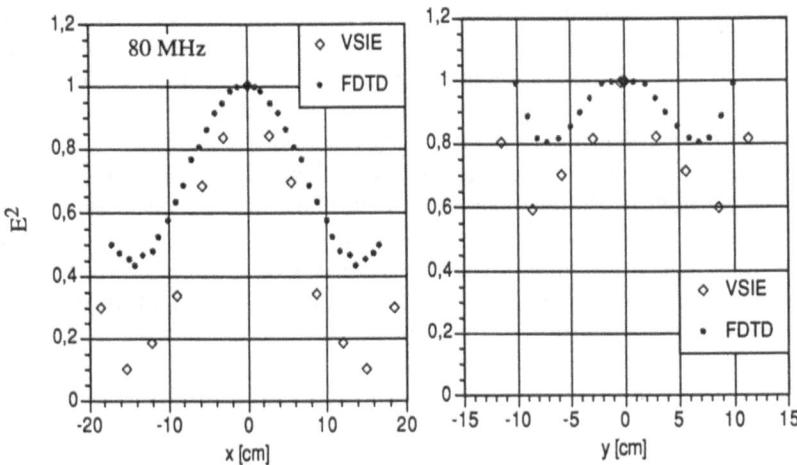

Fig. 1. Comparison of FDTD (*closed symbols*) and VSIE (*open symbols*) for an elliptical phantom at 80 MHz. *Left*, major axis (*X*); *right*, minor axis (*Y*)

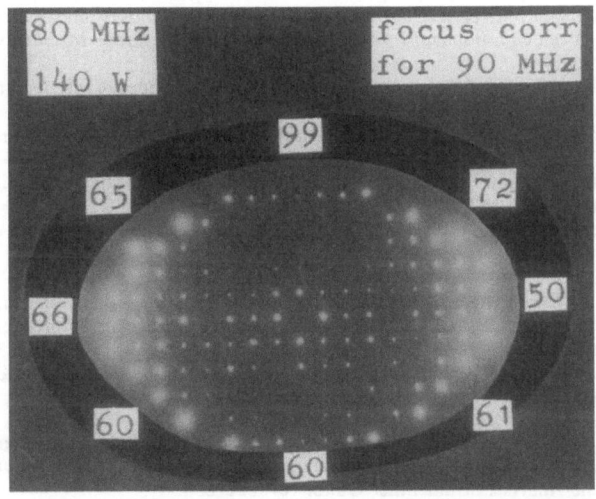

Fig. 2. SAR visualization at 80 MHz by an LED phantom. No qualitative agreement is obtained between calculations (Fig. 1) and measurements

is neither correctly described by the VSIE code (open symbols in Fig. 2, for 80 MHz) nor by the FDTD code, even predicting a qualitatively opposite pattern.

These inconsistencies result, in our opinion, from the fact that a ring applicator acts as a highly resonant cavity with pronounced coupling depending on frequency and lossy medium, especially for symmetric problems (Wust et al. 1991b). These SAR modes arise from reflections at the sharp electrical boundary air/water. A very accurate description of these boundaries as well as inclusion of antenna coupling is demanded for a correct calculation of these modes. The results suggest that both methods in the present implementation might fail for specific test cases, particularly concerning the modeling of sharp electrical boundaries for near field problems in highly resonant geometries.

We note that frequency-dependent SAR phenomena are also accentuated by plastic walls (with low dielectric constant) of common phantoms, either by polarization charges at these walls or by propagation/excitation in the material itself. These questions are under study. Obviously, there is a need for the development of fat-equivalent ($\varepsilon_r = 10\text{--}20$, $\sigma = 0.1$ S/m) phantom materials suitable for the manufacturing of phantom walls.

References

Paulsen KD (1990) Calculation of power deposition patterns in hyperthermia. In: Gautherie M (ed) Thermal dosimetry and treatment planning. Springer, Berlin Heidelberg New York, pp 57–118

Paulsen KD, Lynch DR, Strohbehn JW, (1988) Three-dimensional finite boundary and hybrid element solutions of the Maxwell equations for lossy dielectric media. IEEE Trans Microwave Theory Tech MTT-36: 682–693

Schneider C, van Dijk JDP (1991) Visualization by a matrix of light emitting diodes of interference effects from a radiative four-applicator hyperthermia system. Int J Hyperthermia 7: 355–366

Sullivan DM (1990) Three-dimensional computer simulation in deep regional hyperthermia using the FDTD method. IEEE Trans Microwave Theor Tech MTT-38: 204–211

Sullivan DM (1991) Mathematical methods for treatment planning in deep regional hyperthermia. IEEE Trans Microwave Theor Tech MTT-39: 864–872

Weiland T (1984) On the numerical solution of Maxwell's equations and applications in the field of accelerator physics. Particle Accelerators 15: 245–292

Weiland T (1986) Die Diskretisierung der Maxwell-Gleichungen. Phys Blätter 42: 191–201

Wust P, Nadobny J, Fähling H, Riess H, Koch K, John W, Felix R (1990) Einflußfaktoren und Störeffekte bei der Steuerung von Leistungsverteilungen mit dem Hyperthermie-Ringsystem BSD-2000. I. Klinische Observablen und Phantommessungen. Strahlenther Onkol 166: 822–830

Wust P, Nadobny J, Felix R, Deuflhard P, Louis A, John W (1991a) Strategies for optimized application of annular-phased-array systems in clinical hyperthermia. Int J Hyperthermia 7: 157–173

Wust P, Nadobny J, Fähling H, Riess H, Koch K, John W, Felix R (1991b) Einflußfaktoren und Störeffekte bei der Steuerung von Leistungsverteilungen mit dem Hyperthermie-Ringsystem BSD-2000. II. Meßtechnische Analyse. Strahlenther Onkol 167: 822–830

Wust P, Nadobny J, Seebass M, Dohlus M, John W, Felix R (1992) 3D-computation of E-fields by the volume-surface integral equation (VSIE) method in comparison to the finite-integration theory (FIT) method. IEEE Trans Biomed Eng (to be published)

Part 3

**Advances in Neutron Theory
(Contributions of the EORTC
Heavy Particle Therapy Group)**

Can Relative Biological Effectiveness be Used for Treatment Planning in Boron Neutron Capture Therapy?

R.A. Gahbauer[1], R.G. Fairchild[2], J.H. Goodman[3], and T.E. Blue[4]

Introduction

Single-dose relative biological effectiveness (RBE) values have been determined for the radiations encountered in boron neutron capture therapy (BNCT) [6] and can provide useful guidance for the tolerance to be expected. The difficulty of microdosimetric determination of dose [5], the rapidly varying mix of constituent high- and low-LET radiations with depth, the possible synergistic interaction between high- and low-LET radiations [8], and the strong dependence of biological efficacy on the distribution of boron within the cell are all factors limiting the usefulness of RBEs. Large animal studies are necessary to determine late-effect tolerance. To design, interpret, compare, and apply these studies to clinical use, it may be more practical to divide factors influencing RBE in to two groups: (a) estimated tolerance dose (ETD), which can be inferred from other experience reasonably well; and (b) compound factor (CF), which is much more variable as a function of microdosimetry and boron compound.

We therefore attempted to derive tolerance restrictions from known clinical information about tolerance to high- and low-LET radiations. These are somewhat imprecise, but their numerical uncertainty is small compared to the numerical variation of the compound factor. They can further be verified or adjusted as shown below.

Materials and Methods

Determination of Estimated Tolerance Dose. For reasons discussed extensively elsewhere [2], we anticipate that BNCT with epithermal beams will be used with

[1] Division of Radiation Oncology, Ohio State University, Arthur James Cancer Hospital, 300 W 10th Ave, Columbus, OH 43210, USA
[2] Medical Department, Brookhaven National Laboratory, Upton, Long Island, New York 11973, USA
[3] Division of Neurosurgery, Ohio State University, Arthur James Cancer Hospital, 300 W 10th Ave, Columbus, OH 43210, USA
[4] Division of Nuclear Engineering, Ohio State University, Arthur James Cancer Hospital, 300 W 10th Ave, Columbus, OH 43210, USA

Advanced Radiation Therapy Tumor Response
Monitoring and Treatment Planning
Breit (Editor-in-Chief)
© Springer-Verlag, Berlin Heidelberg 1992

a fractionation scheme employing a minimum of four fractions. Therefore, our first objective is to establish the tolerance of normal brain to four fractions of low-LET radiation. Pezner and Archambeau have used a modified version of Ellis' NSD formula to more realistically reflect brain tolerance [9]. To demonstrate the principle, we use this simple formula, although other formulas can be used:

$$TD = BTU \times N^k \times T^l \tag{1}$$

where BTU = brain tolerance unit, N = number of fractions, T = time in days, $k = 0.45$, $l = 0.03$, and TD = tumor dose. In our discussion, we evaluate the formula for four fractions and a treatment time of 5 days, using a BTU of 1200, which would reflect the upper limit of acceptable risk to normal tissue. Evaluation of this formula suggests a maximum tolerated low-LET dose of 2300 cGy in four fractions in 5 days.

Our second objective, to estimate the tolerance of normal brain to high-LET radiations if only high-LET radiations were used, is more difficult because the experience is more limited, and because varying fractionations and beams with different RBEs have been used. The influence of fractionation on isoeffect is minimal if more than four fractions are used [4]. From clinical information drawn from instances in which more than four fractions were used, we may infer that the tolerance of normal CNS is less than 1000 cGy of high-LET radiations [1, 7]. We apply this limit to any fractionation scheme with more than four fractions of only high-LET radiation. Using the two restrictions given above, the following formula represents the ETD:

$$ETD = D_\gamma + D_h \times 2.3 = 2300 \tag{2}$$

Here D_γ = total dose in cGy for low-LET components, and D_h = total high-LET or particle dose, including components from the $^{14}N(n, p)^{14}C$ and $^{10}B(n, \alpha)^7Li$ reactions and fast-neutron dose. The factor 2.3 [2.3 = TD/1000] is a factor chosen to restrict normal tissue dose to levels of high-LET radiations found acceptable in fast-neutron therapy and can be viewed as taking the function of an RBE. In other words, in this case the estimated tolerance of normal tissue was used to determine RBEs rather than the reverse. The measured single-dose RBE of fast neutrons encountered in BNCT, as well as from the $^{14}N(n, p)^{14}C$ reaction, is around 2, while that from the $^{10}B(n, \alpha)^7Li$ reaction was found to be 2.3 [3, 6]. Increasing the number of fractions would effectively increase our factor (just as RBEs would) as the ETD increases (for 25 fractions ETD = 5600; $5600 = D_\gamma + D_h \times 5.6$). (From Eqs. 1 and 2: the factor 5.6 limits D_h to 1000 cGy, as the RBE would). The ETD (Eq. 2) should be calculated for several depths, at minimum: surface, 3 cm, midline, and blood at 3 cm (divided by protection factor). The treatment time required to reach the ETD at the "hottest" depth becomes the limiting time.

Determination of Compound Factor. In large animal, normal tissue studies, it is then possible to derive the CF with two sets of experiments (dose escalation studies) comparing the same normal tissue endpoints expressed as a function of ETD. The first is in animals treated without boron:

$$D_{1\gamma} + (D_{1N} + D_{1H}) \cdot 2.3 = ETD \tag{3}$$

This experiment also serves to verify or adjust ETD. The second is in animals treated with boron (only one boron tissue level needed):

$$D_{2\gamma} + (D_{2N} + D_{2H} + CF \cdot D_B) \cdot 2.3 = ETD \tag{4}$$

It then follows:

$$D_{1\gamma} + (D_{1N} + D_{1H}) \cdot 2.3 = D_{2\gamma} + (D_{2N} + D_{2H}) \cdot 2.3 + CF \cdot D_B \cdot 2.3 \tag{5}$$

$$CF = \frac{D_{1\gamma} - D_{2\gamma}}{D_B \cdot 2.3} + \frac{D_{1N} + D_{1H} - D_{2N} - D_{2H}}{D_B} \tag{6}$$

where D_N = dose from N(n, p)C, D_H = fast-neutron dose, and D_B = dose from B(n, γ)Li.

Discussion

The biological efficacy of boron is known to be a strong function of intracellular distribution, which is generally unknown or imprecisely known for the compounds being investigated for possible use in BNCT. Problems associated with the definition of dose and the use of RBE in BNCT are discussed elsewhere [5]. To account for unknowns inherent to BNCT, Gabel has proposed a compound factor.

Our formula attempts to relate known information on tolerance to the experiment in BNCT and derives the value of CF with only two sets of experiments. This factor is unique to a given boron compound and epithermal beam combination. For compound development, ETD may help to estimate the therapeutic range. It sets a target range for dose escalation studies, which then will define its value more precisely, as proposed above. The approach outlined should allow the determination of the compound factor with only two sets of experiments, using only one boron tissue level. If the compound factor is not determined, experiments at one boron level would not predict tolerance at another.

References

1. Catterall M, Bloom HJG, Ash DV, Walsh L, Richardson A, Uttley D, Gowing NFC, Lewis P, Chaucer B (1980) Fast neutrons compared with megavoltage X-rays in the treatment of patients with supratentorial glioblastoma: a controlled pilot study, Int J Radiat Oncol Biol Phys 6: 261–266

2. Fairchild R, Bond V, Woodhead A (1989) Clinical aspects of neutron capture therapy. Proceedings of the workshop on boron neutron capture therapy, 1–2 Feb, 1988, Brookhaven National Laboratory, Upton, NY. Plenum Press, New York
3. Fairchild R, Kalef-Ezra J, Saraf S, et al. (1989) Installation and testing of an optimized epithermal neutron beam at the Brookhaven Medical Research Reactor. Proceedings of the workshop on neutron beam design, development, and performance for neutron capture therapy. Massachusetts Institute of Technology, Cambridge
4. Fowler JF (1981) Nuclear particles in cancer treatment. Hilger, Bristol
5. Gabel D, Foster S, Fairchild RG (1987) The Monte Carlo simulation of the biological effect of the ^{10}B (n, α)^{7}Li reaction in cells and tissue and its implication for boron neutron capture therapy. Radiat Res 111: 14–25
6. Gabel D, Fairchild RG, Larsson B, Börner HG (1984) The relative biological effectiveness in V79 Chinese hamster cells of the neutron capture reactions in boron and nitrogen. Radiat Res 98: 307–316
7. Laramore GE, Diener-West M, Griffin TW, Nelson JS, Griem ML, Thomas FJ, Hendrickson FR, Griffen BR, Myrianthopoulos LC, Saxton J (1988) Randomized neutron dose searching study for malignant gliomas of the brain: results of an RTOG study. Int J Radiat Oncol Biol Phys 14: 1093–1102
8. Ngo FQ, Blakely EA, Tobias CA (1981) Sequential exposures of mammalian cells to low- and high-LET radiations. I. Lethal effects following X-ray and neon-ion irradiation. Radiat Res 87(1): 59–78
9. Pezner R, Archambeau J (1981) Brain tolerance unit: a method to estimate risk of radiation brain injury for various dose schedules. Br J Radiat Oncol Biol Phys 7: 397–402

Side Effects of High-Dose Radiation Therapy of Soft-Tissue Sarcoma with 14 MeV DT Neutrons: A Correlation to Irradiated Volume

J. Romahn[1], R. Engenhart[1], B. Hesse[2], G. Gademann[1], K.H. Höver[2], and M. Wannenmacher[1]

Introduction

Soft-tissue sarcomas (STS) are a highly heterogeneous group of malignant tumors of mesodermal origin with some contribution from neuroectoderm. STS are classified on a histogenetic basis according to the adult tissue which they resemble, and the tumors are capable of invasive or destructive growth as well as recurrence and distant metastasis. These tumors may occur anywhere in the body, but the majority arise from the large muscles of the extremities [3]. The most important consideration in determining the patient's prognosis and the treatment strategy is the histological grading [1, 2]. To gain local control a radical surgery is necessary [1, 6, 11, 13], but achievement of safe margins is often limited. Radiotherapy is a potent and well-accepted treatment modality. Even in those patients in whom surgical treatment was not possible, a response of the tumor and significant local control rate following high-dose irradiation has been reported [5]. Radiobiology gave reasons for the use of fast neutrons in STS. Several authors have reported superior results of neutron therapy, compared to photon therapy, especially in those patients with low-grade STS [4, 6, 7, 9–12].

Because of these encouraging results, we stated exclusive neutron therapy to try to improve local control rate. The resulting side effects gave reason for investigating treatment volumes as a possible cause of these effects.

Material and Methods

Since September 1988 we have treated 20 patients suffering from STS solely with fast neutrons, delivered by the 14 MeV DT generator at the German Cancer Research Centre in Heidelberg. The mean maximum neutron dose was 19.06

[1] Department of Radiotherapy, University Clinic for Radiology, University of Heidelberg, Im Neuenheimer Feld 400, 6900 Heidelberg, FRG
[2] Department of Radiology and Pathophysiology, German Cancer Research Center, Im Neuenheimer Feld 280, 6900 Heidelberg, FRG

Advanced Radiation Therapy Tumor Response
Monitoring and Treatment Planning
Breit (Editor-in-Chief)
© Springer-Verlag, Berlin Heidelberg 1992

Gy, ranging from 15 to 20 Gy. The mean tumor-encompassing dose was 15.03 Gy (10–16.27 Gy). The distribution of the administered doses is demonstrated by Fig. 1.

In 17/20 patients the tumor was located in the lower extremity (including groin and buttock). One patient had STS of the neck, and in another patient the tumor was located in the shoulder. One patient was suffering from a sarcoma of the chest wall. All but one patient underwent one or more surgical interventions prior to radiotherapy. Six patients had a complete resection of the tumor (R0) and six a macroscopic complete resection but without histological safe margins (R1). In seven patients a complete resection was not possible, and the patients had been referred to radiotherapy with residual tumor tissue (R2). One patient with a fibrous histiocytoma did not receive a regular tumor resection, as his surgical intervention could be described only as extended biopsy. This patient underwent a regular and complete tumor resection after radiotherapy.

The radiation was delivered via opposed fields in seven patients. In six we used a single port for irradiation of superficial tumor locations. Four patients were treated with moving arc therapy, and in three we had to use more than two fields to obtain a satisfying dose distribution. The moving arc therapy and the three-field arrangements were used for treating eccentric tumors of the buttock and groin. Because of tumor extensions and the limited field sizes of our neutron facility, in nine cases we had to link two ports with a safety margin of 0.5 cm to gain the necessary field lengths.

Using the dose distributions of our treatment plans we calculated the irradiated volumes by planimetry of the areas included by the 50% isodoses. These had been multiplied with the used field lengths. The results were correlated with the rate of radiation-induced complications. Side effects were classified according to the EORTC/RTOG scoring system.

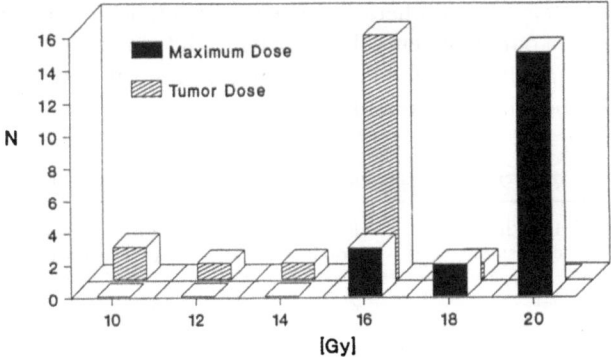

Fig. 1. Distribution of administered single neutron doses

Results

Up to now the mean length follow-up of our series is 16 months, ranging from 5.8 to 31 months. Four of our patients died. Two were locally controlled at time of death; they died because of a progression of lung metastasis. Another patient showed both local and general progression. The fourth patient died because of a small-bowel perforation 5 months after radiotherapy.

In four patients it was not possible to achieve local control. These patients belonged to the R2 group (macroscopic tumor residual after surgery). A deep ulceration in the groin led to a high amputation in one patient, with no clinical evidence of local tumor progress. Pathologists found viable tumor tissue in the former tumor bed after amputation. This patient is still surviving free of tumor. The second patient, suffering from a gross residual tumor mass with signs of a high proliferation rate (GIII), developed the first recurrence 5 months after radiotherapy at the superior border of the irradiated volume. He was treated for a second time but unfortunately developed another recurrence inside the treatment volume. He refused amputation and is surviving now with the local recurrent tumor after 4 months. One patient died of progressive lung metastasis, but her local tumor also showed progress at that time. This patient, with primary tumor location in the neck, developed a cutaneous tumor near but outside the treatment volume. We could not distinguish whether it was a cutaneous metastasis or a local recurrence, but it gave reason for a second irradiation 6 months after first radiotherapy. She has now been controlled locally for 13 months. Three of the four recurrences developed in those patient with length extention by linked fields (Table 1). Four patients developed lung metastasis after treatment; three of them have already died. In one case the metastasis was confirmed prior to radiotherapy. A slow progression was detectable under chemotherapy in this patient, and because of his excellent general constitution a resection of all lung metastases was carried out. The patient has now survived for 15 months free of local recurrence.

Mild to minor side effects of radiotherapy such as subcutaneous fibrosis (grade I/II) were seen in 12 of our 20 patients. These patients did not complain of a significant alteration in quality of life. Two of our patients suffered from stiffness of muscles and subcutaneous tissue. Pain, with maximum 3–6 months

Table 1. Irradiation techniques: recurrences by technique (with and without length extention)

Technique	n	Length extension	Recurrence (total)	Recurrence (in extended field)
Single field	6	2	2	1
Opposed field	7	5	1	1
Moving arc	4	2	1	1
Three field	3	–	–	–

after radiotherapy, was tolerable and showed a good response to mild analgetics. We classified these effects as grade III. We saw six patients with severe
problems, five of them grade IV. Two patients developed severe fibrosis that led
to peripheral neurological symptoms (paralysis of the ischiadic and peroneal
nerves). Both patients underwent neurolysis. One of them had an acute inflammation of the peripheral nerve, exactly that distance lying inside the treatment
volume (confirmed at surgery). These complications were seen 12 and 13 months
after radiotherapy. Two patients developed ulceration of the skin and the
subcutaneous tissue. In both cases the ulceration was combined with local
tumor progression. One ulceration led to the high amputation described above.
Another irradiated skin reaction was seen on the shin of a further patient. This
superficial ulcer originated from a minor traumatic skin lesion and did not show
involvement of subcutaneous tissue. The patient was tumor free, and the ulcer
was treated by dermatoplastic surgery. One patient died of a severe complication. She was suffering with a GIII sarcoma of the buttock. After surgery she had
a prolonged wound heeling and developed a small fistula. Twenty years prior to
the STS she had been treated by hysterectomy and postsurgical irradiation in
Romania for a gynecological carcinoma. We irradiated the tumor bed with a
total dose of 20 Gy(max). Skin did not show any acute reaction; the previously
mentioned fistula healed under therapy. Four months after completion of our
treatment she was admitted to a local hospital with signs of an acute intestine. In
laparotomy the surgeon found a perforation and an inflammatory disease of the
small bowel next to the pelvic wall. The patient died 1 month later of the
complications. We regard this as a grade V side effect. It is important to mention
that three of these six patients, especially the two with subcutaneous necrosis,
had a remarkably prolonged and secondary wound healing after surgery. In
ultrasound examinations during the whole follow-up persistent seroma were
demonstrable (Table 2). Retrospectively we calculated the irradiated volume and
found that volumes included by the 50% isodose ranged from 530 to 6000 cm^3.
The medium irradiated volume was 2500 cm^3. In contrast, we found a medium

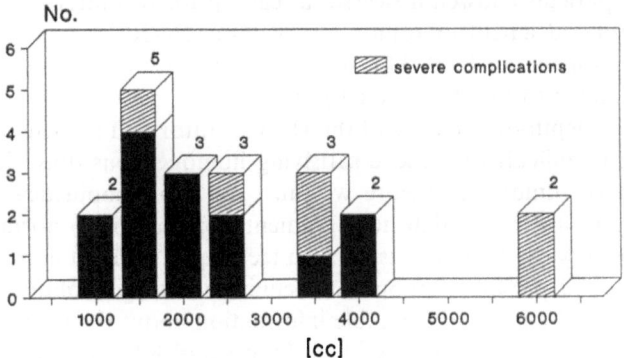

Fig. 2. Effect of increased irradiated volume on the number of severe side effects

Table 2. Severe complication group: list of side effect and the irradiated volumes

Patient	Localization of Side Effects	Delay (months)	Volume (cm³)	$D_{(max)}$ (Gy)	Recurrence	Fistula (before radiation)
A	Small bowel	6	1400	20	–	+
B	Skin	6.4	2300	16	–	–
C	Subcutaneous necrosis	7.7	3300	20	+	+
D	Peripheral nerve	12	6000	18	–	–
E	Peripheral nerve	13.3	3500	20	–	–
F	Subcutaneous necrosis	14.3	6000	20	+	+

irradiated volume of 3750 cm³ (1400–6000) in those six patients showing severe side effects. The distribution is demonstrated by Fig. 2.

Discussion

The incidence of six severe complications in 20 treated patients is high enough to discuss whether the high neutron dose, the large irradiated volume, or the prolonged wound heeling was responsible. As known from the literature [7, 8], irradiated volume has a direct influence on the number of severe side effects. This seems to be a special problem in neutron therapy, because of the higher relative biological effectiveness (RBE) in small fraction sizes. The RBE compares the isoeffect dose of neutrons and ^{60}Co gamma-rays. Because of the typical shape of the survival curves of low-LET radiation RBE increases with smaller fraction sizes. The biological effect at the 50% isodose of photons could be quite different to that of neutrons. This was the reason that we chose irradiated volume as a parameter and not target volume.

We have demonstrated that all the above-mentioned factors are represented in the complication group of our patients. The irradiated volume was larger in this group, and three patients showed abscesses already prior to radiotherapy (Table 2). On the other hand, a neutron tumor dose of about 16–20 Gy is needed to control residual tumor mass [4, 10, 11]. All of our patients who were not locally controlled belonged to the R2 resected group.

Because of the poor depth-dose curves of the DT generator and low-energy cyclotron neutrons it is difficult to achieve satisfying homogeneous dose distributions in these large tumors. Therefore we must use more sophisticated irradiation techniques to achieve a high dose gradient from tumor to normal tissue. But we must be very careful when using such techniques and not enlarge the irradiated volume. This presumes an optimal definition of target volume to avoid local underdosage. We need all available information about the primary tumor location and the location of tumor residuals (in cases of R2 resection). As long as patients are admitted to radiotherapy with a local excision of a large T2

STS without further information, we shall have to use large field sizes, and as long as we have large irradiated volumes. Even a shrinking-field technique is not possible under these conditions without the risk of a local recurrence.

Patients with local infection and secondary heeling should, in our opinion, be excluded from sole neutron therapy. Under the conditions of regular tumor surgery, with an exchange of information among the involved disciplines, and with a careful treatment planning (i.e., moulage, multiple beam irradiation, etc.) it should be possible to prevent severe side effects in radiation treatment of STS with fast neutrons.

References

1. Budach V, Dinges S, Bamberg M, Baumhoer W, Donhuijsen K, Sack H (1990) Neutron boost irradiation of soft tissue sarcomas and chondrosarcomas at the West German Tumor Centre in Essen. Strahlenther Onkol 166: 63–68
2. Costa J, Wesley RA, Glatstein E et al. (1984) The grading of soft tissue sarcomas. Cancer 53: 530–541
3. Enzinger FM, Weiss SW (eds) (1988) Soft tissue tumors, 2nd edn. Mosby, St Louis
4. Laramore GE, Griffeth JT, Boespflug M et al. (1989) Fast neutron therapy for sarcomas of soft tissue bone and cartilage. Am J Clin Oncol 12: 320–326
5. McNeer GP, Cantin J, Chu F et al. (1968) Effectiveness of radiation therapy in the management of sarcomas of the soft somatic tissues. Cancer 22: 391–397
6. Pickering DG, Stewart JS, Rampling R, Errington RD, Stamp G, Chia Y (1987) Fast neutron therapy for soft tissue sarcoma. Int J Radiat Oncol Biol Phys 13: 1489–1495
7. Richard F, Renard L, Wambersie A (1986) Current results of neutron therapy at the UCL, for soft tissue sarcomas and prostatic adenocarcinomas. Bull Cancer 73: 562–568
8. Richard F, Renard L, Wambersie A (1989) Neutron therapy of soft tissue sarcoma at Louvain la Neuve (interim results 1987). Strahlenther Onkol 165: 306–308
9. Romahn J, Engenhart R, Kimmig B, Höver KH, Wannenmacher M (1990) Results of combined photon-neutron-radiotherapy for soft tissue sarcomas. Proceedings of the 2nd European Particle Accelerator Conference, vol 2, pp 53–55
10. Schmitt G, Mills EED, Levin V, Pape H, Smit BL, Zamboglou N (1989) The role of neutrons in the treatment of soft tissue sarcomas. Cancer 64: 2064–2068
11. Schmitt G, Pape H, Zamboglou N (1990) Long term results of neutron- and neutron boost irradiation of soft tissue sarcomas. Strahlenther Onkol 166: 61–62
12. Schwarz R, Krüll A, Schmidt R, Hübener KH (1990) Status report of fast neutron therapy in the department of radiotherapy at the University Hospital Hamburg-Eppendorf. Strahlenther Onkol 166: 72–75
13. Simson MA, Enneking WF (1976) The management of soft tissue sarcomas of the extremities. J Bone Joint Surg 58A: 317–327

Assessment of Tumor Remission Based on Imaging Data (One-, Two-, Three-Dimensional) in Adenoid-Cystic Carcinoma of the Minor Salivary Glands After Neutron Radiotherapy

R. Pötter, G. Kovacs, U. Haverkamp, and I. Loncar

Introduction

In the treatment of salivary gland tumors, in particular adenoid-cystic carcinoma, neutron radiotherapy has been regarded as superior to photon radiotherapy for more than a decade (Catterall and Errington 1987; Griffin et al. 1988b; Henry et al. 1979; Kovacs et al. 1987; Saroja et al. 1987). Nevertheless, sufficient data on tumor control and survival in a considerable number of patients (after a median follow-up period exceeding 5 years) on the effect of histology, stage, tumor size, location, surgical procedure, and radiation dose have not been presented yet. The reported locoregional tumor response rates are based mainly on clinical observations and reveal a high degree of complete remission: 78% (Battermann and Mijnheer 1986), 93% (Catterall and Errington 1987), 73% (Duncan et al. 1987), 85% (Griffin et al. 1988b), 94% (Griffin et al. 1988a), and 79% (Saroja et al. 1987). These complete remissions are followed by only few local recurrences, which results in local control rates slightly inferior to the degree of primarily achieved remission: 66% (78%), 77% (93%), 55% (73%), 67% (85%), 81% (94%), and 63% (79%). Yet, the reported follow-up period is still short (mean 2–3 years). Especially in major and minor salivary gland tumors with deep infiltration and with tumor spread difficult for clinical assessment, the extent of disease as well as the pattern and duration of remission can nowadays be evaluated precisely on the basis of computed tomography (CT) and magnetic resonance imaging (MRI).

As one of the main endpoints in evaluating any treatment in salivary gland tumors is local control, the method of evaluating and reporting the extent of disease, the rate of remission, and the duration of remission must be carefully taken into account. To evaluate the efficacy of neutron radiotherapy in adenoid-cystic carcinoma of the salivary glands, tumor volumes were measured before and after neutron radiotherapy according to their delineation on CT or MRI.

Klinik für Strahlentherapie, Radioonkologie, Westfälische Wilhelms-Universität Münster, Albert-Schweitzer Str. 33, 4400 Münster, FRG

Advanced Radiation Therapy Tumor Response
Monitoring and Treatment Planning
Breit (Editor-in-Chief)
© Springer-Verlag, Berlin Heidelberg 1992

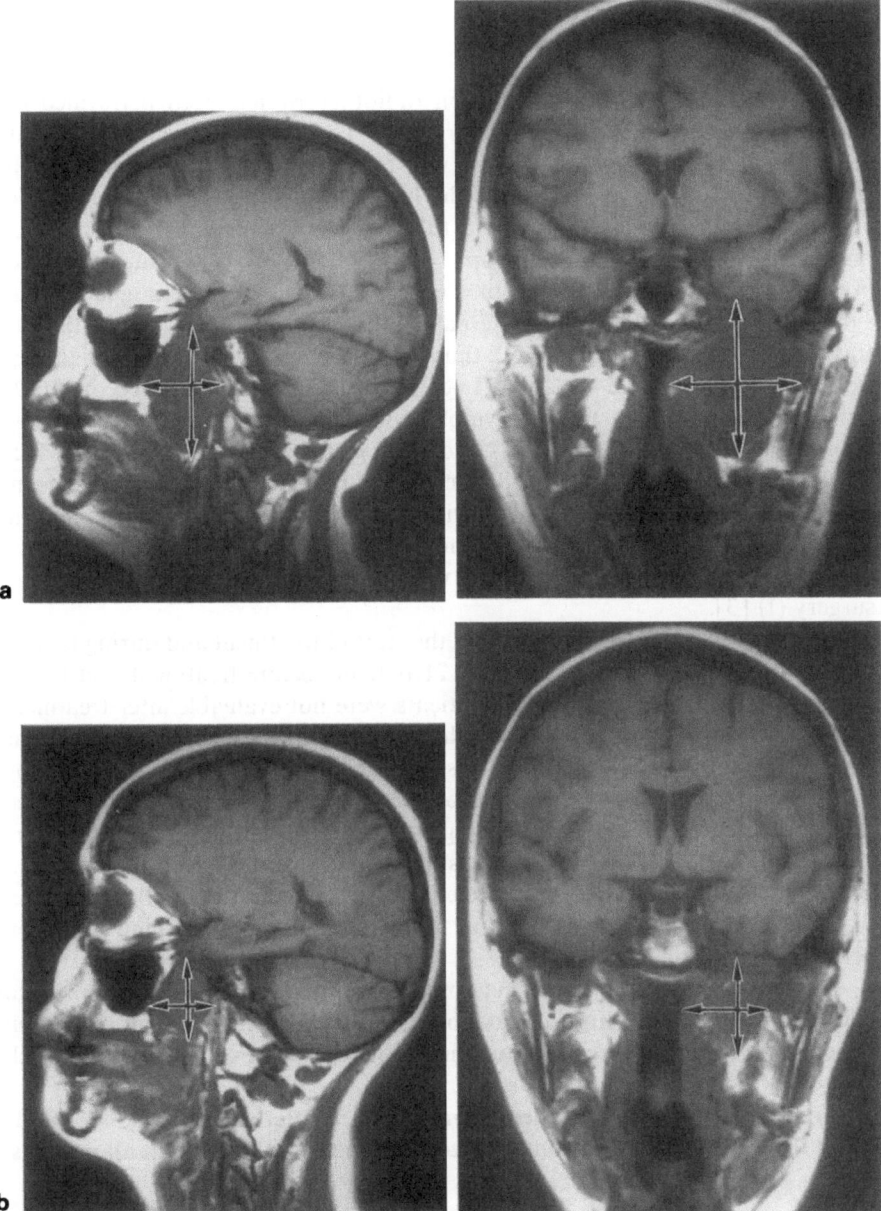

Fig. 1a, b. Inoperable recurrent adenoid-cystic carcinoma in the left fossa infratemporalis in a 51-year-old woman with severe pain. Sagittal and coronal MRI (T1) with measurements of tumor extension before and after treatment in the craniocaudal (CC), anteroposterior (AP), and laterolateral (LL) directions (see Figs. 1, 2 in Pötter et al. 1990). **a** Before neutron radiotherapy: 5.0 cm (CC) × 3.3 cm (AP) × 4.0 cm (LL) (66.0 cm^3). **b** Six months after neutron radiotherapy (15 Gy); complete remission of pain. Considerable tumor shrinkage with residual tissue: 3.2 cm (CC) × 2.2 cm (AP) × 2.3 cm (LL) (16.2 cm^3). Amount of remission by the different assessment methods (see Table 1) is as follows. One-dimensional: 1.8/5.0 cm (CC), 36%; 1.1/3.3 cm (AP), 33%;

Materials and Methods

At the University of Münster neutron radiotherapy has been performed for adenoid-cystic carcinoma since January 1986. To date we have had 27 patients (17 women, 10 men); the mean age was 54 years (19–81). All tumors were confirmed by biopsy. In 20 patients the histological subtype could be defined: solid ($n = 7$), cribriform ($n = 7$), and tubular ($n = 6$). Typical locations when presenting for neutron radiotherapy were the following: paranasal sinuses ($n = 11$), parapharyngeal space ($n = 6$; Fig. 1), base of the tongue ($n = 2$), submandibular gland ($n = 4$), external auditory canal ($n = 1$), orbit ($n = 1$), trachea ($n = 1$), intracanial ($n = 1$); thus the vast majority of tumors originated from the minor salivary glands. Localized disease was observed in 16/27 patients (59%); 5/27 patients had lymph node metastases alone (19%), 8/27 had lung metastases alone (30%), 2/27 had bone metastases alone (7%), and 4/27 had combined metastases (15%). There were 17 patients irradiated for recurrent tumors (numbers in parentheses), 10 within their primary treatment (numbers in square brackets): 9 with inoperable tumors (7) [2], 14 with macroscopic residual disease after surgery (9) [5], and 4 with microscopic residual disease after surgery (1) [3].

All patients had CT or MRI before the start of treatment and during follow-up. Tumor volume was evaluable for 21 patients before treatment and for 16 after treatment (3–9 months). Five patients were not evaluable after treatment because of just having finished it. The tumor volume was measured in the transverse, coronal, and sagittal planes (perpendicular to each other) by taking the longest diameter in each plane on the image of interest (Fig. 1). When multiplying the diameters for assessing the area and volume, corrections were carried out for an approximate adjustment to the geometrical shape if considerable deviations were to be expected. After treatment the smallest diameter that had been achieved was taken in those cases in which imaging had been performed more than once.

Target volume encompassed macroscopic tumor and the region of potential microscopic spread (see Figs. 2, 3 in Kovacs et al., this volume). Regional lymph nodes were irradiated in cases of confirmed involvement or assumed high risk for involvement.

Treatment planning included fluoroscopic simulation and CT- or MRI-based dose calculations by computerized isodose computations in all patients.

(**Fig. 1a, b.** Continued)
1.7/4.0 cm (LL), 43%. Two-dimensional: 9.5/16.5 cm², (CC × AP), 58%; 12.6/20.0 cm² (CC × LL), 63%; 8.1/13.2 cm³ (AP × LL), 61%. Three-dimensional: 49.8/66.0 cm³, (CC × AP × LL), 75%. Based on the identical set of data in this one patient a 42% difference in remission may be reported depending on method of evaluation used (remission evaluation bias). A report based on one-dimensional measurment would claim no change, on two-dimensional measurement partial remission, and on three-dimensional measurment uncertain complete remission

One treatment field was used in 4 patients, two opposed fields in 11, three fields in 7, and four to six fields in 5. In seven patients a specific positioning device and individual shielding for critical structures with standard transmission blocks were used based on beam's eye view imaging from MRI (Kovacs et al., this volume). Bolus material was taken in patients treated for submandibular tumors.

Total dose was 15 Gy at the ICRU point (1989) in 17 patients, 10 Gy in 3 (previous irradiation), and 6–10 Gy in 7 treated with combined modality (40–50 Gy photons) at the start of neutron treatment at the Münster neutron facility (Pötter et al. 1990). The single dose was 1.67 Gy ($n = 20$) and 0.7–1.3 Gy ($n = 7$). The overall treatment time was 3 weeks ($n = 18$), 2 weeks ($n = 2$), and 6–7 weeks ($n = 7$) in combined modality treatment.

Results

The mean tumor diameter before and after neutron therapy in the craniocaudal (CC) direction was 5.7 cm (range 2–8.5 cm) and 3.3 cm (1–5 cm), in the antero-posterior (AP) direction 3.4 cm (1.5–6 cm) and 2.0 cm (1–4 cm), and in the laterolateral (LL) direction 4.6 cm (2–7 cm) and 2.6 cm (1–4 cm), meaning a mean reduction based on these one-dimensional measurements of 42%, 40%, and 44%, respectively. For the area (two-dimensional) the mean reduction in the sagittal, coronal, and transverse projection was 62%, 64%, and 68%, respectively. For the volume (three-dimensional) the mean reduction was 80% (Table 1).

Taking complete remission in its classical WHO definition (disappearance of all known disease; Miller et al. 1981), no complete remission was achieved in the 16 patients with measurable disease before therapy. The mean amount of remission based on one-dimension imaging data (diameter) was 43% (CC, 25%–53%; AP, 17%–67%; LL, 25%–80%), based on two-dimensional imaging data (area) 65% (AP × CC, 38%–83%; LL × CC, 44%–90%; AP × LL, 50%–83%), based on three-dimensional imaging data (volume) 80% (59%–95%) (Table 1, Fig. 1).

Taking the widely accepted WHO criteria for the assessment of remission (Miller et al. 1981), there was a wide range of remission rates, depending on the method of evaluation (Table 2, Fig. 1). Based on one-dimensional measurements no change (or minor change) was found in 50%–63% of cases, whereas based on two-dimensional measurements there was only one case showing no change, and none was seen when relying one three-dimensional measurements. Partial remission increased with the dimensions measured, ranging from 37% to 50% based on one-dimensional measurements up to 100% based on both two- and three-dimensional measurements, in terms of the WHO remission criterion. No complete remission according to the WHO criterion was observed regardless of the method of evaluation (number of dimensions). Introducing the category of

Table 1. What does remission mean? One-, two-, and three-dimensional measurements (means; CT/MRI) in adenoid-cystic carcinomas before and after neutron radiotherapy ($n = 16$)

One-dimensional	CC	AP	LL
Diameter (mean)			
Before (cm)	5.7	3.4	4.6
After (cm)	3.3	2.0	2.6
Remission (mean)			
Absolute (cm)	2.4/5.7	1.4/3.4	2.0/4.6
Relative[a]	42%	40%	44%
Two-dimensional	CC × AP	CC × LL	AP × LL
Area (mean)			
Before (cm^2)	18	23.8	25.6
After (cm^2)	6.8	8.3	9.0
Remission (mean)			
Absolute (cm^2)	11.2/18	15.5/23.8	16.6/25.6
Relative[a]	62%	64%	68%
Three-dimensional	CC × AP × LL		
Volume (mean)			
Before (cm^3)	98		
After (cm^3)	27		
Remission (mean)			
Absolute (cm^3)	71/98		
Relative[a]	80%		

CC, Craniocaudal; AP, anteroposterior; LL, laterolateral.
[a] The mean relative remission is calculated by summing up every single relative remission divided by the total number; this value is not necessarily identical with that obtained by dividing the mean absolute values.

"uncertain complete remission" for a decrease of 75% or more, the assessment of the amount of remission became more precise by subdividing partial remission (Table 2), but the remission rates nevertheless remained dependent on the method of evaluation: partial remission ($\geq 50\% - < 75\%$) based on one-dimensional measurements changed little (ranging from 25% to 50%), whereas a clear decrease — compared to the 100% based on the WHO definition — was seen based on two- and three-dimensional measurements ranging from 69%–75% (two-dimensional), to 25% (three-dimensional; Table 2). Uncertain complete remission ranged from 6%–13% (one-dimensional), over 19%–31% (two-dimensional) to 75% (three-dimensional; Table 2), compared to no complete remission based on the WHO definition.

Taking minimal detectable residual tissue after therapy (up to 1.6 cm longest tumor diameter) as uncertain complete remission, 6/16 patients (38%) met this criterion. Complete and partial continuous local remission was observed in 21/27 patients (78%) based on three-dimensional evaluation. Regarding the 16 patients with macroscopic disease assessable for tumor volume before and after therapy (Table 2) a continuous local partial remission was achieved in 5/8 (one-dimensional, CC), 1/4 (one-dimensional, AP), and 4/5 (one-dimensional, LL), i.e., overall 10/17 (59%); in 7/11 (two-dimensional, AP × LL), 5/10 (two-dimensional, AP × CC), and 7/12 (two-dimensional, CC × LL), i.e., overall 19/33

Table 2. Remission rate by dimensions of evaluation (CT/MRI) in adenoid-cystic carcinomas after neutron radiotherapy ($n = 16$)

	Complete remission (≥ 75%, uncertain)	Partial remission (≥ 50% to < 75%)	No change (< 50%)
One-dimensional			
CC	–	8/16 (50%)	8/16 (50%)
AP	2/16 (13%)	4/16 (25%)	10/16 (63%)
LL	1/16 (6%)	5/16 (31%)	10/16 (63%)
Two-dimensional			
CC × AP	5/16 (31%)	11/16 (69%)	–
CC × LL	3/16 (19%)	12/16 (75%)	1/16 (6%)
AP × LL	5/16 (31%)	11/16 (69%)	
Three-dimensional			
CC × AP × LL	12/16 (75%)	4/16 (25%)	–

CC, Craniocaudal, AP, anteroposterior; LL, laterolateral.

(58%); and in 3/4 (75%; three-dimensional). Continuous uncertain complete
remission was seen in 3/5 (two-dimensional, AP × LL), 3/4 (two-dimensional,
AP × CC), and 2/3 (two-dimensional, CC × LL), i.e., overall 8/12 (67%); and in
7/12 (58%; three-dimensional). The continuous rate of no change based on one-
dimensional measurements was 5/8 (CC), 7/10 (AP), and 6/10 (LL), i.e., overall
18/28 (64%). Based on imaging tumor regrowth was discovered earlier than
based on clinical observation alone.

Mean follow-up was 14 months, ranging from 2 to 46 months. Of the 27
patients 21 survived (78%). Four patients died from disease and two from other
causes; four patients are alive with disease. Of the eight patients with recurrent
disease six had local relapses: three within the treatment volume, three at the
edge of the treatment volume (compare Fig. 2 in Pötter et al. 1990). Five of these
six patients had presented with a tumor size of more than 4 cm in at least one
diameter and a volume exceeding 59 cm^3. A considerable amount of residual
tissue was seen in 4/6 patients. The location was in the paranasal sinuses and the
parapharyngeal space in 5/6 cases.

Discussion

The overall local control rate of 78% in this study is comparable to that in other
reported data (Battermann and Mijnheer 1986; Catterall and Errington 1987;
Duncan et al. 1987; Griffin et al. 1988a, b; Krüll et al. 1990; Saroja et al. 1987).
This is also the case regarding survival rates. In respect to remission rates a
comparison with other reported data based mainly on clinical observations in
parotid tumors (one-dimensional measurements) is rather difficult, as the rate of

complete remission in our series is small based on the evaluation of CT and MRI data.

The method of assessing tumor extension and in particular tumor response remains rather unclear in the reported series. A precise description of tumor extension based on measurement of the longest tumor diameter in one direction was given in the following series: Duncan et al. (1987; $n = 22$) median 3–5.9 cm; Griffin et al. (1988b; $n = 13$) median 6.0 cm, Griffin et al. (1988a; $n = 32$) median 4–6 cm; Saroja et al. (1987; $n = 113$) median 3–5 cm. These reported tumor extensions are comparable to those in our study ($n = 21$) with a mean of 5.7 cm. The rate of complete remission in macroscopically detectable disease based on one-dimensional measurements in these studies is basically different from that observed in our study: 73%, 85%, 94%, 79% versus 0% taking the classical WHO definition and 13% in the AP direction taking the definition of uncertain complete remission. Only the series reported by Saroja et al. described a considerable number of minor salivary gland tumors: in tumors of the oral cavity and oropharynx, which were smaller, local control was 93% and 60%, while in tumors of the maxillary antrum (all > 6 cm) persistent disease was seen in 7/15 (47%) and local control was 27%. Significant residual tissue (< 75% volume reduction, $> 1.6 \times 1.6 \times 1.6$ cm residual tissue) detectable on CT and MRI follow-up studies and assessed by three-dimensional evaluation was seen in 25% of the patients in our series (comparable patient characteristics). The rather low rate of complete remission in our series may be explained by the precise evaluation based on modern imaging techniques. Nevertheless, residual tissue detectable by CT or MRI remains a critical issue. As is well known, it remains impossible to decide from imaging data between scar and viable tumor cells.

In particular, in the large number of patients with initial partial remission — due perhaps to a long volume-halving time (Bessel and Catterall 1983) — a close follow-up with regular imaging is necessary to assess the course of volume shrinkage or the time of regrowth. Residual tissue may shrink or remain as it was, or tumor may regrow from this tissue and result in a clinically detectable recurrence after a longer observation period. Of course, residual tissue detectable after therapy is only one factor influencing treatment outcome, and many other factors such as histology contribute to the definite results.

It should be noted that remission data from other series are comparable with our findings when taking the reduction in volume of over 75% (uncertain complete remission). The number of partial remissions depends considerably on the method and anatomical direction of evaluation, varying between 25% and 75%. These various remission rates must be evaluated from the main endpoint of ultimate local control. Up to now in our small series no clear correlation can be seen between the initial remission rate and the continuous remission rate, even when taking into consideration the large variety in evaluation methods described above. Nevertheless, the local control rate in our patients with detectable disease was 75% and comparable to the reported series but must be confirmed by longer follow-up. Furthermore, it is interesting to note the correlation between initial and continuous remission.

When evaluating and reporting tumor extension and tumor remission data the way in which these data have been obtained must be considered carefully. Otherwise, when not precisely separating data from one-, two-, and three-dimensional evaluations and different directions (CC, AP, LL) within a given anatomical setting, differences regarding the efficacy of a given treatment of up to more than 50% may be claimed using the same set of data. These differences are based then simply on different topographic conditions and different measurement and calculating procedures (Fig. 1; Tables 1, 2). The longest tumor diameter and the greatest perpendicular diameter (WHO criterion, Miller et al. 1981) cannot easily be assessed when relying on imaging, as the conditions for imaging must be taken into account with transverse sections in ultrasound, CT, and MRI, coronal sections or projections in radiography and MRI, sagittal sections or projections in radiography, ultrasound, and MRI, oblique sections or projections in radiography, ultrasound, and MRI, arbitrary sections in ultrasound and MRI. The diameter given by any of these imaging methods is thus the diameter in the chosen projection or section that can be delineated by the chosen method, and which may or may not represent the longest tumor diameter.

Consequently, when judging and reporting the efficacy of different treatment modalities, the method of evaluating and reporting clinical and imaging data must be clearly stated to avoid a complex "remission evaluation bias" (Fig. 1; see Tables 1, 2) which can be overcome only by using a common language and by evaluating initial remission in terms of local control (continuous remission) after an adequate follow-up period. Nevertheless, the most precise methods for the assessment of volume are those based on imaging by ultrasound CT, and MRI, and these are nowadays increasingly available. A sophisticated evaluation can be carried out concerning the onset, extent, and duration of remission serving as a valid and reliable basis for judging the efficacy of different treatment modalities. Nevertheless, the data obtained particularly on volume remission will vary considerably from those known from the period before volume assessment and will have to be evaluated against the final outcome of treatment.

With the "imaging revolution" in planning and response evaluation of cancer treatment a new "common language" must now be found for scientific communication. The still widely cited WHO criterion for reporting results of cancer treatment (Miller et al. 1981), addressing only simple one- and two-dimensional measurement procedures, will have to be reconsidered taking into account the imaging capabilities now available that may provide often more valid and reliable data for judging the efficacy of treatment. For such a common language regarding remission to be substantively valid, the definition of its items must be based on long-term experience with correlation between remission pattern (one-, two-, and three-dimensional) and treatment outcome pattern (evidence of new disease and survival).

References

Battermann JJ, Mijnheer BJ (1986) The Amsterdam fast neutron radiotherapy project: a final report. Int J Radiat Oncol Biol Phys 12: 2093–2099

Bessell EM, Catterall M (1983) The regression of tumors of the head and neck treated with neutrons. Int J Radiat Oncol Biol Phys 9: 799–807

Catterall M, Errington RD (1987) The implications of improved treatment of malignant salivary gland tumors by fast neutron radiotherapy. Int J Radiat Oncol Biol Phys 13: 1313–1318

Duncan W, Orr JA, Arnott SJ, Jack WJL (1987) Neutron therapy for malignant tumours of the salivary glands. A report of the Edinburgh experience. Radiother Oncol 8: 97–104

Griffin BR, Laramore GE, Griffin TW, Eenmaa J (1988a) Fast neutron radiotherapy for advanced malignant salivary gland tumors. Radiother Oncol 12: 105–111

Griffin TW, Pajak T, Laramore GE, Duncan W, Richter MP, Hendrickson FR, Maor MH (1988b) Neutron vs photon irradiation of inoperable salivary gland tumors: results of an RTOG-MRC cooperative randomized study. Int J Radiat Biol Phys 15: 1085–1090

Henry LW, Blasko JC, Griffin TW, Parker RG (1979) Evaluation of fast neutron teletherapy for advanced carcinomas of the major salivary glands. Cancer 44: 814–818

ICRU Report 45 (1989) Clinical neutron dosimetry. I. determination of absorbed dose in a patient treated by external beams of fast neutrons. International Commission on Radiation Units and Measurements. Bethesda, Maryland

Kovacs G, Merkle K, Lessel A, Nemeth G, Kunde D, Vass L (1987) Ergebnisse der Bestrahlung mit verschiedenen Strahlenquellen bei der Therapie maligner Parotistumoren. Strahlenther Onkol 163: 84–89

Krüll A, Schwarz R, Heyer D, Brockmann WP, Junker A, Schmidt R, Hübener KH (1990) Results of fast neutron therapy of adenoid cystic carcinomas of the head and neck at the neutron facility Hamburg-Eppendorf. Strahlenther Onkol 166: 107–113

Miller AB, Hoogstraten B, Staquet M, Winkler A (1981) Reporting results of cancer treatment. Cancer 47: 207–214

Pötter R, Naszaly A, Hemprich A, Haverkamp U, Al-Dandashi CHR, Höver KH, Loncar I (1990) Neutron radiotherapy in adenoidcystic carcinoma: preliminary experience at the Münster neutron facility. Strahlenther Onkol 166: 78–85

Saroja KR, Mansell J, Hendrickson FR, Cohen L, Lennox A (1987) An update on malignant salivary gland tumors treated with neutrons at fermilab. Int J Radiat Oncol Biol Phys 13: 1319–1325

Goals and Achievements of the European Collaboration on Boron Neutron Capture Therapy*

D. Gabel

Introduction

Since 1989 the Commission of the European Communities has funded, through its program Europe Against Cancer, a concerted action European Collaboration on Boron Neutron Capture Therapy. The European Collaboration has two main goals. The first is to initiate clinical trials of glioma at the high flux reactor in Petten at the earliest possible time. The second is to create all necessary conditions to initiate clinical trials of other tumors and treatment at other facilities. This overview summarizes the activities of the European Collaboration toward achieving these two goals.

Tasks Necessary for Consideration of Clinical Trials

The following tasks have been identified as necessary to achieve before clinical trials can begin:

- Design, construction, and installation of an epithermal neutron beam
- Physical and biological characterization of the beam
- Installation of a suitable treatment room with corollary facilities
- Pharmacokinetic and toxicity studies of boronated tumor seekers
- Establishment of a response function for healthy tissue to the treatment intended
- Development of an adequate treatment planning modality.

Beam Development. The high flux reactor of the Joint Research Center of the Commission of the European Communities has been made available to modification for boron neutron capture therapy (BNCT). The reactor is a 45-MW light water swimming-pool reactor. It is used mainly for materials testing. The

Department of Chemistry, University of Bremen, Box 33044, 2800 Bremen 33, FRG
* The work of the European Collaboration on Boron Neutron Capture Therapy is supported by the Commission of the European Communities. Financial support of national agencies and foundations for the individual projects makes this Collaboration possible.

Advanced Radiation Therapy Tumor Response
Monitoring and Treatment Planning
Breit (Editor-in-Chief)
© Springer-Verlag, Berlin Heidelberg 1992

availability of the reactor is very high. One horizontal beam hole of the reactor, the HB11/HB12 hole, can be used for modifications necessary for BNCT. In 1989 a program was started to design an epithermal neutron beam. With Monte Carlo neutron and photon calculations, a filter consisting of Cd (1 mm), Al (150 mm), S (50 mm), Ti (10 mm), and Ar (1500 mm) was devised to yield a beam believed to have suitable properties for BNCT. The irradiation location is approximately 5 m from the reactor core, and consequently the beam has little divergence at the treatment location. For the treatment of glioma it was considered important to utilize to the greatest extent possible all the experience that has been gained with other types of radiation therapy. Therefore, a treatment room has been designed which permits bilateral irradiations of the head; thus a half circle of 2-m radius is available for patient placement. The facility will be able to allow treatment of glioma and other tumors well in excess of 1000 full treatments per year. Treatment will probably be carried out in a series of some five or six fractions.

Preconditions for Therapy

In Europe, BNCT is planned for clinical trial by the end of 1992. Plans call for the treatment of glioma patients with $Na_2B_{12}H_{11}SH(BSH)$ as the boron compound. Before the treatment can be tested, it must be demonstrated that the risk of treatment is low. To achieve this, the tolerance of healthy tissue to BNCT conditions needs to be determined in animals, and the pharmacokinetics of the boron compound in question must be established in both animals and patients.

Healthy Tissue Tolerance. Healthy tissue tolerance will be studied in dogs. The dogs will be given BSH in different amounts, and they will then be exposed to different levels of neutron irradiation. In previous experience of the late 1950s and early 1960s, skin was the most radiosensitive organ. This was due to both the high boron concentration in the skin and the simultaneous use of a thermal neutron beam. With beams of moderate mean energy and using the presently available boron compounds, skin no longer appears to be the dose-limiting healthy tissue. White-matter necrosis may occur with treatment using epi-thermal neutrons, and this will take several months to develop. When this study includes different levels of boron concentration and neutron exposure, opera-tional factors for the effectiveness of a given boron concentration and a given neutron fluence can be derived from a knowledge of the dose components at different depths. These factors will then allow the necessary exposure planning.

Pharmacokinetics of BSH. The pharmacokinetics of the boron compound needs to be known in both the animal model and in man in order to transfer results from the animal study to patients. Therefore, the European Collaboration has placed great emphasis on a thorough pharmacokinetic study of BSH in brain tumor patients. Data on the boron concentration in different tissues and their time dependence are being collected. A number of centers are involved in this study. For BSH, which is presently used in Japan for treating gliomas, no compound-related toxicity was found. Provided that the study on healthy tissue tolerance does not result in unacceptable damage to the tissue exposed, treatment trials for glioma will be able to start toward the end of 1992.

Development of Other Neutron Sources

The construction of a nuclear reactor for BNCT in a hospital environment can be expected to meet considerable difficulties. It is therefore desirable to look into the conversion of existing reactors for BNCT and the construction of accelerator-based neutron sources. Work toward this goal is progressing.

Development of New Tumor Seekers

The future perspectives of BNCT are closely linked to, and indeed dependent on, the development of new and improved tumor seekers. Within the European Collaboration, this aspect therefore has a high priority. Work is being carried out, among other things, on the synthesis of boronated analogues of porphyrins, lipid ethers, and melanoma seekers as examples of low molecular weight tumor seekers, and on growth factors, peptide hormones, and antibodies as examples of high molecular weight tumor seekers. Synthesis will be followed by distribution studies in appropriate test systems, toxicity studies, and pharmacokinetics.

Participating Centers and Internal Structures

In the European Collaboration, over 50 centers from 13 countries in Europe (European Community and COST countries) participate. It is expected that each center will provide funds for its own research through their own grants. The European Collaboration can pay only for costs that are associated with the coordination of the work of the different groups. Because there is no direct competition of the groups for the funds of the European Collaboration, no antagonistic behavior has emerged within the European Collaboration. Indeed, the working atmosphere has been dominated by a high degree of cooperation.

Besides the formal structure of a project leader (D. Gabel, Bremen), assisted by a Project Management Group (D. Chiaraviglio, Pavia; L. Dewit, Amsterdam;

H. Fankhauser, Lausanne; R. Huiskamp, Petten; B. Larsson, Zürich; R. Moss, Petten; P. Schofield, Harwell), no formalized groups have been created to deal with specific tasks. Instead, all members are invited to participate in and suggest meetings and working parties for areas of common interest.

Cooperation with Other Groups

The European Collaboration is determined to maintain a policy of open and free interaction with all other groups interested in BNCT. Thus, the European Collaboration has made available all data and results on, for example, beam design and pharmocokinetics, and it will continue to do so. It has adopted this policy because nothing can be gained from a restricted exchange of information and results. This is even more so because of limited availability and access to suitable neutron sources and because of the impact that successful or unsuccessful therapy trials have on other programs worldwide.

The European Collaboration enters into cooperation and information distribution unconditionally. However, all other groups worldwide are encouraged to do the same, so that maximum benefit can be achieved for patients everywhere.

Acknowledgment. Thanks are due to R. Alberts for skillful and competent organizational and secretarial assistance in the coordination of this project.

Results of Radiotherapy in Soft-Tissue Sarcomas

R. Schwarz[1], A. Krüll[1], M.P. Calamini[1], M. Waller[1], D. Heyer[1], R. Pfeiffer[1],
C. Zornig[2], H.-J. Weh[3], R. Schmidt[1], and K.-H. Hübener[1]

Introduction

Currently, patients with soft-tissue sarcomas are managed by a multimodality
approach. For small low-grade lesions in fleshy parts, treatment will be less than
radical resection alone. For other lesions the treatment will be the combination
of less than radical resection and radiotherapy, and in some patients chemotherapy. A problem remains in local control of inoperable tumors or tumors
with gross residual tumor mass after surgery. A further problem concerns local
control of highly differentiated tumors (G1 and G2). Neutron therapy offers
radiobiological advantages in the treatment of these tumors. From January
1984 to September 1988, 147 patients with soft-tissue sarcomas were treated
with fast neutrons. A current analysis of these patients is presented. A second
analysis will focus 50 patients through January 1990 with neutrons or photons.

Methods and Material

Patients with Soft-Tissue Sarcomas 1984–1988. Over the period from January
1984 through September 1988, 147 patients (72 men, 75 women) with soft tissue
sarcomas were irradiated with fast neutrons of a 14-MeV DT generator at the
University Hospital Hamburg-Eppendorf. Of these, 92 were treated for primary
tumors and 55 for recurrences. The mean age was 51.5 years (range 13–86).
Common histologies were liposarcoma (36 cases), malignant fibrous histiocytoma (27), fibrosarcoma (26), leiomyosarcoma (18), and malignant schwannoma
(13). Grading was evaluable for 135 patients: G1 in 34, G2 in 35, and G3 in 66.
Tumor location was lower and upper extremity (75 cases), head and neck (17),
retroperitoneum (10), or others (45). Staging of the primary tumors showed T1 in

[1] Department of Radiotherapy, University Hospital Hamburg-Eppendorf, Martinistr. 52, 2000
Hamburg 20, FRG
[2] Department of General Surgery, University Hospital Hamburg-Eppendorf, Martinistr. 52, 2000
Hamburg 20, FRG
[3] Department of Medical Oncology, University Hospital Hamburg-Eppendorf, Martinistr. 52, 2000
Hamburg 20, FRG

Advanced Radiation Therapy Tumor Response
Monitoring and Treatment Planning
Breit (Editor-in-Chief)
© Springer-Verlag, Berlin Heidelberg 1992

35 cases and T2 in 108. Metastases to the regional lymph nodes were demonstrable in 11 cases; 43 patients had distant metastases at the time of diagnosis or developed distant metastases during the further follow-up. Nearly all patients had surgery one or several times, ranging from one surgical intervention to 17. The residual tumor classification at the time of radiotherapy was: R0 in 56 cases (38.1%) R1 in 24 (16.3%), R2 in 61 (41.5%), and Rx in 6 (4.3%).

All patients were irradiated with fast neutrons of a 14-MeV DT generator. In general, patients received as a minimum target dose 14.4 Gy DT for postoperative radiotherapy after radical resection: patients with microscopic and macroscopic tumor residuals after surgery received a minimum target dose of 16 Gy DT.

Patients with Liposarcoma 1980–1990. Over the period from January 1980 through January 1990, 50 patients (29 men, 21 women) patients with liposarcoma were irradiated with neutrons and/or photons. Mean and median age was 53 years (range 17–79). Primary tumor was located at the lower extremity in 19 cases, at the upper extremity in 5, at the shoulder in 6, in the head and neck in 7, and in other locations in 13. A pathohistological subclassification could be done in 45 cases. Most of the patients had myxoid liposarcomas (33). Twelve patients had other subtypes such as pleomorphic liposarcoma (5), polymorphic liposarcoma (5), and round cell liposarcoma (2). Grading was evaluable for 48 patients: G1 in 17, G2 in 15, and G3 in 16. Ten patients showed a T1 tumor and 37 a T2. Only two patients showed lymph node metastases and two patients distant metastases at the time of radiotherapy. All patients had one or more surgical interventions before radiotherapy. A total of 111 surgical interventions were performed in these patients. The results of operations could be evaluated in 92% of 111 cases: radical resection (R0) in 37 operations, microscopic tumor residuals (R1) in 17, and macroscopic residuals in 38. Fifty patients received a total of 72 radiation treatments. In 36 cases a primary tumor was treated, in 22 a recurrent tumor, in one patient the locoregional lymph drainage, and in 13 cases distant metastases were irradiated. For calculations, especially Kaplan-Meier plots, radiotherapy for primary tumor took first priority, radiotherapy for recurrences second, and radiotherapy for other reasons third. Patients with G1 and G2 tumors and patients with macroscopic tumor mass were irradiated with fast neutrons: patients with G3 tumors after R0 or R1 resection or patients with distant metastases were irradiated with photons.

Results

Patients with Soft-Tissue Sarcomas 1984–1988. For this analysis data were calculated for survival rates and local control rates. Significance of differences was tested by a two-tailed Wilcoxon test (with $p < 0.01$). Of the 147 patients 108

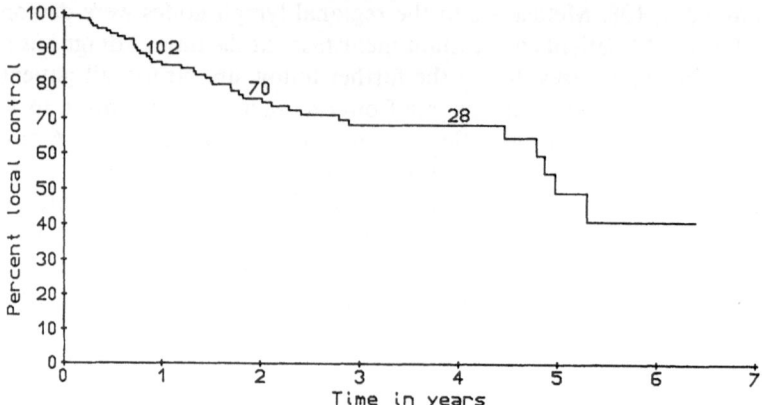

Fig. 1. Local control, all patients

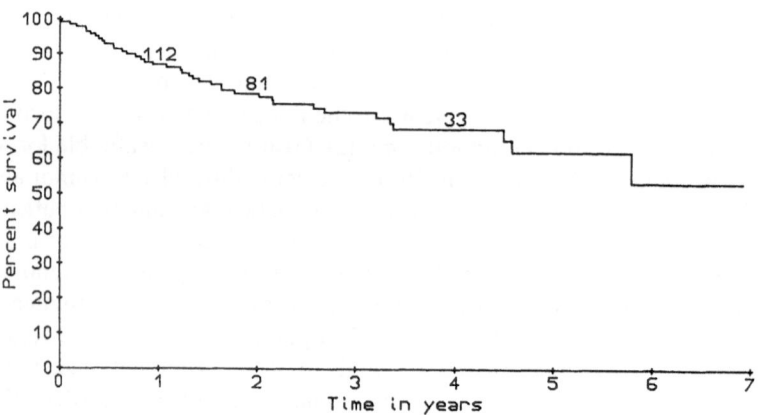

Fig. 2. Probability of survival, all patients

are alive; 25 died with local control, and 14 died with recurrence or progress. Figure 1 shows the probability of survival for all patients. Factors of prognostic value for survival with statistical significance were: tumor situation at the time of neutron therapy (R classification), grade, and the occurrence of distant metastases. Survival rates at 2 years after radiotherapy were 78.5% for all patients: 96.6% in G1 tumors, 93.9% in G2, 66.6% in G3, 93.7% in T1, 74.6% in T2, 89.9% in R0, 86.1% in R1, and 64.4% in R2. Figure 2 shows the probability for local control in terms of tumor situation (radiotherapy for primary tumor or recurrence). Factors of prognostic relevance for local control were: histology and R classification. Liposarcomas showed a significantly lower recurrence rate than other histologies. Local control rates at 2 years after radiotherapy were 75.7% for all patients: 82.4% in grade 1, 85.4% in grade 2, 67.3% in grade 3, 86.5% in T1, 71.1% in T2, 86.0% in R0, 79.5% in R1, and 60.1% in R2.

Patients with Liposarcomas 1980–1990. Median follow-up has been 39 months. Of the 50 patients 43 are under local control. Ten patients died, nine of them from tumor. Two patients developed lymph node metastases and seven distant metastases after therapy. Local control after 2 years was 91.6%, after 3 years 91.6%, and after 5 years 73.3%. Survival rates after 2 years were 85.9%, after 3 years 83.3%, and after 5 years 78.7%. Patients with radiotherapy for primary tumors fared better in terms of local control and survival than patients with radiotherapy for recurrence. Tumor sizes categorized as T1 or T2 and tumor grade are factors of prognostic relevance for local control. Patients with G1 or T2 tumors have a better prognosis. Patients treated with fast neutrons seem to have a better prognosis than those treated with photons.

Discussion

Clinical data from several centers strongly support the combination of radiation with less than radical surgery in the treatment of soft-tissue sarcomas. Nowadays over 90% of all patients with soft-tissue sarcomas are treated by the combination of surgery and radiotherapy. A great problem remains in local control of inoperable tumors or tumors with gross residual tumor mass after surgery. In the group with R2 tumors the local control rate was 57% 2 years after radiotherapy. These preliminary data are in accordance to the published data from other neutron centers [1, 2, 4, 5, 9–14, 16, 17]. A total of 297 patients with macroscopic tumor mass in soft tissue sarcoma were treated with fast neutrons. Of these, 158 (53%) are under local control. Summarizing high-dose radiotherapy with photons or electrons for macroscopic tumor mass, local control rates were about 38% [3, 7, 8, 15, 18] in a total of 128 patients.

Neutron therapy offers special advantages for macroscopic tumor mass, because (a) neutrons are better able to kill hypoxic cells, (b) the damage by neutrons is less readily repaired by the cells, and (c) there is less variation in radiosensitivity across the cell cycle in comparison to photon treatment. Distant metastases in gross tumors and in G3 tumors remain a problem in spite of optimized local control rates and chemotherapy. In many patients distant metastases are the limiting factor for survival.

The analysis shows that patients with liposarcoma may benefit from neutron therapy. This has not been reported before. The effect may be due either to the selection of patients or to a higher dose absorption of neutrons in fatty tissues and therefore in liposarcoma. The difference to other tissues may be up to 15%. Nevertheless, at this time there are no statistically significant differences within the group. Local control rates and survival rates are excellent.

A further problem concerns local control of radioresistant, highly differentiated tumors (G1 and G2). Neutrons may be of advantage for the treatment of these tumors. The existing data are not sufficient to answer this question definitely.

References

1. Batterman JJ, Breur K (1981) Fast neutron radiotherapy for locally advanced sarcomas. Int J Radiat Oncol Biol Phys 7: 1051–1053
2. Cohen L, Hendrickson F, Mansell J et al. (1984) Response of sarcomas of bone and soft tissue to neutron beam therapy. Int J Radiat Oncol Biol Phys 10: 821–824
3. Duncan W, Dewar JA (1985) A retrospective study of the role of radiotherapy in the treatment of soft-tissue sarcoma. Clin Radiol 36: 629–632
4. Duncan W, Arnott SJ, Jack WLJ (1986) The Edinburgh experience of treating sarcomas of soft tissue and bone with neutron irradiation. Clin Radiol 37: 317–320
5. Franke HD (1987) Clinical experiences with treatment of more than 50 patients with fast neutrons (DT, 14 MeV) since 1976 in Hamburg-Eppendorf. In: Lapis K, Eckhart S (eds) Lectures and symposia, 14th international cancer congress, Budapest 1986. Karger, Basel, pp 93–106 (Akademiai Kiado, vol 8)
6. Hall EJ (1988) Radiobiology for the radiobiologist. Lippincott, Philadelphia
7. Leibel SA, Tranbaugh RF, Wara WM et al. (1982) Soft tissue sarcomas of the extremities: survival and patterns of failure with conservative surgery with postoperative irradiation compared to surgery alone. Cancer 50: 1076–1983
8. McNeer GP, Cantin J, Chu F, Nickson JJ (1968) Effectiveness of radiation therapy in the management of sarcoma of the soft somatic tissues. Cancer 22: 391–397
9. Ornitz R, Herskovic A, Schell M, Fender F, Rogers CC (1980) Treatment experience: locally advanced sarcomas with 15 MeV fast neutrons. Cancer 45: 2712–2716
10. Pelton JG, Del Rowe JD, Bolen JW et al. (1986) Fast neutron radiotherapy for soft tissue sarcomas: University of Washington experience and review of the world's literature. Am J Clin Oncol 9: 397–400
11. Pickering DG, Stewart JS, Rampling DG, Errington RD, Stamp G, Chia V (1987) Fast neutron therapy for soft tissue sarcoma. Int J Radiat Oncol Biol Phys 13: 1489–1495
12. Salinas R, Hussey DH, Fletcher G et al. (1980) Experience with fast neutrons for locally advanced sarcomas. Int J Radiat Oncol Biol Phys 6: 267–272
13. Schmitt G, Rassow J, Schnabel K et al. (1984) Radiotherapy of soft tissue sarcomas with neutrons or a neutron boost. Br J Radiol 57: 247–250
14. Schmitt G, Schnabel K, Sauerwein W, Scherer E (1983) Neutron and neutron-boost irradiation of soft tissue sarcomas: a 4.5 years analysis of 139 patients. Radiol Oncol 1: 23–29
15. Tepper JE, Suit HD (1985) Radiation therapy alone for sarcoma of soft tissue. Cancer 56: 475–479
16. Tsunemoto H, Shinroku S, Arai T, Kutsutani Y, Kurisu A, Umegaki Y (1979) Results of clinical trial with 30 MeV d-Be neutrons at NIRS. In: Abe M, Sakamoto K, Philips TL (eds) Treatment of radioresistant cancers. Elsevier/North Holland, Amsterdam, pp 115–126
17. Wambersie A (1982) The European experience in neutron radiotherapy at the end of 1981. Int J Radiat Oncol Biol Phys 8: 2145–2152
18. Windeyer W, Dische S, Mansfield CM (1966) The place of radiotherapy in the management of fibrosarcoma of the soft tissues. Clin Radiol 17: 32–40.

Magnetic Resonance Imaging Based Simulation for Neutron Radiotherapy in Minor Salivary Gland Cylindromas: Primary Experience at Münster University

G. Kovacs*, R. Pötter, U. Stöber, and M. Dittrich

Introduction

The majority of minor salivary gland cancers show a histology of adenoid-cystic carcinoma (Schell et al. 1983). Adenoid-cystic carcinoma (cylindromas) of the minor salivary glands can be found in the oral cavity, nasal cavity, oropharynx, and paranasal sinuses. This type of tumor is not common; the tumors grow very slowly, sometimes over many years. Because of their wide variety of presentations treatment varies depending on the area in which they are found (Laramore 1989). Data in the literature suggest that adenoid-cystic carcinoma in the paranasal sinuses and nasal cavity tend to present with more advanced disease than in other locations (Leafstedt et al. 1971; Goepfert et al. 1983). For adenoid-cystic carcinoma perineural spread is a common feature; the tumor may involve the central area of the nerves and can grow by skipping areas. A normal nerve segment in the histology is no assurance of free margins after surgery. It may grow along the bone without showing bone destruction. Lymph node metastases are less common in patients with origin in the hard palate and paranasal sinuses compared with other sites of origin (Rafla-Demetrious 1970). Adenoid-cystic carcinoma, because of its high grade of differentiation and slow growth, is treated with high-LET radiation treatment. Battermann et al. (1981) measured a relative biological effectiveness for adenoid-cystic carcinoma of 5.7 for a single dose and 8.0 for fractionated radiation.

Reports in the literature suggest a clear advantage for neutron therapy in all types of salivary gland cancer compared with the results of the low-LET radiation (Griffin and Mortimer 1989; Kovacs et al. 1987; Pötter et al. 1991). The technical possibilities of fast-neutron sources used in medicine are different from those of currently used linear accelerators or cobalt machines. Handicaps include the size of the head, field collimation, and some troubles using blocks in the field (except those with multileaf collimator). The aim of our study was to find an irradiation method with our dT 14-MeV isocentric generator, to use this for irradiation of advanced minor salivary gland cancer, and optimally to spare critical organs such as brain stem, eye, etc.

Radioonkologie, Klinik und Poliklinik für Strahlentherapie, Westfälische Wilhelms-Universität Münster, Albert-Schweitzer Str. 33 4400 Münster, FRG
* Klinik für Strahlentherapie (Radioonkologie) des Klinikums der CAU zu Kiel, Arnold-Heller-Str. 9, 2300 Kiel, FRG

Advanced Radiation Therapy Tumor Response
Monitoring and Treatment Planning
Breit (Editor-in-Chief)
© Springer-Verlag, Berlin Heidelberg 1992

Methods and Materials

The size of the head of our isocentric neutron generator allows only 15° gantry rotation under the horizontal plane. In the therapy planning process we must plan with fixed collimator sizes, and if opposed fields, we have a maximal collimator turning for nonquadratic fields of 10°. On the other hand, there are no possibilities for field control neutronograms. Since 1986 we have used fast neutrons (Pötter et al. 1990b) for the treatment of adenoid-cystic carcinoma in 27 patients. Seven of these had tumor with small salivary gland cancer origin infiltrating the base of skull and/or retro-, parabulbar structures. The administered tumor dose was 15 Gy, in one case 10 Gy according to the ICRU reference point. We used a fractionation of 1.67 Gy three times per week. The mean follow-up was 10.5 months. Using the therapy planning method based on magnetic resonance imaging (MRI) described by Pötter et al. (1990a) we tried to find a method to spare the critical structures with the optimization of our therapy.

Results

The method used was a hyperretroflexion of the patient's head. For fixation and reproducibility we used a special table. The degree of the retroflexion is through a laser line, and markers on the skin (minimum of two points for one line) could be easy reproduced (Fig. 1). The usual plans are for two opposed lateral and one or two ventral portals. To spare the critical structures we used 50% transmission

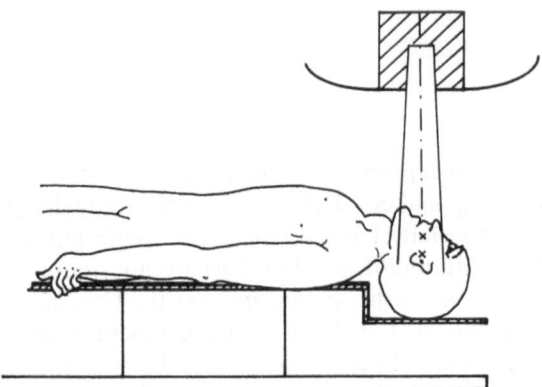

Fig. 1. Patient fixation method with a special table and a laser line (with markers on the skin) in hyperretroflexion of the patient's head

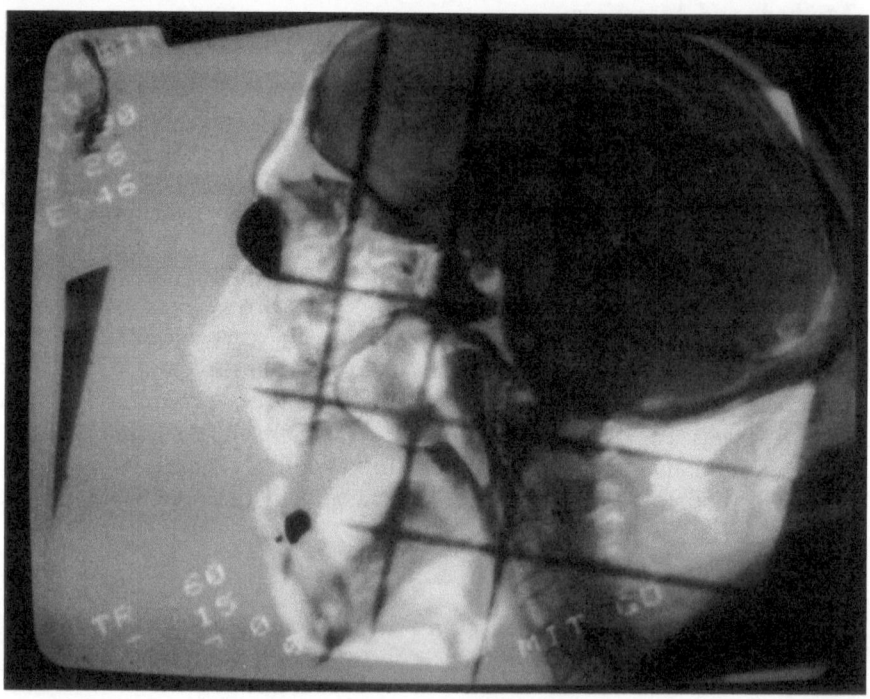

Fig. 2. Image on the screen of the subtrascope: electronic superimposition of lateral simulation film and sagittal MR image in the beam's eye view

standard blocks. After MRI-based treatment planning we checked the simulated portals and the tumor volume on the MR images with the help of the subtrascope. When the target area was in the simulated portals, we administered the simulated fields (Figs. 2, 3).

Discussion

MRI has the best soft-tissue contrast capacity of any imaging modality, and the possibility of multiplanar imaging makes MRI a very useful modality for therapy planning. The restricted technical possibilities of the currently used neutron machines (except those with multileaf collimator) are not optimal for therapy planning. The use of MRI-based therapy planning at the University of Münster and some additional nonconventional patient fixation methods allows a more optimal irradiation technique of retro- and parabulbarly infiltrating small salivary gland cancer.

Follow-up in the seven patients irradiated with the method described above is still relatively short. One patient died with advanced lung metastases after 17

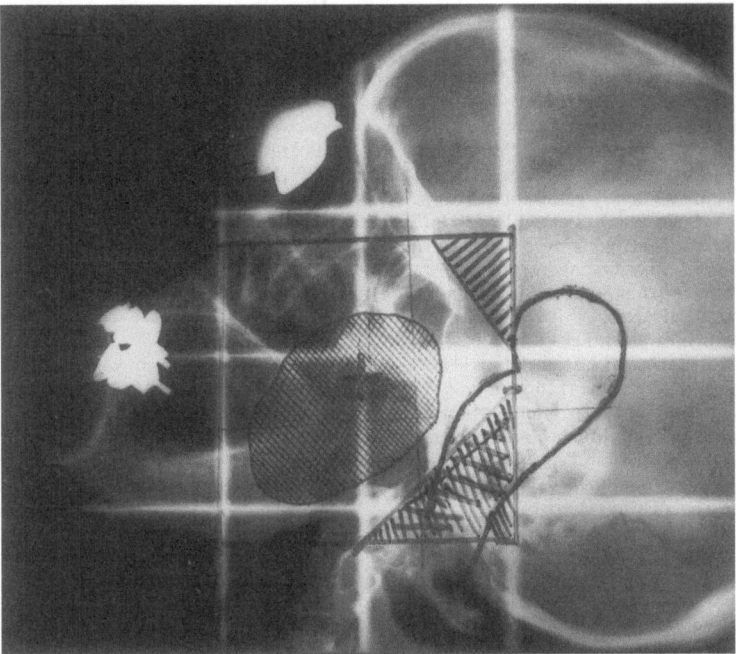

Fig. 3. Simulation film with MRI-assisted delineation of advanced fossa infratemporalis tumor. After checking with the subtrascope correction of the simulated portal and planning of transmission blocks for sparing the critical structures (brain)

months (with a volume reduction of the irradiated primary from 270 cm^3 to 98 cm^3), all the others are alive.

As side effects we observed some depression in all patients (irradiated brain volume?) after the radiation course with a duration of 1–3 months with no need for medication. All the patients had a slightly moderate lymphedema on the portals and a moderate xerostomia. When irradiated, we observed clinical signs of moderate temporomandibular joint fibrosis with no evidence of any functional troubles. In the follow-up no severe late effects were observed. We control the patients through regular clinical and MRI investigations. Further follow-up is necessary to evaluate possible late effects and local control.

References

Battermann JJ, Breur K, Hart Bam et al. (1981) Observations on pulmonary metastases in patients after single doses and multiple fractions of fast neutrons and cobalt-60 gamma rays. Eur J Cancer 17: 539–545
Goepfert H, Luna M, Lindberg R, White A (1983) Malignant salivary gland tumors of paranasal sinuses and nasal cavity. Arch Otolaryngol 109: 662–668

Griffin TW, Mortimer J (1989) Overview of clinical trials and basis for future therapies. In: Laramore GE (ed) Radiation therapy of head and neck cancer. Springer, Berlin Heidelberg New York

Kovacs G, Merkle K, Lessel A, Nemeth G, Kunde D, Vass L (1987) Ergebnisse der Bestrahlung mit verschiedenen Strahlenquellen bei der Therapie maligner Parotistumoren. Strahlenther Onkol 163: 84–89

Laramore GE (1989) Head and neck cancer: a general overview. In: Laramore GE (ed) Radiation therapy of head and neck cancer. Springer, Berlin Heidelberg New York

Leafstedt SW, Gaeta JF, Sako K, Marchetta FC, Schedd DP (1971) Adenoidcystic carcinoma of major and minor salivary glands. Am J Surg 122: 756–762

Pötter R, Heil B, Schneider L, Lenzen H, Al-Dandashi C, Schnepper E (1990a) Magnetic resonance imaging in treatment planning of head and neck tumours including the brain: MRI assisted simulation. Radiother Oncol (in press)

Pötter R, Naszaly A, Hemprich A, Haverkamp U, Al-Dandashi C, Höver K-H, Loncar I (1990b) Neutron radiotherapy in adenoidcystic carcinoma: preliminary experience at the Münster neutron facility. Strahlenther Onkol 166(1): 78–85

Pötter R, Kovacs G, Loncar I, Haverkamp U (1991) Short term results of fast neutron radiotherapy in adenoidcystic carcinoma (Münster 1986–1990) In: Book of abstracts ART91 tumor response monitoring and treatment planning, Munich, 11–13 April, p 185

Rafla-Demetrious S (1970) Mucous and salivary gland tumors. Thomas, Springfield

Schell S, Barkley HT Jr, Chiminazzo H Jr (1983) Treatment of minor salivary gland tumors: MD Anderson hospital data 1/70–2/78. In: Laramore GE (ed) Radiation therapy of head and neck cancer. Springer, Berlin Heidelberg New York

Neutron Therapy of Bladder Carcinoma

C. Kirkove, F. Richard, M. Octave-Prignot, and A. Wambersie

Introduction

Fast-neutron therapy has been used routinely on the cyclotron at the Catholic
University of Louvain in Louvain-la-Neuve since March 1978. This paper
reports the results obtained in bladder carcinoma, including local tumor
control, survival, and radiation-induced side effects. Our data are compared
with those reported in the literature after neutron or conventional photon-beam
therapy.

Materials and Methods

Between 1978 and 1990, 98 patients with invasive bladder carcinoma were
treated with fast neutron beams. A total of 58 could be analysed; among the
others, 7 received an incomplete treatment (less than 35 Gy), 17 had only a
preoperative treatment, 7 had distant metastases at the time of the treatment, 4
presented with a nontransitional cell carcinoma, and 5 were lost to follow-up.
There were 53 men and 5 women. The mean age was 68 years (range 34–85).
Hematuria was the first symptom in 39 patients (67%).

All tumors were classified according to the TNM system and the WHO
malignancy grading system [1]. The urological procedure prior to radiotherapy
was cystoscopy and biopsy in 9 patients, transurethral resection in 37, partial
cystectomy in 8, and cystectomy in 4. Histological examination indicated that 53
tumors were pure transitional cell carcinoma, and 5 were mixed tumors with
epidermoid metaplasia (four patients) or adenocarcinoma (one patient). Twenty
tumors were classified as grade II, 36 as grade III, and the grade could not be
determined in two patients. Twelve patients had T2 tumor, 32 had T3 (24 T3a,
8 T3b), 13 had T4 (12 T4a, 1 T4b), and one had Tx. Based on clinical examination and/or computed tomography, locoregional node involvement was
suspected in nine patients prior to radiotherapy, but none of the 58 patients
showed signs of distant metastases.

Unité de Radiothérapie, Neutron et Curietherapie, Cliniques Universitaires St-Luc, UCL 10/4752,
Avenue Hippocrate 10, 1200 Brussels, Belgium

Advanced Radiation Therapy Tumor Response
Monitoring and Treatment Planning
Breit (Editor-in-Chief)
© Springer-Verlag, Berlin Heidelberg 1992

Due to the limited availability of the cyclotron, patients were treated with a mixed schedule (three neutron and two photon fractions per week). Photon treatments were performed with a 18-MV linear accelerator. Neutrons were generated by 65 MeV protons bombarding a thick beryllium target [2]. The neutron energy was sufficient to achieve a physical selectivity comparable to that of a 10-MV linear accelerator. The daily target-absorbed dose was 0.71 Gy (2 Gy photon equivalent), assuming a neutron relative biological effectiveness of 2.8. A 4 field "box technique" (two parallel opposed anteroposterior fields and two lateral fields) was employed for the irradiation of the whole pelvis, as well as for the boost to the bladder.

Patients were classified into three groups according to doses levels and overall treatment time. Twenty-five patients (treatment A) received whole pelvis irradiation up to 50 Gy equivalent, followed by a boost to the bladder up to 57–66 Gy equivalent. The overall treatment time ranged between 40 and 56 days. In the second group (treatment B), 18 patients were treated by a split course regimen: 30 Gy equivalent on the whole pelvis, then after 3–4 weeks' rest an additional 30 Gy equivalent. The overall treatment time was 66–108 days. The first patients were treated with regimen B (from 1978 to approximately 1983); then the treatment policy was progressively modified, and treatment A was preferred. A last group of 15 patients (treatment C) with advanced tumors and/or in poor condition were not considered suitable for radical treatment and received only 40–54 Gy equivalent over 24–70 days on the whole pelvis.

Statistical analysis was performed according to the method described by Peto et al. [3].

Results

The median follow-up time was 70 months (range 6–152 months). The overall 5-year actuarial survival rate was 35% (SE 9%). Survival curves were calculated according to three parameters: T stage, grade, and treatment technique. As shown in Table 1, T stage and grade were statistically significant prognostic factors. In contrast, the influence of the treatment type did not appear to be of statistical significance, although different survival rates were observed among the three treatment groups (Fig. 1). At 48 months, the overall local control rate reached 21.5%. A better local control was observed for treatment types A and B compared to treatment C (i.e., 15%, 33%, and 0%, respectively). This difference was not statistically significant.

Minimal acute side effects were observed in 14 patients (24%): mild cystitis in 14, diarrhea in 3, and moist dermatitis in 2. Of these 14 patients, 9 were treated by treatment A. Side effects resolved quickly with a conservative treatment in all patients except in one whom cystitis required a 1-week treatment interruption. Late complications occurred in seven patients (12%) mainly in treatment group

Table 1. Estimated 5-year survival rate (multivariate analysis)

Variable	n	Survival	Log rank p
T stage			
T2	12	82%	
T3	32	23%	0.05
T4	13	19%	
Grade			
II	20	59%	
III	36	24%	0.02
Treatment			
A	25	28%	
B	18	51%	0.45
C	15	28%	

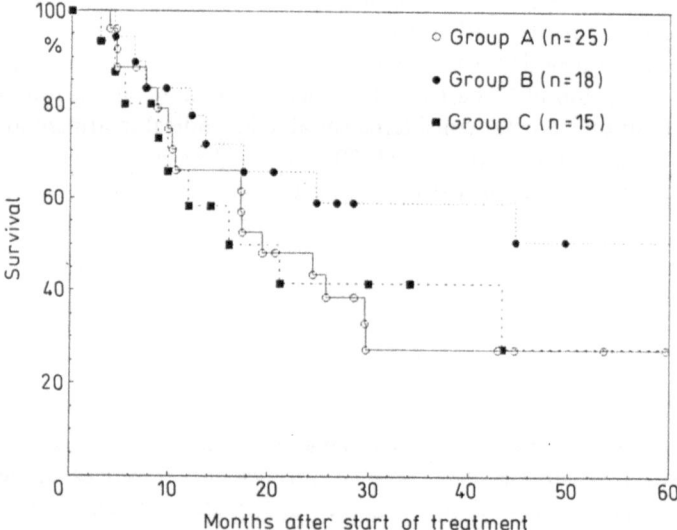

Fig. 1. Actuarial survival by treatment group

B (5/7). They occurred after a median time of 18 months (range 4–60 months). Five patients had a reaction graded as minimal to moderate, and two patients died. Minimal to moderate side effects were as follows: impotence, reduction in bladder capacity, intermittend macroscopic hematuria requiring no treatment, asymptomatic vesical telangectasia, and severe radiation cystitis with frequent hematuria requiring many vesical washings under general anesthesia. In three patients, the symptoms were rapidly followed by a macroscopic recurrence of the tumor. Two patients (2/58) who had received treatment B died free of recurrence. One died 26 months after radiotherapy from a septic episode secondary to a colouretheral fistula and a rectal stricture; he had undergone a salvage cystectomy and received chemotherapy 5 months after irradiation. A second patient died from renal failure after laparotomy for small-bowel occlusion; as this patient had had no abdominal surgical procedure before, one might conclude that the small-bowel occlusion was a consequence of the radiotherapy given 60 months before.

Discussion

In the present series (58 patients) the 5-year actuarial survival rate reached 35%, compared to 24%–31% reported after photon treatment [4–7]. For the T3 tumors (32 patients), a 5-year survival rate of 28% and 22% was observed in treatments A and B, respectively, compared to 15%–39% reported after photon treatment [4–10]. To the extend that a comparison with published series is possible, the 5-year actuarial survival rate obtained with mixed schedule therapy (neutron–photon) was comparable to that obtained with conventional photon treatment. As far as the incidence of late side effects is concerned, comparison is more difficult, mainly because the criteria of long-term toxicity are not identical in the different reported surveys. Treatment-related mortality in the present study was similar to that reported by Salminen [7] in a large series of 203 patients treated with photon beams.

Finally, comparison of our results to those reported by other neutron therapy centers [11–19] (Table 2) shows that the 5-year survival rates are similar, but that the incidence of severe side effects is much lower in our series, as could be expected from the improvement in physical selectivity with higher energy [p(65) + Be] neutrons.

Conclusion

Neutron-beam treatment seems as effective as photon-beam treatment for bladder carcinoma. The high rate of severe side effects observed previously with low-energy neutrons has, however, largely hampered its use. Our observation that with high-energy neutrons there is only a low incidence of major side effects should lead to reconsideration of the role of neutrons in the management of bladder carcinoma. However, further studies are needed to define the subgroup of patients with bladder carcinoma who would most benefit from neutron treatment (predictive tests). Since the incidence of side effects is relatively low, a careful dose-level escalation should be attempted toward optimizing results.

Table 2. Results of fast neutron therapy for bladder carcinoma

Trial, year	n	Stage	Treatment	Bladder dose (Gy)	Survival	Local control	Severe Complications
Amsterdam [11–14]:							
1975–1978	22	Advanced	Neutrons d(14) + T	17–25	23% 2-year	45	32%
1978–1981 (randomized)	24	T4b	Neutrons d(14) + T	17–19		–	12.5%
	6		Photons Co60	50		–	0%
Edinburgh [15, 16]:							
1978–1981 (randomized)	53	T1–T4	Neutrons d(15) + Be	15–16.5	12% 5-year	43	78.3%
	60		Photons 4–6 MV	47.5–55	45% 5-year	43	37.7%
Manchester [17]:							
1978–1981 (randomized)	20	T2, T3	Neutrons d(15) + T	16.5–17	55% 3-year	71	15%
	20		Neutrons d(15) + T	18–18.5	40% 3-year	53	10%
	59		Photons 4–8 MV	52.5–55	42.5% 3-year	46	5%
	8		Mixed beam	49.5–55	37.5% 3-year	62	37%
					NS	NS	
RTOG [18, 19]: 1977–1981	26	B1–D1 (T2–T4)	Mixed Beam (2N–3P)	65–70[a]	12% 5-year	23	27%
	13		Mixed beam + cystectomy	50[a]	31% 5-year	61	30%
					NS		
Present study: 1978–1990	58	T2–T4	Mixed beam: 3N–2P	40–66[a]	35% 5-year	22	12%

[a] Photon gray equivalent.

Acknowledgements. Most of the patients were referred for radiotherapy by Dr. P. Van Cangh (urology surgery unit,UCL St Luc) and Dr. G. Ledent (urology surgery unit, St Pierre Ottignies).

References

1. Union Internationale Contre le Cancer (UICC) (1987) TNM classification of malignant tumours, , 4th edn. Springer, Berlin Heidelberg New York
2. Vynckier S, Pihet P, Flemal JM, Meulders JP, Wambersie A (1983) Improvement of a p(65) + Be neutron beam for therapy at cyclone, Louvain-la-Neuve. Phys Med Biol 28: 685–691
3. Peto R, Pike MC, Armitage P, Breslow NE, Cox DR, Howard SV, Mantel N, Mc Pherson K, Peto J, Smith PG (1977) Design and analysis of randomized clinical trials requiring prolonged observation of each patient. Br J Cancer 35: 1–39
4. Blandy JP, England HR, Evans SJW, Hope-Stone HF, Mair GMM, Mantell BS, Oliver RTD, Paris AMI, Risdon RA (1980) T3 bladder cancer — the case for salvage cystectomy. Br. J. Urol 52: 506–510
5. Shipley WU, Rose MA, Perrone TL, Mannix CM, Heney NM. Prout GR (1985) Full-dose irradiation for patients with invasive bladder carcinoma: clinical and histological factors prognostic of improved survival. J. Urol. 134: 679–683
6. Mameghan H, Fisher R (1989) Invasive bladder cancer. Prognostic factors and results of radiotherapy with and without cystectomy. Br J. Urol. 63: 251–258
7. Salminen E (1990) External beam radiation treatment of urinary bladder carcinoma. An analysis of results in 203 patients. Acta Oncol. 29: 909–914
8. Wallace DM, Bloom HJG (1976) The management of deeply infiltrating (T3) bladder carcinoma: controlled trial of radical radiotherapy versus preoperative radiotherapy and radical cystectomy (first report). Br. J. Urol. 48: 587-594
9. Cummings KB, Taylor WJ, Correa RJ, Gibbons RP. Mason JT (1976) Observations on definitive cobalt 60 radiation for cure in bladder carcinoma: 15-year follow-up. J. Urol 115: 152–154
10. Bloom HJG, Hendry WF, Wallace DM et al. (1982) Treatment of T3 bladder cancer: controlled trial of pre-operative radiotherapy and radical cystectomy versus radical radiotherapy. Second report and review (for the Clinical Trials Group, Institute of Urology). Br. J. Urol. 54: 136-151
11. Battermann JJ, Hart GAM, Breur K (1981) Dose-effect relations for tumour control and complication rate after fast neutron therapy for pelvic tumors. Br. J. Radiol. 54: 899–904
12. Broerse JJ, Battermann JJ (1981) Fast neutron radiotherapy: for equal or for better? Med. Phys. 8: 751–760
13. Battermann JJ (1982) Results of d + T fast neutron irradiation on advanced tumors of bladder and rectum. Int. J. Radiot. Oncol. Biol. Phys. 8: 2159–2164
14. Battermann JJ, Mijnheer BJ (1986) The Amsterdam fast neutron therapy project: a final report. Int. J. Radiat. Oncol. Biol. Phys. 12: 2093–2099
15. Duncan W, Arnott SJ, Jack WJL, MacDougall RH, Quilty PM, Rodger A, Kerr GR, Williams JR (1985) A report of a randomized trial of d(15) + Be neutrons compared with megavoltage X ray therapy of bladder cancer. Int. J. Radiat. Oncol. Biol. Phys. 11: 2043–2049
16. Duncan W, Williams JR, Kerr GR, Arnott SJ, Quilty PM, Rodger A, MacDougall RH, Jack WJL (1986) An analysis of the radiation related morbidity observed in a randomized trial of neutron therapy for Bladder Cancer. Int. J. Radiat. Oncol. Biol. Phys. 12: 2085–2092
17. Pointon RS, Read G, Greene D (1985) A randomized comparison of photons and 15 MeV neutrons for the treatment of carcinoma of the bladder. Br. J. Radiol. 58: 219–224
18. Laramore GE, Davis RB, Hussey DH, Griffin TW, Maor MH, Hendrickson FR, Davis LW, Dupre E (1984) Radiation Therapy Oncology Group phase I–II study on fast neutron teletherapy for carcinoma of the bladder. Cancer 54: 432–439
19. Russel KJ, Laramore GE, Griffin TW, Parker RG, Davis LW, Krall JW (1989) Fast neutron radiotherapy for the treatment of carcinoma of the urinary bladder. A review of Clinical trials. Am J clin Oncol 12: 301–306

Enhancement of the Absorbed Dose in a d(14)+Be Fast-Neutron Beam by ^{10}B Neutron-Capture Therapy*

W. Sauerwein, F. Pöller, J. Rassow, and H. Sack

Introduction

Boron neutron-capture therapy uses the chemical delivery of specific boron compounds to neoplastic tissue in combination with thermal neutrons to produce an enhanced radiation dose in the tumor. The nuclear fission reaction when ^{10}B is irradiated with slow neutrons releases relatively large amounts of high linear energy transfer radiation through its fission products ^{7}Li and stripped helium nuclei. The short range of these particles (approximately 10 μm) theoretically restricts the radiation dose to tumor cells. Because of the rapid attenuation of thermal neutrons in tissue, this treatment modality needs surgical techniques to expose the tumor directly to the thermal neutron beam (Hatanaka et al. 1991). On the other hand, neutrons of all energies become thermalized by their interaction with the target material. Hence, during fast-neutron therapy, low-energy neutrons are present in tissue. Since 1978 a compact cyclotron has been used at the Essen University Hospital for fast-neutron therapy. The neutrons are produced by bombarding a beryllium target with 14 MeV deuterons. The poor depth dose distribution of this beam (median energy 5.7 MeV) limits the treatment of deep-seated tumors (Rassow 1982). An enhancement of the dose at depth could be obtained by neutron-capture reactions if there is a sufficient flux of thermalized neutrons derived from fast neutrons after slowing down in tissue.

Methods

All measurements and calculations were made using cubic phantoms (water or polystyrene) in an axial symmetric geometry. In the phantoms a cubic target volume positioned at the central beam axis simulates a deep-seated tumor. Measurements of γ-dose using thermoluminescence dosimetry 300 have been established to estimate the extent of slowing down of the fast neutrons by a

Radiologisches Zentrum, Universitätsklinikum Essen, Hufelandstr. 55, 4300 Essen, FRG
* This research was supported in part by the Deutsche Forschungsgemeinschaft.

Advanced Radiation Therapy Tumor Response
Monitoring and Treatment Planning
Breit (Editor-in-Chief)
© Springer-Verlag, Berlin Heidelberg 1992

target. The differential γ-dose in a phantom with or without boronated tumor model gives the total dose from the ^{10}B (n, α, γ) ^{7}Li reaction and can be used to calculate the fluence of thermalized neutrons. The exact measurement of the thermal neutron fluence rate in the fast-neutron beam has been made by activation of gold foils (Pöller et al. 1990). This method allows determination of the thermal fluence rate separated from the total fluence rate and has been used to evaluate the influence of various parameters such as phantom depth, phantom material, field size, and ^{10}B concentration. A Monte Carlo model was developed to calculate the distribution of fast, epithermal, and thermal neutrons in a given volume and to determine the dose enhancement by neutron-capture reactions of ^{10}B.

Results

Estimation of the fluence of thermalized neutrons (Φth) using thermolumine-scence dosimetry is 1.5×10^{10} cm^{-2} in polystyrene at a depth of 6 cm at a total energy dose of 1 Gy at the same point. The uncertainty of this method is about $\pm$ 20%. A fluence of 1.42×10^{10} cm^{-2} thermal neutrons was found using the more precise measurements by gold activation under the same conditions. The depth distribution of the thermal neutron fluence rate in water is shown in Fig. 1 comparing measured and calculated values. The influence of the size of the irradiation field is demonstrated in Fig. 2. Fast d(14) + Be neutrons create partially thermalized neutrons by slowing down at each point in the irradiated volume, resulting in a thermal "flux-peaking" at a depth of 6.5 cm (Figs. 1, 2). The attenuation of the thermal neutron fluence rate by neutron capture is shown in Figs. 3 and 4. The thermal neutron fluence rate decreases if the ^{10}B concentration increases. However a selective concentration of 100 ppm ^{10}B in

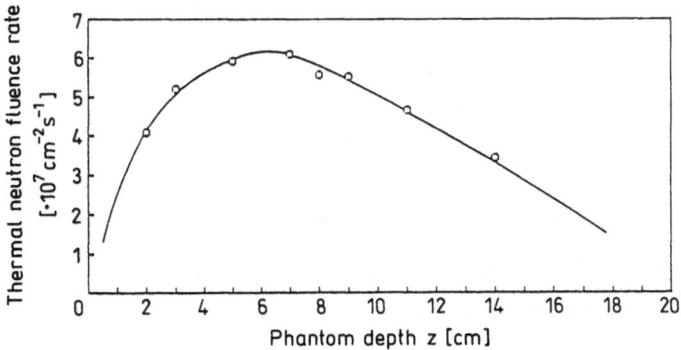

Fig. 1. Depth distribution of thermal neutron fluence rate at the central axis in water (field size 10 × 10 cm). ○, Measured values; *curve*, Monte Carlo simulation

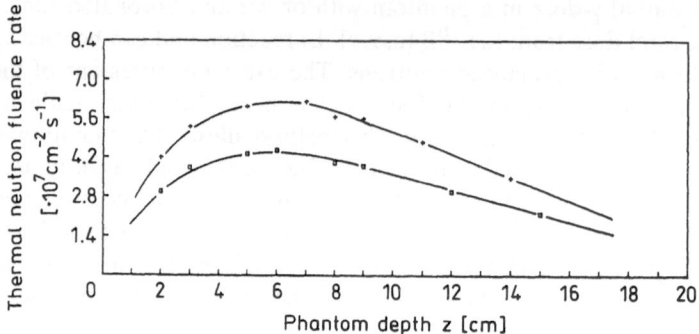

Fig. 2. Depth distribution of thermal neutron fluence rate at the central axis measured in water at two different irradiation field sizes: □, 8 × 8 cm; +, 10 × 10 cm

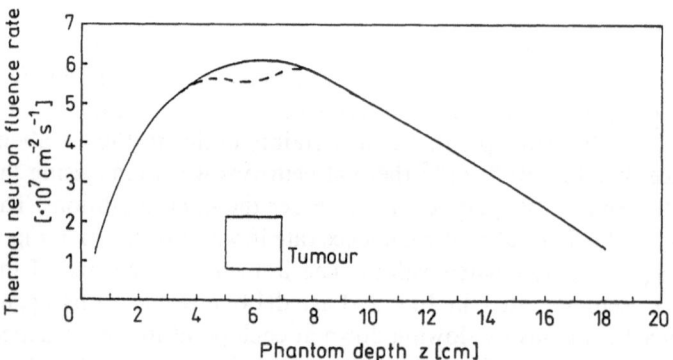

Fig. 3. Depth distribution of thermal neutron fluence rate at the central axis in a water phantom with 100 ppm ^{10}B (*broken line; solid line*, 0 ppm) in a small tumor (2 × 2 × 2 cm) at a depth of 6 cm (field size 10 × 10 cm). *Box*, simulated tumor

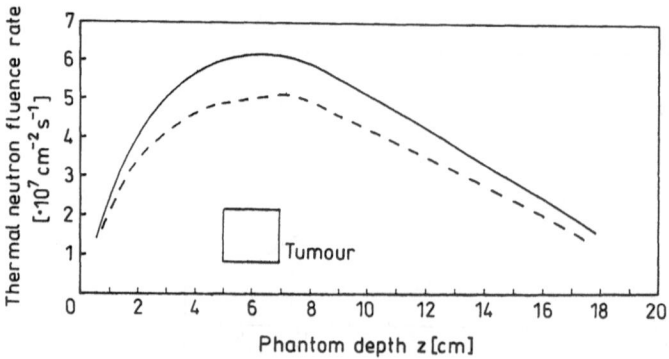

Fig. 4. Depth distribution of thermal neutron fluence rate at the central axis in a water phantom with 100 ppm ^{10}B inside and 100 ppm ^{10}B outside the tumor (*broken line; solid line*, 0 ppm; tumor size 2 × 2 × 2 cm) at a depth of 6 cm (field size 10 × 10 cm)

the tumor (Fig. 3) decreases the thermal fluence rate little (16%). A more realistic situation is illustrated in Fig. 4. A specified ^{10}B concentration exists in normal tissues and in the tumor at the same time. In our example, the depth distribution of thermal neutron fluence rate reaches a nearly flat maximum between 5 and 7 cm of the depth, with a reduction in thermal neutrons of about 18%. Based on the measured fluence rate of thermal neutrons an enhancement of the absorbed dose due to neutron capture can be calculated for a given ^{10}B concentration. Thus, a tumor containing 100 ppm ^{10}B receives at a depth of 6 cm an increase in dose of about 15% when irradiated with the neutron beam of the Essen cyclotron.

Discussion

The depth distribution in the irradiated volume of thermalized neutrons from a fast-neutron beam is different from that of a thermal beam used in conventional neutron-capture therapy (Barth et al. 1990). Fast neutrons slow down to thermal energies at each point in the irradiated volume. Hence in a tumor with a high ^{10}B concentration, the depression in thermal fluence rate due to neutron capture is not significant. Besides the normal neutron-capture therapy effect which requires ^{10}B concentrated in the tumor, the described technique has an additional advantage. The relative contribution of the neutron-capture therapy reactions to the total dose is higher at depth than at the surface even for a homogeneous ^{10}B distribution. Hence the total absorbed dose at depth can be boosted even without a tumor-specific boron compound. Therefore neutron-capture reactions can be used to optimize dose distribution in fast-neutron therapy.

The described enhancement of the absorbed dose does not express the extent of the biological effect. Experiments made in cell culture suggest a higher relative biological effectiveness of the fission products from the ^{10}B (n, α) ^{7}Li reaction than of the d(14) + Be neutrons (Sauerwein et al. 1990). Therefore in a clinical situation a greater therapeutic gain may be obtained than suggested by these physical data.

References

Barth RF, Fairchild RG, Soloway AH (1990) Boron neutron capture therapy for cancer. Sci Am 262: 68–73
Hatanaka H, Yasukochi H, Sano K (1991) Boron neutron capture therapy for brain tumours. In: Abe M, Takahashi M (eds) Intraoperative radiation therapy. Pergamon, New York, pp 153–155

Pöller F, Sauerwein W, Rau D, Wagner FM, Olthoff K, Rassow J, Sack H (1990) Neutronenfluen-zmessungen im d(14) + Be-Neutronenstrahlungsfeld des Zyklotrons in Essen. Strahlenther Onkol 166: 426–429

Rassow J (1982) Medical cyclotron facilities useful tools for clinical therapy, diagnosis and analysis. Proc Int Symp Appl Technol J Rad 1: 47–100

Sauerwein W, Ziegler W, Szypniewski H, Streffer C (1990) Boron neutron capture therapy (BNCT) using fast neutrons: effects in two human tumour cell lines. Strahlenther Onkol 166: 26–29

Mixed-Beam Photon-Neutron Therapy in Recurrences and Nodal Metastases of Head and Neck Cancer

T. Auberger, W. Reuschel, M. Mayr, P. Kneschaurek, P. Lukas, B. Clasen, and A. Breit

Introduction

The therapeutic advantage of fast neutrons in the treatment of advanced low-grade tumors of the salivary glands and nasal cavity, such as adenoidcystic carcinomas, mucoepidermoid tumors, and adenocarcinomas, is well known and confirmed by the literature. Most reports describe local tumor control rates of 67%–85% after therapy with fast neutrons versus 24%–34% after photon therapy [2, 4, 9, 10, 15–17]. In contrast, the effect of fast-neutron therapy in squamous cell carcinoma is discussed controversely, and the results of randomized studies reach from significant advantages to no benefit at all, in comparison to conventional radiotherapy. From the biological point of view the high repair rate and the high share of hypoxic cells in advanced squamous cell carcinomas indicate the use of fast neutrons.

Indeed, the results were encouraging in the first randomized multicenter study with 133 patients reported by Catterall et al. [1], with a local tumor control of 76% after neutron therapy compared with 19% after photon therapy. On the other hand, the results of a European multicenter study published in 1987 by Duncan et al. [3] in which the therapy centers in Edinburgh, Amsterdam, and Essen participated showed no improvement in the neutron arm, whereas the chronic side effects distinctly increased. It must be added that tumors in low stages were often treated in this study. Griffin et al. [8] summarized the results of a large-scale randomized RTOG study with a mixed-beam photon-neutron therapy in 322 patients; they also did not observe significant differences for primary tumors in the local tumor control or in the 2-year survival rate in comparative arms, but they did see a significant difference in the treatment of lymph node metastases, with a complete remission rate of 69% versus 55% [6]. This had no effect on survival. Singular data published by the participating therapy centers also did not show significant differences between mixed-beam therapy and photon therapy alone in respect to primary tumors [11, 13, 14]. In another RTOG study with 35 patients treated with fast neutrons alone, Griffin et al. [7] reported significantly better results in the

Institut für Strahlentherapie and Radiologische Onkologie, Technische Universität München, Klinikum rechts der Isar, Ismaninger Str. 15, 8000 Munich 80, FRG

Advanced Radiation Therapy Tumor Response
Monitoring and Treatment Planning
Breit (Editor-in-Chief)
© Springer-Verlag, Berlin Heidelberg 1992

neutron arm, with a local tumor control of 52% versus 17% in the photon arm. The 2-year survival rate was 25% after neutron therapy and 0% in the photon arm. The poor tumor control after photons is a reason for criticism, but this may have been due to the negative selection of patients admitted to both arms of the study.

It has still not been definitely explored whether there are subgroups which have more benefit from neutron therapy than others. In NIRS in Japan, Tsunemoto et al. [17] reported significant benefit of fast neutrons in the treatment of supraglottic tumors, whereas for glottic and subglottic carcinoma no benefit was noticeable. The results of these various studies are hardly comparable because of the different selection of patients, tumor stages, dosage, and fractionation. For this reason a new phase III study has been initiated by the RTOG, in which the therapy centers of Seattle, Los Angeles, and Houston in the United States and Clatterbridge in Great Britain are participating. In this study, in which 140 patients have been randomized until now, neutron therapy with 20.4 Gy will be compared with photon therapy with 70 Gy [12].

A very poor prognosis is associated with recurrences or lymph node metastases of squamous cell carcinoma after previous radiotherapy because of a minor vascularization of the tumorbed and a selection of resistant cells. One often sees an advanced necrosis. In these cases the tumor response to conventional therapy is even worse than in the first treatment of the primary tumor. In addition, due to the normal tissue reactions to previous therapy an equivalent photon dose to that of the first radiation cannot be delivered, and a palliative dose of 30 Gy tends rather to stimulate tumor growth than to stop it. At our university reactor station in Garching, we concentrate especially on the treatment of these cases.

Materials and Methods

The therapy beam of our reactor is created by a uranium converter plate which can be attached to the reactor core (Fig. 1). We work with a mixed beam which after the filtering process has 75% fission neutrons of an average energy of 2 MeV and 25% photons with an average energy as with a cobalt source. The dose rate is 23 cGy/min; thus for a single dose of 2 Gy we need an irradiation time of approximately 10 min.

Since 1986 we have treated more than 150 patients with recurrences or lymph node metastases after high-dose preirradiation. In 79 patients tumor was located in the head and neck. In 59 (75%) the histologic type was squamous cell carcinoma. Thirteen patients suffered from recurrences of highly differentiated carcinomas, and seven from recurrences of other histologies such as undifferentiated carcinomas and branchiogenous carcinomas. All patients were treated previously by surgery or chemotherapy and single or multiple radio-

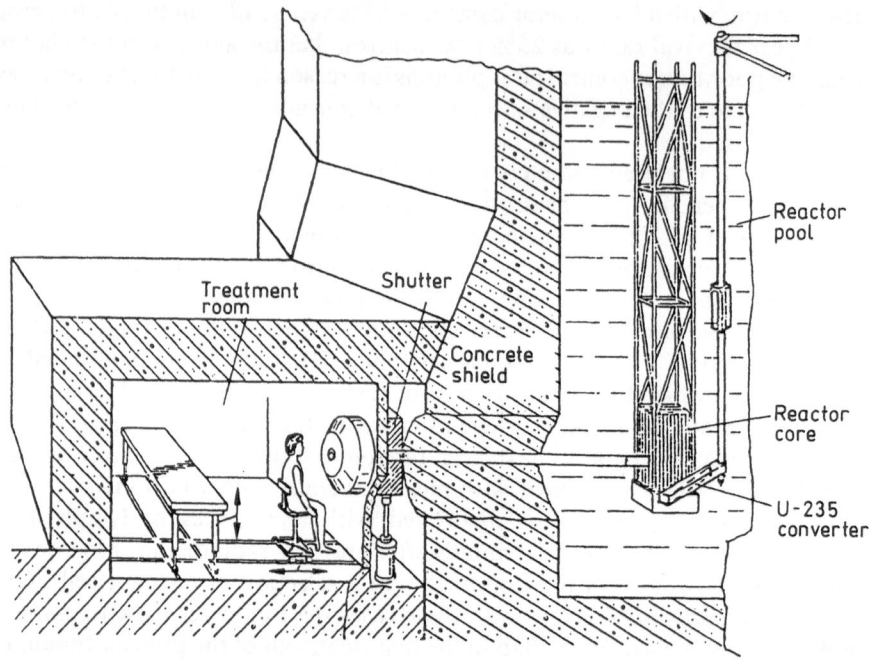

Fig. 1. Diagram of the RENT facility

therapies. In many cases, irradiation doses reached 110 Gy, in some patients even more. The average Karnofsky performance status was 50%. The mean age was over 60 years.

In patients being pretreated with a single radiotherapy with a maximal total dose of 70 Gy, over 6 months ago we combined a photon or electron therapy with a neutron boost. For this mixed-beam therapy we had two treatment schedules. In schedule 1 we delivered 50 Gy photons or electrons and 2–4 Gy of our RENT beam. In schedule 2 we delivered 30 Gy photons or electrons and 6–8 Gy RENT beam. After preceding therapy with higher doses, a palliative treatment (schedule 3) with only 4–8 Gy neutrons with single doses of 2 Gy per fraction was delivered. Total doses and fractions depended on preceding irradiation, the time interval between previous and present therapy, performance status, and age.

Results

Among the 18 patients treated with combined schedule 1 we found complete remission (CR) in 50% 2 months after irradiation; 44% showed partial remission (PR), and no change (NC) was seen in one. In patients treated according to

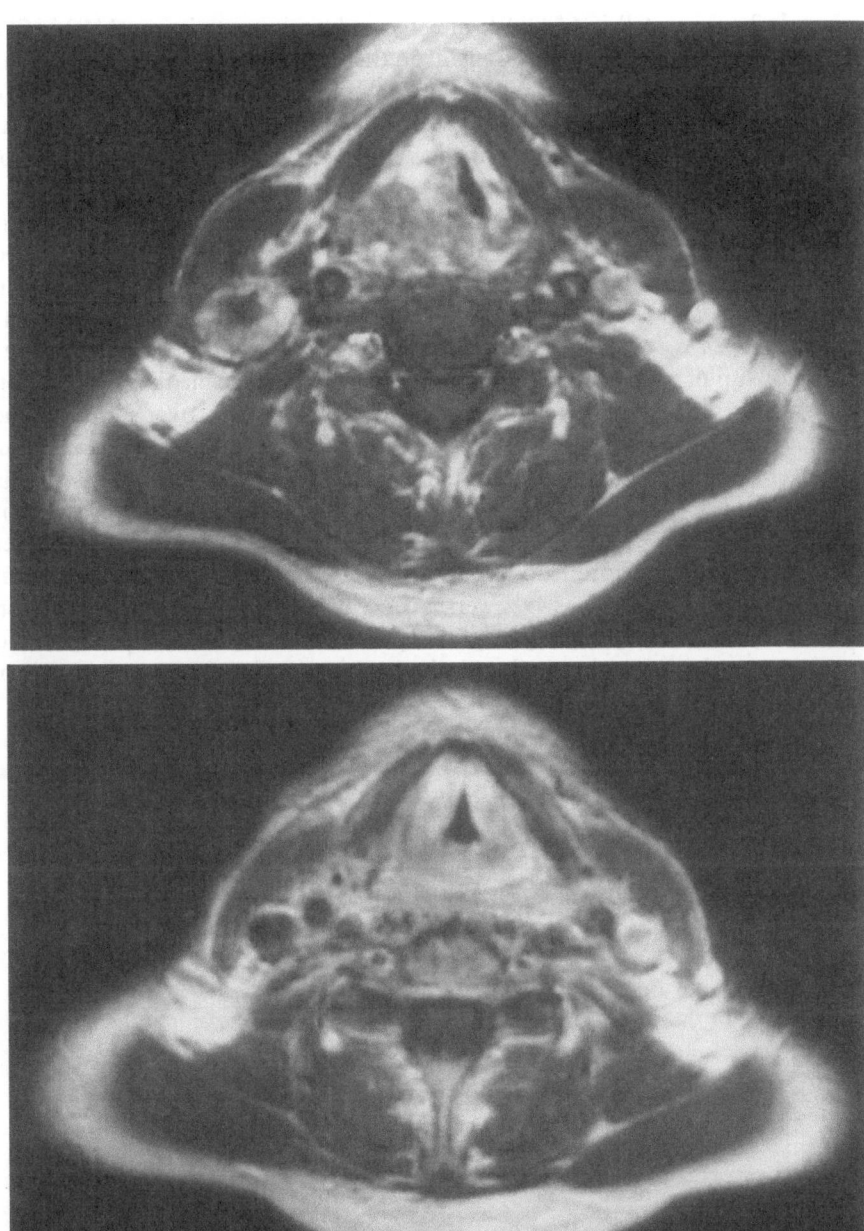

Fig. 2a, b. Axial MR images of a patient suffering from recurrent larynx cancer and consequent pronounced dysphagia. **a** Tumor in the left larynx, infiltrating into the muscle and extending to the contralateral side. **b** Tumor 2 months after combined photon-neutron therapy (schedule 2); no tumor could be seen in MRI. Also in the biopsy no tumor cells were found. The patient has been without relapse for more than 14 months now

schedule 2, we saw CR in 65%, PR in 28%, and a minor remission (MR) in 7% (Fig. 2). As expected, the results of neutron therapy alone were not as good, due to selection of patients with a very poor prognosis and to lower total doses. We found CR in 28%, PR in 59%, and NC in 13% (Table 1). Among those with NC we also saw palliation of symptoms, including alleviation of pain, decrease of compression syndroms, and prevention of exulceration (Fig. 3).

Despite preceding high doses, side effects were small. Moderate cutaneous and mucosal reactions were seen after combined therapy. Frequently we noticed an acute subcutaneous lymphedema and sometimes a moderate soft-tissue pain for some days after neutron irradiation. In 30% of patients we saw no side effects at all (Table 2). We also did not see any fibrosis, but for verification of late effects the follow-up of most patients is not yet long enough. The median observation time was 14 months, but follow-up in some patients was over 3 years. The median survival period was 11–14 months, depending on the treatment arm. The overall survival rates in terms of the Kaplan-Meier calculation — as well as the disease-free survival rates — showed an interesting but not significant difference between the two combined treatment arms, in favor of the higher neutron and lower photon dose (Fig. 4). After combined therapy 2 the local tumor control at 2 years was 49% versus 32% after combined therapy 1. Fission neutron therapy alone was very helpful in palliation; however, as expected, it did not improve the survival rate, due to the low dose and the worse prognosis of this treatment arm.

Table 1. Results 2 months after therapy

	n	CR	PR	MR/NC
Combined therapy 1 (50 Gy + 2–4 Gy)	18	9 (50%)	8 (44%)	1 (5%)
Combined therapy 2 (30 Gy + 6–10 Gy)	29	19 (65%)	8 (28%)	2 (7%)
Neutrons only	32	9 (28%)	19 (59%)	4 (13%)

Table 2. Side effects ($n = 79$)

	Moderate	Strong
Erythema	22	7
Hyperpigmentation	8	3
Madidans desquamation	2	–
Lymphatic edema	13	2
Mucositis	24	4
Pain	7	2
Liquefaction of tumor and exulceration	–	6
Subcutaneous induration	5	–
No side effects	24	–

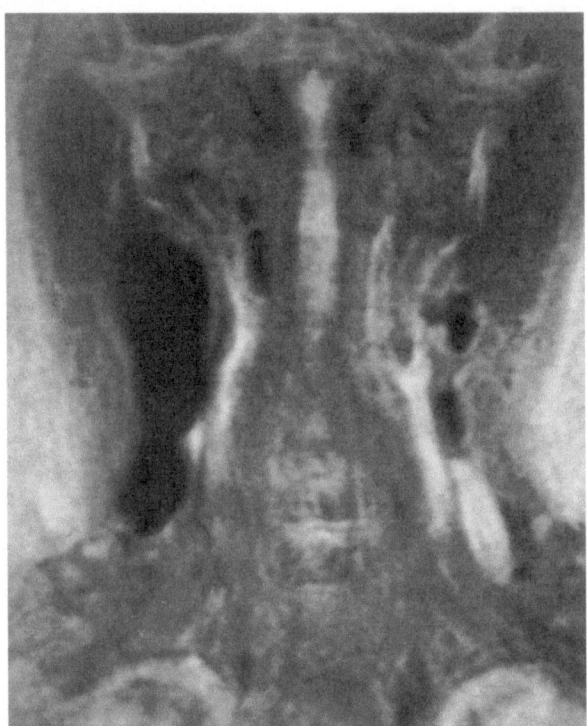

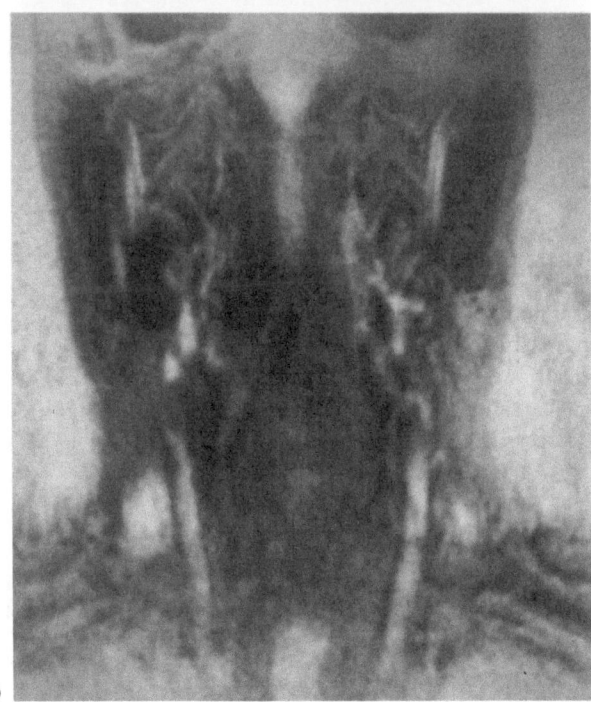

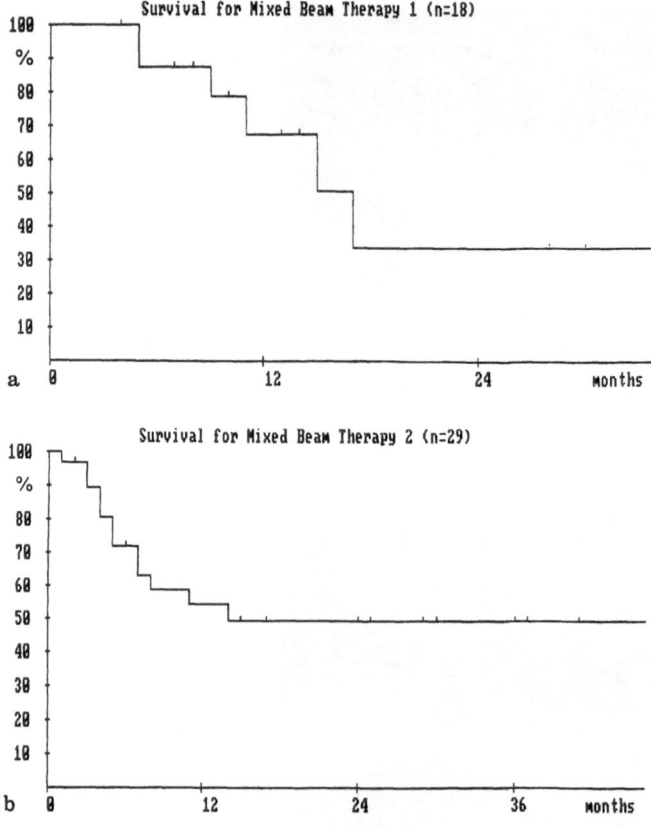

Fig. 4a, b. Survival curves for mixed-beam therapies. **a** Therapy 1. **b** Therapy 2

Conclusion

Unlike some other reports on neutron therapy, our observations show that high response rates and good palliative effect can be obtained with reactor fission neutrons in recurrence of both squamous cell and highly differentiated carcinoma. These are preliminary results based on a retrospective investigation. Prospective studies will be necessary to determine whether an improvement is also possible in survival rates.

Fig. 3a, b. Frontal MR images in inversion echo mode showing a lymph node metastasis of squamous cell carcinoma in the left neck. **a** Before fission neutron therapy with 3 fractions of 2 Gy. **b** Three weeks after the end of therapy partial remission is visible. The area of high signal intensity around the decreased node demonstrates postradiation normal tissue reaction

References

1. Catterall M, Bewley DK (1977) Second report on results of a randomized clinical trial of fast neutrons compared with X or gamma rays in treatment of advanced tumours of head and neck. Br Med J 1: 1642
2. Catterall M, Errington RD (1987) The implications of improved treatment of malignant salivary gland tumors by fast neutron radiotherapy. Int J Radiat Oncol Biol Phys 13: 1313–1318
3. Duncan W, Orr JA, Arnott SJ, Schmitt WJL, Kerr GR (1987) Fast neutron therapy for squamous cell carcinoma in the head and neck region: results of a randomized trial. Int J Radiat Oncol Biol Phys 13: 171–178
4. Errington RD (1986) Advanced carcinoma of the paranasal sinuses treated with 7.5 MeV fast neutrons. Bull Cancer (Paris) 73: 569–576
5. Griffin TW, Davis R, Laramore GE, Hussey DM, Hendrickson FR, Rodriguez-Antunez A (1983) Fast neutron irradiation of metastatic cervical adenopathy. The results of a randomized RTOG study. Int J Radiat Oncol Biol Phys 9: 1267–1270
6. Griffin TW, Davis R, Hendrickson FR, Maor MH, Laramore GE, Davis L (1984) Fast neutron radiation therapy for unresectable squamous cell carcinoma of the head and neck: the results for a randomized RTOG study. Int J Radiat Oncol Biol Phys 10: 2217–2223
7. Griffin TW, Davis R, Laramore GE et al. (1984) Mixed beam radiation therapy for unresectable squamous cell carcinoma of the head and neck: the results of a randomized RTOG study. Int J Radiat Oncol Biol Phys 10: 2211–2215
8. Griffin TW, Pajak TF, Laramore GE, Duncan W, Richter MP, Hendrickson FR, Maor MH (1988) Neutron vs photon irradiation of inoperable salivary gland tumors: results of an RTOG-MRC cooperative randomized study. Int J Radiat Oncol Biol Phys 15: 1085–1090
9. Krüll A, Schwarz R, Heyer D, Brockmann W-P, Junker A, Schmidt R, Hübener K-H (1990) Results of fast neutron therapy for adenoidcystic carcinomas of the head and neck at the neutron facility Hamburg-Eppendorf. Strahlenther Onkol 166/1: 107–110
10. Kurup PD, Hendrickson FR, Cohen L, Awschalom M, Rosenberg I, Ten Haken RK, Mansell J (1982) Radiation therapy utilizing fast neutrons for head and neck cancer — the Fermilab experience. Int J Radiat Oncol Biol Phys 8 (Suppl 1): 103–104
11. Laramore GE (1990) Fast neutron radiotherapy clinical research in the United States: an overview. Meeting of the Heavy Particle Group of EORTC, Münster, 1990
12. Maor MH, Hussey DH, Barkley HT, Peters LJ (1983) Neutron therapy for head and neck cancer. I. A final report of the MDAH-TAMVEC pilot studies. Int J Radiat Oncol Biol Phys 9: 1255–1260
13. Maor MH, Hussey DM, Barkley HT, Peters LJ (1983) Neutron therapy for head and neck cancer. II. Further follow-up on the M.D. Anderson TAMVEC randomized clinical trial. Int J Radiat Oncol Biol Phys 9: 1261–1265
14. Saroja KJ, Mansell J, Hendrickson FR, Cohen L, Lenox A (1987) An update on 113 malignant salivary gland tumors treated with neutrons at Fermilab. Int J Radiat Oncol Biol Phys 13: 1319–1326
15. Schwarz R, Hübener K-H (1988) Ergebnisse der Strahlentherapie bei malignen Tumoren der inneren Nase und der Nebenhöhlen unter besonderer Berücksichtigung der Neutronentherapie. Paper presented at the 19th German Cancer Congress, Freiburg, 1988
16. Tsunemoto H, Morita S, Satho S, Iino Y, Yoo SY (1989) Present status of fast neutron therapy in Asian countries. Strahlenther Onkol 165: 330–336

Subject Index